An Introduction to the
Principles of Disease

SECOND EDITION

John B. Walter, M.D.

Department of Pathology and Department of Medicine
University of Toronto and Toronto General Hospital
Toronto, Ontario, Canada

1982 W. B. Saunders Company

Philadelphia   London   Toronto   Mexico City   Rio de Janeiro   Sydney   Tokyo

W. B. Saunders Company: West Washington Square
Philadelphia, PA 19105

1 St. Anne's Road
Eastbourne, East Sussex BN 21 3UN, England

1 Goldthorne Avenue
Toronto, Ontario M8Z 5T9, Canada

Apartado 26370 – Cedro 512
Mexico 4, D.F., Mexico

Rua Coronel Cabrita, 8
Sao Cristovao Caixa Postal 21176
Rio de Janeiro, Brazil

9 Waltham Street
Artarmon, N.S.W. 2064, Australia

Ichibancho, Central Bldg., 22-1 Ichibancho
Chiyoda-Ku, Tokyo 102, Japan

Library of Congress Cataloging in Publication Data

Walter, J. B. (John Brian)
  An introduction to the principles of disease.

  Includes bibliographies and index.
  1. Pathology. I. Title. [DNLM: 1. Pathology. QZ 4 W232i]
RB111.W15 1982   616.07   81-48329
ISBN 0-7216-9121-8   AACR2

An Introduction to the Principles of Disease   ISBN 0-7216-9121-8

Last digit is the print number: 9   8   7   6   5   4   3   2   1

Preface to the Second Edition

The aim of *An Introduction to the Principles of Disease* is to initiate the student into clinical medicine via the study of pathology. In the past such an approach has been successful in the training of physicians; recently, attempts to deviate from this course have not been particularly popular or successful. Although pathology has often been likened to the basis or roots of medicine, efforts to make students study it in great detail before venturing into clinical medicine have also been unpopular. This lack of enthusiasm for an in-depth study of pathology is quite understandable: Does any tree develop a full root system before embarking on the exciting experiment of sending a shoot toward the sky? Pathology and clinical medicine must be closely associated: This introduction to disease is intended to be no more than a primer in the study of medicine. No prior knowledge of medicine is assumed, but the reader should have had some instruction in biology, chemistry, human anatomy, and physiology.

Part I of this book describes the general principles of disease and the disorders that affect the body as a whole. Part II concentrates on diseases of individual organs. The objective has been to describe important mechanisms of diseases in considerable detail and to omit any reference to rare conditions. This book is not a synopsis of pathology; consequently, readers who are aiming for a degree in medicine will have to graduate to the larger texts of clinical medicine and pathology before attaining their objective.

The complexity and ever-increasing cost of providing medical care have led to a reappraisal of the role of the medical doctor. In the past, it was expected that physicians would assume absolute responsibility for the diagnosis and treatment of their patients. No longer can this view be upheld. Physicians must now rely on the competence of coworkers not trained as medical practitioners, but whose specialized knowledge is of vital importance in the diagnosis and treatment of patients. Nurses, midwives, physical therapists, pharmacists, dentists, and medical technologists are among this group of workers in the health sciences for whom this book has been written.

When studying medicine for the first time, the student meets many new words and concepts. An attempt has been made in this book to define these items when they are first introduced, so that learning can proceed by a series of progressive steps. Little attempt has been made to avoid the specialized terminology of medicine, because this technical language is widely used in medical practice. If used correctly, it acts as a type of shorthand by which medical personnel can express their ideas by either the spoken or the written word. Without learning the language of medicine, one finds it difficult to converse with a physician or to comprehend the medical literature. The medical student and allied health worker must be able to do both.

Five years have elapsed since the first edition was published, and a complete revision of the book has been necessary. The omission of a number of unsatisfactory pictures has allowed 45 new figures to be added. In the main these are of clinical material or gross pathological specimens, since it is felt that a detailed knowledge of the microscopic features of diseased organs is not required of students who do not intend to become pathologists.

The greatest changes have been made in the following chapters: Chapter 9, The Immune Response, a subject that is advancing rapidly; Chapter 30, Diseases of the Respiratory Tract, which now covers chronic obstructive lung disease (COLD) and interstitial pneumonia more adequately than in the previous edition; and Chapter 32, Diseases of the Gastrointestinal Tract, to which sections have been added on the complications of gastrectomy and on the types of gastro-enterocolitis, emphasizing their pathogenesis. Topics that have been expanded or introduced for the first time include: the immunoperoxidase staining technique; introns and extrons; somatic cell hybridization; recombinant DNA techniques; the Ehlers-Danlos syndrome; the floppy valve syndrome; the toxic shock syndrome; diphtheria; non A, non B hepatitis; strongyloidiasis; giardiasis; toxoplasmosis; pneumocystosis; the fetal alcohol syndrome; the Ames test; the role of prostaglandins in thrombosis; obesity; trace elements in metabolism; pericardial disease; Legionnaires' disease; the diffuse neuroendocrine system; vitamin D metabolism; diseases of skeletal muscle; and epilepsy.

The Système International (SI) units have been introduced since they are in common use in many countries, particularly in Europe, and are likely to gain popularity in North America. In the text the conventional units are given first and are followed by SI units in parenthesis. Pathogenic organisms have been named according to the current international nomenclature.* Where abbreviations are used, the first letter of the generic name is followed by the species name in full. When confusion is likely, *e.g., S. aureus* and *S. typhi,* the names are given in full.

The selected readings at the end of each chapter have been updated. These include standard textbooks of pathology as well as journals which are readily available. Among these are some devoted to nursing. These revisions have made it necessary to reset the whole book, and because of a new design, the text is 63 pages shorter than previously.

---

*Skerman, V. B. D., McGowan, V., and Sneath, P. H. A.: Approved lists of bacterial names. International Journal of Systematic Bacteriology, *30*:220–225, 1980.

Acknowledgments

The production of this book would have been greatly delayed and extremely difficult without the cooperation of Churchill Livingstone of Edinburgh; Mr. Robert Duncan has generously allowed me to use material from their publication *General Pathology*, which I coauthored with Dr. Martin Israel. Over 40 illustrations have been taken from this source. A number of illustrations are taken from *Principles of Pathology for Dental Students*, also published by Churchill Livingstone. I thank my other coauthor, Margaret Grundy (née Hamilton), for permitting me to use this material.

I owe special gratitude to those who have given me pictorial material or who have allowed me to modify their original published work. The source of material is detailed in the caption of each figure. I am particularly grateful to Dr. J. B. Cullen for providing additional pictures of autopsy and surgical material from the Toronto General Hospital.

A number of figures (also appearing in *General Pathology*) are of specimens from the Welcome Museum of Pathology, Royal College of Surgeons of England, London; I am grateful to the President and the Council of the Royal College of Surgeons of England for permission to reproduce these illustrations. In accordance with the wishes of the council, each specimen is acknowledged at the end of the caption and the catalogue number of each is indicated. Some specimens are from the Boyd Museum, University of Toronto, and I thank Dr. E. Farber of that institution for permission to use these.

I am indebted to a number of colleagues for providing valuable criticism and for assisting in the areas of their particular expertise: Dr. Dean W. Chamberlain (diseases of the lung), Dr. J. B. Cullen (diseases of the gastrointestinal tract), Dr. Bernice R. Krafchik (diseases of the skin), Dr. Susan Ritchie (diseases of the kidney and liver), and Dr. A. Sima (diseases of the nervous system and muscle). I owe special gratitude to Mrs. Sonja Duda, librarian at the Banting Institute, Toronto, for valuable help in checking and obtaining new references and to my secretary, Mrs. Linda Thoms, for expert typing and secretarial assistance. Members of the Department of Medical Photography and Art at the Toronto General Hospital have provided many of the new pictures. I am particularly grateful to Rasa Skudra for the new art work.

As with many other authors, my greatest debt is to my family, particularly my wife, who has suffered in silence during many evenings.

Finally, it is a pleasure to acknowledge the help of W. B. Saunders Company: in particular, Walter Bailey, who first encouraged me to write this book; Baxter Venable for his help in producing the Second Edition; and Mark Coyle for his skillful editing.

JOHN B. WALTER
Toronto, Ontario, Canada

Contents

Part I
General Pathology

Chapter 1
INTRODUCTION 3

Chapter 2
NORMAL STRUCTURE AND FUNCTION 16

Chapter 3
THE ROLE OF GENETICS IN MEDICINE 39

Chapter 4
CELL AND TISSUE DAMAGE 52

Chapter 5
ACUTE INFLAMMATION 63

Chapter 6
INFECTION 79

Chapter 7
WOUND HEALING 91

Chapter 8
CHRONIC INFLAMMATION 106

Chapter 9
THE IMMUNE RESPONSE 112

Chapter 10
SOME BACTERIAL INFECTIONS—PYOGENIC, ANAEROBIC, MYCOBACTERIAL, AND SPIROCHETAL 143

Chapter 11
MYCOPLASMAL, CHLAMYDIAL, AND RICKETTSIAL INFECTIONS 169

Chapter 12
VIRAL INFECTIONS 173

Chapter 13
FUNGAL INFECTIONS 194

Chapter 14
HELMINTHIC INFECTIONS 200

Chapter 15
PROTOZOAL INFECTIONS 209

Chapter 16
DISORDERS OF GROWTH 217

Chapter 17
NEOPLASIA 228

Chapter 18
IONIZING RADIATIONS AND THEIR EFFECTS 259

Chapter 19
DISORDERS OF FLUID AND ELECTROLYTE BALANCE: EDEMA 269

Chapter 20
DISORDERS OF THE CIRCULATION 280

Chapter 21
SHOCK AND HEMORRHAGE 299

Chapter 22
FEVER AND HYPOTHERMIA 312

Chapter 23
DISORDERS OF NUTRITION 321

Chapter 24
METABOLIC DISORDERS 330

Chapter 25
THE PLASMA PROTEINS: AMYLOIDOSIS 338

Chapter 26
DISORDERS OF THE BLOOD 347

Chapter 27
THE COLLAGEN VASCULAR DISEASES 373

Part II
Diseases of Individual Organs

Chapter 28
DISEASES OF THE HEART 379

Chapter 29
DISEASES OF BLOOD VESSELS 403

Chapter 30
DISEASES OF THE RESPIRATORY TRACT 414

Chapter 31
DISEASES OF THE UPPER ALIMENTARY TRACT 444

Chapter 32
DISEASES OF THE GASTROINTESTINAL TRACT 454

Chapter 33
DISEASES OF THE LIVER 480

Chapter 34
DISEASES OF THE PANCREAS AND THE BILIARY TRACT 496

Chapter 35
DISEASES OF THE KIDNEYS AND URINARY TRACT 502

Chapter 36
MALE REPRODUCTIVE ORGANS 524

Chapter 37
**FEMALE REPRODUCTIVE ORGANS; PREGNANCY
AND ITS DISORDERS** 529

Chapter 38
DISEASES OF THE BREAST 540

Chapter 39
DISEASES OF THE ENDOCRINE GLANDS 550

Chapter 40
DISEASES OF THE BONES, JOINTS, AND MUSCLES 568

Chapter 41

DISEASES OF THE SKIN **591**

Chapter 42

DISEASES OF THE EYE **610**

Chapter 43

DISEASES OF THE EAR **618**

Chapter 44

DISEASES OF THE CENTRAL NERVOUS SYSTEM **622**

INDEX **639**

General Pathology PART I

Introduction CHAPTER 1

After studying this chapter the student should be able to:

- Define the terms sign, symptom, lesion, etiology, pathogenesis, syndrome, idiopathic, biopsy, thoracotomy, and laparotomy.
- List the units of measurement used in microscopy.
- Compare and contrast the techniques and value of light microscopy with those of electron microscopy with respect to (a) resolution, (b) magnification, (c) ease of studying living cells, (d) thickness of tissue sections used, and (e) methods of staining.
- Describe the major steps in the preparation of a paraffin-wax section and the appearance of cells when stained with hematoxylin and eosin (H & E).
- Describe the main uses in pathology of phase contrast and dark ground illumination in microscopy.
- Discuss the advantages that the frozen section technique has over the paraffin-wax technique.
- Describe the techniques of immunofluorescence and compare them with those of immunoperoxidase.
- Give examples of the use of radioactive isotopes in clinical medicine and in experimental pathology.
- Distinguish between cell culture and organ culture.
- Give examples of the types of cells that can be grown in culture and indicate the use of this technique in the study of disease.

Introduction

The majority of persons seeking medical help do so because of some abnormality causing them distress. Often such *symptoms* can be dispelled by simple remedies — quite often by reassurance. Much of medicine is an art, which its practitioners — whether they be doctors, dentists, nurses, or physical therapists — must learn. Nevertheless, there have always been individuals who were not content simply to observe disease and the effects of time-honored remedies upon it. They have attempted to describe and record the abnormalities in their patients in an objective manner; by introducing measurements, they initiated the science called *pathology*.

Disease itself is as difficult to define as is the normal, from which it is a departure. As generally used, the term "disease" is employed to describe a state in which there is a sufficient departure from the normal for *signs* or *symptoms* to be produced. A symptom is an abnormality noted by the patient. A sign is one noted by another observer. The objective variations from the normal are called *lesions*, and although the term generally refers to structural changes, it may also be used to describe functional abnormalities, such as *biochemical lesions* (Chapter 4). The theory of the cause of a disease is its *etiology* and the development of the lesions is its *pathogenesis*. When used strictly, these two terms are quite separate entities, but in practice they are often used interchangeably. Thus, it is commonly said that the cause of a heart attack is blockage of a diseased coronary artery (arteriosclerosis). Nevertheless, the cause of this may be some genetic defect or an abnormality in the diet. Thus, the coronary disease is merely part of the pathogenesis of the whole picture.

The great advances in bacteriology that started at the end of the nineteenth century fostered the concept that each disease had a single cause. To state that the common wart is always caused by a particular virus is true; nevertheless, this is an incomplete statement. It is known that some patients with multiple warts have a deficient immunity that either can be inherited or can be acquired by administration of drugs. Which is the cause of the warts — the virus or the impaired immunity? Present doctrine would still favor the organism, but the genetic or acquired immunological deficiency would be labeled a major predisposing factor. Multiple causes are probably much more common than we think. The doctrine of one cause for one disease has certainly failed to be a profitable concept in the search for the etiology of many common diseases such as cancer, arteriosclerosis, emphysema, and chronic bronchitis. Nevertheless, the concept that each disease is an entity implies a specific cause for each.

To avoid the difficulty of defining disease the term *syndrome* has been introduced. A syndrome is a condition having a defined collection of lesions, signs, or symptoms that are not necessarily always due to the same agent. Thus, Raynaud's syndrome is a condition in which the hands are unduly susceptible to cold, and on exposure become pale, then blue, and finally red and painful. This syndrome can be found in patients with systemic lupus erythematosus (Chapter 27), it may be seen in workers who use pneumatic hammers, and finally it can occur for no apparent reason. When the cause is unknown, the condition is said to be *idiopathic*. Clearly, those conditions that are commonly labeled "diseases," and in which the cause is not known, are difficult to distinguish from syndromes. Indeed, the terms "syndrome" and "disease" are frequently used quite indiscriminately and interchangeably.

Pathology is thus the scientific study of disease. It describes the cause, course, and termination of disease as well as the nature of its lesions. In almost all diseases the lesions are of varying nature and may be morphological, chemical, or functional. Nevertheless, anything that can be measured is within the domain of pathology. The height of the blood pressure, the rate of the heartbeat, and the temperature of the patient are all valued measurements. If they are accurately recorded, they are as scientific as measurements of the size of a nucleus or of the amount of DNA that it contains. The remainder of this chapter is devoted to a brief account of the methods of investigation that can be employed.

Microscopy

The Light Microscope

The application of the compound light microscope to the examination of biological material was one of the most important steps ever taken in scientific medicine. From it stemmed the concept that all living organisms are composed of cells and cell products. The light microscope is now routinely used in the examination of diseased tissue. The study of the changes seen is termed *histopathology*.

The ability to distinguish two closely placed points is called the *resolving power* of the microscope. When light is used, it is limited by the wavelength of the light beam used. With the light microscopes currently available, the resolving power is about 250 nm.* One of the great advantages of the electron microscope is that its resolution is much greater; in fact, it is about 0.5 nm. The maximum magnification obtainable with light microscopes of current design is about 1200. Further magnification is useless, since it merely

---

*1 mm = 1000 μm (micrometers or microns); 1 μm = 1000 nm; 1 nm = 10Å (Ångström units). The present tendency is to dispense with the Ångström unit and use the nanometers (nm) instead. It is useful to remember that most cocci (*e.g.*, *Staphylococcus aureus*) are about 1 μm in diameter, a normal red cell is about 7 μm in diameter, and most nuclei are 5 to 10 μm in diameter.

produces a large image that is indistinct owing to the limited resolution obtainable.

Living tissue is transparent, and the homogeneity in optical density of its components hides its detailed structure. Staining techniques must therefore be employed. Unfortunately, staining almost invariably means that the cells must be dead. Nevertheless, there are two special techniques, having limited specific uses, which can be employed to visualize living cells.

Dark ground illumination relies upon the fact that objects placed in a beam of light may be seen by the light they reflect in much the same way that dust particles are rendered visible by a shaft of sunlight. Using a special substage condenser, this method finds particular application in the demonstration of the organism responsible for syphilis, *Treponema pallidum,* which is regularly demonstrated in venereal disease clinics by this method.

Phase contrast microscopy takes advantage of the different refractive indices of various parts of the cell. These differences are converted into differences in optical density. In this way, living cells can be examined, and the method may be applied in virology where thin sheets of cells in culture can be seen and the effect of viruses on them examined (Figs. 12–4 and 12–7).

Routine Examination of Tissue by Microscopy. The material must be processed and then sectioned into thin slices. The two methods available, the *paraffin section technique* and the *frozen section technique,* are described below. Human tissue for histopathological studies is obtained in two ways:

1. *Biopsy.* This entails the removal of a small piece of living tissue for examination. With skin lesions, this can be done easily under the anesthesia produced by the local injection of 1 or 2 per cent Xylocaine solution. Biopsy through an endoscope is an extension of this method, *e.g.,* bronchoscopy for lung lesions and cystoscopy for bladder lesions. Solid tissues like liver, spleen, and tumors can be examined by needle biopsy; a core of tissue is obtained with this technique. An operation is performed specifically to obtain a biopsy. Thus *thoracotomy* (opening the chest wall) is used to diagnose some diffuse lung lesions not readily examined by needle biopsy. *Laparotomy* (opening the peritoneal cavity) is a necessary prelude to the biopsy of abdominal lesions and is generally followed by some definitive treatment.

2. *Necropsy.* Necropsy provides abundant tissue for histopathological study, but unfortunately postmortem autolysis (Chapter 4) often limits detailed examination.

Paraffin Section Technique. This is the most commonly used routine method of examination. Fresh tissue is placed as soon as possible in *fixative,* generally a 10 per cent solution of formalin. It can remain in this solution for many months without deteriorating. Fixation renders many cell constituents insoluble, and it also inhibits enzymatic action. Blocks no thicker than 2 mm are prepared, *dehydrated* in graded alcohol, *cleared* in xylol, chloroform, or some other solvent that is miscible in both alcohol and wax, *impregnated* with molten paraffin wax, and finally, when cooled, are blocked out or *embedded* in paraffin wax. From the block obtained in this way 5-μm sections are *cut* on a microtome (Figs. 1–1 and 1–3).

When mounted on glass slides the sections must be stained to render tissue components visible. The commonly used stains are *hematoxylin and eosin* (H & E). Hematoxylin is a blue basic dye obtained from the heartwood of a Central American tree. It is oxidized to hematein and mixed with an alum to form a lake. The dye so formed is taken up by acidic substances in the cell. Hence, the nucleus with its nucleic acid content is stained blue. Eosin is a red synthetic acidic dye that binds to basic proteins found for the most part in cytoplasm. H & E stained sections are used routinely for diagnostic purposes.

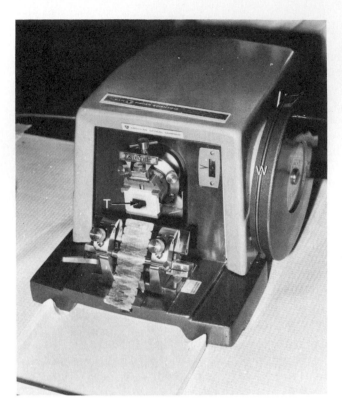

Figure 1–1. The rotary microtome. When the wheel (W) is rotated, the chuck holding the paraffin-embedded tissue (T) moves up and down against the knife. With each rotation the tissue advances 5 μm, and a thin section is obtained. Each section adheres to the previous one so that a ribbon of sections is formed.

Frozen Section Technique.   The *cryostat* is an instrument consisting of a microtome within a refrigerator. Tissue is frozen and cut in this solid state when embedded in a block of ice. The technique has several advantages over the paraffin-wax technique:

1. Frozen sections can be prepared and stained within two or three minutes. Hence, a diagnosis can be given rapidly during the course of a surgical procedure. Some hospital laboratories use this method routinely, so that all surgical material can be examined immediately and the surgeon advised as to the nature of the lesions he encounters and the extent of any disease process, *e.g.*, the extent of the spread of a cancer. The quality of frozen sections does not equal that of the routine paraffin sections, but the technique provides for a rapid diagnosis and often saves the patient from having to be operated on a second time.

2. The paraffin-wax technique removes lipids from cells and tissues. These substances are retained in the frozen section technique and can be stained specifically.

3. Frozen sections contain the active enzymes present in the cell, and these can be detected histochemically.

4. The frozen section technique causes little protein denaturation. Specific proteins, such as antigens and immunoglobulins, can be detected by immunological procedures (Fig. 9–15).

Histochemistry.   H & E and many other staining techniques (*e.g.*, the Ziehl-Neelsen stain) used in histopathology have been discovered empirically. Others have been developed with the intention of demonstrating specific chemicals in the tissue. The technique is called *histochemistry*, and it depends upon specific chemical interactions. A simple example of this technique is the Prussian blue reaction for hemosiderin (Fig. 1–2). Acid is applied to a section and releases Fe^{3+} from hemosiderin, a breakdown product

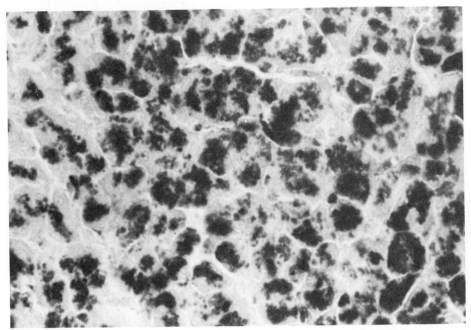

Figure 1–2. Section stained for hemosiderin by the Prussian blue method. The section shows massive deposition of hemosiderin in liver cells. The pigment is stained brilliant blue by this method but appears black in the photograph. The detailed structure of the liver cells is not well shown. This tissue was from a patient with hemochromatosis, a type of cirrhosis of the liver associated with deposition of iron pigments ($\times$ 600).

of hemoglobin. Next potassium ferricyanide is applied; this reacts with the Fe^{3+} to form insoluble ferric ferricyanide.

Enzymes may be detected by applying a suitable substrate to a section and devising methods for visually demonstrating an end-product of the reaction.

The highly specific property of antibodies can be utilized to detect specific proteins within a cell or tissue. Thus, in order to detect a bacterium or a bacterial antigen, an antibacterial IgG antibody is applied to the section. It forms a stable complex with the antigen. If the antibody has been labelled previously with fluorescein, examination of the section under ultraviolet microscopy will reveal brilliant fluorescence at the site of antigen-antibody interaction. In practice a more complex technique is often used. *Unlabelled* antibacterial IgG (of human origin) may be applied to the section and a second fluorescein-labelled antihuman IgG antibody is then applied, thereby forming a type of sandwich. This modification, the multilayered, or sandwich technique, has the effect of amplification of the fluorescence. A supply of labelled antihuman IgG is needed as well as unlabelled specific antibodies to each antigen that is to be investigated. The technique described is termed *immunofluorescence* and is widely used to detect microbial antigens, antibodies (see Fig. 9–15), and complement. A disadvantage of the method is that fresh tissue is generally required since frozen sections must be used. Also, the preparations are not perfect, their quality is often not good, and finally an ultraviolet microscope must be available.

A more recent development is the *immunoperoxidase technique*. The enzyme horseradish peroxidase is used as a label instead of fluorescein. The peroxidase itself is detected by applying a chromogen that is specifically acted upon by the enzyme to produce a stable, colored insoluble product. Diaminobenzidine, or DAB, is commonly used and produces a crisp brown color that does not fade. As with immunofluorescence, a variety of sandwich modifications are utilized. The immunoperoxidase technique has several advantages over immunofluorescence. Tissues embedded in paraffin are used so that retrospective studies can be undertaken. The slides can be stained with H & E so that the section has the appearance familiar to the pathologist since it resembles the sections of his routine work. No special microscope is needed, but the technique is more demanding than immunofluorescence, and as yet pathologists have had less experience with its use and its shortcomings. The technique promises to be the method of the future and has already been used extensively to demonstrate the immunoglobulins, lysozyme, hemoglobin, α_1-fetoprotein, testosterone, and a variety of other hormones, including gastrin and the pituitary hormones.

The Electron Microscope

Transmission Electron Microscope. This instrument resembles the ordinary microscope except that a stream of electrons is used instead of light, and electromagnetic fields replace the glass lenses. The theoretical resolving power is on the order of 0.005 nm. In practice, most instruments have a working resolving power of approximately 0.5 nm, and magnifications of up to 500,000 are possible. The electron microscope has revealed cell structure (*ultrastructure*) in minute detail, but it has many disadvantages. It is expensive and needs constant expert maintenance. The blocks of tissue for electron microscopy must be small (1 to 2 mm in size) and embedded in an epoxy resin (Fig. 1–3). Sections that are 50 to 60 nm thick are cut on a microtome with a glass or diamond knife; the technique is not easy. Finally, the sections are placed on a copper grid and examined in the vacuum of the column of the electron microscope (Fig. 1–4). The tremendous magnification available is impressive, but it does cut down the field of view by a similar dimension. In addition, although the image in the electron microscope can be seen on a fluorescent screen, any detailed examination must be done by taking photographic pictures. Electron microscopy therefore is a highly specialized technique that is very time consuming. It can be used for specific research or diagnostic purposes, but not for routine tissue examination.

Viruses can be seen with ease by the electron microscope; it is in this field that the instrument has really great diagnostic capability. For example, in patients with recurrent ulceration of the genitalia it is important to determine

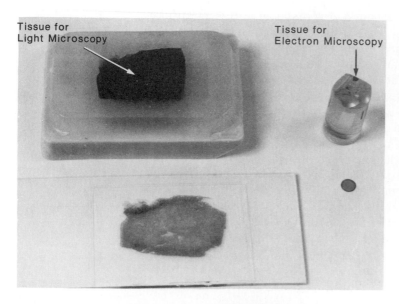

Tissue for
Light Microscopy

Tissue for
Electron Microscopy

Figure 1–3. Comparison of the paraffin wax technique with that of electron microscopy. Top left shows tissue embedded in a paraffin wax block. A section cut on a microtome (see Figure 1–1) has been mounted on a glass 3 × 1 inch slide and stained with hematoxylin and eosin (bottom left). Compare the size of the tissue with the 1 mm block taken for electronmicroscopy and embedded in epoxy resin (top right). After sectioning on a special microtome a number of sections have been floated onto the circular copper grid, which is 3.8 mm in diameter (bottom right). The mesh of the grid is so fine that it cannot be seen with the naked eye.

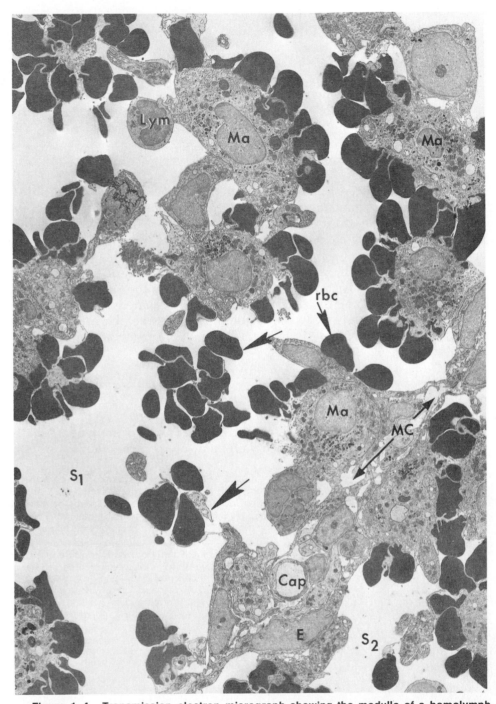

Figure 1–4. Transmission electron micrograph showing the medulla of a hemolymph node of a rat. The tissue was fixed in osmium tetroxide solution, and the section was then treated with lead hydroxide. Since these metals are electron-dense, they are used as stains in electron microscopy.

Hemolymph nodes differ from the usual type of lymph node present in humans in that red cells are present in the sinuses. This picture shows two sinuses, S_1 and S_2, which are separated by a thin medullary cord (MC) containing a capillary (Cap) and macrophages (Ma) to which many red blood cells (rbc) are adherent. In the cytoplasm of the macrophages there are many phagosomes representing degradation products of red cells. In S_1, red cells in groups appear to be free. On closer examination, however, they are partially surrounded by pseudopods of macrophages (large arrows). The medullary cords are covered by sinus endothelial cells (E) between which the macrophages push out pseudopodia to entrap the red cells. The macrophages and lymphocyte (Lym) seen at the top of the picture are in one of the trabeculae that cross the sinus (×2400). (From Nopajaroonsri, C., Luk, S. C., and Simon, G. T.: The structure of the hemolymph node—a light, transmission, and scanning electron microscopic study. Journal of Ultrastructure Research, *48*:325–341. 1974.)

whether or not herpes simplex is the cause (Chapter 12). An electron microscopist can demonstrate the presence of a virus within a few minutes of receiving a swab from a lesion. The precise identification of the virus is performed by culture.

The *high voltage electron microscope* employs a voltage ten times that of the standard electron microscope. Whole cells suitably prepared can be examined, and this has the advantage over thin sections in that the internal structures of the cell are revealed in depth. In this way the microtrabecular lattice of the cytoplasm was discovered (Chapter 2). However, the microscope is not only very expensive but also very large. Current versions are about 30 ft high and weigh 20 tons!

Scanning Electron Microscope.   This instrument works on a different principle from the conventional transmission electron microscope: a very fine beam of electrons is focused to a point and made to scan the surface of a specimen. Secondary electrons scattered from the surface are collected and amplified. The current so generated is used to modulate the brightness of a television tube that is scanned in synchronicity with the electron beam scanning the object. With this method for examining the surfaces of objects, the pictures so obtained have a remarkable three-dimensional appearance (Fig. 1–5). Microorganisms, red cells, the lung, sinuses of the spleen, and the surface of the intestinal mucosa have all been studied with advantage by this technique (Fig. 32–10).

Radioactive Isotopes

Radioactive isotopes are treated by living cells in the same way as the normal elements. Their radiation can be detected by suitable counters, and they may usefully be employed as labels in a wide range of fields. Clinically, the greatest breakthrough in this area has been the introduction of the man-made element *technetium*. This element emits gamma radiation only,

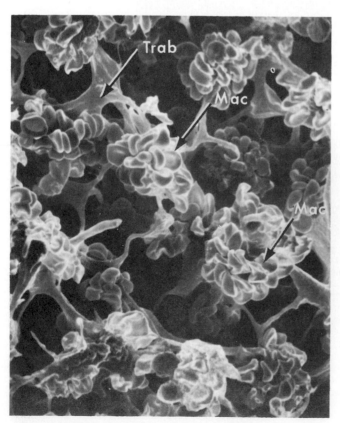

Figure 1–5.   Scanning electron micrograph of a hemolymph node of the rat. Trabeculae (Trab) are seen crossing a sinus. Grapelike groups ot red cells (Mac) are present around macrophages in the medullary sinus. Compare this picture with Figure 1–4, noting the difference in magnification (× 1300). (From Luk, S. C., Nopajaroonsri, C., and Simon, G. T.: The architecture of the normal lymph node and hemolymph node. Laboratory Investigation, *29*:258–265, 1973. © 1973 U.S.-Canadian Division of the International Academy of Pathology.)

Figure 1–6. Bone scan showing tumor of the right tibia in a 15-year-old boy. See Case History 1 for complete description of case.

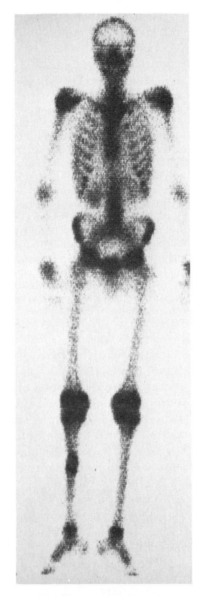

and is therefore safer to use than isotopes that emit other more damaging radiation. It has a half-life of six hours. When injected intravenously with pyrophosphate, technetium is selectively taken up by bone, probably by the osteoid tissue. Using this technique, the whole skeleton can be surveyed, and the method now augments radiography in the detection of bony lesions, particularly tumors (Fig. 1–6). If the technetium is attached to aggregated albumin, it becomes concentrated in the lung; an estimate of blood flow through this organ is then obtained. By various techniques, it is now possible to scan many other organs. It is particularly useful in investigating lesions of the liver and thyroid. In the past, thyroid function has been investigated by estimating the distribution of an administered dose of radioactive iodine, but this has now been replaced by the technetium technique. Many other radioactive techniques are used in medicine; for example, radioactive chromium can be attached to red cells and the length of their survival estimated (Chapter 26). Elements that emit gamma rays or charged particles are termed *radionuclides*, and their widespread use in diagnostic techniques has resulted in the formation of a separate specialty — that of *nuclear medicine*.

CASE HISTORY I (See Figure 1–6). The patient was a 15-year-old boy who complained of pain and swelling of the right leg. About one year prior to seeking medical aid he noticed aching of the leg after skiing or skating. He paid little attention to this, but he noticed the aching gradually became severe and continuous. About three months previously he first noticed a swelling. On examination a slightly tender swelling over the midshaft of the right tibia was the only abnormality detected. A radiograph revealed a bony defect in the region; a provisional diagnosis of primary bone tumor was made. Secondary cancer could have produced a similar picture, but is a very uncommon condition at this age. The figure shows a technetium bone scan; the increased activity in the region of the tumor is obvious. Note also the increased activity over the ends of the long bones, particularly at the knee, wrist, and upper ends of the humeri. This is due to epiphyseal bone growth in this 15-year-old boy. A chest radiograph and a liver scan revealed no evidence of metastatic tumor (see Chapter 17). A biopsy of the tumor revealed osteosarcoma. An above-knee amputation was performed. The boy adapted well to the procedure but shortly afterwards developed a wound infection from *Staphylococcus aureus*. Three months after the amputation a sinus was excised, and a 2-inch section of femur was removed so that a better stump could be fashioned. The wound healed well, and the patient was able to walk. He remains well 14 months after diagnosis. Nevertheless, the prognosis must be guarded, since less than 20 per cent of patients survive for more than five years following treatment. This case illustrates two other important features: (1) Noninvasive investigations such as a bone scan are carried out before invasive procedures such as biopsy. (2) Radical surgery for malignant disease should never be undertaken without first obtaining a definite tissue diagnosis.

Autoradiography

Radioactive isotopes can be used at a microscopic level. If a section of tissue is placed on a photographic film for a suitable time, subsequent photographic development will reveal the site of isotope localization as a series of black grains. This principle is often applied in experimental pathology; for example, it is found that tritiated thymidine (thymidine containing tritium, the radioactive isotope of hydrogen) is incorporated into DNA in the same way as ordinary thymidine. DNA synthesis and therefore mitotic activity can be investigated by this technique (Fig. 1–7).

Tissue Culture

Tissues of various types can be cultured outside the body with comparative ease. Growth commonly occurs on the surface of glass or plastic, and tissues can be grown in test tubes, medicine-flat bottles, or the surface of a coverslip.

There are two types of tissue culture:

Cell Culture. If isolated cells of an organ or tissue (or portions of a tissue) are placed in a tissue culture medium, individual cells grow as a flat sheet on the surface of the container. This is an extremely important technique in virology, because viruses can be grown in the cultivated cells (Chapter 12). Its use for other purposes, such as in cancer research, is limited, because the cells are growing in a highly artificial medium and often do not carry out the specific functions of the organ from which they were isolated. Nevertheless, cell culture has found many uses. *Fetal cells from amniotic fluid* (obtained by amniocentesis, see Chapter 3) can be cultured in order to detect chromosomal abnormalities or specific enzyme defects, *e.g.*, that found in Tay-Sachs disease.* Likewise, cells from individuals with known inherited

---

* In Tay-Sachs disease there is an abnormal accumulation of lipid in cells, particularly nerve cells, owing to a lysosomal enzyme defect. Affected infants suffer from mental retardation and blindness. The disease is inherited as an autosomal recessive trait. It is particularly common among Ashkenazi Jews, in whom it has been estimated that approximately 1 in 30 are carriers, being heterozygous for the abnormal gene. Prenatal diagnosis of this severe disease is generally held to be a good indication for therapeutic abortion. Carriers of the trait can be identified by estimating the level of the specific enzyme in the serum. Married couples in which both partners are carriers can be advised as to the likelihood of producing an affected child (Chapter 3).

Figure 1–7. Autoradiograph of a mitotic figure in a squash preparation of the root tip of an onion fed with tritiated thymidine.

A, Photographed at the level of the section to show the chromosomes. *B,* The same cell photographed at the level of the photographic emulsion. The labeled thymidine has been taken up by the cell and incorporated into DNA. Note how the silver dots correspond to the chromosomes. This technique is used to locate the sites of DNA synthesis during the period when the labeled thymidine was available (×3200). (Photographs courtesy of Dr. P. B. Gahan.)

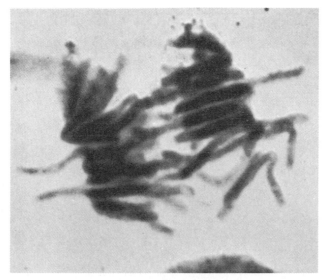

A

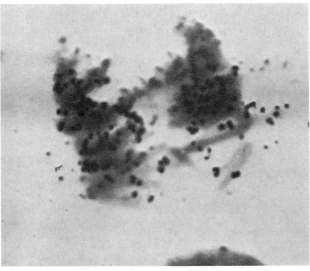

B

disease can be studied in the laboratory in order to unravel the biochemical defect responsible for their condition. Short-term *lymphocyte culture* is used extensively in chromosomal analyses (Chapter 3).

Normal cells are difficult to maintain in culture, because with repeated subculture they invariably die. Efforts to establish a permanent *cell line* consisting of a single *clone** are invariably unsuccessful, and even fibroblasts, which grow relatively easily, die out after 50 to 60 generations. Normal cells have a finite life span.

Sometimes a change occurs in a culture (termed *transformation*) after which the cells can be subcultured indefinitely. These potentially immortal cells develop into malignant neoplasms if grafted into a suitable host. Transformation may occur spontaneously (presumably by mutation) or as a

---

*A clone is a group of cells of like hereditary constitution that has been produced asexually from a single cell. The word is derived from the Greek *klon,* meaning a cutting used for propagation.

result of a viral infection. Thus *lymphoblastoid cell lines* have been obtained by transforming human lymphocytes with the Epstein-Barr virus.

The best known example of a permanent cell line is that of the *HeLa cell*. This was derived from a carcinoma of the uterine cervix of *Helen Lane*, a patient after whom the cell line was named.

Somatic cell hybridization is a technique whereby two dissimilar cells are allowed to fuse to produce a single hybrid cell. The two cells may be from the same individual or from completely separated species, *e.g.,* man and mouse. This technique has been used extensively in genetic mapping (Chapter 3) as well as in the production of monoclonal antibodies using hybridomas (Chapter 9).

Organ Culture.   A fragment of tissue is grown on a grid, so that there is no cellular outgrowth, but histologically the organ is kept as normal as possible. Limb buds, eye rudiments, and bones have been studied while growing in an artificial medium, and their differentiation has been observed.

Chemical and Physical Analysis of Biological Materials

Chemical technology has now advanced to the stage at which it is possible to analyze substances as complex as the insulin molecule and the ribonuclease molecule, the latter containing 124 amino acid residues. X-ray diffraction techniques have revealed the complex folded structure of a large molecule such as myoglobin. Apart from these research applications, modern methods of chemical analysis combined with automation now make it possible to estimate a large number of chemical substances in the small quantity of body fluids, *e.g.,* blood. With the SMA-12 Auto Analyzer, which is routinely used, it is currently possible to estimate 12 substances from a single sample of blood, *e.g.,* sodium, potassium, chloride, blood urea nitrogen, glucose, etc.* In many centers, this biochemical analysis (*biochemical profile*) is now performed routinely in much the same way that the pulse has been taken and the blood pressure recorded for many years.

The separation and identification of proteins have been greatly facilitated by the technique of electrophoresis, which is illustrated in Figure 25–1.

As more and more complex techniques become available and adapted to medical use, there is a tendency to regard patients as objects for the academic exercise of investigation and scientific treatment. Batteries of investigations are ordered and abnormalities are treated. This can lead to disastrous results, because every test has its limitations: experimental errors, biological variations, and significance under particular circumstances, all of which must be taken into consideration. The patient must be treated as an individual and not dehumanized by the modern medical center. Too often one hears of a patient failing to respond to treatment and then dying. The truth is that the wrong treatment was applied through miscalculations on the part of the medical attendants, or that no effective treatment was available. Blame the practice of medicine but not the patient!

Review Questions

1. Describe the basis for the use of hematoxylin and eosin as histological stains. How would you expect the following cells to appear when stained with H & E?
    (a) Mature red cells, which have no nuclei, and have cytoplasm that contains basic proteins.
    (b) Reticulocytes, which are young red cells but differ in that the cytoplasm also contains threads or strands rich in ribonucleic acid (RNA).

---

*The others usually estimated are serum glutamic-oxaloacetic transaminase (SGOT), lactic dehydrogenase (LDH), alkaline phosphatase, bilirubin, calcium, phosphate, and uric acid.

(c) Plasma cells, which are nucleated, and whose cytoplasm contains basic protein as well as some RNA.

(d) Thyroid cells, whose cytoplasm contains basic protein but very little RNA.

2. The fate of ingested potassium iodide is to be investigated. A number of rats are given a dose of radioactive iodine in the form of potassium iodide. How would you attempt to follow the absorption, utilization, and excretion of the labeled iodine?

3. The frozen section technique is an essential component of a modern laboratory service. Discuss the use of this technique from the viewpoint of the surgeon, the patient, and the pathologist.

4. Define the following terms: (a) biochemical profile, (b) histopathology, (c) histochemistry, (d) resolution, as applied to microscopy.

5. Outline the methods available for the demonstration of a specific protein (*e.g.,* IgM) in the cytoplasm of a cell.

Selected Readings

Champion, R. H., Gillman, T., Rook, A. J., and Sims, R. T.: An Introduction to the Biology of the Skin. Oxford, Blackwell, 1970. Note, in particular, Chapter 4, "Some Tinctorial and Cytochemical Methods," which is a simple account of the principles underlying the action of common fixatives and stains.

Ham, A. W.: Histology. 8th ed. Philadelphia, J. B. Lippincott Company, 1979. Chapters 1 and 2 elaborate on many of the topics covered in this chapter.

Leeson, C. R., and Leeson, T. S.: Histology. 4th ed. Philadelphia, W. B. Saunders Company, 1981. Note, in particular, the introduction, which provides basic information on microscopy, tissue preparation, examination of sections and stains.

Taylor, C. R.: Immunoperoxidase techniques: practical and theoretical aspects. Archives of Pathology and Laboratory Medicine, *102*:113–121, 1978.

Normal Structure and Function

After studying this chapter the student should be able to:

- Distinguish epithelial cells from connective tissue cells with respect to their structure and function.
- Describe the structure of the plasma membrane and list its functions.
- Draw a diagram of a typical epithelial cell and include its nucleus, nucleolus, mitochondria, lysosomes, glycogen granules, endoplasmic reticulum, and Golgi apparatus.
- Describe the important functions of each of the organelles.
- Relate the structure of DNA to chromosomes and genes.
- Draw a diagram to show how the information of DNA is utilized in the formation of protein.
- Describe how gene action is controlled.
- List the information that can be learned about the chromosomes and their arrangement from an examination of:
  - (a) nuclear morphology
  - (b) the Barr body
  - (c) the Y body
- Describe the two components of the endoplasmic reticulum and relate them to lysosomes and the Golgi apparatus in terms of both structure and function.
- Describe the distribution of reticuloendothelial cells and their functions.
- Describe the components of the ground substance.
- Describe collagen fibers with respect to their
  - (a) distribution in the body
  - (b) appearances under the light microscope and the transmission electron microscope
  - (c) relationship to reticulin
  - (d) chemical composition
  - (e) formation

- Describe the cell cycle and the phases of mitosis

Introduction   The human body is formed from the division of a single cell, the fertilized ovum. The process of division, *mitosis*, is described later in this chapter. It results in the formation of two daughter cells, each of which closely resembles the original. Nevertheless, as division follows division, the daughter cells exhibit new or altered structure and function. This process is called *differentiation* or *maturation*. The first evidence of differentiation in the mass of cells of the developing embryo is the formation of three distinct germ layers. An outer layer of cells forms the *ectoderm*, while a tube develops within the mass and the cells lining it form the *endoderm*. This tube forms the basis of the future alimentary canal and organs that bud from it — lungs, liver, pancreas, and others. The *mesoderm* consists of cells lying between ectoderm and the endoderm.

The primitive cells of each germ layer can differentiate along two separate lines — forming either epithelium or connective tissue.

Epithelial cells cover surfaces (*e.g.*, skin) or line cavities (*e.g.*, the mouth); in these situations they are essentially protective in function. Covering epithelia may also perform a secretory function: the intestinal and respiratory epithelia, for instance, secrete mucus (Figs. 2–1 and 2–2).

In addition to covering surfaces, the secretory type of epithelium may be arranged to form solid glands. Thus, during development hollow buds of endodermal cells form masses that subsequently differentiate into liver, pancreas, and salivary glands. Likewise, buds from the ectoderm form sweat glands and breast tissue. The secretory cells are arranged around a central cavity to form acini into which the secretion is poured (Fig. 2–3). From here the secretion passes into collecting ducts and reaches the epithelial surface from which the gland originated. In some glands the connection with the epithelial surface is lost, the duct disappears, and secretion takes place directly into the blood stream. Such secreting organs are the *endocrine glands;* even in these, although no secretion is collected into ducts, acinar spaces may be formed. This configuration is clearly seen in the normal thyroid (Fig. 39–4). A feature common to all epithelial cells is that they are closely contiguous with one another. This structural feature is evident on light microscopy, and even under the electron microscope the cells appear to be separated by only a thin layer of electron-dense material that is about 15 nm in width.

Connective tissue, or *mesenchymal, cells* are the other cell type present in the body. They are usually widely separated from each other by a zone containing ground substance in which fibers are embedded. *Collagen fibers*

Figure 2–1. Small intestine. This photomicrograph shows part of the muscle coat (M) covered by the mucosa. Between the muscle coat and the mucosa there is a layer of loose connective tissue called the submucosa (Sm). The picture is typical of a slide prepared by the paraffin-wax technique and stained with hematoxylin and eosin (× 50).

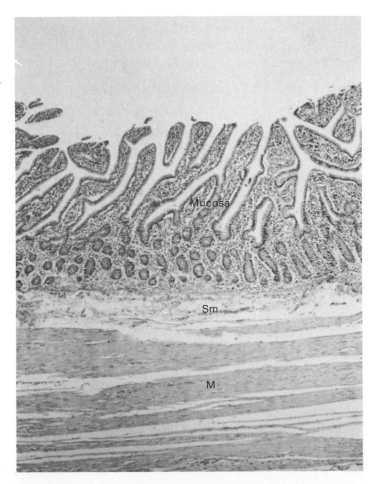

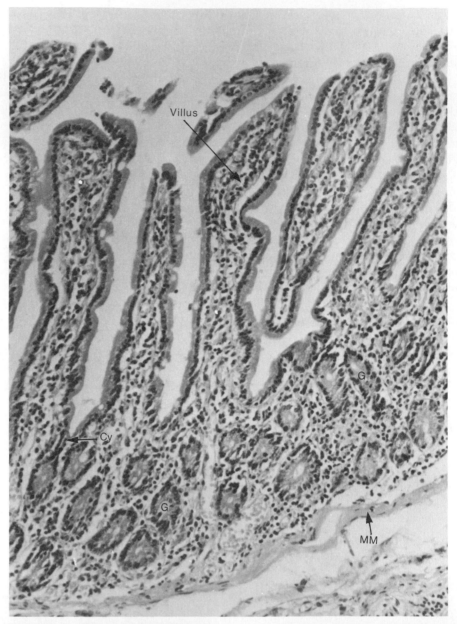

Figure 2–2. Mucosa of the small intestine. The mucosa is covered by an epithelium composed of a single layer of tall columnar cells, some of which secrete mucus. The absorptive surface is increased by the folds, or villi, that project into the lumen of the gut. Simple tubular glands (G) open into the crypts (Cy). Beneath the epithelium, the mucosa consists of connective tissue containing thin fibers of collagen, associated fibroblasts, and blood vessels. There is a sparse infiltration by small round cells, most of which are lymphocytes or plasma cells. It is not possible to identify individual cells at this magnification. The thin layer of muscle of the mucosa, the muscularis mucosae (MM), is seen in the lower part of the picture (× 200).

are the most abundant, but in some areas (*e.g.,* the walls of large arteries) *elastic fibers* are also present. This type of connective tissue — typified by tendon, bone, cartilage, and fibrous tissue — is primarily supportive in function. Other connective tissue cells have been endowed with specialized cytoplasm either for *contraction* (muscle fibers) or for *conduction* (nerve cells). It should be noted that while much of the body's connective tissue is derived from mesodermal cells, the mesoderm is also capable of differentiating into epithelium. The kidney and the gonads are mesodermal in origin, and

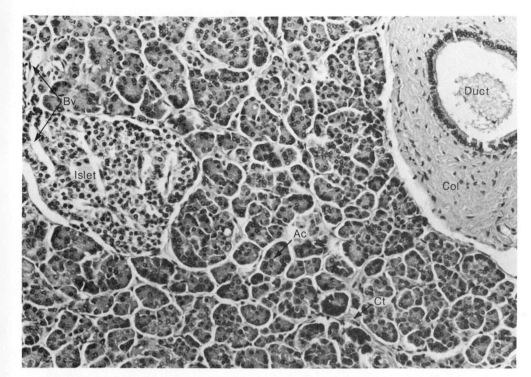

Figure 2–3. Normal pancreas. The exocrine portion of the gland is composed of secretory epithelial cells arranged in groups or acini (Ac), each of which has a central lumen into which the secretion is poured (the lumina cannot be seen at this magnification). Secretion is collected into small ducts, and these drain into larger ducts and finally into a main pancreatic duct. The endocrine portion of the gland forms a small portion of the pancreas and is represented in this figure by one islet of Langerhans, which has no acini or duct. The connective tissue of the gland is represented by small blood vessels (Bv) and a collagenous stroma, scanty between the acini, but more obvious around the duct (Col) (× 250).

yet they are epithelial in structure. The ectoderm and endoderm tend to differentiate into epithelia; even here, however, there are exceptions. Some of the muscle of the eye is of ectodermal origin. Most of the nervous system, including its glial connective tissue, is derived from ectoderm. Only the microglia are mesodermal.*

The study of the embryological origin of cells and tissues is of some importance in pathology in explaining certain curious phenomena. Thus, in some diseases of the breast, gland structures are found that closely resemble those of the apocrine sweat gland (Chapter 38). Both sweat glands and breast tissue have a common ectodermal origin. Likewise, tumors can be found in the anterior lobe of the pituitary that closely resemble those found normally in the jaw or skin. The pituitary gland, teeth, and epidermis all have a common ectodermal origin.

The process of differentiation, by which cells become highly specialized, is sometimes accompanied by loss of ability to divide. Thus, neurons are highly specialized and are quite incapable of mitosis as they become differentiated. Nevertheless, in other tissues — liver cells, for instance — the power to divide is never lost. What is lost during the process of maturation is the ability to differentiate along different lines. The fertilized ovum is *totipotent,* *i.e.,* capable of producing all the tissues of the body, and its immediate daughter cells have a similar capability. Separation of cells at this early stage

---

*Because nervous tissue and muscle are so different from ordinary connective tissue, some authorities describe four basic tissues: epithelial, connective, nervous, and muscular. This further subdivision serves little purpose in pathology.

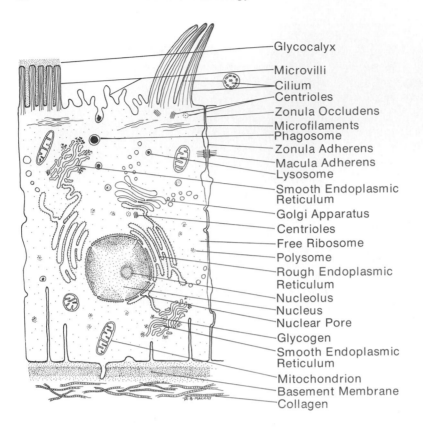

Glycocalyx
Microvilli
Cilium
Centrioles
Zonula Occludens
Microfilaments
Phagosome
Zonula Adherens
Macula Adherens
Lysosome
Smooth Endoplasmic Reticulum
Golgi Apparatus
Centrioles
Free Ribosome
Polysome
Rough Endoplasmic Reticulum
Nucleolus
Nucleus
Nuclear Pore
Glycogen
Smooth Endoplasmic Reticulum
Mitochondrion
Basement Membrane
Collagen

Figure 2–4. Diagram of a hypothetical typical epithelial cell. (Drawn by Margot Mackay, Department of Art as Applied to Medicine, University of Toronto.)

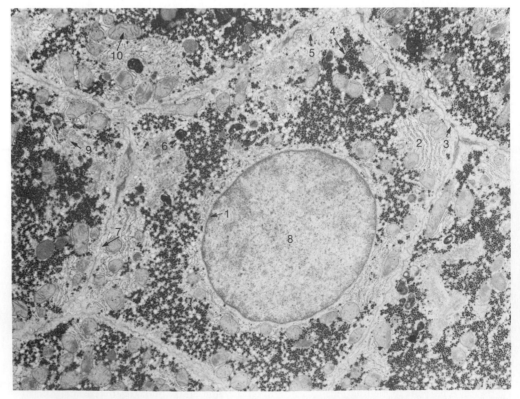

Figure 2–5. Survey of normal human liver. (Courtesy of Dr. Y. C. Bedard.) Parts of six cells are shown (× 10,000). Compare this with Figure 2–4. See Review Questions, No. 4.

results in multiple fetuses with consequent identical twins, triplets, and other such multiple births.

The cells of the body show considerable diversity of structure and function, yet each is remarkably independent. Each receives a supply of oxygen and foodstuff from the blood stream, with which it must produce its own structural components and secretions. Each cell must also release the energy required for mechanical, chemical, or electrical work. It is therefore not surprising that all cells are built upon a similar plan (Fig. 2–4).

The number of chemical reactions known to occur inside the cell is so great that it would be difficult to understand how these could proceed in a structure that appears, under the light microscope, to be so simple. The electron microscope has changed all this; the cell's appearance has been changed from a barren wilderness to that of a structure resembling a large industrial city with its factories, warehouses, streets, and powerhouses (Fig. 2–5).

STRUCTURE OF THE NORMAL CELL

The Cell or Plasma Membrane

Each cell is surrounded by a *cell or plasma membrane,* which is composed of a complex protein-lipid combination (Fig. 2–6). The plasma membrane is not a rigid structure and its movement allows for phagocytosis, a process whereby prolongations of the cell surround particles and envelop them to form a vacuole in which the contents are digested. Likewise, motility of cells is a function of plasma-membrane movement. This is well illustrated by the ameboid movement of the white blood cells.

At the ultrastructural level, small invaginations of the cell membrane can become nipped off to form vesicles called phagosomes. In this way, small quantities of fluid may be imbibed by a process known as endocytosis.

The cell membrane has other important functions. It contains specific antigens by which the body is able to *recognize* its own cells and tolerate them. The cells from another individual are regarded as aliens and are attacked (see Chapter 9). The cell membrane is also concerned with *adhesiveness,* which is a factor that induces cells of like constitution to stick together. This property can be well demonstrated experimentally: if the cells of an embryo are separated from each other and then are allowed to come together again under suitable conditions, like cells tend to aggregate to reform organs and tissues. This affinity that cells have for their own kind must be an important mechanism in the development and maintenance of the architecture of multicellular animals. But not all cells behave in this manner. The mature cells of the blood do not stick to each other, and the lack of adhesiveness exhibited by cancer cells allows them to wander off and infiltrate freely into the surrounding tissues. This characteristic allows cancer cells to spread and kill.

The cell membrane acts as an *exchange surface* across which cell constituents are interchanged with those of the extracellular fluids. Thus, the cell membrane acts as a chemical barrier as well as a mechanical one, and it is this function that is responsible for the maintenance of the characteristic

Figure 2–6. Diagrammatic representation of the plasma membrane. The membrane is shown as a double layer of phospholipid molecules with their hydrophilic (water-loving) ends pointing outward and their hydrophobic (water-hating) ends facing inward. Globular proteins are partially or completely embedded in the lipid. This concept of a fluid lipid bilayer with embedded protein was described by Singer and Nicolson (Science, *175:*720, 1972). (Drawn by Margot Mackay, Department of Art as Applied to Medicine, University of Toronto.)

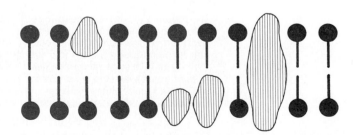

chemical composition of the interior of the cell. Potassium, magnesium, and phosphate ions are present in high concentration in the cytoplasm. In contrast, the extracellular fluids are rich in sodium, chloride, and bicarbonate ions. The cell membrane is able to extrude sodium ions and thereby allows the potassium to accumulate within the cell. This mechanism, which is sometimes known as the *sodium pump*, requires energy. The integrity and normal functions of the cell membrane are therefore important factors in maintaining this special chemical composition of the cell substance. Another interesting feature of the cell membrane is the presence of areas of so-called *cell*, or *surface*, *receptors*. It is to these areas that viruses become attached, and it is at these sites that many substances such as drugs and toxins act. An interesting application of the receptor concept is the supposition that many hormones react with specific receptors on their target cells. The interaction appears to activate an enzyme that leads to the formation of adenosine 3':5'-cyclic monophosphate, usually referred to as *cyclic AMP*. This substance triggers a sequence of events specific for that cell and leads to its response associated with the hormone. Cyclic AMP is therefore regarded as a *second messenger* acting within the cell (Fig. 2–7).

One fascinating aspect of cell receptor function deserves mention. It has been found that opiate (morphine) receptors are present in certain areas of the central nervous system. It seems that the brain can manufacture substances (called *endorphins*) that have a morphine-like action and are normal chemical transmitters within the brain. This helps to explain how the appreciation of pain can vary according to circumstances. A cut finger in the kitchen can be extremely painful, and yet during the heat of battle a whole limb can be lost almost without notice.

The Cytoplasm   The *cytoplasm* is that part of the protoplasm not included in the nucleus. It is filled with a delicate three dimensional web or lattice of thin, intercommunicating filaments that form the *microtrabecular meshwork* (Fig. 2–8). In the spaces between the meshwork there is the watery portion of the cytoplasm. The cytoplasm is further subdivided into many compartments by membranes that closely resemble the cell membrane in structure. The most

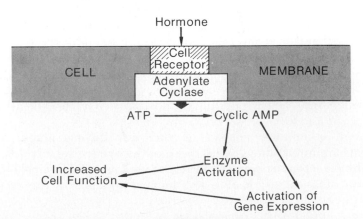

Figure 2–7. The second-messenger concept. Many hormones act first by becoming attached to specific receptor sites on the membranes of target cells. Thus, adrenal cells have receptors that "recognize" adrenocorticotropin. The enzyme adenylate cyclase is activated in the cell membrane and passes into the cytoplasm where it catalyzes the formation of cyclic AMP, which acts as a second messenger. In some cells it leads to enzyme activation. Thus, in the liver, phosphorylase is activated and leads to the formation of glucose from glycogen. This is a mechanism by which epinephrine causes the release of glucose from the liver cell. Cyclic AMP appears to act also by stimulating the expression of genetic information. It may therefore be regarded as a type of chemical switch that turns on the cell to perform specific functions. (Drawn by Anthony J. Walter.)

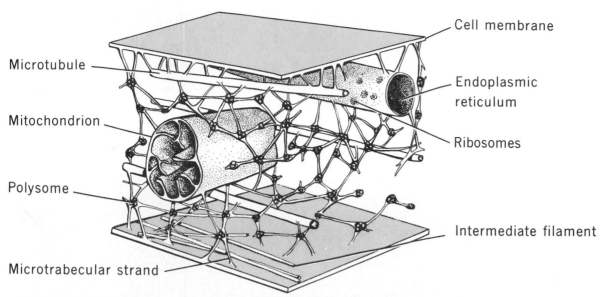

Cell membrane

Microtubule

Endoplasmic reticulum

Mitochondrion

Ribosomes

Polysome

Intermediate filament

Microtrabecular strand

Figure 2–8. The microtrabecular lattice. In this drawing the microtrabecular lattice is seen to occupy the substance of the cytoplasm. It has attachments to other structures (endoplasmic reticulum, mitochondria, and other organelles), and at points of junction groups of ribosomes are gathered together to form polysomes. The concept of the microtrabecular lattice has been derived from examination of cells by high voltage electron microscopy. There is some doubt as to whether the lattice seen is the result of artifact or whether it is a real structure perhaps modified by artifact—as indeed are all structures seen in preparations of tissue for both electron microscopy and light microscopy. (Drawing by Rasa Skudra, Department of Medical Photography and Art, Toronto General Hospital, Toronto. Modified from Porter, K. R., and Tucker, J. B.: The ground substance of the living cell. Scientific American, *244*:59, 1981.)

extensive subdivision is effected by the endoplasmic reticulum. The cytoplasm also contains other membrane-bound structures or *organelles, e.g.,* mitochondria and lysosomes. Furthermore, the cytoplasm contains thin tubular structures (microtubules) and various types of filaments. All these structures are bound together by the fine filaments of the microtrabecular meshwork in which they are suspended, much in the same way as a blade of grass or a fly is suspended when caught in a mass of cobwebs. The simile is not exact, however, because the filamentous and tubular elements of the cell's internal structure are not rigid; they can contract, or be rapidly removed and reformed during movement both of the cell itself and of its internal structures such as secretory granules, chromosomes, etc.

Endoplasmic Reticulum

This consists of a series of membranes that enclose an intercommunicating series of tubes and vesicles (Fig. 2–9). In most areas, ribosomes are attached to the endoplasmic reticulum, which therefore appears rough; this part is known as the granular or *rough endoplasmic reticulum.* Ribosomes appear as granules 15 nm in diameter, contain ribonucleic acid (RNA), and play a very important part in cell metabolism; it is in relation to them that protein synthesis occurs. Some of the ribosomes are not attached to endoplasmic reticulum but appear to be lying free in the cytoplasm. They often form small aggregates *(polysomes)* attached to the microtrabecular lattice. These polysomes are concerned with the formation of protein that is retained within the cell for its own requirements. Protein produced for export is synthesized in the rough endoplasmic reticulum. It passes into the Golgi apparatus and is packaged to form secretory granules, which move to the cell surface to discharge their contents by the process of *exocytosis* (Fig. 2–12).

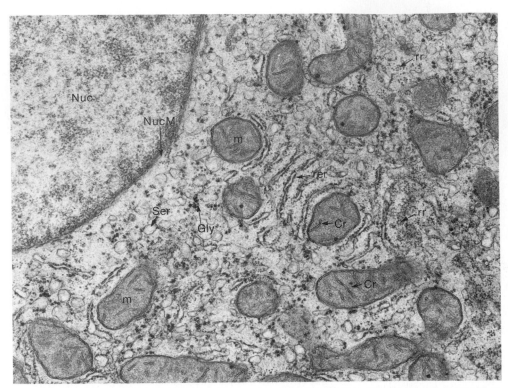

Figure 2–9. Liver cell showing part of its nucleus (Nuc) and cytoplasmic organelles. Mitochondria (m) with their cristae (Cr) are shown along with rough endoplasmic reticulum (rer) to which are attached ribosomes. Smooth endoplasmic reticulum (Ser) is associated with glycogen granules (Gly). Some ribosomes appear free in the cytoplasm and are forming rosettes (rr). Note also the nuclear membrane (NucM) surrounding the nucleus ($\times$ 40,000). (Photograph courtesy of Dr. Y. C. Bedard.)

The endoplasmic reticulum and its associated ribosomal granules cannot be distinguished in the ordinary "paraffin" sections used in routine pathology. The ribonucleoprotein content, however, can be distinguished by its basophilia (cells having an affinity for basic dyes) with hematoxylin. It follows that the cytoplasm of cells actively engaged in protein synthesis appears mauve or blue in H & E sections.

In some cells the endoplasmic reticulum also forms a complex lattice of tubules that have no attached ribosomes and therefore appear smooth (Fig. 2–10). The functions of this part of the cell are less clearly defined, but *smooth endoplasmic reticulum* appears to be related to detoxification of drugs as well as to the synthesis of steroid hormones. It should be noted that the membranes of the smooth and rough endoplasmic reticulum are continuous with each other, with the outer lamina of the nuclear membrane, and perhaps also with the cell membrane.

Mitochondria
These rod-shaped bodies have a characteristic appearance (Fig. 2–9); their complex internal structure is a reflection of their function. They contain all the enzymes of the Krebs cycle and of the terminal electron transport system. The Krebs cycle, illustrated in Figure 2–10, is a system whereby the products of carbohydrate, fat, and protein metabolism are oxidized to produce energy. This process requires oxygen and is therefore called *aerobic respiration* or *oxidative phosphorylation*, since the energy is stored in the form of high-energy bonds of adenosine triphosphate (ATP). The energy can be released by the breakdown of ATP and utilized whenever the cell performs any kind of work. The mitochondria are therefore the powerhouses of the cell

Figure 2–10. Outline of the metabolic pathways involved in energy production. The entire process in the oxidation of glycogen to CO_2 and H_2O can be considered as occurring in two phases. The first, which requires no oxygen (anaerobic), results in the formation of pyruvate and is known as *glycolysis.* If oxygen is not available pyruvic acid is converted into lactic acid. The second phase, which requires oxygen (aerobic), is known as the *Krebs cycle.* Products of carbohydrate, fat, and protein metabolism are fed into the Krebs cycle, and the energy generated ultimately appears in the form of ATP. The hexose monophosphate shunt is shown on the right as an alternate pathway and results in the formation of ribulose 5-phosphate. This is an aerobic process and is important in the metabolism of white cells and red cells. Various genetic defects are known that result in hemolytic anemia or incompetent polymorphs, which are unable to destroy bacteria. (Key: NAD, nicotinamide adenine dinucleotide; $NADH_2$, dihydronicotinamide adenine dinucleotide; Pi, inorganic phosphate; ADP, adenosine diphosphate; ATP, adenosine triphosphate.)

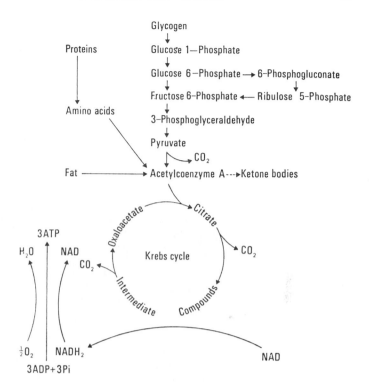

and are among the first structures to be affected when adverse conditions prevail. An interesting feature of mitochondrial structure is that these bodies also contain some DNA, which appears to replicate during cell division. Some people have held it to indicate that mitochondria originated from symbiotic bacteria.

These are round, membrane-bound bodies containing lytic enzymes that are active at a low pH (Figs. 2–11 and 2–12). Acid phosphatase and various proteolytic enzymes come into this group. The lysosomes cannot normally be seen in paraffin sections, but in certain cells (polymorphonuclear leukocytes, for instance) the lysosomes are visible as the characteristic granules. Particles ingested by a cell during the process of phagocytosis appear as membrane-bound bodies, and fusion with lysosomes results in these vacuoles' acquiring digested enzymes (see Fig. 5–4). Lysosomes are therefore important as a source of the enzymes necessary for digestion of phagocytosed material. Likewise, when parts of a cell wear out or are damaged, they also are enclosed in lysosomal bodies. Such lysosomes containing remnants of degenerate cell structure are called *cytolysosomes,* or *autophagocytic vacuoles.* Release of lysosomal enzymes from dead cells plays an important part in the digestion of dead material. The enzymes may also activate mediators of acute inflammation (Chapter 5). Under some circumstances lysosomal enzymes, particularly those derived from neutrophils, can cause severe tissue damage (see Arthus reaction, Chapter 9).

Lysosomes

The Golgi complex, which is best developed in glandular cells and is usually situated close to the nucleus on the side nearest to the lumen, consists of a series of flattened sacs and small vesicles. The Golgi complex appears to be responsible for packaging proteins in membrane-bound vacuoles. Thus, in secreting cells, such as those in the pancreas, secretions formed in the endoplasmic reticulum collect in the Golgi complex, and the vesicles so

Golgi Complex (Golgi Apparatus)

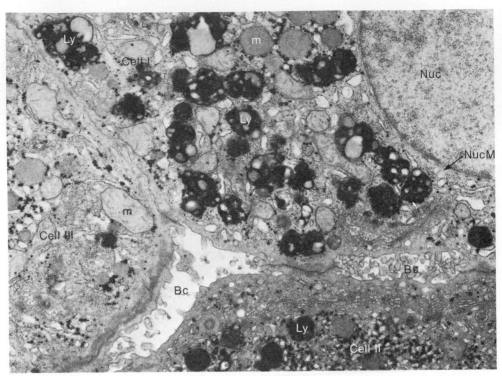

Figure 2–11. Liver showing bile canaliculi. Parts of three adjacent liver cells are shown; between them are the bile canaliculi (Bc), which ultimately drain into the bile duct. Short, irregular microvilli are seen projecting into the lumen. One liver cell contains numerous lysosomes (Ly). Also shown are parts of one nucleus (Nuc) with the double-layered nuclear membrane (NucM), and mitochondria (m) (×17,500). (Photograph courtesy of Dr. Y. C. Bedard.)

formed are then discharged onto the cell surface. Likewise, lysosomes are probably assembled in the Golgi complex, and the completed packages of enzymes are pinched off as membrane-bound organelles (Fig. 2–12).

Lipoprotein synthesis occurs in the Golgi complex, and its vacuoles can migrate to the cell surface and fuse with the cell membrane. Damaged membrane can be replaced and new membrane formed.

Other Structures   High-resolution electron microscopy has revealed many other structures in the cell cytoplasm. Among these are small tubular structures called *microtubules,* which in some cells appear to act as an internal skeleton and to give the cell rigidity. These structures are called *neurotubules* in the axons of nerve cells; possibly, these microtubules act as means of transport from one part of the cell to another. Microtubules form the spindle in mitosis and are components of cilia. Thus, they are concerned with movement. In addition to the microtubules, filaments of various types are found. Some contain myosin (15 mm diameter) or actin (6 mm in diameter) and are concerned with cell movement. Others are intermediate in size (10 mm in diameter) and are called *intermediate filaments.* The composition of these filaments varies with each cell type. For example, in the epidermal cells they form tonofilaments and are composed of keratin, a protein that finally forms the hard, horny outer layer of the skin.

Other structures seen in cells are glycogen granules, fat droplets, and specialized granules in secreting cells. As refinements in the electron microscope have allowed for increased resolution, further structures have been described. In many instances their function is poorly understood, but there is

Figure 2–12. The Golgi complex (Golgi apparatus) and its possible functions. This diagram depicts the Golgi complex as a series of flattened sacs from which numerous vacuoles arise. Some vacuoles contain secretory material that has been synthesized in the endoplasmic reticulum. Some vacuoles appear to be empty and travel to the cell surface, where their membranes fuse with the cell membrane. Other vacuoles contain lytic enzymes and become primary lysosomes. These fuse with autophagosomes or heterophagosomes to form secondary lysosomes. Undigested material remains in residual bodies. (Drawn by Margot Mackay, Department of Art as Applied to Medicine, University of Toronto.)

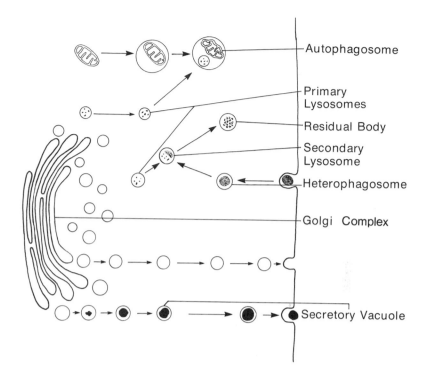

Autophagosome

Primary Lysosomes

Residual Body

Secondary Lysosome

Heterophagosome

Golgi Complex

Secretory Vacuole

little doubt that in due course, the ultrastructure of cells will prove to be very complex — as complex as life itself.

The Nucleus

Situated within the cell and enclosed by a membrane is the nucleus, an important structure because it contains in chemical form the coded information that is handed down from one cell to its progeny and from one generation to the next. The chemical that performs this function is deoxyribonucleic acid (DNA). Like the RNA of the cytoplasm, this substance is basophilic in H & E–stained sections, and the nucleus invariably stains deep blue. This blue material was named *chromatin* before the discovery of DNA, and the term is still convenient and in common use.

Chemical Structure of DNA

The chemical structure of DNA is well known. It is a polymer composed of a long chain of monounits or nucleotides. Each nucleotide consists of a base combined with deoxyribose sugar and phosphate. The common bases are either purines (adenine and guanine) or pyrimidines (cytosine and thymine). As a result of x-ray diffraction studies, Watson and Crick proposed a structure that fits remarkably well with our concept of DNA as a self-replicating genetic material (Fig. 2–13).

Role of Nucleic Acids as Genetic Material

The DNA of the nucleus contains genetic information that is passed via RNA into the cytoplasm where it is used in the manufacture of proteins — often enzymes — of exact composition. The word *gene* is used to describe a hypothetical unit of heredity for any single characteristic. Genes are an expression of the information contained within the DNA molecule. The order of the bases in DNA constitutes the genetic code, a sequence of three bases designating a single amino acid. A type of RNA (messenger RNA, or "mRNA") is manufactured in the nucleus in the presence of DNA-dependent RNA polymerase. This process is called *transcription*, and the mRNA is modeled after one of the polynucleotide chains of DNA, which acts as a template. The base sequence of the RNA is complementary to that of DNA, *i.e.*, cytosine

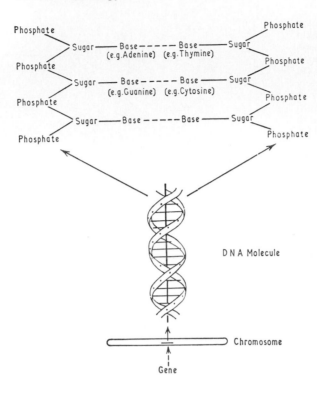

Figure 2–13. Suggested chemical structure of DNA. The two polynucleotide chains are united by their bases, the order of which constitutes the genetic code. (After Watson, J. D., and Crick, F. H. C.: Nature (London), *171*:737, 1953.)

corresponds with guanine, uracil corresponds with adenine, etc.* This mRNA passes into the cytoplasm and becomes associated with a group of ribosomes (a polysome). Here protein synthesis occurs. Each triplet, or codon, of the RNA base order codes for one amino acid. As the ribosomes "read along" the RNA molecule, successive amino acids are added to an ever-increasing polypeptide chain. In this way, a protein of exact composition is built up. The actual addition of each amino acid is effected by another type of RNA (transfer RNA, or "tRNA"), a separate form of which exists for each of the amino acids. This process is described as *translation*, for the code of the DNA finally appears legible in the form of a polypeptide chain (Fig. 2–14).

Thus, the genetic code of DNA consists of codons that determine the insertion of particular amino acids in the peptide chain. The sequence of the codons is collinear with the sequence of amino acids. Codons responsible for an entire peptide chain form a group called a *cistron*. It is believed that a number of cistrons are grouped together to form a larger unit, the *operon*, which is described below. The actual code has been investigated by various means. Synthetic polyribonucleotides have been prepared and can act like mRNA in cell-free preparations containing ribosomes, suitable substrates, and a source of energy. Thus, a polynucleotide containing only uridine (poly U) leads to the formation of a polypeptide containing only phenylalanine. Hence the code for this amino acid is "UUU."

Control of Gene Action

It is evident that each newly created cell of the body contains the necessary information for the manufacture of every protein of which the body is composed. That all cells do not do so at all times is evidence that there is some very adequate control mechanism. For example, erythroid cells man-

---

*When DNA replicates, the double helix unwinds and each strand acts as a template for the formation of a new strand. Thus, cytosine pairs with guanine, and adenine pairs with thymine. In the formation of single-stranded mRNA, thymine is replaced by uracil.

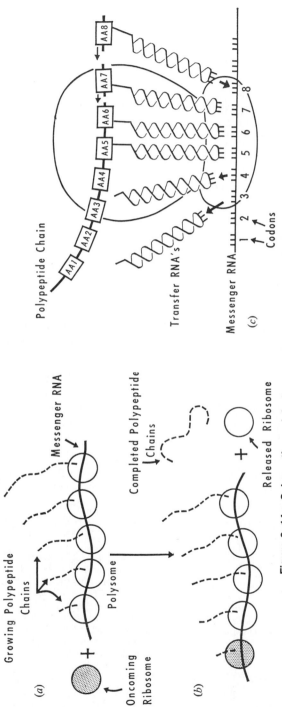

Figure 2–14. Schematic model of protein synthesis. In (a) and (b) a long single-stranded molecule of messenger RNA (mRNA) is seen associated with a group of ribosomes to form a polysome. As each ribosome moves along the mRNA, an ever-growing polypeptide chain is produced. In (c) a single ribosome is depicted as a combination of two particles of unequal size. The sequence of bases of the mRNA forms triplets, or codons, which for the sake of clarity are drawn as groups of three upright lines. Each molecule of transfer RNA (tRNA) is composed of a long thread bent on itself to form a helical structure. At one end of the molecule there is a particular amino acid (AA1, AA2, etc.), and at the other end, where it is bent on itself, there are three unpaired bases that form an anticodon. Each codon of the mRNA is "recognized" by a corresponding anticodon of a tRNA. In this way specific amino acids are added to the polypeptide chain in a specific linear sequence determined by the mRNA, which is itself modeled on the nuclear DNA. (Drawn by the Department of Art as Applied to Medicine, University of Toronto, after Warner, J. R., and Soeiro, R.: New England Journal of Medicine, 276:613, 1967 and Nirenberg, M. W.: The Living Cell. San Francisco, W. H. Freeman & Company, 1965. Reprinted by permission from the New England Journal of Medicine.)

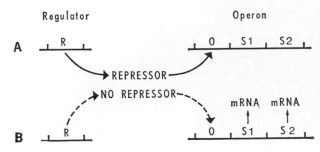

Regulator   Operon

Figure 2–15. The regulator-operator hypothesis. *A,* The regulator gene (R) forms a repressor substance that acts through the cytoplasm to repress the operator gene (O). When O is thus inhibited, the structural genes (S1 and S2) in its operon cannot form mRNA. *B,* If the regulator gene cannot form repressor substance, or if the repressor does not reach the operator gene, the operator is *derepressed* and S1 and S2 are then able to produce mRNA. (Redrawn from Thompson, J. S., and Thompson, M. W.: Genetics in Medicine. 2nd ed. Philadelphia, W. B. Saunders Company, 1973. The hypothesis is that of Jacob, F., and Monod, J.: Journal of Molecular Biology, *3*:318, 1961.)

ufacture hemoglobin, and plasma cells form immunoglobulin. Nevertheless, it is not surprising that under abnormal circumstances cells produce substances that are alien to their accustomed products. It is for this reason that a tumor of the lung can produce hormones normally produced only by the pituitary. Many examples of this phenomenon will be seen later.

Some genes lead to the production of either enzymes or proteins used in the metabolism of the cell. These are termed *structural genes*. It has been found that a group of genes can be closely linked together and can either function together or be completely repressed, *i.e.*, no mRNA is produced. Figure 2–15 illustrates a simple scheme based on the hypothesis of Jacob and Monod. Each group of genes, or operon, is controlled by a closely associated gene called the *operator gene*. This itself is regulated by another gene, the *regulator gene*, which through its own mRNA leads to the formation in the cytoplasm of a protein (repressor substance), which suppresses the operator gene. The regulator gene may itself be inhibited, and in that event, the operator is derepressed, the genes of the operon are allowed to act, mRNA is produced, and protein synthesis proceeds. The complexity of gene action is apparent when it is appreciated that in every cell, every gene is under continuous control and is so regulated that the requirements of the body are met. This applies not only during adult life but also during the complex processes of development. The ovum provides an excellent example of how protein synthesis can be inhibited, only to be switched on suddenly by the event of fertilization.

The structure of the gene and the processes of translation and transcription described above are applicable to bacteria but not to animals, including man, in which the details are far more complex. In humans there is much more DNA present in the chromosomes than appears to be necessary to encode for all the proteins that are present in the body. The length of DNA

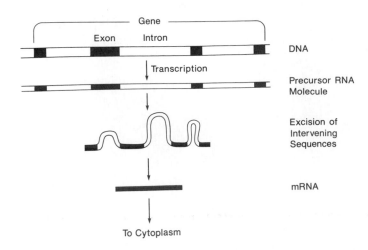

Figure 2–16. Transcription of genetic information. Diagrammatic representation of a gene, showing exons and introns. After the formation of a precursor RNA molecule, the intervening sequences coded by the introns are excised, and mRNA is assembled before being passed into the cytoplasm for translation. (Drawing by Rasa Skudra, Department of Medical Photography and Art, Toronto General Hospital, Toronto.)

containing information for one protein is not continuous but is broken up into segments (called *exons*), which are separated by long stretches of other intervening DNA (called *introns*). The RNA transcribed in the nucleus may be ten times or more longer than is needed for translation in the cytoplasm. The cell removes this excess RNA and splices the remainder to form mRNA (Fig. 2–16). The function of the excess nucleic acid is not known. Some probably provide signals that say in effect "start here" or "stop here." What other messages, if any, there are in these silent areas of DNA is not known. The subject is of more than academic interest. Current research wherein human DNA is recombined with bacterial DNA requires detailed knowledge of the structure of the DNA that contains the necessary information for one gene together with its regulatory switches (Chapter 3).

The DNA molecules are not lying free in the nucleus but are contained in long threads called *chromosomes*. Each resting somatic cell contains a definite number of chromosomes, the diploid or 2N number. This corresponds to the normal amount of DNA. In humans, the diploid number is 46; of these, 23 are derived from each parent. Two chromosomes, which are related specifically to sex, are called the *sex chromosomes*. One is considerably larger than the other and is called an X chromosome, whereas the smaller one is the Y chromosome. Females have two X chromosomes; males have one X and one Y. The remaining 22 pairs are identical in appearance in both sexes and are called the *autosomes*.

Chromosomes

Each resting somatic nucleus contains a constant number of chromosomes (the diploid number, which is twice the haploid number). Certain exceptions to this condition are found. As a person ages, some cells of the liver contain more chromosomes than normal. When a cell contains three or more times the haploid number of chromosomes, the condition is termed *polyploidy*. Thus, some liver cells have large nuclei containing 92 chromosomes. A similar event occurs in tumor cells.

During the period between cell divisions, the chromosomes are present in the nucleus as long, drawn-out threads. These are not visible as such when the light microscope is used, but in some areas along the thread there is sufficient coiling for the condensation of material to render these areas visible as basophilic chromatin dots in the nucleus. Such chromatin is thought to represent regions of the chromosomes that are condensed and relatively inert metabolically. The remainder of the nucleus is lightly stained and the chromatin appears dispersed. The actual morphology of the nucleus varies considerably from one cell to another, and an assessment of function can be made from nuclear structure. Thus, in active cells, *e.g.*, cancer and nerve cells, the nucleus contains little condensed chromatin and is described as "vesicular." In inactive cells, such as small lymphocytes and spermatozoa, the condensed chromatin occupies much of the nucleus, which consequently is deeply basophilic and small.

Some very large cells, *e.g.*, megakaryocytes of the bone marrow, contain many nuclei and are called *multinucleate giant cells*.

Apart from DNA, the nucleus contains RNA, and some of this may appear as a separate structure called the *nucleolus*. This structure is particularly prominent in cells that are active metabolically. Nucleoli are therefore prominent features in the nerve cells and in many cancer cells.

The Barr Body.   Dr. Murray Barr first noticed a discrete mass of chromatin in the nuclei of cells from a female animal — a mass that was not present in the nuclei of the male. This can be easily demonstrated in the human by examining suitably stained cells scraped from the buccal mucosa; it appears as

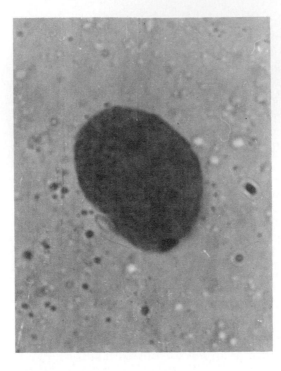

Figure 2–17. The Barr body. Nucleus of a cell from female buccal mucosal smear showing the sex chromatin mass on the nuclear membrane. (Photograph courtesy of Dr. Nigel H. Kemp.)

a demilune on the nuclear membrane (Fig. 2–17). This chromatin can be shown to be formed by an X chromosome that is tightly condensed and mostly inactive. The normal female has two X chromosomes, and one of these is extended and active, while the other forms the Barr body. This hypothesis was first proposed by Dr. Mary Lyon, and it appears that the inactivation of one of the X chromosomes is random and occurs in each cell in early embryonic life. Hence, in the normal female about one half of the cells carry an active maternal X chromosome, while the other half carry an active paternal X chromosome. The inactive chromosome divides later than other chromosomes during cell division, and its descendants follow the same pattern. It occasionally happens that an individual has more than two X chromosomes, and in these cases the number of Barr bodies seen in a cell is equal to the total number of X chromosomes less one. Examination of the buccal smear is an important investigation in cases of chromosomal abnormality. Cells possessing a Barr body are also called *chromatin positive*.

The Y Body. The Y chromosome selectively takes up the dye quinacrine hydrochloride, which has the property of fluorescing strongly under ultraviolet light. If the smear of buccal mucosal scraping or peripheral blood is stained

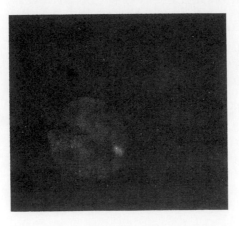

Figure 2–18. The Y body. Nucleus from a normal male cell stained with quinacrine hydrochloride and examined under ultraviolet light. The bright fluorescent dot represents the Y chromosome. (Photograph courtesy of Dr. Peter K. Lewin.)

with this dye, a bright fluorescent dot in the nucleus indicates the presence of a Y chromosome (Fig. 2–18).

This system of cells is found widely scattered throughout the body, and its components all share an ability to become phagocytic. Not only do they phagocytose coarse particles, but they also are able to abstract highly diluted dyes when injected into the blood stream. It was by this technique that this group of cells was first delineated by Aschoff, who called it the *reticuloendothelial system* (RES). The RE cells are closely associated with lymphocytes, with which they are sometimes grouped together as the *lymphoreticular system.* More recently the term *mononuclear-phagocyte system* has been proposed. The name alludes to the structure and function of its constituent cells. The term reticuloendothelial is misleading because neither the endothelial cells lining the ordinary blood vessels nor the reticular cells belong to it. Reticular cells are closely associated with reticulin fibers, which they are thought to produce. These are described later in the chapter. The fibers form a supporting network in many organs such as the lymph nodes, spleen, and liver. Reticular cells closely resemble histiocytes, but the two are probably quite distinct because reticular cells are only feebly phagocytic. Nevertheless, it is difficult to distinguish between these two types of cells morphologically; it is probable that both cell types are derived from stem cells.

There are two groups of RE cells:

Fixed Cells.   These comprise cells that line the sinuses of certain organs, notably the liver (Kupffer cells), spleen, bone marrow, and lymph nodes (sinus-lining, or littoral, cells), and also the resting *histiocytes* that lie in the various connective tissues of the body. Those in the central nervous system are called microglia.

In most tissues it is assumed that there are primitive multipotential cells that when suitably stimulated can differentiate into reticular cells, histiocytes, hematopoietic cells, and probably other more specialized connective tissue cells such as fibroblasts. These *stem cells* are poorly defined morphologically, and indeed they may differ in appearance in different organs. In the bone marrow they are believed to resemble lymphocytes.

Mobile or Wandering Cells.   These are the blood monocytes.

Whenever there is a local pathological process in a tissue, such as an infection or tissue damage, reticuloendothelial cells migrate to the area, become phagocytic, and in this form are called *macrophages* (Fig. 2–19). The majority of these cells are derived from the blood monocytes, but a variable number are probably also derived from local tissue histiocytes. It should be noted that the other phagocytic cells of the body, the neutrophil granulocytes of the blood, are not included in the RE system by definition. This is because they cannot perform the same type of phagocytosis generally associated with the RE system.

The ground substance varies in consistency from an amorphous gel forming the translucent material of hyaline cartilage to the glairy fluid found in the synovial joint cavities. It is in the molecular meshes of the ground substance that the extracellular, or interstitial, fluid is contained. This fluid constitutes about one third of the total water and lies between the blood vessels and the cells. It contains many electrolytes in a concentration similar to that of plasma as well as small uncharged solute materials such as oxygen, carbon dioxide, urea, and glucose, which are being conveyed either for cellular metabolism or for excretion. In addition, the ground substance contains the following:

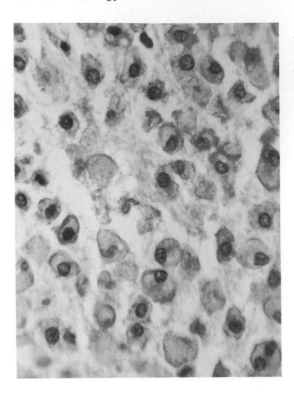

Figure 2–19. Macrophages. Section from an area of brain damage showing many macrophages that are engaged in removing dead brain tissue. The cells have abundant cytoplasm (× 500).

Glycoproteins.   These are proteins that contain a firmly bound component of carbohydrate.

Mucoproteins.   These are loose combinations of protein with acid mucopolysaccharides; the latter consist of polymers of hexose sugars containing amino groups. The best-known acid mucopolysaccharide is hyaluronic acid. The mucoproteins are largely responsible for the viscosity of the intercellular ground substance. The enzyme hyaluronidase, which is produced by streptococci, depolymerizes hyaluronic acid and renders the ground substance more watery. This may play some part in the spread of infection by streptococci. The special property of hyaluronidase can be used in therapy. If fluid has to be injected into the subcutaneous tissues, *e.g.,* in a young child, the addition of hyaluronidase facilitates the penetration of saline as well as its subsequent absorption.

Collagen   Collagen fibers constitute about one third of the body's protein. They form the scaffold in all tissues and are the chief component of such tissues as fascia, dermis, cornea, and tendon. They give these structures tensile strength. Collagen accounts for about 90 per cent of the organic matrix of bone, and in this situation is adapted for the deposition of bone salts. At least five different types of collagen are known, and these differ in the amino acid sequence of their constituent polypeptide chains (see below). They differ also in their distribution within the various tissues of the body.

The collagens and ground substance are synthesized by fibroblasts and by similar cells such as are found in tendon, cornea, bone, and cartilage.

Light-Microscopic Appearance of Collagen.   The first formed collagen consists of fine branching fibers called reticulin (Fig. 2–20). These fibers are demonstrated by silver impregnation methods and are not seen in ordinary H & E sections. In many organs of the body, collagen formation stops at this stage, and the reticulin forms a scaffold for the parenchyma (*e.g.,* liver, spleen, and lymph nodes). In the connective tissues proper, the fibers become

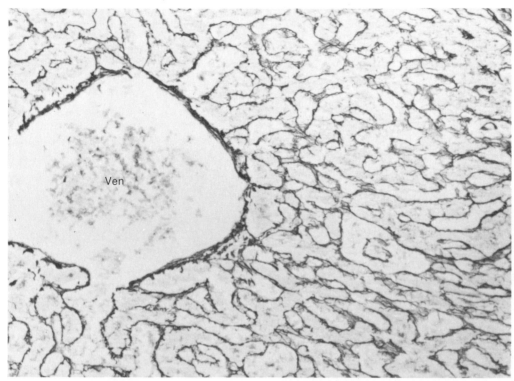

Figure 2–20. Reticulin fibers in liver. This section of liver has been stained by a silver technique; only reticulin fibers, which are stained black, can be seen clearly. The spaces between the reticulin fibers are occupied by hepatocytes and sinusoids that drain blood into a venule (Ven).

enlarged and are then called collagen fibers. They lose their affinity for silver but readily take up eosin and can be stained specifically with aniline dyes combined with phosphotungstic acid (Mallory's trichrome stain).

Under the electron microscope both reticulin and collagen fibers are seen to be composed of fibrils having a characteristic cross-banding with a periodicity of about 64 nm (Fig. 2–21).

Composition of Collagen. The basic unit of collagen is a molecule called *tropocollagen*. This consists of three polypeptide chains, each coiled on itself. The three coiled chains are wound around a common axis like a three-stranded rope. It is thus a coiled coil! The tropocollagen molecules are bound to their lateral neighbors with a quarter overlap, so that the periodicity so characteristic of collagen is produced (Fig. 2–22). Seven chemically different types of polypeptide chains are known, and it follows that by various combinations of three molecules different types of tropocollagen, and therefore collagen, can be formed.

Collagen is characterized by its high content of glycine (33 per cent), proline, and hydroxyproline (the latter two together constituting about 22 per cent). Hydroxyproline is an amino acid that is not found to any extent in other proteins; an estimation of the amount of it in hydrolysates of tissue may therefore be used to measure the amount of collagen present.

The formation of collagen is a complex affair involving the formation of the three polypeptide chains in the rough endoplasmic reticulum and the subsequent winding together to produce mature tropocollagen. For this process to take place, vitamin C is necessary. The tropocollagen finally passes into the extracellular tissues and a variety of bonds are formed so that the collagen, from being a soluble solution of tropocollagen, is converted first into reticulin fibers, then into collagen fibers, and finally into adult, mature, tough collagen tissue.

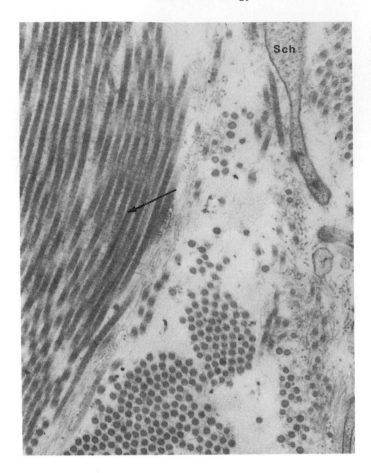

Figure 2–21. Section of collagen fibrils in a peripheral nerve. The fibrils show the characteristic cross-banding (arrow), which is best seen where the fibrils are cut longitudinally. Part of the cytoplasm of a Schwann cell (Sch) is also shown (× 12,000). (Photograph courtesy of Dr. N. B. Rewcastle.)

Elastic Fibers   Elastic fibers are found in large blood vessels, in the lung, and to a lesser extent in many other tissues. On light microscopy they stain deep red with eosin and can be specifically demonstrated by staining with orcein, which renders them black. Elastic fibers are quite different from collagen; they have a different electron microscopic appearance and a different chemical composition. There is some debate as to how elastic fibers are formed as well as evidence that they can be produced by both fibroblasts and smooth muscle cells.

CELL DIVISION   Before cell division occurs, the DNA molecules unwind, and each half acts as a template for the manufacture of the corresponding half. In this way, the amount of DNA is doubled. The chromosomes divide and become double structures called *chromatids;* these are joined together by a single *centromere.* The chromosomes become coiled along their whole length, thereby becoming shorter, thicker, and therefore visible. The cell has now entered the first phase of mitosis — *prophase.* Meanwhile, two centrioles have migrated,

Mitosis

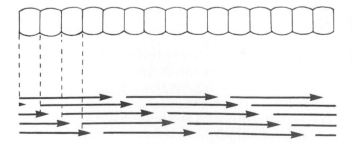

Figure 2–22. Formation of collagen fibril. Diagram to illustrate how the lateral arrangement of tropocollagen molecules, depicted as arrows, results in the formation of banded collagen fibril. (Drawn by Anthony J. Walter.)

Figure 2–23. The cell cycle. DNA reduplication occurs during the synthesis (S stage). This is followed by a short resting stage (G₂) before the cell enters mitosis. Following division the daughter cells may enter the second resting stage (G₁) before recommencing DNA synthesis. Other daughter cells can pass into a resting phase (G₀) and after a period can either re-enter the cell cycle or become differentiated and cease to be capable of mitosis.

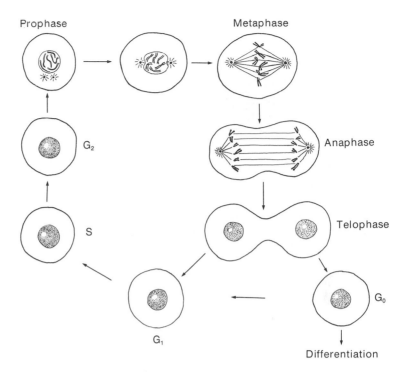

one to each pole of the cell, and microtubules develop in association with them. Each centriole looks like an *aster*, or star (Fig. 2–23).

The nucleoli and the nuclear membrane disappear next, and the cell enters into *metaphase.* By this time, the centrioles are at opposite poles of the cell, and their associated microtubules enter the nuclear region where the split chromosomes become arranged along an imaginary equatorial plate that bisects the cells. The microtubules are attached to the centromeres, and in this way the spindle is formed.

During the next phase, *anaphase*, each set of chromatids, now again called chromosomes, is pulled by the microtubules of the spindle to either pole of the cell. The final stage *(telophase)* involves division of the cytoplasm of the cell, and reconstitution of the nuclear membrane of each daughter cell.

It can readily be understood how during mitosis each chromosome reduplicates itself exactly, and the two daughter cells contain an identical quota of nuclear material. Each DNA molecule is also reduplicated exactly. Should an error occur during mitosis such that an abnormality of the DNA is produced, the process is called a *somatic mutation.* Presumably, this is related to an abnormal sequence of the bases in the DNA molecule.

In the testis and ovary, the process of cell division is more complex and is called meiosis. The process results in cells containing only half the number of chromosomes (the "N," or haploid number, *i.e.*, 23 in man) and half the amount of DNA. These cells develop into gametes — either sperm or ova. With fertilization the diploid number of chromosomes (46) is restored.

Meiosis

During meiosis, the chromosomes become paired off into 23 pairs, with one of each moving into each of the daughter cells. Which chromosome of each pair migrates into which daughter cell is random; thus, the total number of possible combinations is extremely great. Furthermore, during the complex process of meiosis, portions of one chromosome sometimes move and are replaced by corresponding portions of the homologous chromosome. This is termed *crossing over,* and together with the random distribution of each of the pairs of chromosomes within a single gamete is responsible for the tremendous variation that is seen in the progeny of individuals produced by sexual reproduction.

It sometimes happens that during meiosis a pair of chromosomes fail to separate and both are drawn into one daughter cell. This is called *nondisjunction,* and it results in one gamete having an extra chromosome while the other is deficient. Sometimes fragments of chromosomes are lost (by a process called *deletion)* or become attached to another chromosome (by a process called *translocation*). If two breaks occur in the same chromosome, the ends may join together to form a ring chromosome. Chromosomal breaks that result in deletion, translocation, or the formation of ring chromosomes can be induced by the action of ionizing radiation, by certain drugs, and by viruses. It is of interest that it is these same agents that are capable of causing cancer.

The next chapter deals with some of the effects of genetic errors and chromosomal abnormalities.

Review Questions

1. How would you attempt to determine the number of cells in a whole liver? How could its total content of collagen be estimated?

2. Apart from fertilizing ova, spermatozoa have only one major function: to travel several centimeters as fast as possible with their inactive genetic material. Can you relate this function to their structure?

3. Write a brief account of the formation and functions of ATP in a cell.

4. Name the structures numbered 1 to 10 in Figure 2–5.

5. Examine Figure 2–2. The epithelial cells covering the villi are thought to arise in the crypts by mitosis. From there they migrate along the surface of the villi and are cast off finally from the tip. How would you attempt to confirm this movement and to measure the time taken for a cell to migrate from the crypt to the tip?

6. How many types of RNA are there in a cell? Indicate their main functions.

7. The genes that control the formation of the enzyme glucose-6-phosphate dehydrogenase (GPD) are situated on the X chromosome. If you were able to culture cells from various parts of a normal human female, would you expect every cell to manufacture GPD? Explain the reasoning behind your answer.

Selected Readings

Baserga, R.: The cell cycle. New England Journal of Medicine, *304*:453–459, 1981.
Fawcett, D. W.: The Cell. 2nd ed. Philadelphia, W. B. Saunders Company, 1981.
Fox, C. F.: The structure of cell membranes. Scientific American, *226*:30–38, 1972.
Grant, M. E., and Prockop, D. J.: The biosynthesis of collagen. Parts I, II, and III. New England Journal of Medicine, *286*:194–199; 242–249; 291–300, 1972.
Ham, A. W.: Histology. 8th ed. Philadelphia, J. B. Lippincott Company, 1979.
Lazarides, E.: Intermediate filaments as mechanical integrators of cellular space. Nature, *283*:249–256, 1980.
Leder, P.: Discontinuous genes. New England Journal of Medicine, *298*:1079–1080, 1978.
Leeson, T. S., and Leeson, C. R.: Histology. 4th ed. Philadelphia, W. B. Saunders Company, 1981.
Pastan, I.: Cyclic AMP. Scientific American, *227*:97–105, 1972.
Porter, K. R., and Tucker, J. B.: The ground substance of the living cell. Scientific American, *244*:56–67, 1981.
Prockop, D. J., Kivirikko, K. I., Tuderman, L., and Guzman, N. A.: The biosynthesis of collagen and its disorders. New England Journal of Medicine, *301*:13–23; 77–85, 1979.
Ross, L. M.: The cell. *In* Clinical Symposia (Ciba), *26*:4–35, 1974.
Weinstein, R. S., and McNutt, N. C.: Cell junctions. New England Journal of Medicine, *286*:521–524, 1972.
Wilson, R. W., and Elmassin, B. J.: Endorphins. American Journal of Nursing, *81*:722–725, 1980.

The Role of Genetics in Medicine

CHAPTER 3

After studying this chapter the student should be able to:

- Define the terms gene, locus, allele, heterozygote, penetrance, expressivity, homozygote, phenotype, genotype, and polymorphism.
- Draw diagrams to illustrate the mode of inheritance of a disease inherited as
    - (a) an autosomal dominant
    - (b) an autosomal recessive
    - (c) an X-linked dominant
    - (d) an X-linked recessive
- Give at least one example of each type of inheritance.
- Describe the biochemical defect, the effects of the abnormality, and the mode of inheritance of the following genetic diseases:
    - (a) galactosemia
    - (b) phenylketonuria
    - (c) sickle cell disease
- Describe the chromosomal abnormality and the outstanding clinical features of each of the following:
    - (a) the most common type of Down's syndrome
    - (b) Klinefelter's syndrome
    - (c) ovarian dysgenesis
    - (d) cri du chat syndrome
- Describe the nature of plasmids and indicate their importance in relation to
    - (a) bacterial resistance to antibiotics
    - (b) gene cloning
- List the investigations that can be performed on amniotic fluid to detect fetal abnormality. Give examples of the types of defects that may be found.

The study of medicine has largely revolved around the effects of adverse external agents. The great discoveries made in bacteriology, virology, and immunology at the end of the last century strengthened the belief that each disease had a specific cause and that often this cause was a particular external agent — frequently a living organism. As diseases of obviously infective origin have been recognized and brought under control, it has become clear that some diseases have no simple cause and are probably due to many agents acting simultaneously. Inherited diseases were certainly recognized in the past, but they were often regarded as being uncommon. Inherited traits were believed to result from a merging of parental traits, and in this climate of thought the discoveries of Gregor Mendel were passed over and ignored for 25 years. Mendel himself followed the course of many other successful yet frustrated investigators: he abandoned research and became an administrator.

Today we realize that disease has two major bases. It is the result of the interplay between inherited genetic constitution on the one hand and the environment on the other. This chapter is mainly concerned with the first of these components.

THE GENETIC BASIS OF DISEASE

Mendel's laws of inheritance have laid the foundations of the science of genetics and are of great importance in the understanding of many disease processes. He postulated that a particular characteristic is determined by a pair of factors, now called *genes*, each of which is situated at a particular site (or *locus*) on one of a pair of chromosomes. Such genes, forming a pair, are called *alleles*. An individual with a pair of similar genes is called *homozygous*, whereas if the genes are dissimilar, he is *heterozygous*. The genetic make-up of an individual is called the *genotype*, and the effect that is produced is called the *phenotype*.

It is basic in modern genetics to assume that genes occur in pairs, that one of each pair is received from each parent, and that the genes remain unchanged through many generations. The simplest approach to the mode of inheritance of a particular characteristic — for example, a disease — is to consider that the condition is due to a *single-gene disorder*. The gene may be either *dominant* or *recessive*. A dominant gene produces its effect both in the heterozygote and in the homozygote. Recessive genes, on the other hand, produce their effects only in the homozygous condition. Genes occupying an intermediate position are described later. Sometimes a particular locus on a chromosome can be occupied by one of many possible genes. An example of this type is illustrated below with the explanation of ABO blood grouping.

Dominant Genes

A simple example of inheritance of a dominant gene is shown by reference to the ABO blood grouping. The allelic genes that can occupy one locus are "A," "B," or "O".

A homozygous individual who has two *A* genes (genotype *AA*) has on his red cells the blood group substance "A" (phenotype group A). Likewise, the heterozygote *AO* is also phenotypically blood group A because *A* gene is dominant, whereas *O* is recessive. The *B* gene, like the *A* gene, is dominant, and both are described as *codominant*. The possible blood groups in this system are shown below.*

GENOTYPE	*PHENOTYPE*
AA	**A**
AO	**A**
OO	**O**
BB	**B**
BO	**B**
AB	**AB**

Thus, the six genotypes produce only four recognizable blood groups. A person of blood group "A" may be genotype *AA* or *AO*. It is not easy to distinguish between these two genotypes by an examination of the individual himself, but the genotype can be deduced from the family pedigree. It should be noted that the occurrence of two or more genetically different classes of individuals with respect to a single trait is known as *polymorphism*. The blood groups provide an excellent example of this, but many others are known. For example, there are many genetically determined variants of plasma proteins, hemoglobin, and enzymes.

The mode of inheritance of a dominant disease is illustrated in Figure 3–1. It should be noted that:

---

*The ABO blood groups are more complicated than this. For example, *O* is an amorph, and subgroups of A are known.

Figure 3–1. Transmission of a disease inherited as a dominant trait. One pair of chromosomes is shown for each individual, the black chromosome being the one carrying the defective gene. Each person inheriting the defective gene will have the disease. Each member of the next generation has a 50 per cent probability of inheriting the disease.

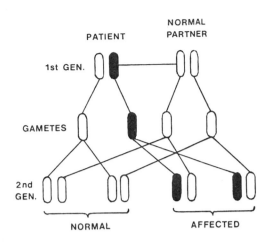

1. The disease appears in every generation or else it dies out. The occasional instance of poor penetrance (discussed later in this chapter) and the occurrence of a new mutant provide exceptions to this rule. If the disease greatly reduces the breeding potential of the affected person, it follows that most cases encountered will be sporadic and due to new mutations.

2. Unaffected members do not pass on the disease (see "Penetrance and Expressivity" later in this chapter).

3. The affected members are usually heterozygous, and if the breeding partner is normal, the chances of his offspring being affected are 50 per cent.

4. Males and females are equally liable to be affected.

Huntington's chorea, achondroplasia, osteogenesis imperfecta, and multiple neurofibromatosis (Fig. 3–2) are examples of diseases inherited as dominant traits.

Diseases Inherited as Recessive Traits

Frequently, these are severe and reduce the breeding potential of the affected person. The mode of transmission is shown diagrammatically in Figure 3–3. The following features should be noted:

1. The birth of an abnormal child is usually the first indication of the condition.

Figure 3–2. Multiple neurofibromatosis (von Recklinghausen's disease). This patient appeared normal at birth except for the presence of several irregularly shaped pigmented macules (café-au-lait spots). The skin lesions shown in the picture began to appear at about 13 years of age. The patient, who is now 60, has thousands of soft skin nodules, many of which are pedunculated. Microscopically these show neurofibromas. The disease is named after von Recklinghausen, who gave the first good account of the disease in 1882. The patient was an orphan and has three children. One daughter is similarly affected, but the others apparently have escaped the disease.

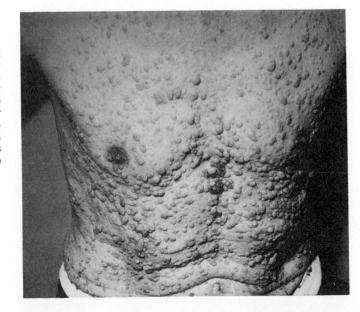

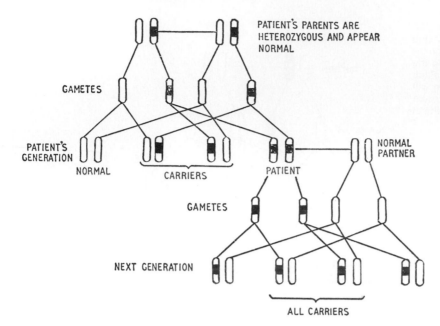

Figure 3–3. Transmission of a disease inherited as a recessive factor. The patient is homozygous and therefore expresses the disease. Both parents are heterozygous and consequently appeared normal. All the patient's offspring are heterozygotes and thus carriers of the trait.

2. As with other mendelian characters, the chances of additional members of the family being affected or passing on the trait can be calculated. Thus, the chances of the next child being affected are one in four. One half of the offspring will be heterozygous and carriers of the trait. If the affected individual mates with a normal partner, all of the progeny will be carriers.

3. The seriousness of producing carriers should not be overemphasized. It has been estimated that we all carry harmful genes that usually remain hidden for generations. A particular gene is liable to be more frequent in a particular family; the danger of close intermarriage is therefore evident. The incidence of defective offspring is much higher in consanguineous matings (those between close relatives) than when the parents are not related.

Some of the best-known diseases inherited as recessive traits are galactosemia, albinism,* phenylketonuria, and cystic fibrosis of the pancreas (see Fig. 30–8).

Sex-Linked Genes.   A gene is said to be sex-linked when it is localized on an "X" or "Y" chromosome. Usually the gene is recessive and is situated on the X chromosome. The most famous disease to be inherited as a sex-linked recessive is hemophilia, which is illustrated in Figure 3–4.

Sex-linked dominant traits are recognized but are rare. Affected females convey the gene to half their sons and daughters, whereas affected males transmit it only to their daughters. Since there can be no male-to-male transmission, there is therefore an excess of female victims. Hemolytic anemia due to glucose-6-phosphate dehydrogenase deficiency is an example of this type of inheritance.

Other Features of Gene Expression   Not all human inherited disease can be explained in terms of simple dominant or recessive gene action. There are many complicating factors:

Penetrance and Expressivity.   It may happen that a trait, although

---

*In albinism the pigment-producing cells (melanocytes) are defective and fail to produce pigment. The transparency of the irides combined with the lack of retinal pigment causes the eyes to appear pink. The hair is white and the skin pale. The white mouse is an example of the typical albino. In the human couterpart there is some pigment formed, so that the hair is a very pale yellow and the eyes are blue.

Figure 3–4. Mode of transmission of a disease inherited as an X-linked recessive Mendelian factor. A common example of such a disease is hemophilia. The abnormal gene is situated on an X chromosome and therefore produces its effect in the male but not in the female except in the very rare event of her being homozygous. The patient's daughters are all carriers of the disease, and his sons are all normal. There is never any direct male-to-male transmission; the disease is perpetuated by the females in the family.

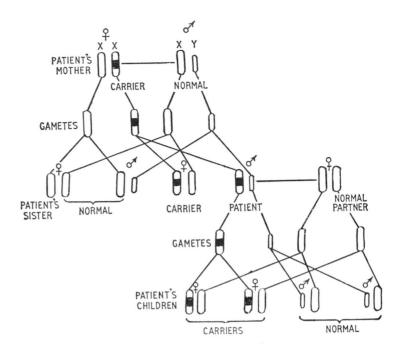

apparently dominant, occasionally misses a generation. The trait is said to exhibit *reduced penetrance*. Another complication is seen in some families in which a dominant gene produces a variable effect. Some individuals who possess it have a severe disease, whereas others have a minor defect (known as *forme fruste*) of the disease. In this instance the trait is said to exhibit *variable expressivity*. Clearly, penetrance and expressivity are closely related, but while penetrance is defined in terms of an all-or-none effect, expressivity is variable.

Intermediate Inheritance. When the heterozygote differs from either homozygote, the inheritance is described as *intermediate*. A good example is sickle cell disease. The homozygote who has two sickle cell genes has the fully developed sickle cell anemia, whereas the heterozygote carrying one defective allele and one normal allele has the mild sickle cell trait — a state intermediate between the disease and the normal. This condition is described in more detail later in the chapter.

Other complicating factors are recognized in human disease. Sometimes several nonallelic genes interact in complex ways; in other instances, a particular trait appears to be the result of many genes acting in various ways. Thus, in the inheritance of intelligence and height there is no simple explanation of the means of inheritance, and it is assumed that many genes are involved. Likewise, some diseases, such as systemic hypertension, obesity, and diabetes mellitus, appear to fall into this group. This type of inheritance is termed *multifactorial*. The precise mechanisms involved are difficult to analyze because there are the additional complicating effects of environmental agents acting in concert with the inherited tendency.

Linkage. Mendel's observation that non-allelic genes are sorted independently at meiosis applies only if the genes are on different chromosomes or, if on the same chromosome, when the loci are far apart. If the genes are close to each other they do not sort independently but are transmitted to the same gamete. This is termed *linkage*. In one form of linkage, the genes are on one of the sex chromosomes, as previously described.

Linkage has been used as the explanation of many facts of inheritance that are not explicable in terms of a single-gene defect or of multifactorial inheritance. Thus it is known that the ability to mount an immune response is related to genes at the *Ia* locus, which is closely linked on chromosome 6 with the major histocompatibility genes, particularly HLA-D (Chapter 9). For example HLA-B7 and HLA-D$_{W2}$ tissue antigens are associated with multiple sclerosis, and over 95 per cent of patients with ankylosing spondylitis are HLA-B27 type.

It is evident that the total genetic material of an individual (the *genome*) can affect the person in many subtle ways. Genes can interact with each other either to cancel each other out or to produce an additive effect. They also determine how the body reacts to external events, particularly in respect to the immune response in relation to susceptibility to infection, hypersensitivity, or the development of an autoimmune disease. Presumably, such interactions and associations explain how particular characteristics are associated with certain diseases, although they are not themselves the obvious cause. The association of a particular disease with a particular ethnic group, *e.g.*, diabetes mellitus and pemphigus vulgaris with Jews, or with sex, *e.g.*, goiter in women and cancer of the lung in men, is an example of this.

Mode of Gene Action   With the discovery of chromosomes and DNA it was logical that attempts should be made to equate genes with segments of the DNA molecule. The first clue came with the description of some diseases characterized by a deficiency of a single enzyme. These genetically determined biochemical lesions, or *inborn errors of metabolism*, to use a term coined by Sir Archibald Garrod over 50 years ago, are a group of diseases in which the individual lacks one particular enzyme. An excellent example of this is the disease *galactosemia*. Babies with this defect lack an enzyme that converts galactose to glucose. The galactose or its metabolites, derived from the lactose in milk, accumulate in the blood and interfere with the development of the brain, the eyes, and the liver. Mental defect, cataracts, and cirrhosis of the liver are the results of this simple biochemical defect. It should be noted that the effects of this enzyme deficiency can be averted by eliminating lactose from the diet. If a child with galactosemia is fed a lactose-free diet, development proceeds normally. The ethics of condemning a person to a lifelong artificial diet might, however, be questioned. Nevertheless, this example illustrates the interrelationship between a genetic defect and an external agent — in this instance, a particular chemical in the diet.

A second example of this type of disease is *phenylketonuria*. Between 3 and 5 persons per 100,000 of the population exhibit this condition, which commences shortly after birth and is characterized by retardation of mental development. The disease is due to the absence of an enzyme that converts the amino acid phenylalanine to tyrosine. Hence, with a normal diet an affected baby develops a high blood level of phenylalanine and its keto derivatives. These cause brain damage, which can be largely averted by the administration of a diet low in phenylalanine. Early diagnosis, by finding phenylalanine or its derivatives in the urine, is therefore very important. The condition is inherited as a mendelian autosomal recessive trait; 1 per cent of the population are heterozygotes, and the condition can be detected by the administration of a test dose of phenylalanine, when the blood level rises. This does not occur in a normal individual. This detection of heterozygotes has a practical value. If a married couple are both carriers, their chance of producing an affected child is 25 per cent. They can be warned of this risk. This is just one example of the kind of information offered in *genetic counseling*.

Hemoglobinopathies.   The translation of the mysterious gene action into concrete chemical terms was first achieved successfully with a group of diseases in man known as the hemoglobinopathies, in which an abnormal form of hemoglobin is manufactured. The globin of the hemoglobin molecule is a protein of known amino acid sequence. In certain individuals, usually of African ancestry, the hemoglobin contains an abnormal globin in which valine replaces the usual glutamic acid in the sixth position of one of the two polypeptide chains of the molecule. Presumably, this is due to an error in one codon of one section of the DNA molecule. Homozygous individuals manufacture the abnormal hemoglobin S, which renders their red cells liable to distort to a sickle shape at low oxygen tensions. These abnormally shaped red cells are easily removed from the circulation and are quickly destroyed, with the result that the patient becomes severely ill with sickle cell anemia. Heterozygous individuals suffer from a mild anemia and are said to have the sickle cell trait. Their red cells contain both normal hemoglobin A and the abnormal hemoglobin S.

Many other diseases are known in which the body synthesizes an abnormal form of a protein — either a structural protein such as hemoglobin or an enzyme. These diseases are grouped together as the *molecular diseases*. Presumably these have arisen by mutations. If the product of the mutant gene differs little from the previous substance, the gene probably becomes part of the gene pool of the population. This is probably the mechanism whereby genetic polymorphism arises. Thus, there are 22 variants of the enzyme glucose-6-phosphate dehydrogenase and at least 150 variants of hemoglobin. In some cases, the mutant provides a definite advantage over the pre-existing gene and presumably will eventually replace the original. In the case of the sickle cell gene, it is believed that those who have the sickle cell trait possess an increased immunity to infection with malaria. It is evident that although sickle cell anemia is a lethal disease, the sickle cell trait provides an advantage to those who possess it and live in a tropical climate where malaria is endemic.

Genetic Mapping and Genetic Engineering

Since genes form part of the DNA molecule, it should be possible to locate exactly where each is situated, not only in which chromosome but exactly on which part of the DNA molecule. Various techniques have been developed to attain this knowledge.

Somatic Cell Hybridization

It is possible to fuse together two cells of different origins to form a single hybrid cell. Thus a mouse and a human cell hybrid can be obtained. When these cells divide in culture there is a tendency for the human chromosomes to be eliminated so that cell lines, or clones (Chapter 1), can be obtained that possess a complete complement of mouse chromosomes but only a few, possibly a single, human chromosome. By studying the properties of these hybrid cells it is possible to allocate a gene to a particular chromosome. Thus, only hybrid cells containing a human X chromosome are capable of producing human type glucose-6-phosphate dehydrogenase (G6PD). The human type enzyme can be differentiated from mouse G6PD by electrophoresis (Chapter 25). It may be deduced that the gene coding for this enzyme is situated on the human X chromosome.

Gene Cloning

Before describing the techniques and importance of gene cloning it is necessary to describe the properties of plasmids.

Plasmids.   Plasmids are small particles found in bacteria that consist of a circular double strand of DNA. They have no outer protein coat and therefore have a simpler structure than viruses. Plasmids may exist in the bacterial cells as separate entities that replicate independently of the cell, or their DNA may become incorporated into the single molecule of DNA that constitutes the bacterial chromosome. In the latter event the plasmid DNA becomes part of the genome of the bacterium and replicates when the cell divides. Plasmids are known to be of importance in several respects. It has been found that some bacteria undergo a process called *conjugation*, in which two cells closely approximate to each other and exchange genetic material. This is a primitive type of sexual reproduction. Only bacteria that contain a particular fertility factor (termed *F factor*) are able to undergo conjugation; this F factor is a plasmid. A second important role of plasmids (originally called *R factor*) is the transfer of bacterial resistance to antibiotics. Some plasmids contain DNA that so alters the host's metabolism that the organism is resistant to antibiotics; the effect may be brought about by excluding the antibiotic from the bacterium, by destroying the antibiotic, or by circumventing the effect that the antibiotic has on the cell's metabolism. Transfer of a plasmid from one bacterium to another is one way in which antibiotic resistance can develop. Thus, an antibiotic-resistant *Escherichia coli* can have its information transferred to a pathogen such as one of the salmonellae. Furthermore, a plasmid may have many DNA components that render the bacterium resistant to a whole range of antibiotics. In this way resistance to many antibiotics can develop quite suddenly. Although bacterial antibiotic resistance can occur by mutation of the bacterial chromosome itself, it is likely that plasmid transfer is a more common mechanism. In recombinant DNA research plasmids play a major part (see below). As yet plasmids are not known to play any part in human disease, but it is possible that similar agents exist and are responsible for extrachromosomal genetic mechanisms. It has been suggested that slow viruses (Chapter 12) are agents of this nature, but this is at the moment speculation. The presence of plasmids and other extrachromosomal genetic nucleic acids indicates that simple mendelian inheritance is by no means the only way by which a cell can acquire genetic information.

The Process of Gene Cloning. Various bacterial enzymes termed *restrictive endonucleases* have the property of splitting the DNA molecule at a specific site where there is a particular sequence of bases. Over 40 of these highly specific enzymes are known. By using one or more of them a DNA molecule can be split into a number of fragments that can be separated (e.g., by electrophoresis). In order to locate a particular gene it is necessary to use a probe, *e.g.*, a specific mRNA that corresponds to the gene under examination. The mRNA is labelled with a radioactive marker so that the fraction of DNA containing the desired gene can be identified and spliced into a plasmid that has been opened by the same restrictive endonuclease (Fig. 3–5). This plasmid is inserted into a bacterium that when cultured can produce large quantities of the gene DNA and its product for analysis.

This and similar recombinant DNA techniques, sometimes termed *genetic engineering*, have great practical as well as commercial possibilities; in the future, bacterial cultures will no doubt be used to produce human polypeptides and proteins — hormones, interferon, etc. The transfer of information by plasmids has been described above. Bacteriophages have also been used for a similar function. This type of genetic engineering is as yet in its infancy and, like all techniques, can be used for good or ill. Since it is possible to insert foreign DNA into organisms, the new man-made bacteria might well be capable of producing devastating epidemics, either by accident or by design in warfare.

It is possible to insert DNA into mammalian cells. A virus may be used as the carrier, or the DNA may be directly injected into the nucleus. In the future

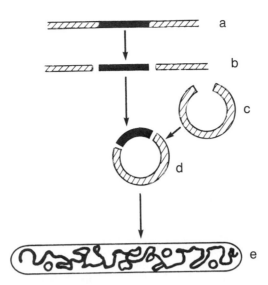

Figure 3–5. Gene cloning. (*a*) Portion of foreign DNA with segment containing the gene depicted in solid black. (*b*) DNA molecule cleaved by restrictive endonuclease. (*c*) Circular DNA molecule of plasmid opened by the same restrictive endonuclease. (*d*) Segment of foreign DNA inserted into the plasmid's DNA. (*e*) Host *Escherichia coli* with plasmids. The plasmids may multiply independently of the bacterial DNA as shown here, or they may become incorporated into the single strand of DNA that constitutes the bacterial chromosome. (Drawing by Rasa Skudra, Department of Medical Photography and Art, Toronto General Hospital, Toronto.)

it may be possible to take cells from a patient with a genetic defect, insert the appropriate normal gene, and return the cells to the patient.

The techniques described in Figure 3–6 have made it possible to study chromosomes as a routine investigation. Certain individuals have been found to have more than 46 chromosomes, while others have fewer. Abnormalities in the shape or form of individual chromosomes have also been noted. These abnormalities may be considered under two headings: (1) alteration in *number* of chromosomes and (2) alteration in *structure* of chromosomes.

Diseases Associated with Gross Chromosomal Abnormalities

Although the finding of chromosomal abnormality is regarded as uncommon, it is now apparent that those cases detected in postnatal life represent only the residue of a much larger group of abnormal zygotes. About one half of the fetuses spontaneously aborted in the first three months of pregnancy have chromosomal abnormalities, one of the commonest being *triploidy* (the cells

Figure 3–6. Human chromosomes at metaphase. Lymphocytes from the blood of a normal woman were grown in culture for 72 hours before colcemid (a colchicine derivative) was added. This chemical inhibits spindle formation so that mitoses are halted at metaphase. Two hours later a hypotonic solution was added to make the cells swell. The dispersed chromosomes were then stained with Giemsa after they had been pretreated with trypsin. This technique brings out the banding of the chromosomes.

The mitosis shown contains 46 chromosomes, each of which is a divided structure joined by a centromere. The individual chromosomes can be cut out with scissors and arranged in pairs as shown in Figure 3–7. Such an arrangement is called a karyotype. (Photograph courtesy of Dr. H. A. Gardner, Division of Cytogenetics, Toronto General Hospital.)

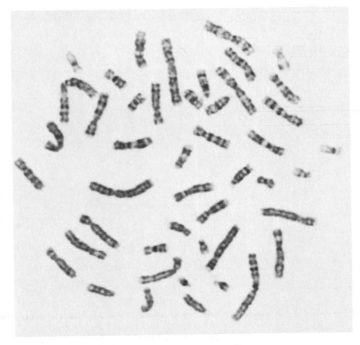

having 69 chromosomes). It has been estimated that about one third of the results of conception are aborted spontaneously and that gross genetic errors are a major cause of this (Fig. 3–7).

CASE HISTORY I.   (See Figure 3–7). A 26-year-old woman gave birth to a stillborn male child at 41 weeks of gestation. Before birth there was clinical evidence of a small head, which was confirmed at ultrasonic examination. No fetal heart was heard during the three days prior to delivery.

The infant showed many abnormalities, the most striking of which was a single eye, containing two lenses, in the center of the forehead. The brain was underdeveloped and exhibited many severe abnormalities. An attempt was made to culture fetal skin cells, but no growth could be obtained. This was not unexpected, since the fetus showed obvious signs of autolysis. However, placental tissue was viable and grew well in culture; photographs of several mitoses were obtained. One of these was arranged as shown in Figure 3–7. The chromosomes are arranged in pairs and are numbered 1 to 22 in order of length, position of the centromere, and banding characteristics. With good technique it is possible to identify each chromosome. When this identification is not possible, the pairs of chromosomes are then arranged into seven groups, A to G, excluding the X and Y chromosomes.

Alteration in Number of Chromosomes

Additional Chromosomes.   The commonest example of this abnormality is when there is one extra chromosome. This condition is called *trisomy*, and the best known example is trisomy 21. The individual has 47 chromosomes

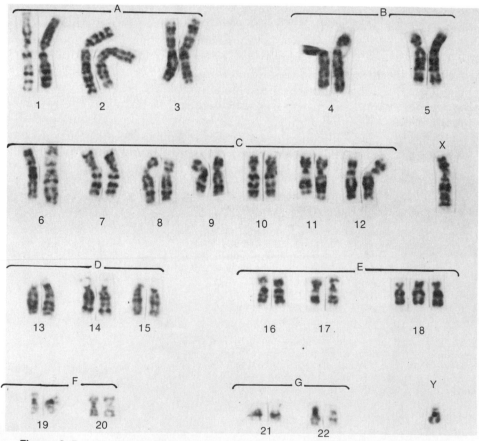

Figure 3–7. Karyotype showing trisomy 18 from a stillborn male with cyclopia. The karyotype is that of a cell with 47 chromosomes. It is evidently from a male, since there is a Y chromosome. The anomaly must therefore be of fetal origin, since the mother had a normal 46,XX karyotype. The additional chromosome No. 18 arose by nondisjunction; its manifestations were incompatible with postuterine life. (From Lang, A. P., Schlager, M., and Gardner, H. A.: Trisomy 18 and cyclopia. Teratology, *14*:195–203, 1976.) For a more complete description, see Case History I.

and may be either male or female. The condition is *Down's syndrome*, otherwise known as mongolism (Fig. 3–8). This is always accompanied by mental defect, and the condition is quite common since such affected children are produced with an incidence of approximately 1 in every 600 live births. Trisomy of other autosomes is known but is much less common.

The presence of additional sex chromosomes is not uncommon. Certain individuals are found to have an extra "X." Some are apparent males, have the genetic constitution 47,XXY, and have chromatin-positive cells. They have small testes that fail to develop at puberty; there is little facial hair; they may have a female type of breast development (gynecomastia); and they are sterile. These features become evident at puberty; the condition is known as *Klinefelter's syndrome*. Another group of patients have the karyotype 47,XXX and are females, usually with normal secondary sex characteristics and sometimes with mental defect.

In the 47,XYY syndrome, the patients appear as normal males, but in some instances the subject is abnormally tall and exhibits a criminally aggressive temperament. Nevertheless, other individuals with this anomaly appear normal.

Reduction in the Number of Chromosomes. The loss of an autosome is incompatible with postuterine life. In those cases where such a state has been described, a small chromosome is involved, and it seems likely that the chromosome is in fact present but has become attached to some other chromosome, *i.e.*, it has been translocated.

The sex chromosomes are less vital for survival, and deletion of one is quite compatible with life. In about 1 in every 3000 births, a female is produced with the karyotype 45,XO. The condition, which is known as *ovarian dysgenesis*, becomes obvious at adolescence when the ovaries fail to function normally, ovulation does not occur, and menstruation is absent

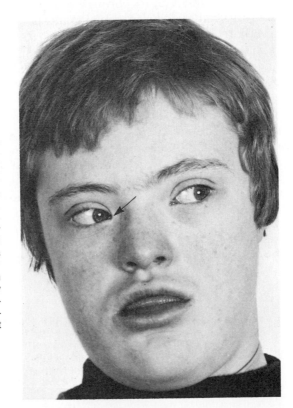

Figure 3–8. Down's syndrome. This patient exhibits the typical facial appearance of persons having the syndrome. Note the large tongue protruding from the mouth. Particularly characteristic is the presence of an epicanthal fold, which is best seen on the right side (arrow). This is a fold of skin that covers the medial angle of the palpebral fissure and gives the eyes an appearance that superficially resembles that of an Oriental. Down's syndrome can generally be recognized at birth, with the diagnosis being confirmed by chromosomal analysis. The mortality is high during the first few years of life, death being related to respiratory infection, congenital heart disease, or leukemia. Dwarfism is common and mental deficiency invariable. Mothers over the age of 35 years are more likely to give birth to an affected child than younger women. (Photograph courtesy of the Department of Clinical Illustration, Birmingham Dental School, Birmingham, England; supplied by Margaret C. Grundy.)

(primary amenorrhea). Such individuals tend to be short because of stunted growth and are sterile. Often they have a number of other abnormalities such as webbing of the neck and a shieldlike chest with widely spaced nipples. Abnormalities of the cardiovascular system are common — in particular, coarctation of the aorta — and the eponym *Turner's syndrome* is applied. These unfortunate females are chromatin-negative, since only one X chromosome is present.

Abnormalities of Chromosome Structure

The recent developments of chromosomal staining have revealed that some individuals have chromosomes differing somewhat from those of the average person. In many instances, these abnormalities are either individual or racial variations and are of no known significance. Any gross abnormality of an entire autosome appears to be incompatible with postuterine life. A number of syndromes have been described in which part of an autosome is missing. For instance, the short arm of chromosome 5 is missing in a syndrome in which the infant exhibits mental defect and cries with a whimpering noise resembling that of a cat in distress (cri du chat syndrome).

So far only one acquired disease has been found to have any consistent chromosomal abnormality. This is chronic myelocytic leukemia, in which the abnormal white cells lack one arm of chromosome 22, usually called the *Philadelphia chromosome*.

Avoidance of Genetic Defects

Genetic counseling will dissuade some high-risk couples from procreation, but once conception has occurred, the only course open may be the induction of abortion. Removal (by *amniocentesis*) and testing of amniotic fluid can be employed for the prenatal detection of fetal abnormality. The supernatant of the fluid can be examined biochemically and checked for the presence of virus. The amniotic cells (of fetal origin) can be examined for the presence of the X and Y chromatin. They can also be cultured for biochemical investigation and chromosomal analysis. These investigations can usually be completed between the sixteenth and twentieth week of gestation. If a defect is found, an abortion can be performed safely at this time. Whether or not to adopt this course also depends on moral and legal factors. In the future, genetic engineering may offer an alternative approach.

ACQUIRED DISEASE

Many human diseases are acquired in postnatal life as a result of the action of external factors. The effects of physical and chemical agents, living organisms, and dietary deficiencies are the common causes of these *acquired diseases*. It should be remembered that the developing fetus is also sensitive to environmental factors, and the tragedies that followed administration of thalidomide to pregnant women bear witness to the extreme sensitivity of the fetus under some circumstances. Intrauterine events may produce defects that are present at birth *(congenital)* but are not inherited, since no genetic mechanism is involved. Inherited diseases may be congenital, *e.g.*, achondroplasia, but they may also appear later on in life, *e.g.*, polyposis coli (Chapter 32). The time of onset of a disease gives no indication as to whether the cause is environmental or genetic.

Review Questions

1. A mother and her child both have the blood group AB. What are the possible genotypes of the father?

2. A patient with galactosemia mates with a heterozygous carrier of this disease. What are the chances that they will have a clinically unaffected child? Will all such children be carriers?

3. Deaf-mutism is inherited as an autosomal recessive trait. Two deaf-mutes marry and have ten children, all of whom have normal hearing. This is not an isolated example of this occurrence. Account for the birth of the children with normal hearing.

4. A man with hemophilia and glucose-6-phosphate dehydrogenase deficiency (inherited as an X-linked dominant trait) has a son. What are the chances that he will have:
   - (a) hemophilia only
   - (b) glucose-6-phosphate dehydrogenase deficiency only
   - (c) both of the above defects
   - (d) neither of the above defects

5. Describe the potential value of being able to culture bacteria that contain human genetic material.

6. Two phenotypically normal parents have a child with phenylketonuria.
   - (a) What is the genotype of each of the parents?
   - (b) What is the probability of the next child also having phenylketonuria?
   - (c) What is the probability of a normal child of these parents being a carrier of phenylketonuria?

Selected Readings

Anderson, W. F., and Diacumakos, E. G.: Genetic engineering in mammalian cells. Scientific American, 245:106–121, 1981.

Cohen, S. N., and Shapiro, J. A.: Transplantable genetic elements. Scientific American, 242:40–49, 1980.

Emery, A. E. H.: Elements of Medical Genetics. 4th ed. Berkeley, University of California Press, 1975. A short, up-to-date account of the subject.

Grobstein, C.: The recombinant-DNA debate. Scientific American, 237:22–33, 1977.

Leading Article: HL-A antigens and rheumatic diseases. British Medical Journal, 1:238, 1975.

Novick, R. P.: Plasmids. Scientific American, 243:102–127, 1980.

Rosenberg, L. E., and Kidd, K. K.: HLA and disease susceptibility: a primer. New England Journal of Medicine, 297:1060–1062, 1977.

Sergovich, F.: Human cytogenetics. In Raphael, S. S.: Lynch's Medical Laboratory Technology, 3rd ed. Philadelphia, W. B. Saunders Company, 1976, pp. 1352–1452.

Thompson, J. S., and Thompson, M. W.: Genetics in Medicine. 3rd ed. Philadelphia, W. B. Saunders Company, 1980. Written for medical students, this book emphasizes the statistical aspects of inheritance.

Valentine, G. H.: The Chromosome Disorders. 3rd ed. London, William Heinemann Ltd., 1975. An excellent, easy-to-read, short account of chromosomal disorders.

Cell and Tissue Damage

After studying this chapter the student should be able to:

- Describe the concept of a biochemical lesion as a cause of cell damage, and give three examples of such lesions.
- Differentiate between cell death, autolysis, and necrosis.
- List the effects that chemicals can have on liver cells.
- List the events that can lead to cell damage.
- Define the terms ischemia, hypoxia, and infarction.
- Describe the effects of hypoxia on a cell.
- Describe the pathogenesis of fatty change in the liver.
- Give examples of the value of serum enzyme determinations in the diagnosis of
  - (a) liver disease
  - (b) heart disease
- Define the term "gangrene."
- Describe the pathogenesis of gangrene in the
  - (a) intestine
  - (b) mouth
  - (c) limbs
- Describe hyaline degeneration and elastosis as applied to collagen.
- Contrast necrobiosis with hyaline degeneration.
- List the conditions in which excess ground substance accumulates in a tissue.

The importance of the cell as the basic unit of the body has been recognized since the microscope was first applied to the analysis of biological material. This is scarcely surprising, because simple forms of life like the ameba consist entirely of one cell. Just over 100 years ago Virchow published his textbook on cellular pathology; since then our concept of many diseases has centered on abnormalities in cellular behavior or appearance. The cells of any particular organ or tissue usually closely resemble each other, and it is not surprising that a sick cell such as one from the liver is the essential component of a sick liver; likewise, this "sickness" at the cellular level produces a particular clinical syndrome called liver failure. The advent of electron microscopy has greatly increased our knowledge of cellular changes in disease and has further strengthened the concept that abnormalities in cellular appearance and behavior are the building blocks from which disease entities are built. Nevertheless, a morphological view of cellular behavior has its limitations. The application of chemical techniques has considerably widened our views. At a cellular level the techniques of histochemistry allow us to identify particular chemicals within cells. Furthermore, chemists have exerted a quite different influence on the study of disease by adopting another approach. Instead of concentrating on the individual cell or its organelles, they have turned their attention to specific chemical reactions. Thus, with respect to the metabolism of galactose, most cells can be regarded as behaving in a standard way. The disease *galactosemia* is characterized by a defect in an enzyme that converts galactose to glucose. Deficiency of this enzyme produces a disease leading to microscopic changes in cells that are particularly dependent on this chemical reaction during development. As described previously, the brain, the lens of the eye, and the liver are most severely affected. This second approach to the study of a pathologic condition has been of immense value both in the delineation of disease processes and in the treatment of individual patients. Ultimately, the broad concept of "biochemical disorder" must be reduced to a cellular level. In some instances this has already occurred, and it is convenient, therefore, to consider some examples of cellular damage caused by lesions of known chemical mechanism.

Biochemical Lesions

The concept of a biochemical lesion was first advanced by Sir Rudolph Peters and was based on the observation that pigeons subjected to a thiamine-deficient diet developed severe neurological symptoms, such as convulsions, and ultimately died. In spite of the severity of the disease, no abnormality could be detected by histological examination of the brain. The cells looked normal, but they were not functioning properly. Thiamine was found to be one of the factors necessary for the conversion of pyruvate to acetyl coenzyme A. This is an important mechanism in the feeding of the Krebs cycle (Chapter 2). Hence, thiamine deficiency impairs energy production, and this affects the nerve cells, which have a high metabolic requirement. Biochemical lesions can be deliberately induced in cells by feeding them with agents that closely resemble metabolites. Thus, cells fed with 5-fluorouracil respond to the agent as if it were uracil, but the abnormal end-product blocks other essential processes. This deliberate sabotage of cellular metabolism has been called *lethal synthesis* by Peters and has been used with some success in the treatment of malignant disease. Another example of lethal synthesis is the action of chemotherapeutic agents on bacteria. Thus, sulfonamides are treated as para-aminobenzoic acid by some bacteria. This ultimately blocks cellular metabolism. Likewise, penicillin blocks cell-wall synthesis, thus rendering the bacteria extremely fragile and easily destroyed by osmotic effects.

Patterns of Cell Reaction

Lethal synthesis is but one way in which chemicals can affect our bodies. Indeed, it is instructive to list the mechanisms whereby chemicals, by being metabolized themselves, affect the metabolism of the cell. The liver has attracted the attention of most investigators, and this is not surprising because the organ occupies a key position in dealing with exogenous agents, the majority of which are ingested. Several reaction patterns can be recognized:

Pattern 1. Harmless Reaction. The majority of chemicals are metabolized to harmless products, often being conjugated with glucuronic acid and subsequently excreted.

Pattern 2. Metabolic Imbalance. A few chemicals produce an imbalance in the cells during their metabolism. Thus, the methionine analogue ethionine induces ATP deficiency by excessive trapping of adenine. Lethal synthesis, described above, is another example of this mechanism. A similar mechanism may explain the liver damage produced by ethanol. Knowledge of the metabolic imbalance produced by a chemical is potentially very useful information, because if a deficiency can be identified it may be remedied and cell damage averted.

Pattern 3. Activation to Toxic Metabolites. Some chemicals are metabolized to highly reactive derivatives (free radicals, see below), which then cause cellular damage. Often the active derivative of a drug can be trapped by sulfhydryl-containing compounds such as glutathione. Depletion of glutathione may thus be a predisposing factor to liver damage, and increasing the supply of glutathione may protect the liver against toxic compounds. This has found practical application. Patients who take an overdose of acetaminophen (an analgesic sold as paracetamol, Tylenol, Campain, Exdol, etc.) may develop severe or even fatal liver damage. N-acetylcysteine, a glutathione substitute that combines with the hepatotoxic acetaminophen metabolite, is an effective antidote.

Pattern 4. Induction of Enzymes. Some chemicals can induce the formation of detoxifying enzymes, and this may be manifested microscopically as proliferation of smooth endoplasmic reticulum (Fig. 4–1). Thus, phenobarbital induces the increased formation of the enzyme that also conjugates bilirubin and allows this compound to be excreted harmlessly. The drug is therefore used in the treatment of hemolytic disease of the newborn (Chapter 33).

Pattern 5. Carcinogenesis. Many carcinogens, *e.g.*, the nitrosamines, are thought to be converted into active products that then lead to the poorly understood changes that result in tumor initiation (Chapter 17).

Exogenous chemicals are not the only damaging agents or adverse circumstances that cells encounter. They are also subjected to endogenous chemicals (sometimes generated by antigen-antibody interactions), nutritional deficiencies, and physical agents. When the effects of these agents are detrimental, they may lead to morphologically recognizable changes that traditionally have been described as the *cellular degenerations*. More realistically they can be regarded as *adaptive changes*. When the adaptation is successful, the cell can recover — this is *reversible cell injury*. However, if the adaptation is not successful the changes are indeed degenerative, since

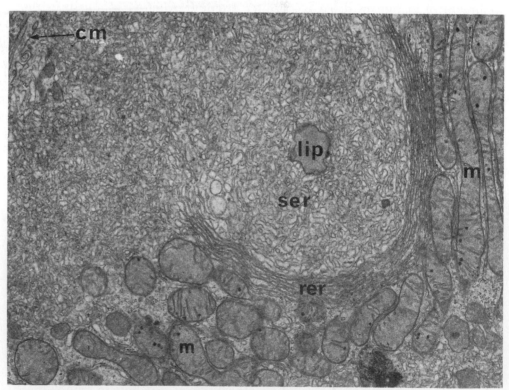

Figure 4–1. Proliferation of the smooth endoplasmic reticulum (ser) in the periphery of a rat liver cell following the administration of ethionine. Phenobarbital can produce a similar change. The proliferated vesicles of the agranular reticulum are tightly packed and well demarcated from the rough endoplasmic reticulum (rer), which can be identified by the ribosomes studded on the membranes. Mitochondria (m) are elongated. (Other abbreviations: cm, cell membrane; lip, lipid droplet.) Tissue was stained by lead hydroxide (× 15,750). (Photograph courtesy of Dr. Katsumi Miyai.)

they represent *irreversible cell injury* and their occurrence is the prelude to cell death.

At this point it is convenient to list the causes of cell damage.

Causes of Cèll Damage

Internal Events

Genetic error — enzyme defects (see galactosemia)

Deprivation of essential chemicals such as hormones, vitamins, and oxygen

Loss of blood supply — deficient blood flow through a part is described as *ischemia,* and the effect is diminished supply of oxygen (*hypoxia*)

Hypersensitivity reactions

External Events

Physical — heat, cold, trauma, and radiation

Chemical — poisons and lack of oxygen

Microbial — microbial invasion and effects of toxins

Pathogenesis of Cell Injury

The mechanism of cell injury varies greatly according to the causative agent. Damage due to hypoxia and chemicals has been studied most extensively.

Hypoxic Injury.   In hypoxic cells there is a reduction in aerobic respiration (oxidative phosphorylation), which reduces ATP production. This has many consequences, *e.g.:*

1. Active cells cease to function. *e.g.,* heart muscle ceases to contract.

2. Anaerobic glycolysis leads to the production of pyruvate and subsequently lactic acid (see Fig. 2–10).

3. The sodium pump (Chapter 2) is impaired. Sodium is retained in the cell and potassium escapes from it. The cell undergoes acute swelling as fluid accumulates in the sacs of the endoplasmic reticulum. The cell indeed becomes water-logged.

4. Ribosomes become detached from the rough endoplasmic reticulum and protein synthesis is reduced.

These changes are all reversible. However, if hypoxia continues there occurs a *point of no return* from which recovery is impossible, and the cell dies. This is accompanied by great swelling of the mitochondria, fragmentation of cell membranes (endoplasmic reticulum, etc.), and increased permeability of the outer cell membrane. The nuclear changes are described later. At some point the cell must be regarded as "dead," but there are no morphological or biochemical markers by which this event may be pinpointed. Following death the lytic lysosomal enzymes act on cell components and the process of self-digestion or *autolysis* takes place.

The degree of ischemia that leads to cell death varies from one tissue to another. Thus, 3 to 5 minutes is sufficient to cause neurons to die, whereas the liver undergoes irreversible damage after 1 to 2 hours.

Chemical Injury.   Some chemicals, *e.g.,* the toxins of *Clostridium perfringens,* directly interact with phospholipids of cell membranes and cause damage. In most instances, however, it is thought that the chemicals are metabolized (usually in the smooth endoplasmic reticulum) to form *free radicals.* These are electrically uncharged atoms or groups of atoms that are chemically highly active. The process is complex, but often the free radicals are powerful oxidants and act on lipids (*lipid peroxidation*). In particular, cell membranes are damaged. The oxidant free radicals can be neutralized by vitamin E and sulfhydryl compounds (such as cysteine and glutathione). As noted previously these substances are being used to counter the effects of some poisons.

Effects of Cell Injury

Some of the electron microscopic changes have already been described. Of greater practical importance in human pathology are the light microscopical and gross changes. Two major groups are described:

1. **Cellular Swelling.** Many types of injury produce waterlogging of the cell. The cytoplasm has a ground glass appearance or contains vacuoles. The terms *cloudy swelling* and *vacuolar degeneration* have been used to describe these changes. If the swelling is extreme, *hydropic degeneration* is used. It may proceed to cell rupture and death (Fig. 4–2).

2. **Accumulation of Fat (Fatty Change).** Normally no stainable neutral fat (triglyceride) can be seen in cells except for fat cells in adipose tissue. Damaged liver cells often show small droplets of neutral fat in their cytoplasm, and ultimately the droplets fuse together to form one large globule that pushes the nucleus to one side (Figs. 4–2 and 4–3). The mechanism of this *fatty change* in liver cell damage is as follows: Fat stored as triglyceride is mobilized from the adipose stores and carried to the liver in the form of free fatty acid. This is taken up by the liver, converted into phospholipid, combined with protein to form lipoprotein, and finally passed into the blood stream (Chapter 25). In liver cell damage there is impaired protein production, so that the fatty acids accumulate within the cell and are converted into triglycerides, which accumulate as droplets or globules within the cytoplasm. In the past this change has often been called "fatty degeneration," but this term is not strictly accurate since fat can also accumulate in the liver under other circumstances. Thus, in starvation an excessive quantity of neutral fat is mobilized from the fat stores and carried to the liver, which, being unable to deal with the excess, forms triglyceride, so that lipid accumulation occurs (Chapter 23). Fatty change is also seen in other organs, *e.g.*, the heart muscle in patients with severe anemia.

Other Changes Seen in Damaged Cells. Many other changes have been

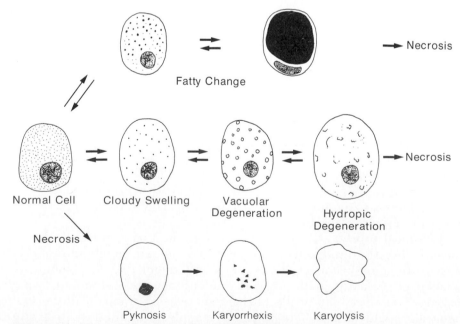

Figure 4–2. Changes that may follow cell injury. Mild injury can cause either fatty change or water-logging. These changes are reversible, but if the injury continues, the cell may die. Necrosis follows.

Severe injury may kill the cell rapidly; the nuclear changes of pyknosis, karyorrhexis, and karyolysis indicate necrosis. These changes become evident about 12 hours after cell death and are not reversible. (Drawing by Margot Mackay, Department of Art as Applied to Medicine, University of Toronto.)

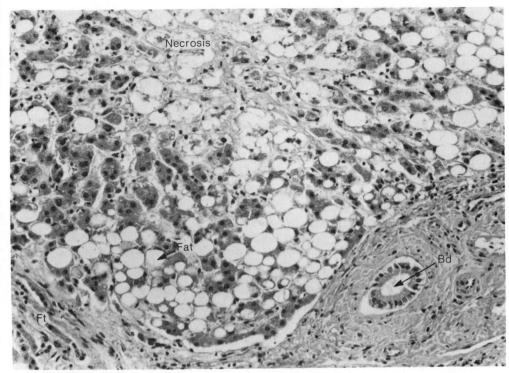

Figure 4–3.   Alcoholic liver disease. The liver is severely damaged. Some cells show fatty change, the lipid in each cell appearing as a clear intracellular globule (Fat). Other cells are necrotic, and the structure of the liver lobule has collapsed. In the area of necrosis the reticulin fibers will be replaced by collagen fibers. Such a change to fibrous tissue (Ft) has already occurred in another area as a result of a previous episode of necrosis. The amount of fibrous tissue around a bile duct (Bd) is increased (× 250).

described. In *hyaline degeneration* of cells an eosinophilic, homogeneous material (called hyaline) accumulates in the cytoplasm. The best example of this is the accumulation of *alcoholic hyaline* seen in liver cells following a period of alcoholic debauchery. Hyaline droplets are found in the renal tubular cells in cases of severe proteinuria (Chapter 35).

At the electron microscopical level many changes have been described. Sometimes localized areas of a cell appear to become degenerate, and the term "focal cytoplasmic degeneration" has been applied. These degenerate areas may be cast off from the surface or sometimes included in membrane-bound structures that fuse with lysosomes. These membrane-enclosed structures containing lytic lysosomal enzymes are called *autophagosomes* or *cytolysosomes,* and an increase in their number is an indication of cell injury.

There are many diseases in which there is an accumulation of some material within the cell owing to a specific enzyme defect. Thus, absence of an enzyme necessary for glycogen metabolism results in accumulation of glycogen (*glycogen storage diseases*). Also there are other conditions in which lipid or mucopolysaccharide accumulate within the cells. These conditions are all rare and are generally inherited as autosomal recessive traits.

Cell Death and Necrosis

Cell death is difficult to define in precise terms, but in practice it may be regarded as having occurred whenever a cell is incapable of further division or of continuing its normal synthetic functions.

The appearance of the dead cells varies according to the cause of the injury. If the cells are killed suddenly as a result of physical or chemical trauma, they show no changes initially other than those directly attributable to the agent concerned, *e.g.*, disruption in electrical injuries and the effects of freezing or burning.

Cells less severely damaged — for instance, by poisons — may develop biochemical lesions that first progress to changes associated with waterlogging and fatty change. As noted previously, these changes as detected by light microscopy are cytoplasmic and in themselves do not indicate cell death.

In a dead cell respiration ceases, but glycolysis proceeds for a while; as a result, there is the production of lactic acid and a drop in the pH. The synthetic activities of the cell stop, but the lytic destructive processes resulting from released lysosomal enzymes continue. As a result of this, the cell undergoes a process of self-digestion (*autolysis*) and within a few hours shows morphological changes by which cell death can be recognized. This process is called *necrosis*, which may be defined as the *circumscribed death of cells or tissues with structural evidence of their death. Necrosis and cell death are therefore not synonymous.*

The microscopic changes of necrosis affect the whole cell. The cytoplasm generally becomes homogeneous — often brightly eosinophilic. At the same time the nucleus shows changes that are pathognomonic of necrosis. Sometimes the nucleus becomes intensely dense-staining, and this is known as *pyknosis.* The pyknotic nucleus either breaks up into fragments (*karyorrhexis*) or becomes indistinct as the nuclear material is digested (*karyolysis*). The importance of these nuclear changes cannot be overemphasized, because it is by their recognition that the pathologist can diagnose necrosis. Autolysis also occurs after the death of the whole individual, and the term *postmortem change* is applied to this process. The microscopic changes can closely mimic those of necrosis, but of course there is no accompanying vital reaction such as inflammation (see discussion later in this chapter).

Diagnosis of Necrosis by Biochemical Means

A diagnosis of the occurrence of necrosis is frequently of great clinical importance. When areas of heart muscle, pancreas, liver, or brain are dying, the patient's life is often in jeopardy. As necrosis occurs, various soluble substances such as enzymes diffuse out of the cells and are absorbed into the blood stream, where their detection is an aid to clinical diagnosis. Some important examples of this response may be listed. The serum glutamic oxaloacetic transaminase (SGOT), hydroxybutyrate dehydrogenase (HBD), and lactate dehydrogenase (LDH) are all raised after myocardial infarction, since these enzymes are found in high concentrations in heart muscle. An elevation of serum glutamic pyruvate transaminase (SGPT) and LDH is found after liver cell necrosis, such as in viral hepatitis. Some enzymes can be separated into separate fractions by electrophoresis. These separate fractions, each having a similar biochemical activity, are termed *isoenzymes;* specific isoenzymes occur in particular organs. In the case of the LDH, LDH_1 and LDH_2 are released from the heart muscle, whereas LDH_5 is of hepatic origin (Fig. 4–4).

Types of Necrosis

Coagulative Necrosis. In most tissues the process of necrosis entails the denaturation of cytoplasmic proteins, causing the tissue to become firm and somewhat opaque. The process resembles the change seen in the white of an egg on boiling.

Denaturation often releases active side-chains of the molecules, which are then available for binding to dyes such as eosin. As noted previously, eosinophilia is a useful sign of cell death, and this is particularly helpful when one is looking for early signs of tissue necrosis. Thus, the patient who dies of a

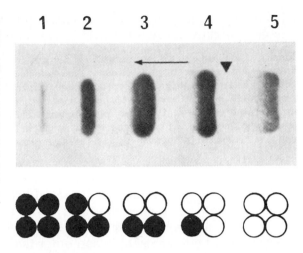

Figure 4–4. The lactate dehydrogenase (LDH) activity of serum is shown as five component isoenzymes separated by electrophoresis. LDH_1 is the fastest component and has traveled farthest in the direction of the arrow toward the anode. In the lower part of the diagram each molecule is depicted as a tetramer made up of varying combinations of either H polypeptides (closed circles) or M polypeptides (open circles). The H and M chains are determined by separate genes. (After Latner, A. L.: Journal of Clinical Pathology, 24, suppl. (Association of Clinical Pathology), 4:8–13, 1970.)

heart attack may show increased eosinophilia of the heart muscle fibers, indicating the early changes of an infarct (see below). Likewise, in patients suffering a cardiac arrest, the detection of eosinophilia in brain cells is a useful, reliable indication of permanent cerebral damage. In practice, of course, these changes are seen only at necropsy.

The increased binding capacity of necrotic tissue is also a factor in causing calcification. Necrotic tissue sometimes takes up calcium salts and becomes calcified. This response, which is termed *dystrophic calcification,* is quite frequently see in necrotic tumor tissue. Since calcium can be detected easily by radiography, its detection has been utilized in diagnosis. In some cancers of the breast, characteristic flecks of calcium deposition can be seen even before the tumor can be palpated. The degenerate tissue of tuberculous lesions also commonly calcifies, as does the material found in atheroma.

A common cause of necrosis is sudden deprivation of the blood supply to the part. The process is called *infarction* and is common in the heart, kidneys, and spleen. These infarcts show the typical changes of coagulative necrosis. Microscopically, in addition to nuclear changes of pyknosis, karyorrhexis, or karyolysis another feature is noteworthy. The general architecture of the tissue may still be recognizable, even though its constituent cells are dead and their nuclei have disappeared. This is called *structured necrosis,* and the appearance has been likened to that of a city of the dead. In other examples of coagulative necrosis, in which there may be no residual structure at all, the effect is called *structureless necrosis;* it is the characteristic change seen in tuberculosis (see "Caseation," Chapter 10).

Colliquative Necrosis.   In the central nervous system, necrotic tissue undergoes softening and liquefaction, so that either the tissue collapses or a cyst is formed. Liquefaction is seen as a secondary event in other tissues when there is suppurative infection (see "Suppuration," Chapter 5) and following caseation in tuberculosis.

Acute Inflammation.   Necrotic tissue excites an inflammatory response, which is followed by a phase of demolition and healing. The appearance of the acute inflammatory response, including an infiltration of polymorphs, is an important feature of most necrotic tissues and is a useful microscopic change that helps to distinguish necrosis from postmortem change. Thus, if an area of apparently necrotic cardiac muscle is surrounded by a zone of acute inflammation, the lesion may be safely diagnosed as an infarct. Likewise, the appearance of degenerate renal tubules associated with much edema and

Further Changes in Necrotic Tissue

separation of tubules indicates premortem tubular necrosis, not a postmortem change. The acute inflammatory reaction is followed by a phase of demolition, as evidenced by the presence of many macrophages. If much lipid is present in the tissue, or if adipose tissue becomes necrotic, these macrophages contain multiple fine fat droplets and are called *foam cells*. This is a striking feature when necrosis affects brain or fatty tissue, such as in the breast. Sometimes macrophages fuse to form giant cells; these are described later in the section on granulomas (see Chapter 8). An important clinical effect of the acute inflammatory response is fever. This is caused by the release of pyrogens from polymorphs and macrophages (Chapter 5). Thus, fever is encountered in patients with myocardial or pulmonary infarction, and its presence does not necessarily indicate infection.

Gangrene.   Sometimes the dead tissue is invaded by saprophytic protein-splitting anaerobic bacteria, which cause its decomposition with the production of hydrogen sulfide and other foul-smelling substances. There is blackening of the area because of the formation of iron sulfide from the iron of decomposed hemoglobin. This *necrosis with superadded putrefaction is called "gangrene,"* which is an old clinical term that was applied to any black, foul-smelling area in continuity with living tissue.

Clostridial Gangrene.   The putrefactive bacteria are usually the clostridia of intestinal origin. Therefore, necrosis of the bowel, particularly of the large intestine, is often followed by gangrene. These putrefactive bacteria are of little importance in themselves, because they live on dead tissue and do not invade or harm the living tissues. Nevertheless, gangrenous lesions always contain pathogenic bacteria that invade tissues and cause further destruction. It follows that gangrene is a very serious condition and is fatal unless treated expeditiously.

Gangrene Due to Other Organisms.   Some putrefactive bacteria are also pathogenic, *e.g.*, certain strains of anerobic streptococci and members of the family *Bacteroidaceae.* The latter includes the well-known member *Fusobacterium fusiforme,* which is often found in company with a spirochete (*Borrelia vincentii*).

These putrefactive organisms are frequently found in the mouth and are the cause of ulcerative gingivitis, which is often seen following neglect; it is known as "Vincent's infection" or "trench mouth." A more serious gangrenous lesion occasionally affects the soft parts of the face and leads to great tissue destruction. It used to be described in debilitated children, particularly following measles, but it is now extremely rare in civilized countries.

This same group of anaerobic putrefactive organisms is also found in the vagina and is occasionally responsible for gangrene of the uterus following badly conducted labor or ill-performed abortion.

Gangrene of the Limbs.   All the examples of gangrene so far mentioned are "wet." There is progressive tissue destruction, and unless effective treatment is instituted without delay, death results. A similar type of wet gangrene occurs in the limbs. It is usually due to sudden blockage of the main arterial supply and is not infrequently a complication of diabetes mellitus. Generally the legs are affected, rather than the arms.

Dry Gangrene.   If the blood supply to a limb is slowly occluded, the tips of the digits become black and necrotic and at the same time undergo desiccation. This drying of the part greatly impedes bacterial growth, and infection with pathogenic organisms is minimal. The condition therefore slowly extends until a point is reached where the blood supply to the limb is adequate. A line of demarcation develops, and the dead tissue is discarded by a process of spontaneous amputation. This condition is called *dry gangrene,* but since the amount of putrefaction is minimal, the term is somewhat of a misnomer. The process is, in fact, mummification of an infarcted portion of a limb.

Gas Gangrene.   This condition is due to invasion by pathogenic clostridia and is described in more detail in Chapter 10.

Degenerations in the fibrovascular connective tissues are common and form as heterogeneous a group as do those affecting cellular parenchymal tissues.

Degenerations of the Connective Tissues

Fibrosis.   In those organs in which collagen formation stops at the reticulin stage, damage seems to stimulate the maturation of the fibers to ordinary fibrous tissue. The term *fibrosis* is used to describe this response. Good examples are the fibrosis seen in cirrhosis of the liver (Chapter 33) and the fibrosis of lymph nodes draining areas of chronic infection.

Changes in Collagen

Ehlers-Danlos Syndrome.   This syndrome constitutes a group of inherited diseases in which collagen can be unduly stretched with ease, due probably to an abnormality in the cross-linkages between collagen fibrils (Chapter 2). Mild forms of this syndrome are not uncommon, and subjects are "double jointed," being able to hyperextend their joints. In more severe forms of the syndrome the hypermobility of skin and joints produces the "Indian rubber men" of the circus ring.

Hyalinization.   "Hyaline" is a term used to describe any glassy, eosinophilic, acellular tissue. Intracellular hyaline has been described previously. Amyloid may be described as hyaline until its true nature is recognized. As generally used, however, the term hyalinization is applied to a change in collagenous tissue when it becomes acellular and homogeneous. The changes are seen in the collagen of old scars, in the fibrous tissue of chronic inflammatory lesions, in the walls of small blood vessels in hypertension, in atheroma, and in "fibroid" tumors of the uterus. Hyalinized collagen has the normal staining properties of collagen, and it appears very inert and stable.

Elastosis of Collagen.   Following prolonged exposure to ultraviolet light, the dermal collagen changes in such a way that it takes on some of the staining properties of elastic tissue. This gives the skin the familiar wrinkled, aged look in those fair-skinned individuals whose occupation or pleasures have resulted in excessive sun exposure.

Necrobiosis.   Sometimes collagen becomes eosinophilic and weak and breaks up. This is a characteristic feature of rheumatoid arthritis, and the degenerate collagen excites a chronic inflammatory reaction (Chapter 40). Necrobiosis in collagen is sometimes described as "fibrinoid necrosis," but this term is also used in other contexts. Thus, the blood vessel walls in malignant hypertension show necrosis and marked eosinophilia. This latter change is probably different from the necrobiosis of rheumatoid arthritis and represents degeneration of the vessel wall as well as infiltration with fibrin.

Sometimes the connective tissues show an excessive accumulation of ground substance, which appears as a basophilic pool of structureless material. This overhydration of ground substance is sometimes a physiological event and appears to be under hormonal control. Thus, the colorful swelling of the sexual skin of the baboon and the enlargement of the cockscomb of the rooster are in large part due to this change. A similar change occurs in myxedema (Chapter 39).

Changes in the Ground Substance

Sometimes the accumulation of excessive ground substance is associated with degeneration of the connective tissue fibers. Such a condition is called *myxomatous degeneration.* A good example of this is seen in the aorta when weakness in the vessel wall may cause rupture and consequent dramatic effects. A similar change in the heart valve leaflets leads to a floppy valve and regurgitation — generally mitral regurgitation.

There is a group of genetically determined diseases involving an abnormality in the metabolism of mucopolysaccharide (the *mucopolysaccharidoses*). These diseases are usully accompanied by skeletal deformities and sometimes by corneal opacity. The best known member of this uncommon group of diseases is *Hurler's syndrome*, which, because of the grotesque appearance of the head of its sufferers, is also known as "gargoylism."

Review Questions

1. How would you prove that a patient, under the situations listed below, had had a myocardial infarct:
   (a) during life; use biochemical tests
   (b) at necropsy; use microscopic examination of the heart.

2. Describe the circumstances under which lysosomal enzymes are activated in a cell.

3. Describe the changes caused by an excessive intake of alcohol (ethanol) that can be seen in liver cells. What happens to the reticulin framework of the organ, and what are the possible end results?

4. Compare and contrast the causes and end results of dry gangrene of a limb with those of wet gangrene.

Selected Readings

Peters, R. A.: Biochemical Lesions and Lethal Synthesis. Oxford, Pergamon Press, 1963.

Prescott, L. F., Park, J., Ballantyne, A., et al.: Treatment of paracetamol (acetaminophen) poisoning with N-acetylcysteine. Lancet, 2:432–434, 1977.

Robbins, S. L., and Cotran, R. S.: Pathologic Basis of Disease. 2nd ed. Philadelphia, W. B. Saunders Company, 1979. See in particular Chapter 2, "Cell Injury and Cell Death," as a source of further information.

Walter, J. B., and Israel, M. S.: General Pathology. 5th ed. Edinburgh, Churchill Livingstone, 1979. Chapters 4 and 5 give greater details of the topics covered in this chapter.

Acute Inflammation CHAPTER 5

After studying this chapter the student should be able to:

- Define the following terms: hyperemia, vasodilatation, opsonization, chemotaxis, surface phagocytosis, macrophage, ulcer, and slough.
- Describe the vascular changes of acute inflammation and relate these to the formation and composition of inflammatory edema.
- Describe the cellular components of the inflammatory exudate; outline the mechanisms involved in their accumulation; and indicate the role of each type of cell.
- List the variations of the acute inflammatory reaction and give examples of each.
- List the possible local sequelae of an acute inflammation.
- Describe the process of suppuration.
- Describe the triple response.
- List the important chemical mediators of acute inflammation and indicate their probable role.

The body's reaction to injury is complex, for it involves not only a generalized response, which is described in Chapter 21, but also a localized response, which has several components. The initial local reaction is concerned mainly with changes in the connective tissues. The blood vessels dilate and, by becoming more permeable, allow white cells and plasma to leak into the affected area. This reaction is termed "acute inflammation" and is familiar to anyone who has ever experienced a boil. It is characterized by four cardinal signs, which were originally described by Celsus in the first century A.D. These signs are *rubor, tumor, calor,* and *dolor,* which indicate that the area is *red, swollen, warmer* than the surrounding tissues, and *painful.* Since an inflamed part is often held still, loss of function has been added as a fifth sign of acute inflammation.

Inflammation is extremely common in clinical practice, and it is convenient to use the suffix *-itis* to denote its presence. Thus, tonsill*itis* is inflammation of the tonsils. In itself, this is not a complete diagnosis, for it does not indicate the cause. There can be tonsillitis due to streptococcal infection or tonsillitis due to infectious mononucleosis or to other viral infections.

Causes of Acute Inflammation

The causes are the same as those of tissue injury:

Physical Agents. *Traumatic injury,* such as cutting and crushing, may cause inflammation. Cuts of the skin become inflamed after several hours and are then more painful than at the time of their infliction. *Thermal* and *freezing injuries* cause typical acute inflammation, and the blisters that form in the skin in both conditions bear witness to the leakage or exudation of plasma from the blood vessels. *Ultraviolet light* and *ionizing radiations* (sunburn and radiation burns) are other physical causes.

Chemical Agents. When introduced into the tissues most chemicals cause inflammation. This may be severe, as with a wasp sting, or minimal, as with the introduction of a stainless steel prosthesis, such as in total hip replacement surgery. Consequently, the problem in reconstructive surgery has been to find substances that cause no reaction at all.

Infarction.   The necrosis that results from obstruction of circulation to an area is termed *infarction* (Chapter 20).

Living Organisms.   Inflammation is a feature of many infections, such as when a staphylococcal infection causes a boil. Note that the inflammation is a response to tissue damage rather than to the organism itself. In some infections, such as syphilis and typhoid fever, the invading organisms cause little immediate damage and therefore little immediate inflammation.

Antigen-Antibody Reactions.   The IgE antibodies render tissues susceptible to the action of antigen, so that damage is done. Another method by which immunoglobulins can cause damage is by the formation of immune complexes. Sensitized lymphocytes can cause damage in several ways, including the release of damaging cytotoxic lymphokines. These topics are described in Chapter 9.

Changes in Acute Inflammation

Inflammation can be studied in the living animal by observations of thin tissues. The mesentery of the rat, the stretched-thin tongue of the frog, and the rabbit-ear–chamber (Chapter 7) have all been used to observe the changing events of inflammation.

The Vascular Response

Although most tissues are liberally provided with capillaries, the limited supply of blood that normally reaches the part is carefully distributed, so that at any one time only some vessels contain a stream of blood. Indeed, there is a central or *thoroughfare channel,* and during inactivity much blood passes through it directly from the arterioles to the venules (Fig. 5–1). During activity the thoroughfare channel closes, and blood is diverted to perfuse the tissues in response to their increased metabolism. In addition, there is arteriolar dilatation, which increases the total volume of blood available. In acute inflammation the response is similar. There is arteriolar dilatation so that more blood passes into the part. The precapillary sphincters open, so that the capillaries become distended and blood ceases to flow through the preferential channel (Fig. 5–1*B*). This increased content of blood is termed *hyperemia* and is the reason why the inflamed part appears red. The skin, being normally cooler than the arterial blood, becomes warmer because of the increased flow. Dilatation of blood vessels (*vasodilatation*) is thus a characteristic feature of acute inflammation.

Changes in Blood Flow.   In a normal tissue, blood in the arterioles travels so fast that one cannot discern individual cells. In the large tortuous venules, on the other hand, the cells can be seen to occupy the central or axial part of the stream and are separated from the endothelial lining by a clear zone of plasma (*plasmatic zone*). This arrangement is dictated by physical laws and has the advantage of reducing the viscosity of blood. In acute inflammation, plasma leaks from the vessels, and the blood consequently becomes more viscid; the lubricating action of the plasmatic zone is impaired, and the stream slows down. This process is termed *stasis*. Meanwhile, two other important changes occur. The endothelial cells become swollen, and electron microscopy shows that the spaces between adjacent cells become widened, thereby permitting plasma and cells to pass between them. At the same time, white cells move into the plasmatic zone and stick to the altered vessel wall. This adhesion is highly characteristic of acute inflammation and is best seen in the venules. At first, the cells adhere for a short time, and then they either roll gently along the endothelial lining or get swept back into the blood stream. Later, however, the cells become more firmly adherent and line

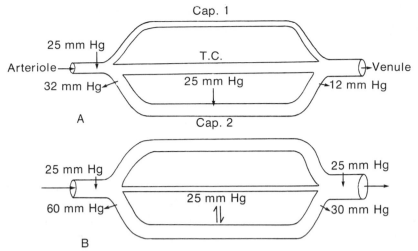

Figure 5–1.   Diagrammatic representation of the vascular bed in normal tissue (A) and in acutely inflamed tissue (B). In the normal resting tissue much of the blood passes from the arteriole to the venule directly through the thoroughfare channel (T.C.). One capillary is closed (Cap. 1), while some blood passes through the other capillary (Cap. 2). The hydrostatic pressure at the arteriolar end of the capillary is 32 mm Hg and at the venous end is 12 mm Hg. These forces tend to drive fluid out of the vessel and are countered by the osmotic pressure of the plasma proteins—about 25 mm Hg. The interstitial extravascular fluid normally contains very little protein. Hence, fluid tends to leave the vessel at the arteriolar end and to be reabsorbed at the venous end.

In an inflamed tissue (*B*) the arteriole is dilated, the thoroughfare channel is closed, and both capillaries are dilated by the increased blood flow. The hydrostatic pressure at each end of the capillary is increased as shown. Plasma proteins have leaked from the vessels so that their concentration in the interstitial tissue fluid approximates that in the plasma. The osmotic effect of the plasma proteins tending to drive fluid into the vessels is thereby neutralized. Fluid is exuded along the entire length of the capillary, therefore, and is ultimately halted by a rise in tissue tension. (Drawing by Margot Mackay, Department of Art as Applied to Medicine, University of Toronto.)

the endothelium, forming masses that may even block the lumen. This phenomenon is known as *pavementation of the endothelium* and is the prelude to the emigration of the white cells from the blood stream into the interstitial tissue spaces.

The most characteristic feature of acute inflammation is the formation of an exudate that has both a fluid and a cellular component.

The Fluid Exudate.   Under normal conditions the vascular endothelium is virtually impermeable to the plasma proteins, and the fluid that escapes from the vessels has a low protein content; on reaching the interstitial tissues, it either returns to the venules or is gathered by the lymphatics and returned to the circulation. In acute inflammation the increased vascular permeability allows the plasma proteins to leak through the vessel wall, causing the osmotic pressure effect of the plasma proteins to be lost. An increased volume of fluid therefore leaves the vessels, and this forms the inflammatory exudate (Fig. 5–1*B*). A useful method of investigating this phenomenon is to tag the blood albumin either with a dye such as trypan blue or with a radioactive isotope of iodine. The accumulation of tagged albumin in the interstitial tissues of an area of inflammation then becomes an index of the change in vascular permeability. This type of investigation indicates that increased permeability occurs in three phases:

1. *Immediate Transient Phase.*   This lasts about 30 minutes, affects venules, and is largely mediated by histamine (page 75).

2. *Immediate Prolonged Phase.*   The exudation starts immediately and persists. It appears to be due to direct damage to vessels.

Formation of the Exudate

3. *Delayed Prolonged Phase.* In this phase it is thought that both capillaries and venules are affected both by direct injury and by chemical mediators.

There is another factor that plays an important part in the formation of the inflammatory exudate: one of the first detectable changes in experimental lesions is an alteration in the ground substance, causing it to become more fluid. The effect of this increased fluidity is to allow the exudate to diffuse into surrounding tissues more readily and thereby to prevent an immediate rise in tissue tension. Nevertheless, the tissue tension eventually increases, thereby limiting the amount of exudate formed, because it tends to drive fluid back into the venules. The increased tissue tension is one important factor in the causation of pain. It follows that inflammation in a densely compact tissue or in an enclosed space causes severe pain. This is well illustrated by the pain that is experienced in infections of the pulp of a finger, an acne pustule on the nose, and acute osteomyelitis where the marrow is encased in unyielding bone.

The fluid leaving the blood vessels in acute inflammation has almost the same composition as plasma, and it contains antibacterial substances (such as complement) as well as specific antibodies. If present in the plasma, drugs and antibiotics also appear in the exudate. The importance of the early administration of therapeutic agents is obvious when one recalls that these agents are merely carried to the inflamed area in the exudate and are in no way concentrated there. Furthermore, the fluid in the exudate is in a state of flux, since it is in equilibrium with the circulating plasma. Therapeutic agents must therefore be administered continuously if their concentration is to remain at a therapeutic level in the area of inflammation.

The fluid of the exudate has additional effects. It dilutes any irritating chemicals and bacterial toxins that might be present. The fibrinogen in it is converted into fibrin by the action of tissue factor (Chapter 26), and a *fibrin clot* forms. This fibrin forms a fine network of fibers and has three main functions:

1. It forms a *union* between severed tissues.
2. It forms a *barrier* against bacterial invasion (Chapter 6).
3. It aids *phagocytosis* (discussed later in this chapter).

The Cellular Exudate. The white cells adhering to the endothelium of blood vessels soon push pseudopodia between adjacent endothelial cells, penetrate the basement membrane, and emerge on the external surface of the vessel. This remarkable process is called *emigration of the white cells;* for the most part, neutrophil polymorphonuclear leukocytes* predominate during the early phases of an acute inflammatory response. The gap that is left by the emigrating white cell soon closes behind it, although sometimes a few red cells escape at the same time. A variable number of lymphocytes and monocytes also leave the blood vessels. Figure 5–2 shows the typical appearance of an acutely inflamed tissue. The fixed tissue cells are separated by edema, and fibrin threads can be seen bathed in the edema fluid. Numerous white cells — for the most part polymorphs — are seen lying within the fluid exudate.

The movement of white cells into the interstitial tissues of an inflamed part appears to be a purposeful event, but it is obvious that the cells are not capable of independent, thoughtful action and that there must be some mechanism by which they are enticed from the vessels into the area of damage. It

---

*These cells are commonly called "PMNs," "polys," or "polymorphs." The abbreviation *polymorph* is used frequently in this book.

Figure 5–2. Acute appendicitis.
This section was taken through the wall of an acutely inflamed appendix. The smooth muscle cells (Musc) are separated by inflammatory edema, and the whole area is heavily infiltrated by inflammatory cells, mostly polymorphs (Poly). Macrophages (Mac) and red cells (RBC) are also present in the exudate (× 600).

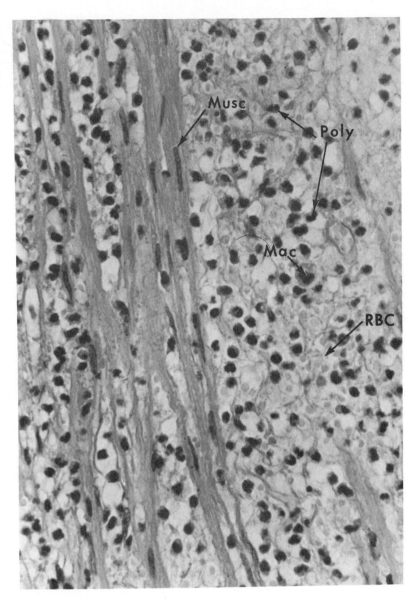

is generally believed that the attraction is of a chemical nature. Directional movement of cells in response to a chemical gradient is well known in biology and is called *chemotaxis*. An example of this movement is seen in the reproduction of the fern. The spermatozoids of the male are attracted by malic acid produced by the female germ cells.

A great deal of research has gone into the identification of the chemicals responsible for chemotaxis in acute inflammation in humans. Both polymorphs and monocytes have been shown to be attracted *in vitro* to a number of agents (Fig. 5–3), such as starch and certain bacteria. Other chemotactic agents are antigen-antibody complexes and dead tissue. These function only if complement is present and activated (Chapter 9). The activated trimolecular complex $C\overline{567}$ and the anaphylatoxins C3a and C5a are the chemotactic agents.

One of the characteristic features of the inflammatory exudate is that in the initial stages polymorphs predominate, but as time goes by, these are replaced by monocytes. One explanation of this phenomenon is that polymorphs, having a very limited life span (probably a few hours), soon die off,

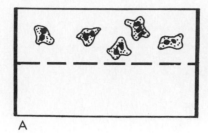

A

Figure 5–3. The Boyden chamber for detecting chemotactic activity. The Boyden chamber consists of two tissue culture chambers placed one on top of the other and separated by a membrane of 3 μm pore size (*A*). A suspension of polymorphs is placed in the upper chamber, and the test substance is placed in the lower. The number of cells that migrate to the lower surface of the filter is a measure of the chemotactic effect (*B*).

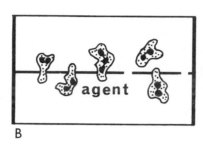

B

leaving the long-lived mononuclear cells to replace them. Until recently it was thought that all agents attracting polymorphs also attract monocytes and that the change in population of the inflammatory exudate could be explained on the basis of a slow, steady recruitment of monocytes in the face of rapid destruction of polymorphs. It is now known that this is an oversimplification of the process and that the immune response plays a part (Chapter 9). Thus, the reaction of antigen with IgE appears to release a chemotactic factor that specifically acts on eosinophils — cells that are prominent in certain allergic inflammations and in parasitic infections. Another important source of chemotactic agents is derived from sensitized lymphocytes. When these cells are acted upon by specific antigens, they release a number of factors called *lymphokines*. These have not been clearly defined, but some appear to have a specific chemotactic effect on polymorphs, eosinophils, or monocytes.

Lymphocytes are found in areas of inflammation, particularly during the healing process. In certain instances they are the predominant cell in the early phase of acute inflammation; viral infections and acute dermatitis are good examples in which this occurs. The mechanism of their accumulation is not known, because no definite chemotactic agents have been found that affect these cells. As noted above, lymphocytes can release lymphokines; they may therefore play several roles in acute inflammation.

Functions of Cellular Exudate: Phagocytosis

Polymorphonuclear Leukocytes. The main function of these cells is *phagocytosis*. They ingest bacteria and other foreign particles (Fig. 5–4). Phagocytosis is aided by two mechanisms:

1. *Opsonization.* Opsonins are proteins present in the plasma that coat organisms and cause them to be more easily phagocytosed. Some opsonins appear to be quite *nonspecific* and are present in all normal individuals, whereas others (*immune opsonins*) are antibodies that are *specific* for the particular organisms that excited their formation. It follows that phagocytosis is more marked in the inflammation of an individual who has been immunized against the particular infecting organism. Phagocytes possess Fc and C3 receptors that enable them to recognize and adhere to organisms coated with antibody or complement (Chapter 9).

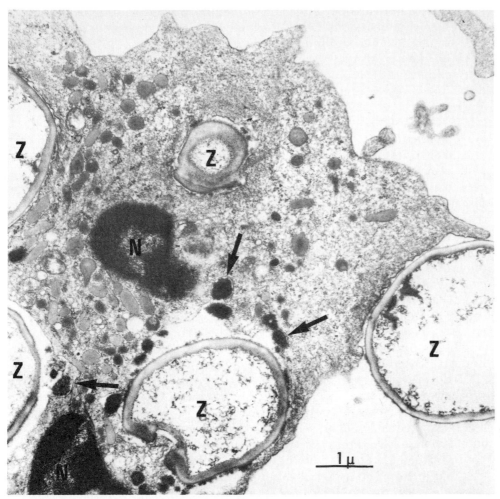

Figure 5–4. Phagocytosis. A human peripheral blood polymorphonuclear leukocyte that has been exposed to zymosan particles (Z). Two lobes of its nucleus are seen (N), but they are not connected in this section. At the right is a particle that has been bound to the cell but has not yet been ingested. In the lower portion of this picture are zymosan particles in phagocytic vacuoles. Lysosomes surround the particles and have degranulated into the vacuoles (arrows). Bacteria are treated in a similar manner and may later be destroyed (×21,500). (Courtesy of Dr. Sylvia Hoffstein and Dr. Gerald Weissmann, New York University Medical Center.)

2. *Surface Phagocytosis.* The fibrin clot of the inflammatory exudate provides a network on which polymorphs can trap organisms. This method of phagocytosis can occur in the absence of opsonins and is presumably of value to the individual who is not immune.

Polymorphs show loss of their granules following phagocytosis. The granules are, in fact, lysosomes; they fuse with phagocytic vesicles and their lytic enzymes enter the common sac where digestion proceeds (Fig. 5–4).

Polymorphs release various chemicals following phagocytosis. These include *lysosomal enzymes,* which play a part in the digestion of dead tissue during the phase of healing as well as endogenous *pyrogen,* which is a major factor in the pathogenesis of the fever that accompanies any acute inflammation other than the most trivial.

The way in which organisms are killed by polymorphs and macrophages is complex and incompletely understood. The energy for phagocytosis is derived from glycolysis, and the lactic acid produced by this anaerobic process is bactericidal. Nevertheless, bactericidal activity is dependent mainly on oxidative reactions, with glucose being oxidized via the hexose monophosphate shunt (see Fig. 2–10). Hydrogen peroxide appears to be one of the vital bactericidal agents produced as a result of this.

The details of polymorph activity in acute inflammation have been stressed because these cells play a vital role in the body's defenses against many infections. Patients with a low neutrophil count (*e.g.,* due to bone marrow aplasia or acute leukemia) often develop severe gingivitis or pharyngitis, and subsequently die of overwhelming infection. Furthermore, there are a number of rare but interesting diseases in which polymorph function is defective. In the "lazy leukocyte syndrome" there are defective movement and chemotaxis. In the more common *chronic granulomatous disease* there is defective bactericidal activity following normal phagocytosis of bacteria. The disease affects boys (it is an X-linked recessive trait) and is characterized by repeated bacterial infections, often staphylococcal.

Macrophages. The monocytes that accumulate in the area of acute inflammation are highly phagocytic; as with the polymorphs, their ingestion of virulent organisms is aided by opsonins. The monocytes are termed *macrophages* when they show morphological evidence of having phagocytosed material within them. Thus, the monocyte may be regarded as a resting cell that circulates in the blood. Once it enters an area of inflammation, it enlarges, becomes highly phagocytic, and is then termed "a macrophage." Another important function of the macrophage is that it appears to play a part in the initiation of the immune response (Chapter 9).

The macrophage also acts as a secretory cell in that it releases many substances, particularly when engaged in phagocytosis. These include endogenous pyrogen, complement components, lysozyme, elastase, collagenase, and plasminogen activator, as well as substances that stimulate lymphocytes and fibroblasts. The importance of the secretory function of the macrophage is not fully known, but it is evident that this cell plays a vital role in inflammation and in the processes of healing that follow. Its role in defense against infection is complex and does not appear to rest entirely on activities relating to scavenger function.

Variations of the Acute Inflammatory Reaction

Although all examples of acute inflammation have many features in common, some types have been categorized on the basis of some particular gross or microscopic feature — often the type of exudate. The categories are useful for descriptive purposes and are commonly used, but the differences are of no fundamental importance.

Serous Inflammation. In inflammation of serous sacs and loose tissues such as the subcutaneous tissues around the vulva, scrotum, and eyes, the fluid component of an inflammatory exudate exceeds the cellular one, because the limiting factor of increased tissue tension is absent. There results a large accumulation of inflammatory edema, which is termed *serous inflammation.*

Fibrinous Inflammation. Fibrin formation is an obvious feature of inflammation in the lungs and on the surface of the serous membranes. Thus, it forms a well-marked feature of pericarditis and peritonitis (Fig. 5–5). Fibrinous inflammation of this type is often accompanied by an accumulation of serous fluid; thus, the term "sero-fibrinous inflammation" is an apt one.

Hemorrhagic Inflammation. The blood-stained exudate indicates severe vascular damage and bleeding. It is seen in the lungs following phosgene poisoning and in acute influenzal pneumonia. Hemorrhagic inflammation is encountered in vasculitic lesions, *e.g.,* those of gonococcal septicemia (Fig. 10–2) and the Arthus reaction (Chapter 9). Acute hemorrhagic pancreatitis provides another example (Chapter 34).

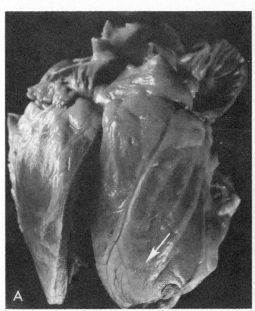
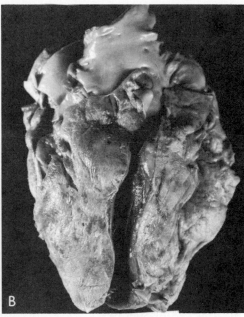

Figure 5–5. Acute pericarditis. Two hearts have each been opened in the routine way at necropsy. *A,* Heart from 24-year-old female who had been diagnosed as having systemic lupus erythematosus. In spite of treatment, the patient developed the nephrotic syndrome and died of renal failure. At necropsy the pericardial sac contained 60 ml of straw-colored clear fluid; in some areas overlying the left ventricle, the pericardium was covered by a thin layer of fibrinous exudate (arrow). Elsewhere the pericardium is thin, shiny, and normal-appearing. This is an example of a serofibrinous inflammation. *B,* Heart from patient who had been operated on for cancer of the stomach but in whom the area of surgery had become infected. At necropsy pus was present in the left pleural space (thoracic empyema or pyothorax). Infection has spread to the pericardial sac, which also contained thick pus. The pericardial surface of the heart is seen to be covered by a thick, shaggy inflammatory exudate. Compare with *A.*

Catarrhal Inflammation. This is seen when a mucus-secreting mucous membrane is involved in an acute inflammatory reaction. There is some destruction of the epithelial cells and a profuse mucus secretion from those cells that remain as well as from the underlying glands. The common cold provides an excellent example of this type of inflammation.

Pseudomembranous Inflammation. This type of reaction is encountered on mucosal surfaces and describes the formation of a pseudomembrane, consisting of necrotic epithelium and inflammatory exudate, that covers the surface and is tightly adherent to it in the initial stages of its formation. The reaction is characteristic of diphtheritic lesions of the tonsils or pharynx. If an attempt is made to remove the gray membrane, bleeding results. Pseudomembranous colitis is described in Chapter 32.

Gangrenous Inflammation. Gangrene occurs in inflammation when the dead tissue is invaded by putrefactive organisms (Chapters 4 and 10).

Suppurative Inflammation. Inflammation resulting in the formation of pus is described later in this chapter.

Certain inflammations do not show the usual neutrophil polymorph response. Sometimes *eosinophils* are plentiful — particularly with inflammations produced by parasitic worms and with some allergic conditions, such as hay fever. *Lymphocytic infiltration* is frequent in inflammatory lesions produced by viruses, even in the early stages. It is also a feature of acute inflammation in many skin diseases. Occasionally *macrophages* are the predominant cell in the inflammatory response (see "Pathogenesis of Typhoid Fever," Chapter 6). This variation in cellular response is probably brought about by the actions of various chemotactic agents.

Variability of the Cellular Exudate

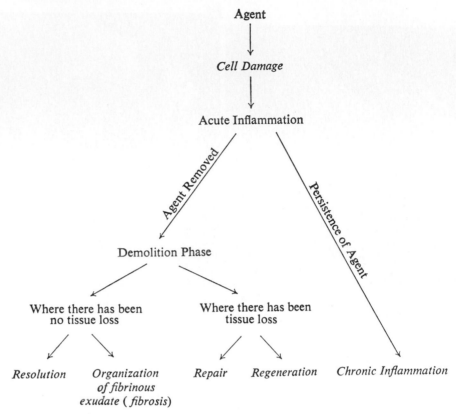

Figure 5-6. The local sequelae of acute inflammation.

Local Sequelae of Acute Inflammation

The changes following acute inflammation are shown in Figure 5–6 and depend upon two major factors: (1) the amount of tissue damage sustained; and (2) whether or not the causative agent remains in the body.

Resolution

In acutely inflamed tissues in which cellular damage has been relatively slight and reversible, necrosis does not occur. If the causative agent is eliminated by the inflammatory reaction — for instance, the pneumococcus in lobar pneumonia — or if the agent itself acts only once, such as in acute sunburn, the acute inflammatory reaction terminates by resolution (Fig. 5–7). The polymorph cellular infiltrate is replaced by macrophages that engulf degenerate fibrin, red cells, polymorphs, and any other dead tissue that remains. Some of the fluid exudate returns to the blood in the venules, but most of it is carried away by the lymphatics to the regional lymph nodes, where reticuloendothelial cells remove cellular debris before the fluid is returned to the circulation. With the removal of the inflammatory exudate and subsequent return of the macrophages to the lymphatics, the tissue is restored to its normal, previous state. *Resolution is the term applied to the process by which the tissue returns to normal following acute inflammation.*

Organization of Exudate

Occasionally the inflammatory exudate is not removed expeditiously enough, and it becomes invaded by granulation tissue and converted into scar tissue. It is a very common event to find fibrous adhesions between the visceral and parietal layers of the pleura. These are the organized remnants of some previous pleurisy. Likewise, fibrous adhesions are very common in the abdomen. They may occur around a site of previous inflammation such as an inflamed appendix, or they can follow surgery. Such adhesions make subsequent surgery more difficult; they can render it impossible to undertake sterilization by ligating the fallopian tubes through a peritoneoscope.

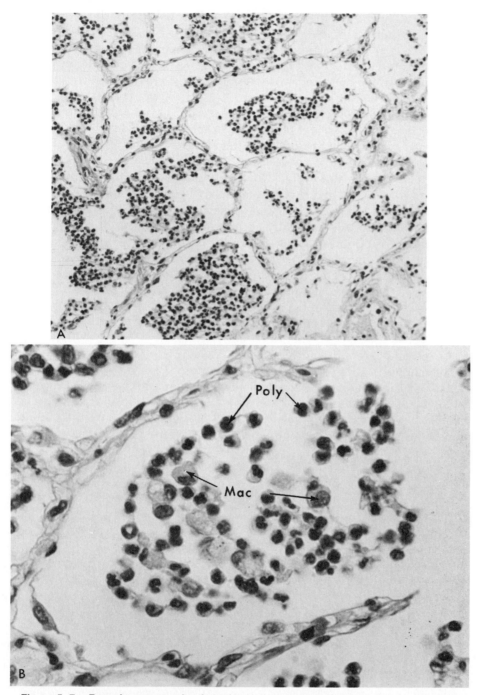

Figure 5–7.   Bronchopneumonia. *A,* Instead of containing air, the alveoli are filled with inflammatory exudate, the cellular component of which is the most obvious. An inflamed lung such as this is airless (*consolidated*); the condition is called pneumonia (× 250). *B,* Higher magnification of one alveolus from the same case as *A.* The cellular exudate contains many macrophages (Mac) in addition to the polymorphs (Poly). The pneumonia is beginning to resolve (× 600).

When the noxious agent produces much necrosis of the tissue involved, **_Suppuration_**
resolution is impossible. If the exudate contains many polymorphs, the center
of the inflammatory lesion becomes a cavity filled with a liquid containing
dead tissue and numerous polymorphs, which are now called *pus cells.* The
fluid is referred to as *pus,* and an inflammation with this type of response is
termed *suppurative.* An agent causing this type of reaction is termed *pyogenic,* and a typical example of such an infection is a boil caused by *Staphylococ-*

cus aureus. The hair follicle and adjacent dermis undergo necrosis, and a small sac of pus is formed. The necrotic tissue in an area of suppuration softens by virtue of the proteolytic lysosomal enzymes of the polymorphs as well as by autolysis mediated by the tissue's own enzymes. The creamy fluid is contained in a cavity called an *abscess* (see Fig. 44–4), and surrounding this there is a *pyogenic membrane,* which at this stage consists of inflamed and necrotic tissue with much fibrinous exudate and polymorph infiltration. The pus itself is composed of (a) leukocytes, some of which are dead; (b) other components of the inflammatory exudate, such as edema fluid with fibrin; (c) organisms, many of which are alive and can be cultured; and (d) tissue debris, such as nucleic acids and lipids. The pus tends not to remain at the site of its formation but rather to track in the line of least resistance until a free surface is reached. Then the abscess bursts and discharges its contents spontaneously. In clinical practice this is usually anticipated by surgical drainage, because until the pus has been evacuated, healing is much delayed. If drained, an abscess heals by granulation tissue, but if the causative agent persists, chronic inflammation ensues. This response is considered in later chapters.

If, as occasionally happens, the abscess is not drained and remains localized or sequestered in the tissues, its walls become organized into dense fibrous tissue, and the pus undergoes thickening, or *inspissation.* It develops a porridgelike consistency and eventually calcifies.

When an acute suppurative inflammation involves an epithelial surface, the covering is destroyed and an ulcer is formed (Fig. 5–8). An *ulcer* is a term used to describe a localized defect of a covering or a lining epithelium. In the first instance the floor of the ulcer is covered by necrotic tissue and acute inflammatory exudate; this layer is called a *slough* and is at first adherent, because the dead tissue has not yet become liquefied. Eventually, however,

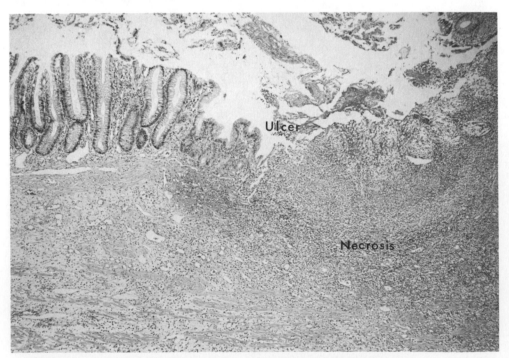

Figure 5–8. Suppurative appendicitis with mucosal ulceration. The wall of the appendix shows the changes of acute inflammation. Edema separates the muscle fibers, and there is a heavy infiltration by polymorphs, which cannot be identified at this magnification. On the right there is necrosis. The overlying epithelium has been cast off, thereby leaving an area of ulceration. This is an example of suppurative inflammation with ulceration of a mucous membrane (× 60).

the slough becomes detached, and the ulcer heals by the processes of repair and regeneration, as described in Chapter 7. Alternatively, the ulceration may persist and become chronic (see Fig. 7–3).

The other sequela of acute inflammation is progression to a state of chronicity. This occurs whenever the cause of tissue damage persists. In essence, chronic inflammation is a condition in which the causative agent persists, and the persisting acute inflammation is combined with healing and repair proceeding side by side.

Chronic Inflammation

Inflammation may be defined as *the reaction of the vascular and supporting elements of a tissue to injury, provided the injury has not been severe enough to destroy the area, and results in the formation of a protein-rich exudate.* Acute inflammation is mainly a vascular phenomenon and cannot occur in an avascular tissue like the cornea. The reaction is usually beneficial but may not be so under all conditions. The inflammatory cells, particularly macrophages, can themselves spread infection; this is a feature of tuberculosis. Furthermore, inflammatory edema may in some situations endanger life. Thus, in acute laryngitis the patient, particularly if it is a young child, may asphyxiate. Inflammation must be regarded as a mechanism that has evolved to protect the individual from a wide range of hazards. On the whole, it is a beneficial reaction; under certain circumstances the reaction itself becomes a hazard.

Conclusion: Definition of Inflammation

The apparent uniformity of the acute inflammatory response — regardless of its cause — has led many investigators to presume that the changes are mediated by chemical agents that are formed when the tissue is damaged, rather than being caused directly by the injury itself. The search for these mediators has a practical as well as a theoretical objective. If these chemical substances could be identified, antagonistic drugs might be designed and administered to prevent or modify the acute inflammatory response.

The Chemical Mediators of Acute Inflammation

At first, it appeared that the major mediator in acute inflammation was histamine. This is a simple amine of the amino acid histidine; if it is injected into the skin, it produces a reaction that is very similar to that produced by injuring the skin mechanically.

The Triple Response.   Shortly after a firm stroking of the skin, a *red line* appears that is due to capillary dilatation. Soon after this, a more diffuse and widespread *flare* appears surrounding the red line. This results from arteriolar dilatation. Finally, a swelling or a *wheal* appears at the site of the red line, and this is due to exudation of fluid through the altered vascular wall (Fig. 5–9). This triple response of the red line, flare, and wheal was first noted by Sir Thomas Lewis to be very similar to the local changes that follow an injection of histamine. Indeed, there is little doubt that injury to the skin releases histamine from mast cells and that histamine is responsible for the phenomenon of the triple response. It now appears that histamine is the important mediator of the early phase of acute inflammation. Antihistaminic drugs have been developed, and their administration, while blocking the early phase of exudation, is without effect on the prolonged phases. Histamine is especially important in inflammation having a type I allergic basis (Chapter 9), and antihistaminic drugs are of some value in the treatment of hay fever. Nevertheless, in the acute response to most infections, histamine appears to play little part. Antihistamines are therefore of limited value in practice.

Histamine

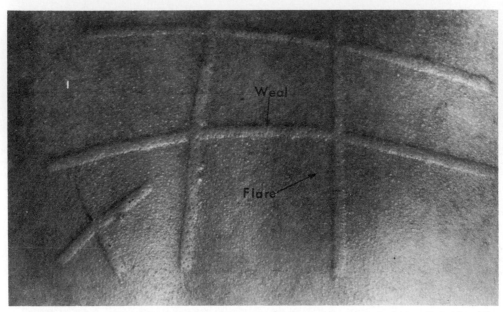

Figure 5–9.   The triple response. This game of tick-tack-toe was started on the skin of the back about three minutes before the photograph was taken. Red lines developed and were soon replaced by well-marked weals. The response is more marked in this subject than in the average person, but the ability to write on the skin in this way is not uncommon and is termed *dermatographism.* It is generally asymptomatic as in this 21-year-old female.

The Kinins

The blood contains an enzyme called *kallikrein,* which exists as a precursor *(prekallikrein)* and can be activated under certain circumstances (Fig. 5–10). The kallikrein acts on a plasma protein *(kininogen)* and produces a polypeptide called *bradykinin.* This was so named because it causes a slow contraction of guinea pig small intestine *in vitro.* Bradykinin is an extremely potent chemical that causes an increase in vascular permeability and is chemotactic to white cells. It causes pain and clearly is a good candidate for being a mediator of acute inflammation. There is good evidence that bradykinin is formed following injury; as with histamine, however, it seems that its role is limited strictly to the early phase of acute inflammation. Tissues become refractory to the prolonged action of both bradykinin and histamine; therefore, neither can be mediators of the prolonged phases.

Biologically Active Cleavage Products of Complement

Complement can be activated not only by antigen-antibody interaction but also by tissue damage. A number of fragments of complement, *e.g.*, C5a and C3a, can release histamine from mast cells. Likewise, there is a chemotactic component $C\overline{567}$ (Chapter 9).

Biologically Active Components of Polymorphs

Although inflammation can occur in the absence of polymorphs, these cells can release vasoactive compounds that may play a part in the inflammatory reaction. Among these are lysosomal enzymes that can activate kallikrein and indirectly can lead to the formation of bradykinin. In addition, they can lead to local tissue destruction. This is an important mechanism in the pathogenesis of immune-complex reactions.

Prostaglandins

The prostaglandins are a group of long-chain fatty acids that were first identified in human semen. They are highly active pharmacologically and cause vasodilatation and smooth muscle contraction. When injected into the skin, they cause a well-marked vasodilatation that lasts for some hours. It is believed that an important effect of the prostaglandins is their potentiation of

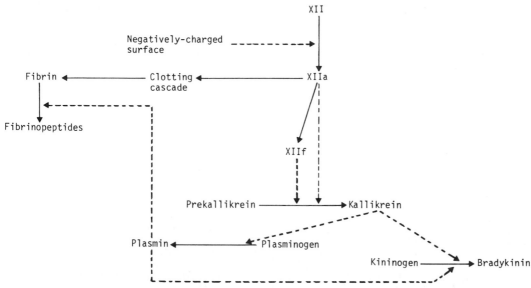

Figure 5–10. The current hypothesis for the activation of the kinin system. Note the central role of Hageman-factor (factor XII) activation which initiates clotting, fibrinolysis, and kinin formation. Factor XIIa has a major role in initiating the clotting cascade but a minor one in activating prekallikrein. Factor XIIf, on the other hand, has as its major action the activation of prekallikrein to kallikrein. Note that activation of the Hageman factor also initiates the clotting cascade. Kallikrein also functions as a plasminogen activator and the plasmin so formed not only digests fibrin but also can convert kininogen to a kinin (bradykinin). Transformations are depicted as solid lines, while enzymatic actions are shown as interrupted lines.

the action of kinins in increasing vascular permeability. The prostaglandins may therefore be significant mediators of acute inflammation, either by a direct action or, more likely, by regulating or *modulating the effect of other mediators.* Prostaglandins can be synthesized in human platelets — an action that is inhibited by aspirin. Here then may be a clue to the action of this well-used but poorly understood anti-inflammatory agent.

Many other agents (*e.g.*, lactic acid and lymphokines) have been suggested as chemical mediators of acute inflammation, but their relative importance is not known. Indeed, the number of chemicals that have been suggested as mediators of acute inflammation is now so large, and their interrelationship is so complex, that it is not possible to give any clear account of their role in acute inflammation. One cannot but agree with Ryan and Majno — the inflammatory "soup" is so complicated that no single individual can claim to know how the dozens of components relate to each other or how they change during the evolution of the inflammatory response. There has been a tendency to stress the uniformity of the inflammatory reaction regardless of its cause, but this uniformity may be more apparent than real. There can be little doubt that bacterial toxins can also initiate or modify the inflammatory response; in particular, clostridia produce toxins that are capable of acting directly on blood vessels and increasing their permeability. Recent observations of the details of the vascular response to injury have revealed that it is a multiphased response with both early and delayed components affecting capillaries and venules. The precise changes vary according to the type of injury and the species of animal involved. It is therefore hardly surprising that no single common chemical mediator is involved. So far, much research has been directed to the vasodilatation and increased vascular permeability of acute inflammation caused by trauma and chemical agents. The much more com-

Conclusion

plex cellular changes and the intricacies of infection have been largely neglected.

Review Questions

1. Describe the four cardinal signs of acute inflammation; explain how they occur.

2. An irritant solution is accidentally injected into one pleural cavity. Predict the possible results of this injection.

3. Describe the origin and functions of the macrophage in acute inflammation and its sequelae.

4. Describe the morphological types of acute inflammation that might be encountered in the peritoneal cavity. Name some likely causes of the inflammation.

5. Describe the possible role of complement in the pathogenesis of acute inflammation.

Selected Readings

Elattar, T. M. A.: Prostaglandins: physiology, biochemistry, pharmacology and clinical applications. Journal of Oral Surgery, 7:175, 1978.
Hurley, C. V.: Acute Inflammation. Edinburgh, Churchill Livingstone, 1972.
Leading article: Mechanisms of eosinophilia. Lancet, 2:1187–1188, 1971.
Ryan, G. B., and Majno, G.: Acute inflammation. American Journal of Pathology, 86:183–276, 1977.
Stossel, T. P.: Phagocytosis: The department of defense. New England Journal of Medicine, 286:776–777, 1972.
Weissmann, G. (Ed.): Mediators of Inflammation. New York, Plenum Press, 1974, 205 pp.
Ward, P. A.: The inflammatory mediators. Annals of the New York Academy of Sciences, 221:290, 1974.
Zweifach, B. W., Grant, L., and McCluskey, R. T. (Eds.): The Inflammatory Process, 2nd ed. New York, Academic Press, Inc., 1974. This reference book, now in three volumes, covers many facets of the inflammatory response in considerable depth.

Infection CHAPTER 6

After studying this chapter the student should be able to:

- Define the difference between intoxication and infection and give two examples of each.
- Distinguish between an endogenous infection and an exogenous infection.
- Describe how organisms are transmitted to the body.
- Define what is meant by a zoonosis and give some examples of the condition.
- Discuss the role of arthropod vectors in the spread of human infections.
- Discuss the importance of hospital infections.
- Describe the body's defenses against infection by using the skin, the intestine, and one other mucosal surface as examples.
- Discuss the three major patterns of infection, using as examples infection by:
  - (a) *Staphylococcus aureus*
  - (b) *Corynebacterium diphtheriae*
  - (c) *Salmonella typhi*
- Describe the various avenues through which infection can spread.
- List the factors that are of importance in predicting whether a particular infection will spread.
- List five examples of opportunistic infection.

From the moment of conception, the human body is exposed to microorganisms, some of which can produce lethal effects. Intrauterine development is rarely complicated by infection; the main microbial assault occurs after birth. Organisms can cause disease in two ways: either they gain access to the tissues of the host, multiply, and cause *infection,* or they manufacture powerful toxins that are subsequently introduced into the body and cause an *intoxication.*

Intoxication

Staphylococcal food poisoning provides an important example of an intoxication. If staphylococci of a suitable strain are allowed to grow for a few hours in a sample of food, the unfortunate victim who eats it will subsequently develop an acute attack of enteritis with accompanying diarrhea and vomiting. This reaction occurs even if the food is cooked, because even though heat kills staphylococci, it does not inactivate the toxin. It is obvious that anyone with a staphylococcal skin lesion, such as a boil, should not be allowed to handle food. Another example of intoxication is *botulism*, which fortunately is very rare. It occurs after food contaminated with *Clostridium botulinum* is eaten, when sufficient time has elapsed for the organism to grow and produce its toxin. Most outbreaks have been due to the ingestion of home-canned food in which the sterilizing process has been inadequate to destroy the highly resistant spores of the organism. When food containing toxin is ingested, the toxin is absorbed into the blood stream and affects the nervous system — apparently by interfering with acetylcholine release at nerve endings. Paralysis results, and in many instances it is progressive and fatal.

Sources of Infection

The most important method whereby microorganisms cause disease is by their *invasion of and multiplication in the living tissues of the host*. This is the definition of *infection*, and organisms capable of producing it are termed pathogens. An infection can be acquired from several possible sources:

Congenital Infection

Infection of the fetus via the placenta is a rare event. Rubella, toxoplasmosis, and syphilis are the best known examples.

Endogenous Infection

If the source of infection is from within the person himself, the infection is termed *endogenous*. Endogenous infections usually occur when the organism leaves its normal habitat. Thus, intestinal organisms cause wound infection and urinary tract disease. Nasopharyngeal organisms cause bronchopneumonia when they migrate down to the lower respiratory tract.

Exogenous Infection

Infection acquired from the external environment is termed exogenous. The organisms may be derived from the following sources:

Patients.   In diseases that run an acute or self-limiting course, the source of infection is a patient. Tuberculosis, whooping cough, measles, and influenza provide examples.

Carriers.   In the case of some other diseases *carriers* play a major role. A carrier harbors the organisms but does not exhibit any clinical disease. The carrier state may follow a clinical attack of the disease (*convalescent carrier*), or a subclinical attack *(contact carrier)*. Streptococcal, staphylococcal, pneumococcal, and meningococcal infections, diphtheria, typhoid fever, bacillary dysentery, and poliomyelitis provide examples.

Infected Animals.   Some pathogens are primarily a cause of animal disease but occasionally infect humans. Such an animal disease is called a *zoonosis*. Bovine tuberculosis, salmonella food poisoning, rabies, and psittacosis are good examples. Likewise, *Leishmania tropica* is a zoonosis among desert gerbils and is occasionally transmitted to humans by the bite of a sand fly (Chapter 15).

Soil.   A number of organisms live in the soil and contaminate wounds. Some are derived from feces (the clostridia, Chapter 10), while others are soil saprophytes (see maduromycosis, Chapter 13).

Transmission of Organisms to the Body.   The exogenous organisms that cause infection may be injected directly into the host by the bite of an insect or through an injury, but more often they are first deposited on the surface of the body, which is thereby contaminated. Contamination may or may not be followed by infection.

The following modes of transmission are important:

Physical Contact.   The causative agents of syphilis, gonorrhea, and other venereal diseases pass from one individual to another by *direct contact*. So also do staphylococci when they are transferred from the hands of one person to the skin surface or wound of another. The transfer of organisms from one individual to another may be by *indirect contact* through fomites, *i.e.,* clothing, bedding, cups, and other articles that are contaminated by an infected person or a carrier and subsequently handled by another individual. This mode of transfer applies to hardy organisms (staphylococci and coliforms) that can withstand drying for some hours.

Inhalation.   Although it is commonly stated that many respiratory infections are "spread by droplets," it is doubtful whether this is true. Droplets are formed during talking, coughing, and sneezing when air passes over a mucous membrane covered by saliva or over tracheal or nasal secretions. The *large droplets,* over 0.1 mm in diameter, settle to the ground within a few seconds and have a limited range. The *small droplets* rapidly evaporate to leave droplet nuclei that are small and may contain some organisms. It is thought that these may be the means whereby certain viruses, *e.g.*, measles and chickenpox, are spread.

It is more likely that respiratory diseases are caused by the inhalation of dust derived from dried contaminated secretions. These secretions may be on handkerchiefs, clothing, bedding, floors, etc., and on drying become converted into dust, which can easily be stirred by movement of any sort, such as walking, dressing, or bedmaking. Airborne transfer of organisms is particularly important within enclosed areas. This therefore applies to hospital wards and operating rooms, where all efforts should be made to keep dust to a minimum. Avoidance of unnecessary movement and adequate ventilation within an operating room are important procedures designed to reduce wound infection.

Ingestion.   Food is a common vehicle of transmission of organisms and can be contaminated in a variety of ways:

Flies can carry organisms from feces, on which they feed, to human food, on which they alight so readily. This is one way in which typhoid fever, bacillary dysentery, amebiasis, poliomyelitis, and hepatitis A are transmitted. *Food handlers* who are carriers of intestinal parasites (*e.g.*, helminths, *Entamoeba histolytica,* and salmonellae) are another source of contamination. The use of human feces as fertilizer may directly contaminate vegetables.

Milk may contain bacteria because the animal itself is diseased; for example, brucellosis in goats and bovine tuberculosis in cows may be transmitted to man via the milk of these animals. Salmonella infections of fowls are passed on in their eggs. Contamination of water supplies is an important means of transmission of some infections, such as cholera and typhoid fever.

Role of Arthropod Vectors.   Insects (which together with spiders constitute the phylum of arthropods) play a variety of roles in the transmission of certain infective organisms to humans. There may be direct transfer as when feces are transferred to food on the hairy legs of house flies. Of greater importance is the transfer of those organisms that are present in the blood of infected individuals; these can be spread by the bite of one of the blood-sucking arthropods such as the mosquito (malaria and yellow fever), flea (plague), louse (epidemic typhus fever), tick (Rocky mountain spotted fever), mite (typhus), or tsetse fly (trypanosomiasis).

The actual mode of infection varies. The organism may be injected into the next victim via the insect's saliva (malaria), or it may be passed in the feces. In the latter event the organism is inoculated by the scratching of the victim.

Hospital Infection (Nosocomial Infection)

Whenever human beings live together in confined quarters, there is always the danger that there will be carriers of pathogenic organisms. Although not suffering from clinical illness themselves, they may pass on the organisms to others who succumb to the infection because of their reduced resistance. In turn, they further transmit the disease. This process is called *cross-infection;* in the past there have been many examples of epidemics of meningococcal meningitis and dysentery occurring in nurses' homes, army camps, and other places housing large numbers of people.

In hospitals it is not uncommon for patients to acquire severe infections from their environment; this is hardly surprising, because many patients are debilitated and their resistance to infection is lowered. Furthermore, surgical incisions provide a ready avenue for the invading bacteria. Extensive burns are particularly liable to become infected, and such patients should be isolated from possible sources of infection. This is termed *reverse isolation*.

A particularly unfortunate feature in hospitals is that the staff acquire pathogenic organisms from their patients, become carriers, and further disseminate the organism. Often, the strain is one that is resistant to the antibiotics in common use in that particular hospital. The infection is therefore all the more serious.

In the past, streptococcal infections have been serious, particularly in maternity wards. Identification of the strain of organism involved and a subsequent search for the source of infection has usually incriminated microbes in the throats of a few members of staff. The exclusion and treatment of such carriers and general measures designed to improve aseptic techniques have usually brought such epidemics to a halt. Penicillin therapy is very effective in streptococcal infections, since resistant organisms do not occur. It follows that outbreaks of streptococcal hospital infection are not a problem at the present time.

The staphylococcus has, on the other hand, attained a much more prominent position. Outbreaks of postoperative wound infection are not uncommon, and the methods of control that proved effective with streptococcal outbreaks are quite inadequate. Often the majority of the staff are found to be carriers, and in addition the hospital itself — the floors, air-conditioning system, and patients' bedclothes — is also contaminated with a virulent strain of staphylococcus. Although human carriers provide the reservoir, the hardy staphylococcus often infects patients by indirect means: for instance, in airborne dust particles. The problem of control is not easy; indeed, there is no simple answer to an outbreak of staphylococcal wound infection.

Other organisms that sometimes cause hospital infection are the coliform groups, particularly the *Proteus* species, and *Pseudomonas aeruginosa*. As with the staphylococcus, the transfer of these organisms is usually indirect — via dust, contaminated articles, and fomites. The source of organisms is often a patient with urinary-tract infection who contaminates his immediate environment—bed clothing, urine bottle, and other articles with which he has contact.

The Body's Defenses Against Infection

It is evident that the body surfaces are commonly contaminated by pathogenic organisms. Whether infection follows depends upon two factors: (1) the mechanical integrity of the body surface; and (2) its powers of removing organisms, *i.e.*, its powers of *decontamination*.

The protective mechanisms vary greatly from one tissue to another. Some examples will be considered below; others will be described under individual organs.

Mechanical Integrity of Body Surfaces

The mechanical strength of the epidermis with its tough outer layer of keratin is an important defense mechanism. Intact skin appears to be completely impervious to invasion by organisms, and it is only after injury that infection is established. Excessive sweating may macerate the keratin layer and render it incapable of repelling organisms. For this reason, skin infections are very common in the tropics, and boils are frequently seen in moist areas like the axillae (armpits). Boils are also common on the buttocks, a condition presumably related to the trauma of continual pressure in the sitting posture. Likewise, yeast infections (ringworm and candidiasis, see Chapter 13) are generally encountered between the toes, in the groin, in the axillae, or under pendulous breasts.

In other areas, the integrity of the covering epithelium is of less importance in repelling infection. Thus, in the mouth, esophagus, and stomach minor trauma causing superficial ulceration is common, and yet infection rarely occurs. In these situations the underlying connective tissue seems to have some special ability to prevent infection. The nature of this local immunity is not understood, but without it, every dental extraction would present a severe hazard, for not only is the underlying fibrous tissue exposed, but also the socket penetrates deeply into the bone of the jaw. In other situations, exposed bone is readily infected, and yet osteomyelitis in the jaw is very uncommon following dental extraction.

Pathogenic organisms that are deposited on a body surface are generally removed expeditiously. Contamination is followed by decontamination. In the case of the skin, this can be readily demonstrated by deliberately contaminating the hands with hemolytic streptococci and subsequently estimating their rate of disappearance by taking swabs at regular intervals. The organisms are often removed or destroyed within two or three hours.

Decontamination

The mechanisms of decontamination vary with each individual surface and can be considered under three headings: *mechanical, biological,* and *chemical.*

Mechanical.   The surface keratin flakes of the skin are continually being rubbed off. This shedding carries away any surface organisms. Mucous membranes have a covering of fluid, and its movement has a washing effect that tends to remove organisms. The flow of tears over the conjunctiva, the upward moving sheet of mucus of the respiratory tract, the flow of saliva in the salivary ducts, and the flow of urine in the urinary tract are all mechanical methods that serve to wash away any organisms that have alighted on the surface. If this flow of fluid is diminished or impeded, then infection soon follows.

Biological.   Most body surfaces are not sterile but are contaminated by organisms constituting the *resident flora.* This flora is characteristic of each particular surface. In the case of the skin, it includes *Staphylococcus albus* and diphtheroids. In the mouth, alpha hemolytic streptococci *(Streptococcus viridans)* predominate. In the large intestine on the other hand, bacteroides, coliforms, and enterococci abound. These organisms, constituting the resident flora, are so adapted to their environment that they do not normally cause infection. In fact, they provide protection to the host by producing antibiotic substances and by competing with other organisms for essential foodstuffs. If the resident flora is upset by antibiotic therapy, subsequent contamination by pathogenic organisms can lead to infection. This is sometimes seen when potent broad-spectrum antibiotics are administered by mouth. The flora of the intestine is so altered that an acute, fulminating — sometimes lethal — gastroenteritis can result from infection with *Clostridum difficile* or *Staphylococcus aureus. Candida albicans* can likewise cause a troublesome stomatitis and pruritus ani.

Chemical.   The various secretions that are found on each body surface often contain chemicals that destroy unwanted pathogens. The chemicals vary from one tissue to another. In the stomach, the hydrochloric acid is of great importance and destroys many pathogens such as pneumococci and streptococci. The stomach also forms an important defense mechanism for the respiratory tract, since pathogens present in the expectorated mucus are destroyed when this is swallowed.

Two other antibacterial substances are noteworthy in body secretions. *Lysozyme* is an enzyme present in many secretions and is capable of removing the cell wall of some bacteria. This was first described by Fleming, who is better known for his discovery of penicillin. The other important chemical agent is immunoglobulin (see IgA, Chapter 9).

Patterns of Infection

The relationship between a host and its invading pathogens is a complex one. Three main patterns will be described: (1) *Invasive organisms producing local damage;* (2) *toxic organisms;* (3) *invasive organisms producing little local damage.*

Invasive Organisms Producing Local Damage. Some infecting organisms produce toxins that, by causing local tissue destruction, excite an acute inflammatory reaction. *Staphylococcus aureus* is an example of an organism that produces such an infection; in the skin, this response can vary from a mild *folliculitis* involving the superficial part of a pilosebaceous follicle to a *boil* involving the whole hair follicle apparatus and leading to abscess formation. Local spread of infection leads to involvement of the subcutaneous tissues so that a *carbuncle* is formed (see Fig. 10–1). Spread into the lymphatic vessels leads to inflammation of the tissues around these vessels *(lymphangitis)*. When these vessels are superficial, the inflammation appears as red streaks under the skin. When organisms reach the regional lymphatic nodes, there is swelling and tenderness of the nodes as evidence of *lymphadenitis*. Finally, the organisms may penetrate the barrier of the lymph nodes and enter the blood stream via the thoracic duct. The local tissues and the inflammatory reaction form the *first defense against infection,* and the *lymph nodes form the second,* but it is in the blood stream that the third and most effective defense mechanism is encountered. This is the *reticuloendothelial system.* The cells of this system have the property of being able to phagocytose circulating organisms, and frequently they destroy them. If the cells of the reticuloendothelial system are capable of destroying such organisms, the presence of organisms in the blood is of both short duration and little consequence. It sometimes happens that during the course of an infection blood is taken for culture and organisms are grown. The presence of these organisms in the blood is termed *bacteremia,* and it signifies the presence of a positive blood culture in the absence of any marked symptoms.

Sometimes organisms engulfed by the reticuloendothelial system are not destroyed but are allowed to proliferate in the cytoplasm of the cells. This situation occurs when immunity is low and results in vast numbers of organisms being produced in the cytoplasm of the reticuloendothelial cells. When these cells undergo necrosis, the organisms and their toxic products are released into the blood stream. The blood culture is again positive, but on this occasion the patient is gravely ill. Such a condition is known as *septicemia*. It indicates a positive blood culture and a complete overwhelming of the defenses of the body. It is therefore a grave condition that frequently proves fatal.

Toxic Organisms. Some organisms manufacture extremely potent exotoxins that produce local tissue damage. In addition, these toxins can enter the blood stream and cause damage at distant sites. An excellent example of this type of infection is diphtheria. When the causative organism, *Corynebacterium diphtheriae,* alights on a tonsil, it proliferates and produces diphtheria toxin. This leads to local tissue necrosis and a local acute inflammation, recognized clinically as a sore throat. The tonsils are covered by a layer of necrotic epithelium and exudate, which is called a *pseudomembrane.* Surrounding edema can be so severe that life is threatened by involvement of the larynx. However, the more frequently dangerous effects of diphtheria are related to the effects of disseminated toxin. Damage to nerves can cause paralysis, *e.g.,* of the palate, and damage to the heart leads to a toxic myocarditis and heart failure. It should be noted that the manifestations of diphtheria are entirely due to the exotoxin. The organisms themselves are not invasive, but remain on the surface of the tonsils or on the pharyngeal wall (Chapter 10).

In tetanus there is a similar pattern of disease. Spores of the organism are introduced into a wound, germinate if circumstances are favorable, and produce tetanus exotoxin. This agent is absorbed both via perineural spaces and directly into the blood stream. When the toxin reaches the central nervous system, its actions lead to violent spasms of skeletal muscles and ultimately to paralysis and death. Once again the organisms remain localized, but the disease is attributable to the effects of exotoxin. Gas gangrene is another example of an infection with a toxic organism (Chapter 10).

Invasive Organisms Producing Little Local Damage. Some organisms appear to produce little or no local tissue damage and therefore no inflammatory response at the site of entry. Such organisms can proliferate rapidly and spread throughout the body via the lymphatics and ultimately via the blood stream. Infection with this type of organism is common, and the manner by which lesions are produced can be understood by a study of the disease typhoid fever.

Pathogenesis of Typhoid Fever. The pathogenesis of mouse typhoid (infection with *Salmonella typhimurium*) has been studied in considerable detail. By analogy, the sequence of events in man is as follows.

Typhoid fever is contracted by the ingestion of food or water contaminated with *Salmonella typhi*. The organisms reach the lumen of the intestine and are taken up by phagocytes on its mucosal surface. In the cytoplasm of these cells the organisms are carried into the mucosa itself and then to the local lymphoid tissue (Peyer's patches). Scarcely any local tissue damage occurs, and little or no inflammation ensues. The organisms multiply, and some pass on through lymph vessels to the mesenteric nodes and finally the blood stream via the thoracic duct. In this way a bacteremia develops and the phagocytic cells of the reticuloendothelial (RE) system engulf them. However, since the bacteria are pathogens they are able to live and multiply in the RE cells; by about the tenth day the parasitized cells undergo necrosis and cause the blood stream to be flooded with large numbers of bacilli. This is the end of the *incubation period* (usually 10 to 14 days), and the patient becomes seriously ill with septicemia (Fig. 6–1).

The *septicemic phase* lasts about a week and is characterized clinically by a progressive rise in temperature, by constipation, and by severe constitutional symptoms. The mind becomes clouded, coma ensues, and death may occur. Diagnosis rests on one's obtaining a positive blood culture.

The next phase of the disease is marked by the onset of diarrhea associated with ulceration of the small intestine and by the appearance of organisms in the feces. The bacilli reach the gut via the bile, which is heavily contaminated as a result of passage of bacteria from the RE cells of the liver. The ulceration occurs over the inflamed Peyer's patches and is accompanied by enlarged mesenteric lymph nodes. In both the ulcers and the lymph nodes there is an accumulation of macrophages; polymorphs are conspicuously absent. At this stage the two most dreaded complications are intestinal hemorrhage, and intestinal perforation leading to peritonitis. The most likely explanation of these events is that following the initial infection the local lymphoid tissue of the gut becomes sensitized to the organisms or their products, and that subsequent contact with the organisms produces damage. The sensitizing antibodies are presumably produced locally, because the blood level of antibodies detectable as agglutinins does not rise until later in

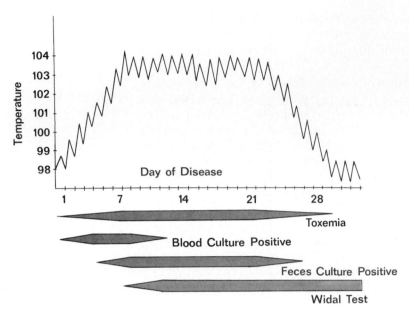

Figure 6–1. Chart correlating the clinical course of a typical case of untreated typhoid fever with the principal methods of bacteriological diagnosis. Note the step-ladder rise in temperature during the first week. (Drawing by Anthony J. Walter.)

the course of the disease. During the second week of typhoid fever, diagnosis depends upon finding the organism in the feces. The characteristic *rose spots* appear in crops between the seventh and twelfth days. They are small red papules seen on the skin of the trunk and are due to bleeding secondary to an acute vasculitis comparable to the lesions of gonococcal bacteremia (Chapter 10).

Typhoid fever therefore represents an infection by a highly invasive organism in which tissue damage appears to be produced by some type of antigen-antibody interaction. Since antibody production takes 10 to 14 days to begin, it follows that symptoms do not occur until after the organism has spread widely. The incubation period is therefore long and contrasts with the short incubation period of diseases caused by invasive organisms that produce direct local tissue damage, *e.g.*, staphylococci and streptococci.

Toward the end of the second week of typhoid fever, antityphoid antibodies appear in the blood, and their titer subsequently rises. These antibodies are usually detected as agglutinins; the test employed is referred to as the *Widal reaction* (see Fig. 9–8). Since a rising titer of agglutinins is particularly significant in the diagnosis, a specimen of blood should be taken early in the course of a suspected case of typhoid fever so that its titer of antibodies can be compared with that of later samples. This method of confirming the diagnosis of an infective illness is particularly useful in viral disease, since the infective agent is often difficult to isolate once the disease is clinically apparent. The method is also of use if the virus laboratory is not immediately at hand.

During the third week of typhoid fever the patient gradually recovers, the diarrhea abates, and the temperature returns to normal. Nevertheless, even with chloramphenicol therapy there is a relapse rate of 10 to 20 per cent — the blood culture again becomes positive and symptoms, including the rose spots, return.

Other invasive organisms produce a disease similar in overall pattern to that of typhoid fever. In syphilis there is widespread dissemination of organisms, and a local ulcer does not appear for three to four weeks (Chapter 10). In many viral infections (*e.g.*, smallpox and measles), widespread dissemination of the organisms occurs before the onset of the characteristic disease. Once again, the incubation period tends to be about two weeks. It is interesting that in many instances the ability of the organisms to spread is inversely proportional to their ability to produce immediate local tissue damage. Thus, staphylococci produce local inflammatory lesions but tend to remain localized, whereas the organism of syphilis produces no immediate damage yet is highly invasive.

Other Patterns of Infection.   Many other patterns of infection can be recognized. Some organisms can produce a local lesion with minimal inflammation such that the incident goes unnoted. This is a *subclinical* infection. Some organisms can enter into a symbiotic state with their hosts — either permanently or between phases — when they cause damage. An example of the latter type of infection is the common coldsore due to the herpes simplex virus. The virus causes the characteristic blisters of the skin; between attacks, however, it resides in the ganglion of a sensory nerve supplying the part. A special group of virus infections (oncogenic viruses) is known that will produce tumors; these are described in Chapter 17. It is evident that infection proceeds according to many different patterns, and the situation is further complicated by the fact that one particular strain of organism can, under different circumstances, produce different types of infective illness. Thus, *Streptococcus pyogenes* can on the one hand produce a relatively minor local infection in the form of a sore throat, but under other circumstances (*e.g.*, when it is introduced into a cut sustained while a necropsy examination is performed) can lead to a fulminating septicemia. Likewise, the herpes simplex virus can remain as a latent infection in some individuals, while in others it causes coldsores, pneumonitis, or encephalitis. It may even be a major factor in the etiology of cancer of the uterus.

Following is a summary of the ways in which infection can spread (Fig. 6–2):

Spread of Infection

The natural cohesion of tissues tends to prevent the spread of organisms. Nevertheless, the tissue fluids are in constant motion because of movement of the part, and organisms are carried in any stream of fluid that may be present. Since muscular activity causes considerable fluid movement, the time-honored treatment of inflammation is to rest the part. Two features should be noted. First, the actual motility of the organism appears to play no part in the spread of infection. Thus, *Clostridium tetani* is a motile organism, but the infection (tetanus) is a localized affair. Second, the degree of local spread is inversely proportional to the amount of damage produced by the organism. Damage leads to an inflammatory reaction, and this is often an efficient local

Spread by Continuity: Direct Spread

Figure 6–2. Diagram illustrating the sequence of events that can follow the spread of infection.

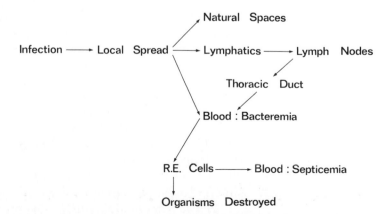

defense mechanism. Thus the deposition of fibrin sometimes appears to be important in walling off an infection; for example, fibrinous adhesions prevent the spread of infection from an acutely inflamed appendix (Chapter 32).

Local spread can occur in an entirely different way. Some organisms are ingested by phagocytes and are transported by these cells. This is an important means of spread in tuberculosis and almost certainly occurs in other infections.

Spread by Natural Channels   If local spread implicates a natural passage, infection may extend by this route. The following examples are important:

Peritoneum.   Infection may spread rapidly throughout the peritoneal space from a localized lesion. Acute appendicitis is therefore serious, because following perforation of the organ, the entire peritoneal cavity can become infected. A large surface is involved, and there is rapid absorption of toxic substances, causing the patient to become severely ill. Likewise, infection can spread throughout the pleural cavity, the subarachnoid space, the pericardium, or a joint space.

Infection can also spread along tubes, such as the bronchi (with bronchopneumonia and tuberculosis), the ureter, and the gut.

Lymphatics.   In acute inflammation the lymphatic vessels are held wide open by the increased tissue tension. The permeability of the vessel walls is increased and so also is the flow of lymph. Invading organisms that gain access to the lymphatics are carried to the nearest lymph node where, for a time at least, they are held up by the local reticuloendothelial cells. Lymphangitis and lymphadenitis are characteristic of certain types of infection, *e.g.*, streptococcal and tubercular infections.

Blood Stream.   There are several ways by which organisms enter the blood stream. These will be elaborated on in the following sections.

Direct Invasion of Blood Vessels.   A few organisms may invade the blood vessels during the course of any local infection. The infection may itself be quite trivial, but the adjacent blood vessels can be ruptured by trauma, thereby allowing organisms to enter. Gingival infection or abscesses related to the apices of the roots of teeth are common lesions in which this invasion occurs. Such spread of infection often follows dental extraction, scaling of teeth, or even chewing hard food. When small numbers of organisms enter the blood stream in this way, they are rapidly removed by the reticuloendothelial system, and the bacteremia that occurs causes no symptoms. An exception to this is bacteremia caused by one of the gram-negative bacilli of the coliform group. In this instance, the patient sometimes has rigors and develops a fever. This is occasionally seen in the bacteremia that follows passage of a catheter up the urethra.

Bacteremia cannot be dismissed as a completely inconsequential event. Under certain circumstances, it can lead to serious sequelae.

Metastatic Lesions.   Experimentally it can be shown that when an animal has a bacteremia, histamine injected at any site will precipitate a local infection by the organism concerned. Trauma has a similar effect. It is believed that this is the origin of acute osteomyelitis. A child who happens to have a staphylococcal bacteremia and traumatizes a limb then develops an acute infection of the bone (Chapter 40). Another danger of a bacteremia is that the organisms can be filtered off by the kidneys, and if there is a simultaneous obstruction of the outflow of urine, a kidney infection (*pyelonephritis*) results. A further hazard of bacteremia is that the organisms may colonize a damaged heart valve and cause endocarditis (Chapter 28).

Septic Thrombophlebitis.   When infection spreads to a vein, its walls become inflamed and thrombosis occurs. The condition is called *throm-*

buphlebitis. If the thrombus is invaded by a pyogenic organism, it may soften and parts of it become detached, leading to the condition of pyemia (Chapter 20).

Spread from the Lymphatic System.   Organisms that are not held up in the tissues at the site of entry or in the lymph nodes reach the venous circulation via lymphatic ducts. This has already been described in the instance of typhoid fever.

Along Nerves.   This is not a common route of infection and in fact is restricted to some viruses, such as the virus of rabies.

The following sections include a summary of the factors that determine whether a particular organism is likely to spread from the site of infection or to remain localized.

Factors Determining Localization or Spread of Infection

Virulence.   Within each species of organism there are many different strains, each with differing virulence. For example, there are many strains of staphylococci, and some of these are associated with particularly severe infection. Likewise, some strains of diphtheria bacilli produce more exotoxin than do others.

Factors Involving the Organisms

Dose.   A large dose of organisms tend to produce a more severe infection than a small dose.

Portal of Entry.   This is a most important factor, because some organisms will cause infection only if administered by a particular route. For example, *Vibrio cholerae* can be injected subcutaneously without harm, but if it is swallowed, it causes cholera. Likewise, many of the coliform organisms produce no damage in the intestine, but cause infection if introduced into the urinary tract.

Synergism.   The combined effect of two organisms may be more severe than the effect of either acting alone. Staphylococcal infection of a wound, for example, can precipitate the onset of gas gangrene (Chapter 10).

Products of the Organism.   The toxic products of organisms can presumably aid their infection. They act in many ways; some destroy tissue locally. Leukocidins damage white cells and hyaluronidase depolymerizes the ground substance, whereas streptokinase aids in the lysis of fibrin by activating plasmin (Chapter 20).

General Factors.   The *general state of health* of the host is important. Patients who are starved or who suffer from chronic debilitating diseases like chronic nephritis and diabetes mellitus are less capable of resisting infection. The factors involved are complex and probably involve both humoral factors (*e.g.*, a low complement level) and an impaired activity of phagocytes.

Factors Involving the Host — Host Resistance

The Immune State.   This involves both nonspecific factors like complement and the presence of specific antibodies of acquired immunity. Defective B or T cell function can render the individual highly susceptible to infection (Chapter 9).

Low White Cell Count.   Infections occur more readily and spread more widely whenever the neutrophil polymorphonuclear leukocyte count is low, as in agranulocytosis or acute leukemia.

Abnormal White Cells.   Occasionally patients are encountered in whom there is an inherent defect in white cell function. These patients tend to suffer from repeated bacterial infections that commence in childhood. Specialized techniques are now available for investigating the phagocytic and bactericidal activity of polymorphs.

Local Factors.   The presence of necrotic tissue is an important predisposing cause of local infection. Foreign bodies and chemicals that cause necrosis are therefore harmful. Another important factor is the local blood supply. Ischemia of any origin, by impairing the local inflammatory reaction, is detrimental to the body's efforts at repelling infection. Infection and ulceration can follow quite trivial injuries to the legs of patients who have varicose veins or suffer from arteriosclerosis. Likewise, tetanus can sometimes follow the local injection of epinephrine (which causes contraction of the blood vessels) if a dirty needle is used.

Opportunistic Infections

It is now apparent that some organisms that in the past have been considered to be avirulent can cause infection under certain circumstances. This is called *opportunistic infection* and may occur when either local or general factors operate in favor of the organism.

Abnormal Local Conditions.   Prosthetic heart valves provide an admirable site for infection with a wide range of organisms, including rickettsiae and fungi, which normally do not produce endocarditis. Another example is related to the use of broad-spectrum antibiotics. As noted previously, these drugs can so alter the flora of the gut that fulminating gastroenteritis can be caused by *Staphylococcus aureus*. Secondary infections stemming from alteration of the microbial flora by antibiotic therapy are usually called *superinfections*.

Immunologically Suppressed Patient.   The administration of glucocorticoids and anticancer drugs, particularly to patients with malignant disease of the reticuloendothelial system (*e.g.*, Hodgkin's disease), can create conditions favorable to opportunistic infections. Thus, it is not uncommon for such patients to die of infections by fungi that in normal people rarely cause infection. Furthermore, organisms (*e.g.*, *Candida*) that commonly produce a local infection can become widely disseminated in the immunologically suppressed patient (Chapter 13).

Conclusion

The traditional division of organisms into pathogens and nonpathogens, while serving a useful purpose under most circumstances, is an artificial separation. Before deciding whether an organism is causing a particular infection one must consider the organism in relation to the circumstances of a particular patient. In the ongoing battle between man and microbe there are no simple rules for distinguishing friend from foe.

Review Questions

1. Explain the following complications of untreated or inadequately treated typhoid fever: (a) suppurative parotitis; (b) bronchopneumonia; (c) boils; (d) pyelonephritis; and (e) typhoid osteitis and periosteitis.

2. Give examples of infections that result from the obstruction of a natural passage.

3. The incubation period of diphtheria is 2 to 7 days, whereas that of typhoid fever is about 10 days. Based on your knowledge of the pathogenesis of the two diseases, account for this difference.

4. Why is a wound infection with *Staphylococcus aureus* of greater importance than one due to *Streptococcus pyogenes*?

5. When placed in reverse isolation, a patient is protected from organisms that are carried by visitors, including the attending medical and nursing staff. Give some examples of patients who should be placed in reverse isolation and indicate the reason for doing this.

Selected Readings

Leading article: What makes bacteria pathogenic? Lancet, 2:266, 1972.
Youmans, G. P., Paterson, P. Y., and Sommers, H. M.: The Biologic and Clinical Basis of Infectious Diseases. Philadelphia, W. B. Saunders Company, 1975. Chapter 2, "Characteristics of Host-Bacteria Interaction: External Defense Mechanisms," elaborates on many of the topics covered in this chapter.

Wound Healing CHAPTER
7

After studying this chapter the student should be able to:

- Compare the process of axial regeneration in amphibians with that of healing in humans.
- Describe the differences between repair and regeneration.
- Compare wound contraction with cicatrization.
- Describe how wound contraction can be measured experimentally.
- Describe the mode of formation and the components of granulation tissue.
- Describe how an incised skin wound heals and compare it with the healing of a skin wound with separated edges.
- List the important causes of slow wound healing.
- List the important complications of wound healing.
- Describe the main features of healing in liver, kidney, tendon, and muscle.
- Compare and contrast healing in the peripheral nervous system with healing in the central nervous system.
- Describe the nature of chalones and indicate the role that they might play in the processes of wound healing.

Sustaining injury is one of the inevitable tribulations of life. It follows that the individual's ability to heal wounds is one of the fundamental processes in pathology. The term "wound healing" is taken to include all those reparative processes that result from the inflammation caused by the infliction of tissue damage.

Introduction; Definition of Terms

The types of injury include not only obvious traumatic damage such as that caused by a surgical incision or a stab wound but also the tissue damage produced by heat, freezing, radiation, infection, chemical toxins, ischemia, and the results of damaging antigen-antibody interaction. The process of healing has obvious survival value for the individual, and has therefore been highly developed in all forms of life. Nevertheless, it differs from one species to another as well as from one tissue to another within the same individual.

In insects, amphibians, and crustaceans, the ability to replace lost parts has long been known and is truly remarkable. Thus, if the lens of the eye of a salamander is removed, a new lens develops from the adjacent iris. Other well-known examples of regeneration are the regrowth of the amputated limbs of insects and newts and of the claws of lobsters. The process whereby whole limbs are re-formed is well developed in lower forms of life; it is complex and resembles embryonic development or asexual reproduction. The process is termed *axial regeneration* by zoologists and has been intensively studied in the hope that it might provide some clues to our understanding of healing in humans. Following the amputation of the arm of a newt, the stump rapidly becomes covered by a layer of epidermal cells while the underlying connective tissue cells dedifferentiate to form a mass of primitive cells that form a *blastema*. Its cells multiply rapidly in an avascular field in the first instance. Later there is vascularization and differentiation: bone, muscle, tendon, nerves, and blood vessels are produced in a coordinated manner such that there is accurate replacement of the limb that was lost. No matter what the level of the original amputation, only the distal parts are replaced. Thus, after a forearm amputation the wrist and hand are re-formed, but never an elbow. This rule of *distal transformation* has been summed up by the trite description "hands from elbows, but never elbows from hands."

Wound Healing in Humans

In humans the cells adjacent to the area of damage fail to dedifferentiate, and no blastema comparable to that described above is formed. The healing process has two aspects:

Contraction. This is the process whereby the size of the wound decreases during the first few days following the infliction of the wound.

Replacement of Lost Tissue. In this process, migration of cells as well as division of adjacent cells provides extra tissue to fill the defect. This can be accomplished in two ways:

Repair. This is a process by which the lost specialized tissue is replaced by granulation tissue, which later matures to form scar tissue. It is an inevitable end-result when the surviving specialized cells do not possess the ability to proliferate.*

Regeneration. This term is applied to the process by which the lost tissue is replaced by a tissue similar in type. Thus, when liver cells have been damaged, more liver tissue is produced by a proliferation of the surrounding undamaged specialized cells. Regeneration occurs when the damaged tissue is composed of labile or stable cells. *Labile cells*, also called continuous replicators, undergo division throughout life to replace those that are lost through differentiation or desquamation. Most protective or covering epithelia fall into this group. *Stable cells*, also called discontinuous replicators, rarely divide under normal circumstances but are able to proliferate if suitably stimulated. Glandular tissue such as liver, kidney, and endocrine glands falls into this category.

It should be noted that there is no dedifferentiation of cells as occurs in the axial regeneratiion of amphibians. Indeed, the only human counterpart to this situation is seen in the healing of bone fractures. Here connective tissue cells — osteoblasts, fibroblasts, etc. — do dedifferentiate to form a blastema that is capable of redifferentiating to form fibrous tissue, cartilage, or bone (Chapter 40).

Before the coordinated process that occurs during simple skin wound healing is described, it is convenient to describe *wound contraction* and *granulation tissue formation*. These are two components of the process that can be studied experimentally and can be quantitated.

Wound Contraction

This is a dynamic process that can be studied in the experimental animal by excising a small, circular, full-thickness disk of skin from the back or flank. Figures 7–1 and 7–2 show the result of such an experiment. The size of the wound is measured at regular intervals; after an initial period of two to three days, there follows a phase of rapid contraction, which is largely completed by the fourteenth day. New tissue formation is not included, since the measurements are made from the original wound edges. The importance of wound contraction is illustrated in Figure 7–2. It can be seen that with good contraction a small scar is produced, while with inadequate contraction a large scar results, with all the cosmetic and functional complications that follow.

Much experimental work has been carried out with a view to understand-

---

*The term repair is also used in pathology to describe the process whereby damaged molecules are restored to normal. Thus, a section of a DNA molecule damaged by ultraviolet light can be excised and replaced by a normal segment by a process of repair.

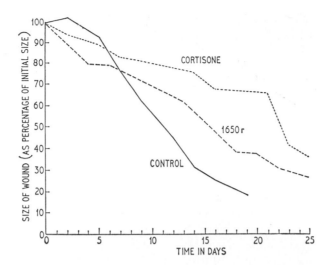

Figure 7–1. Graphic representation of wound contraction in the rat. Three groups of animals were used; a standard 1-cm excised wound was made on the back of each animal. One group of animals was given a daily injection of cortisone acetate. Another received one dose of a 1650r x-ray immediately after infliction of the wound; the third group acted as the control. Each wound was measured daily, and the average wound area within each group was calculated. The graphs show that both irradiation and cortisone administration caused considerable delay in wound contraction.

ing the process of wound contraction so that it may be brought under control when necessary. It is generally agreed that the contractile force resides in the new granulation tissue that forms around the circumference of a healing wound. This has been called the *picture frame area*. Although the mechanism is not fully understood, it appears that contraction of the myofibroblasts of granulation tissue plays a role in this process.

Wound contraction can be inhibited by the systemic administration of glucocorticoids and by the local application of ionizing radiation. Mechanical factors, such as tethering of the wound edges, are also effective in preventing contraction. This is well illustrated by the large chronic ulcers that occur around the ankle in patients with venous stasis (Fig. 7–3). Dense, fibrous tissue fixes the wound edges to the periosteum of the tibia, and healing results in very extensive scar tissue formation. The scar is covered by thin (atrophic) epidermis and is liable to ulcerate with subsequent injury — even quite trivial injury.

Granulation tissue is formed by the proliferation and migration of surrounding connective tissue elements. In the first instance, it is composed of *capillary loops* and *myofibroblasts,* together with a variable number of inflammatory cells. Initially, granulation tissue is highly vascular, but with the passage of time it becomes avascular scar tissue. The manner of its formation can be studied experimentally in various ways. A convenient method is by

Granulation Tissue Formation

Figure 7–2. Diagram showing how contraction accelerates the healing of a wound and produces a small scar. Note that in actual practice a circular wound invariably shows considerable distortion in shape by the time healing is complete. (Drawing by Anthony J. Walter.)

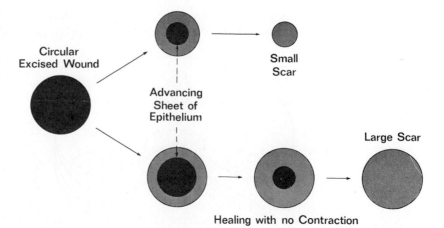

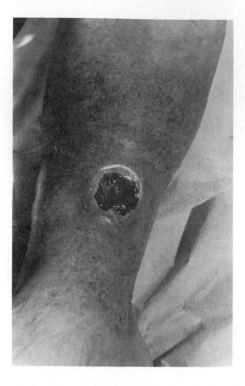

Figure 7–3. Chronic leg ulcer in patient with varicose veins. The ulcer is almost circular and is covered by a dark blood-stained slough. A thin layer of regenerating epidermis is beginning to grow across the ulcer bed. The surrounding skin is thickened as a result of edema and fibrosis of the dermis. It is firmly tethered to the underlying muscle sheaths and bone. Hence, there can be no contraction in such an ulcer. The discoloration of the skin is due to the deposition of blood and hemoglobin-derived pigment (hemosiderin). There is also increased melanin pigmentation of the epidermis.

observations of the rabbit ear–chamber, which is illustrated in Figures 7–4 to 7–7.

Buds of endothelial cells grow out from existing blood vessels at the wound margin, undergo canalization, and form a series of vascular arcades by joining with their neighbors. At first the new-formed vessels all appear similar and have a thin wall consisting of only endothelium. These vessels leak protein readily, so that the fluid bathing the area consists virtually of plasma and forms an admirable nutrient medium. Very soon differentiation occurs: some vessels acquire a muscular coat and become arterioles, while others form thin-walled large venules. Some persist as part of the capillary bed, while the remainder disappear as the granulation tissue steadily becomes modified.

At the same time that the vessels grow into the clot, fibroblast-like cells around the wound margin multiply and accompany the vascular invasion. Thus, the clot is converted into a living vascular granulation tissue, and the process is called *organization*. The cells have in the past been termed "fibroblasts," but they differ from the fibroblasts seen in other situations. The cells have contractile elements in their cytoplasm and have therefore been renamed myofibroblasts. These cells can contract and by doing so cause

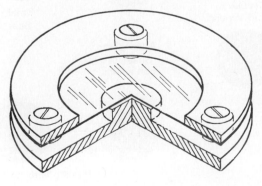

Figure 7–4. Diagrammatic representation of one type of rabbit ear–chamber with wedge cut out to show its construction. The chamber is composed of a Perspex base plate that has a raised central table and three peripherally arranged pillars. The coverslip consists of a disc of mica supported at the edge by a ring of Perspex. The coverslip is placed upon the three pillars and is held in position by screws that are inserted into threaded holes in the pillars. The height of the pillars is such that the gap between the top of the table and the mica is 50 to 100 μm. (Drawing by S. P. Steward.)

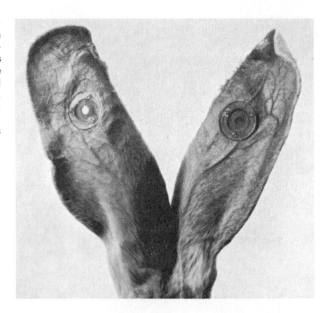

Figure 7–5.   Two rabbit ear-chambers in position. The one in the left ear shows the clear central area in which observations are made. In the chamber on the right, the area of the central table is still filled with blood clot. (From Blair, G. H., van den Brenk, H. A. S., Walter, J. B., and Slome, D.: Experimental study of effects of radiation on wound healing. In D. Slome (Ed.): Wound Healing. New York, Pergamon Press, 1961, pp. 46–53.)

wound contraction. At first, the cells are large and plump and have in their cytoplasm the endoplasmic reticulum necessary for the formation of collagen. Hence, collagen fibrils steadily form around cells that become thin and elongated and finally resemble the inert fibrocytes of adult tissue. The myofibroblasts are also responsible for the formation of ground substance.

Lymphatic vessels grow into the maturing granulation tissue in much the same way the blood vessels do. The two sets of vessels do not anastomose, and the lymphatics form blind-ended channels. At the same time, there is an ingrowth of nerve fibers so that not only do blood vessels acquire an autonomic nerve supply but also the tissue regains sensation.

As maturation proceeds, there is a general remodeling of granulation tissue. Some vessels undergo atrophy and disappear, whereas others exhibit thickening of their coats and eventual obliteration of the lumen. This process of devascularization and collagen formation eventually results in the formation of an avascular scar.

Healing of Skin Wounds

Skin wounds are so common that one takes it for granted that they will heal. Nevertheless, the process by which this occurs is by no means well understood. Following is a description of the healing of two separate types of wound.

Healing of a Clean, Incised Wound with Apposed Edges

This process is sometimes described as *healing by primary intention*, and it is the desired result in all healing surgical incisions. Little tissue is lost, and the separated skin edges are brought together by the use of sutures, clips, or tape.

Bleeding occurs immediately after injury and a small amount of blood clot forms in the wound area. An acute inflammatory reaction follows, and the fibrinous exudate helps to join the cut margins of the wound together.

Epithelial Changes.   Within 24 hours of injury, the epithelial cells from the adjacent epidermis migrate into the wound and slide between the inert dermis and the overlying clot (Fig. 7–8). A continuous layer of epidermal cells soon covers the surface, and overlying this is a crust or scab of dried clot. During the next 24 hours these epidermal cells invade the space where connective tissue will eventually develop. In this way, spurs of epidermal cells are formed not only in the area of incision but also along the tracts of any

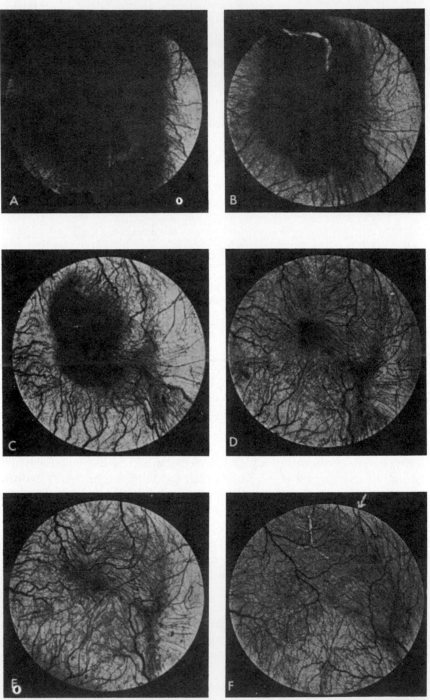

Figure 7–6.   Granulation tissue formation in the rabbit ear–chamber. Photographs taken at the following times after the insertion of the chamber: *A*, 9 days. *B*, 12 days. *C*, 17 days. *D*, 21 days. *E*, 24 days. *F*, 44 days. At 9 days vessels are seen to be invading the dark clot in the center, and by 24 days organization is complete. The large tortuous vessels are venules; the arterioles are more difficult to see at this magnification. The arrow in *F* indicates an arteriole that divides almost immediately. Note how by 44 days changes have occurred in the course of many blood vessels, although the original pattern of certain venules can still be recognized on the left-hand side of the picture. A lymphatic vessel is now visible at the top of the chamber (× 8.5).

Figure 7–7. The growing edge of granulation tissue in a rabbit ear–chamber. The rapidly moving stream of blood in the capillary loops at the top produces a streaked effect, and individual red cells cannot be distinguished; in the right-hand vessel, white cells are adherent to the endothelium and appear as transparent globules. In the lower half of the picture, the capillary buds, which contain plasma with few cells, show no flow. Rouleaux formation is seen in one of the capillary buds.

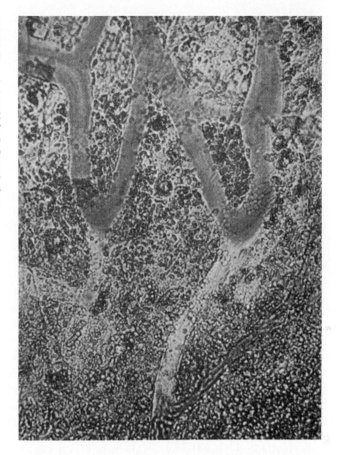

sutures that have been inserted. These epidermal cells are derived from the cut epidermis and from any severed hair follicle or sweat-gland cells.

Connective-Tissue Changes.   Following the initial acute inflammatory reaction, the edema subsides and the polymorphs are replaced by monocytes. These cells, which become phagocytic and perform a scavenger function, are then called *macrophages.* This *demolition phase* is an essential prelude to the organization that follows.

Organization.   By about the third day, the area of the wound is invaded by granulation tissue from the adjacent subepithelial layers. The major part of this ingrowth occurs from the subcutaneous tissues, since there is little or no contribution from the dense, inert reticular dermis.

Soon after the granulation tissue appears, collagen formation commences. At first this appears as reticulin fibers, but these later mature into collagenous bundles. This collagen is of vital importance to the wound, because it forms the main connecting tissue between the originally divided skin. The amount of collagen can be assessed subjectively by examining sections of wounds. A more accurate method is to measure the amount of hydroxyproline in hydrolysates of wound tissues. By this technique it can be shown that the *tensile strength* of a wound during the first month is proportional to the amount of collagen formed. The tensile strength can be measured experimentally by excising the entire wound area and applying a disrupting force across the wound. The force needed to cause separation of the wound edges is measured, and from this information it is possible to calculate the amount of energy necessary to disrupt the wound. Such measurements are not of purely academic interest, because the strength of a wound is of prime importance when one considers the way in which surgical incisions heal. Were it not for the tensile strength of a laparotomy wound, this common surgical incision could burst open and the abdominal contents would spill out to the exterior. This is an occasional catastrophe following surgery; it is often fatal. A remarkable experimental finding is the fact that the tensile strength of a wound continues to increase for many months, long after the total amount of collagen has ceased to increase. It is thought that the formation of new bonds between adjacent collagen bundles accounts for this phenomenon (Chapter 2).

The granulation tissue that is formed in a healing wound appears to prevent excessive epithelial migration into the wound. The epithelial spurs noted peviously soon undergo degeneration and are replaced by granulation tissue. Only the surface epithelial cells persist, and these divide and differentiate so that a multilayered covering of epidermis is re-formed. It first covers a vascular granulation tissue, so that the wound has a pink color. Gradually, devascularization occurs; the scar shrinks in size and changes in color from red to white.

In the healing of a simple incised wound, it therefore appears that the epithelial cells are first stimulated to divide, and they then migrate into the wound. The stimulus for the epithelial growth and migration is not known. Experimentally it has been noted that cells in tissue culture continue to divide until they have established contact with similar cells, at which point mitosis stops. This process is termed *contact inhibition*. The epithelial cells appear to excite a connective tissue response; this results in the formation of granulation tissue, which in its turn prevents excessive epithelial migration into the wound. The presence of epithelial ingrowths along a suture tract explains why granulation tissue is formed in this situation. It is a common finding that if stitches remain *in situ* for three days or more, their site is marked subsequently by small punctate areas of scarring that remain permanently. It is to avoid these ugly punctate marks that surgeons often use tapes to hold skin edges together. A subcuticular stitch is used to hold the wound together while healing proceeds. It should be noted that puncture wounds due to injections do not form such scars, because the wound is not held open, and therefore no epithelial invasion occurs.

Healing of a Wound with Separated Edges (Healing by Secondary Intention)

When the edges of a wound are not approximated or when there is extensive tissue loss, either by direct trauma or following infection, a large defect is present that has to be corrected. Since the main bulk of tissue to perform this service is granulation tissue, this type of healing is sometimes

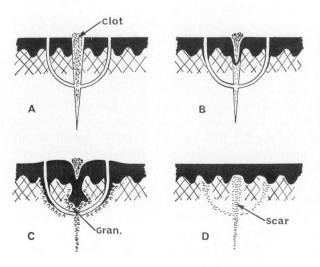

Figure 7–8. **Diagrammatic representation of the healing of an incised wound held together by a suture of which the track alone is shown.** A, The wound rapidly fills with clot. B, Shortly afterward, the epithelium migrates into the wound and down the suture tracks. C, Epithelial spurs are formed, and granulation-tissue (Gran.) formulation proceeds. D, The suture has been removed, and scar tissue remains to mark the site of the incision and the suture tracks. The epithelial ingrowths have degenerated.

known as *healing by granulation*. The term, however, is a poor one, since it wrongly implies that granulations are not formed in a simple incised wound. The difference between primary and secondary intention healing is quantitative, not qualitative.

In healing by secondary intention, the wound edges are widely separated so that healing has to proceed from the base outward as well as from the edges inward. From a practical point of view, healing of a well-approximated incised wound is fast and leaves a small, neat, linear scar. Healing of a wound with separated edges is slow and results in a large distorted scar. The difference lies in the type of wound and not in the type of healing. The following account of the healing of a large uninfected wound is illustrated in Figure 7–9.

1. There is an initial inflammatory reaction affecting the surrounding tissues, and the wound area is filled with a coagulum consisting in part of inflammatory exudate and in part of blood clot. This coagulum dries on its surface and forms a scab or crust.

2. The wound contracts, as has aleady been fully described. This process is important, because it reduces the size of the wound and the amount of tissue that has to be produced to fill in the gap.

3. The epidermis adjacent to the wound shows mitotic activity, and the epithelial cells migrate into the wound as a thin tongue that grows between the pre-existing viable connective tissue and the central area of coagulum, which includes some necrotic epithelium and connective tissue. The epithelial cells secrete a fibrinolytic enzyme that aids their penetration between the fibrinous crust and the viable connective tissue.

4. Demolition follows acute inflammation, and the clot in the center of the wound is invaded and replaced by granulation tissue. This grows from the subcutaneous tissues at the edge of the wound; it is believed that this zone is responsible for wound contraction. Granulation tissue is also formed in the base of the wound, the amount depending upon the nature of the area and its vascularity.

When the wound is viewed with a magnifying glass, the surface (under the scab, if one is present) is deep-red and granular, the capillary loops forming elevated mounds. It is very fragile, the slightest injury causing bleeding. It is this granularity that is responsible for the name *granulation tissue*. The covering of a wound by granulation tissue serves an important protective role, because it has the ability to withstand bacterial infection. Under experimental conditions, organisms introduced into a recent wound are likely to cause infection. However, if the wound is first allowed to granulate, infection does not occur. Thus, granulation tissue forms a temporary protective layer until the surface is finally covered by epithelium.

5. The migrating epidermis covers the granulation tissue. A mushroom-shaped scab is thus formed with a central attachment that finally becomes nipped off.

Figure 7–9. Diagram illustrating the healing of an excised wound. The wound is rapidly filled with clot. *A,* Epithelium soon migrates in from the margins to undermine the clot, which dries to form a crust. *B,* Granulation tissue (Gran.) grows into the wounded area and is most profuse around the circumference where it is derived from the subcutaneous fat. *C,* Epithelial ingrowth continues, and spurs are produced; these, however, do not persist. *D,* The end-result is a scar covered by epidermis that lacks rete ridges. During the healing process, contraction has taken place so that the final scar is considerably smaller than the original wound.

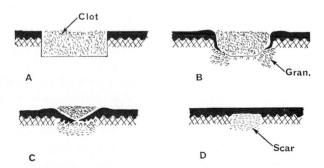

6. The regenerating epidermis becomes thicker and re-forms the multicellular layer of epidermis. This epidermis tends to be abnormally thin and lacks the normal rete ridges. Although cells from hair follicles and sweat glands can contribute to the re-formation of epidermis, these structures themselves are not re-formed. The healing of epidermis falls into the category of regeneration, but the regeneration is imperfect, because in man none of the appendages are replaced.

A scar differs from normal skin in many respects. The epidermis is thin and lacks hair follicles and sweat glands. Melanocytes are not re-formed in normal numbers, and the area therefore appears hypopigmented. The underlying scar tissue consists mainly of collagen, but its arrangement is quite different from that of the structured dermis.

Factors Influencing Wound Healing

The ability of wounds to heal is of fundamental interest in the practice of surgery. Surgeons must pay great attention to anything that could influence the healing process. It would be desirable to analyze the factors that influence repair according to whether they affect granulation tissue formation, collagen production, contraction, or some other process. Unfortunately, this is rarely possible, since we are ignorant about many of these fundamental processes. In practice, the factors affecting wound healing may be divided into two groups: those that act locally, and those whose influence is general.

Local Factors

Blood Supply. The normal blood supply varies greatly from one part of the body to another. The scalp and face have an excellent blood supply, and wounds there heal quickly. It is possible to remove stitches on the third day without having the wound gape, provided undue traction is not applied. The skin of the leg has a poor blood supply and wounds there heal much more slowly.

Pathological changes affecting the blood vessels have an enormous effect on wound healing. Patients who have varicose veins or atheroma in the leg vessels show very slow healing: trivial injuries can lead to ulceration, which takes many months to heal. Other causes of poor blood supply are local pressure and chronic inflammation. *Bed sores* are caused by local pressure, which is also a factor in their poor healing. Likewise, *chronic inflammation* is liable to be accompanied by endarteritis obliterans, ischemia, and slow healing. An excellent example of this is x-ray dermatitis, in which ulceration is notoriously slow to heal. Finally, the slow wound healing of old age is in part related to a poor circulation.

Continued Tissue Breakdown and Inflammation. Any condition causing continued tissue breakdown leads to persistent inflammation, and this delays the completion of the healing process. The most important examples are *infection,* the presence of a *foreign body* or irritant chemical, and *excessive movement.*

Infection. If a simple incised wound becomes infected, the two edges do not become adherent, and the wound tends to gape. Furthermore, the infection may result in tissue destruction, causing healing to proceed, in effect, by secondary intention.

Foreign Bodies and Other Irritants. The presence of a foreign body in a wound may delay healing, either as a result of its direct irritant properties or by encouraging infection. The overenthusiastic use of irritating antiseptics may cause considerable damage and may delay healing. The use of potent antiseptic and antibiotic agents was once popular in the local treatment of wounds, but it is now appreciated that they frequently do more harm than good. Sometimes hypersensitivity develops and leads to extensive inflammation. A good example of this is the acute allergic contact dermatitis that can follow the use of ointments containing neomycin.

Movement.   It is a time-honored dictum that injured parts should be kept at rest. Movement delays healing because the edges of the wound are continually disrupted, and this damages the delicate granulation tissue, leading to repeated injury and consequently to inflammation.

Adhesion to an Underlying Bony Surface.   By anchoring the wound edges, this adhesion prevents contraction.

Direction of the Wound.   Skin wounds made in a direction parallel to the crease lines of the skin heal faster than those made at right angles to them. Skin incisions made across the lines tend to gape, and their healing is delayed. Therefore, when one plans a surgical incision, these lines should be taken into consideration. Incisions parallel to or in the crease lines heal more readily than those in other directions, and the scars are less visible.

The Presence of a Large Hematoma.   Some blood clot is always present in a wound, but a large hematoma should be avoided. Its presence favors infection, and in any case the space caused by its presence leads to delayed healing and to the formation of a large scar.

General Factors

Age.   Wound healing is fast in the young and is generally of normal rate in old age unless there is some associated debilitating disease or ischemia.

Nutrition.   Animals starved of protein show poor wound healing and defective collagen formation. This abnormality can be corrected by the administration of proteins containing methionine and cystine.

Vitamin C Deficiency.   Vitamin C is essential for the formation of collagen (Chapter 2). Animals deficient in this vitamin therefore show poor wound healing. Wound contraction is normal and so are epithelial regeneration and granulation tissue formation. The abnormality is in the absence of normal collagen formation, and the wound is therefore very weak. Capillaries are unduly fragile and bleeding occurs. Although overt scurvy is uncommon in civilized countries, minor degrees of vitamin C deficiency are not infrequent in patients on a marginal intake of the substance, and in those who are stressed.

The Role of Zinc.   The addition of zinc salts to the diet of rats has been shown to promote wound healing. The mechanism of this is not known, but the oral administration of zinc sulfate has been tried in man and claimed to accelerate wound healing. These claims have not been substantiated by all workers, and the role of zinc in healing of human wounds remains problematic.

Glucocorticoids.   The administration of excessive amounts of these steroids delays wound contraction and the formation of granulation tissue.

Temperature.   It is the general experience that wounds of the exposed parts heal more slowly in cold weather. Experiments on animals that hibernate have lent some support to this observation.

Complications of Wound Healing

Infection.   Wounds form a ready avenue for the invasion of pathogenic bacteria. All the techniques of aseptic surgery are devoted to preventing infection of surgical wounds.

Delayed Healing.   Any of the factors mentioned above — either local or general — may produce delayed healing.

Wound Dehiscence.   The bursting open of a wound is described as *dehiscence.* It occurs when stress is applied before the wound has healed sufficiently. It is a particularly serious complication of an abdominal incision, because it results in the exposure of the abdominal contents to the outside atmosphere. Quite apart from delayed healing due to infection and the other factors just considered, another important contributing element is increased intra-abdominal pressure, such as is caused by heaving coughing.

Cicatrization.   Scar tissue tends to contract in an erratic way such that the wound becomes greatly distorted. This process is quite different from contraction, because it occurs as a late event and appears to be due to some change in the dense avascular collagenous scar tissue. The mechanism is not understood. Cicatrization is a frequent complication in the healing of skin following extensive burning. It produces great deformity and can immobilize joints in the affected area. Cicatrization involving hollow viscera such as intestine, esophagus, or urethra is an important cause of stenosis.

Keloid Formation.   Occasionally, an excessive amount of collagen results in the appearance of a raised nodule of scar tissue called a *keloid*. The precise cause of this is not known, but keloid formation is particularly common in young women (particularly if they are pregnant) and in Blacks. Keloids are found most frequently in the region of the neck and shoulders. They are especially frequent after burns. One should be particularly wary of performing nonessential surgery on patients who are prone to develop keloids. Thus, the removal of a small nevus for cosmetic purposes can result in the formation of a large ugly keloid, far more disfiguring than was the original lesion. The treatment is quite unsatisfactory, because removal is followed by even more keloid formation. Postoperative radiotherapy can be given in an effort to prevent this.

Weak Scars.   If the scar tissue is subjected to continuous strain, it may stretch. Incisional wounds may therefore bulge and, in the abdomen, produce incisional hernias.

Healing in Specialized Tissues

It is generally stated that the greater the degree of specialization of a tissue, the less well developed are its powers of regeneration. Certainly, nerve cells are highly specialized and are incapable of division, but degrees of specialization in the cells are as difficult to define as are degrees of specialization among human beings. Is a liver cell more or less specialized than a simple unstriped muscle fiber? Liver cells show remarkable powers of proliferation and yet perform functions of which they alone are capable. Similarly, it is impossible to compare the degree of specialization of the different types of epithelium, each of which has its own particular characteristics. It seems likely that the power of regeneration is best developed in those organs and tissues that are most liable to injury and the replacement of which has survival value for the individual and for the species.

Regeneration in Epithelial Tissues

All covering epithelia show good regeneration power. They are repeatedly subjected to trauma, and the integrity of the surface therefore depends upon the ability of the cells to regenerate. The re-formation of the squamous epithelium of epidermis has already been described in the healing of skin wounds, and a similar regeneration is seen in the mucosa of the mouth, the intestine, the respiratory tract, and the urinary tract.

The solid epithelial organs show varying regenerative capacity. In the liver it is quite remarkable; if three quarters of the liver of a rat is resected, there is such active division of the remaining cells that within a few weeks the organ is restored to its original weight. Its anatomical shape is different, but normal liver lobules are formed in relationship to new blood vessels and bile ducts. In man, regeneration of liver cells is seen following any type of necrosis, provided the patient survives. The end-result of this regeneration varies widely, depending on the type of necrosis (see Chapter 33 for a consideration of this important subject). Kidney tubules show excellent regenerative capacity, and in patients with extensive tubular necrosis (as occurs in shock) it is common for regeneration to result in complete recovery, provided the patient does not die in the acute phase. This type of renal disease is therefore most eligible for treatment by dialysis (artificial kidney), since the ultimate prognosis is good. If entire nephrons or glomeruli are destroyed, there is no replacement.

As a general rule, specialized connective tissues show good regeneration if circumstances are favorable. The *mesothelial lining* of the peritoneum and other serous cavities is readily re-formed from exposed underlying connective tissue cells, which take on the form and function of flattened mesothelium. Were it not for this, abdominal surgery would be hazardous. One can leave extensive areas of tissue exposed in the abdominal cavity, and they will be rapidly covered by newly formed mesothelium: adhesions do not form, unless healing is complicated by infection or by the presence of irritants such as suture material or the talc or starch in glove powder. Likewise, synovial cells are readily re-formed. With cut *tendons* regeneration is good, provided the severed ends are carefully approximated and are held in good position. It is important that the ends be meticulously sewn together; otherwise, the space between them becomes organized and ultimately union is by scar tissue. Since scar tissue is relatively weak, it will stretch. *Unstriated muscle* shows little regenerative capacity, and destroyed muscle tissue is replaced by scar tissue. Thus, if the patient has a deep penetrating gastric ulcer, even though it may heal, scar tissue remains for life to indicate the site of the previous ulceration. *Heart muscle,* unfortunately, shows no regenerative capacity either, and patients who suffer extensive myocardial necrosis are forever destined to have a scar replacing the pre-existing muscle. With *striated voluntary muscle,* the situation is somewhat more variable, and under good conditions striated muscle can regenerate, so that a clean surgical incision through a voluntary muscle will ultimately unite and no scar tissue will remain to indicate the site of previous surgery.

Regeneration in Connective Tissues

Adult nerve cells are unable to divide, and therefore when part of the brain or spinal cord is destroyed, no new neurons are produced. The common "stroke" therefore inevitably results in the formation of scar tissue (Chapter 44). When the axons of the nerve cells are damaged, the situation is quite different, because the body of the cell itself is not directly affected. The effects vary according to whether the axon is in the peripheral or central nervous system.

Healing in Nervous Tissue

Peripheral Nervous System.   Following the section of a nerve fiber, the corresponding nerve cell shows degenerative changes. Sometimes the cell dies, but more usually it recovers. The severed axis cylinder itself becomes irregular in shape, and by 48 hours has broken up. With myelinated nerves the surrounding myelin shows fragmentation, and the Schwann cells enlarge, proliferate, and become phagocytic. These changes are known as *wallerian degeneration,* and they affect the nerve fiber distally to the point of section and proximally up to the first node of Ranvier. The original nerve becomes replaced by a mass of Schwann cells. From the proximal portion of the cut axon numerous neurofibrils sprout out and are seen to invaginate into the cytoplasm of the Schwann cells. They push their way distally through the Schwann cells at a rate of about 1 mm per day. Many of the fibrils lose their way and degenerate, but one may reach an appropriate end organ and persist to form the definitive replacement axon. It is evident that accurate apposition of the cut ends of the nerve is of vital importance in facilitating this process. The final process involves the re-formation of the myelin sheath by the Schwann cells as the regenerating nerve axon matures and increases in diameter.

The functional end-result of nerve damage depends on various factors. If the axons are damaged but the nerve trunk itself is not severed, an excellent result may be expected. When the nerve is severed, careful suturing and avoidance of infection are important. Functional recovery is more complete when a pure motor or a pure sensory nerve is cut. Recovery from section of a mixed nerve — like the median nerve — is often poor, and this is presumably because motor nerves often find themselves arriving at sensory nerve endings and vice versa.

Central Nervous System.   In the central nervous system the oligodendroglia takes on the functional and anatomical function of the Schwann cells in relation to the axons. For reasons that are not clear, regeneration of long axon tracts does not occur. In some experiments on mammals a limited degree of regeneration has been reported, but with humans, when long tracts such as the corticospinal and spinothalamic tracts have been destroyed, no effective regeneration occurs. Degenerating tissue is phagocytosed by macrophages, and the area becomes replaced by a type of granulation tissue. Unlike the granulation tissue of ordinary connective tissue, the proliferating cells are astrocytes rather than fibroblasts. The end-result is a glial scar containing astrocytes with their matted processes but with relatively little collagen and few fibrocytes.

Mechanisms of Repair and Regeneration

When one considers that in a healing wound there is cell and tissue proliferation proceeding at a rate exceeding that seen in most malignant tumors, it is humiliating to admit how little we know of the mechanisms involved.

The injury must initiate a signal that induces cell proliferation. In labile and stable tissues this seems to have the effect of recruiting cells from the G_0 phase into the cell cycle. Experimental work has provided some insight into the mechanisms involved by suggesting that *stimulating substances* are formed. In tissue culture experiments it has been found that a number of factors stimulate cell growth. These include polypeptides, hormones like insulin, factors released by monocytes that stimulate fibroblasts, and other factors released from platelets that stimulate both smooth muscle and fibroblast proliferation. Proteolytic enzymes (such as trypsin) alter the cells' plasma membrane such that the cells are stimulated to divide. What role, if any, these substances have in the mechanism of wound healing is not known.

An alternative hypothesis is that each tissue normally produces a *specific inhibiting substance* (called a *chalone)* that is responsible for inhibiting mitotic activity. It is postulated that destruction of an area of tissue leads to a lack of the specific chalone locally, and this results in proliferation of adjacent cells so that the original bulk of tissue is restored. Unfortunately, the nature of these chalones is not well understood, nor is it known whether they play any role in wound healing.

Another approach to the explanation of wound healing focuses on the part played by mechanical physical factors. It has been noted that cells in tissue culture continue to divide and move on a surface until they establish contact with similar cells, at which point movement stops. This is called *contact inhibition.* Also, in tissue culture, growth tends to stop when a certain mass of tissue is produced. This appears to be dependent upon the density of cells present and has been termed *density-dependent regulation of growth*. Whether this is due to some direct cell-to-cell interaction or to the local production of communicating chemicals from one cell to the other is not known.

It is evident that our knowledge of the phenomenon of wound healing is woefully deficient. We understand neither the signal that starts the process of healing nor the mechanisms that control and maintain it. Failure to identify the mechanism by which normal tissue homeostasis is maintained is particularly disappointing, since any understanding of the major disorder of cell division (cancer) must surely be related to a knowledge of the normal controlling mechanisms of cell growth.

Review Questions

1. A surgeon opens the abdominal cavity and removes a portion of small intestine that is 1 meter long. The cut ends of the gut are sutured together by an end-to-end anastomosis. Describe the healing processes that take place in the intestinal wall.

2. It is claimed that a new compound, when given by a daily injection, has a beneficial effect on the healing of a skin wound. Describe how you would attempt to prove this in a group of experimental animals.

3. A patient receives a severe burn over one shoulder. It involves an area approximately 20 cm in diameter. What are the possible local complications?

Selected Readings

Baserga, R.: Multiplication and Division in Mammalian cells. Biochemistry of Disease, Vol. 6. New York, Marcel Dekker, 1976.

Bucher, N. L. R.: Experimental aspects of hepatic regeneration. New England Journal of Medicine, 277:686–696; 738–746, 1967.

Editorial: To heal the wound. Lancet, 1:84, 1973.

Editorial: Zinc in human medicine. Lancet, 2:351–352, 1975.

Forrester, J. D.: Mechanical, biochemical, and architectural features of surgical repair. Advances in Biological and Medical Physics, 14:1–34, 1973.

Gabbiani, G., Hirschel, B. J., Ryan, G. B., Statkov, P. R., and Majno, G.: Granulation tissue as a contractile organ. Journal of Experimental Medicine, 135:719–734, 1972.

Holley, R. W.: Control of growth of mammalian cells in the cell culture. Nature, 258:487–490, 1975.

Houck, J. C. (Ed.): Chalones. Amsterdam, North-Holland Publishing Company, 1976.

King, G. D., and Salzman, F. A.: Keloid scars. Surgical Clinics of North America, 50:595–598, 1970.

Leading Article: Understanding hepatic regeneration. British Medical Journal, 282:1412–1413, 1981.

Ordman, L. J., and Gillman, T.: Studies in the healing of cutaneous wounds. Parts I and II. Archives of Surgery, 93:857–882; 883–928, 1966.

Peacock, E. E.: Biologic frontier in the control of healing. American Journal of Surgery, 126:708–713, 1973.

Rytömaa, T.: The chalone concept. International Review of Experimental Pathology, 16:155–206, 1976.

Walter, J. B.: Wound healing. Journal of Otolaryngology, 5:171–176, 1976.

Weinbren, K.: Problems in restoration of the liver. *In* Illingworth, C. (Ed.): Wound Healing. London, Churchill Livingstone, 1966, pp. 69–77.

Chronic Inflammation

After studying this chapter the student should be able to:

- Define chronic inflammation.
- Enumerate the causes of chronic inflammation.
- Give examples of chronic suppurative inflammation and describe the microscopic appearance of a pyogenic membrane.
- Define the term granuloma and describe the three types of the tuberculoid variety.
- Discuss the role of healing in relation to the tissue reaction seen in chronic inflammation.
- Discuss the role of the immune response in relation to the cause of chronic inflammation and in terms of the tissue response seen.
- Discuss the general effects of chronic inflammation and relate these to the reticuloendothelial system.

Definition   When an irritant substance that has caused acute inflammation persists locally, it leads to *chronic inflammation,* which may be defined as a *prolonged process in which destruction and inflammation are proceeding at the same time as attempts at healing.*

The tissue response to injury has been divided into three phases: (1) *acute inflammation,* which is characterized by vascular and exudative phenomena; (2) *demolition,* which is accomplished by macrophage activity; and (3) *healing,* the final phase, by which lost tissue is replaced by the combined processes of repair and regeneration. Pathologically, chronic inflammation is a mixture of the effects of tissue damage, acute inflammation, demolition, and healing.

Causes of Chronic Inflammation   Any cause of tissue damage can, if it persists, lead to chronic inflammation. Three main groups can be recognized:

1. **Infections.**   The body has a limited ability to destroy certain organisms, *e.g.,* the tubercle bacillus and *Treponema pallidum.* Infection with these agents therefore commonly leads to chronic inflammation (Fig. 8–1). Moreover, if local or general conditions impair the body's defenses, an organism that usually produces a self-limiting acute inflammation may persist to cause a chronic one. Thus, *Staphylococcus aureus,* which can produce a boil that generally heals rapidly, can also produce chronic inflammation in some situations, such as in the bone marrow (see "Chronic Osteomyelitis," Chapter 40). Any of the causes of delayed healing may so turn the scales against the host that there develops the "frustrated healing" that chronic inflammation has so aptly been called.

2. **Insoluble Particulate Irritants.**   Silica and asbestos are examples of irritant particles that the body cannot easily remove. Inhalation of such substances leads to persistent chronic inflammation of the lungs (see "The Pneumoconioses," Chapter 30).

3. **Hypersensitivity.**   The development of hypersensitivity is an important factor in chronic infective diseases, of which tuberculosis is the proto-

Figure 8–1. Tuberculous pericarditis. The patient was a 22-year-old man who had had pulmonary tuberculosis for 5 years. The specimen shows the opened pericardial sac, in which the heart is seen to be covered by a thick fibrinous exudate. Over the apex there is a layer of blood clot due to recent hemorrhage. The parietal pericardium is greatly thickened and is also covered by fibrinous exudate and blood clot. (EC 12.1. Reproduced by permission of the President and Council of the R.C.S. Eng.)

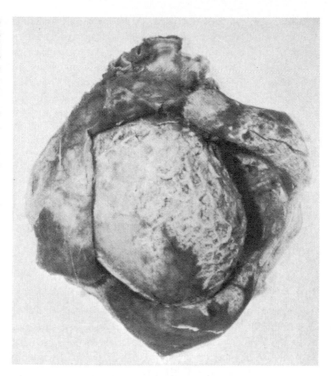

type. Much of the chronic damage produced by persisting tubercle bacilli is mediated by damaging antigen-antibody interactions. There is also a group of diseases in which damaging antibodies are produced against the body's own tissues. This group of autoimmune diseases is typified by rheumatoid arthritis.

Chronic inflammation is encountered in all organs of the body; many examples will be described later. Pathologically, these inflammations share certain features. All consist of varying mixtures of the basic pathological reactions previously described as acute inflammation, demolition, and healing (Table 8–1). The reaction encountered under any particular circumstance

Types of Chronic Inflammation

TABLE 8–1. COMPONENTS OF CHRONIC INFLAMMATION

COMPONENT	TISSUE RESPONSE
Acute Inflammation	Polymorph Infiltration Edema Fibrin
Demolition	Macrophage Formation Epithelioid Cell Formation Giant Cell Formation
Healing 　Repair	Granulation Tissue 　Blood vessels 　Fibroblasts 　Collagen 　Neuroglia in CNS
Regeneration	Epithelial Overgrowth Specialized Connective Tissue 　Overgrowth
Immune Response	Lymphocytes Plasma Cells Eosinophils

consists of varying mixtures of these three basic ingredients. Cells involved in an immune response are often added to this mixture and contribute to the variety of the tissue response to chronic irritation.

Chronic Suppurative Inflammation. Suppuration is frequently followed by chronic inflammation if the causative agent is not removed or if the pus is not adequately drained. A chronic abscess consists of a central cavity filled with pus and lined by a pyogenic membrane. The latter consists of granulation tissue heavily infiltrated with neutrophils and a variable number of lymphocytes, plasma cells, and macrophages. Examples of this type of lesion are seen in the lung following bronchopneumonia, in chronic osteomyelitis, and in a chronic brain abscess (Fig. 44–4). The term *empyema* denotes a collection of pus in a cavity. Thus, in *empyema thoracis* there is pus in the pleural cavity. This condition often becomes chronic, especially if the pus is inadequately drained. Empyema thoracis follows the rupture of a lung abscess into the pleural cavity, and in preantibiotic days it was high on the list of the complications of pneumonia.

Granulomatous Inflammation. In some types of chronic inflammation the predominant cell is the macrophage. By tradition, an inflammation showing a heavy macrophage infiltration is called *proliferative*, in contrast to the exudative lesions of suppuration. This concept was based on the supposition that the macrophages were derived from local histiocytes by mitosis. In fact, most of them are derived from blood monocytes, but the term "proliferative" is still retained. Since the accumulation of macrophages can produce a tumorlike swelling, and since there is an underlying mass of granulation tissue, the term "granuloma" is in common use.

Diffuse Type of Granulomatous Inflammation. Under some circumstances, the macrophage infiltration is diffuse, causing a nearly uniform enlargement of the tissue, perhaps with some areas of nodularity. This type of reaction is uncommon, but it is seen typically in lepromatous leprosy.

Tuberculoid Type of Granulomatous Inflammation. Under certain circumstances, macrophages enlarge, lose their phagocytic activity, develop eosinophilic cytoplasm, and are so closely applied to their neighbors that individual cell borders cannot be defined other than by electron microscopy. The cells then somewhat resemble the epithelial cells of the epidermis and are therefore called *epithelioid cells*. Epithelioid-cell formation is accompanied by a tendency for the cells to be arranged in groups rather than in diffuse sheets. The formation of groups of epithelioid cells is characteristic of the reaction to the tubercle bacillus. An inflammation characterized by the formation of groups of epithelioid cells is traditionally called a *tuberculoid reaction* (see Fig. 10–3).

When macrophages encounter insoluble material, they frequently coalesce to form giant cells (Fig. 8–2). This response is seen around exogenous foreign bodies, *e.g.*, catgut, silk, talc, and plastic sponges. Coalescing macrophages are also seen around endogenous debris such as dead bone, cholesterol crystals, and uric acid crystals (in gout). They are formed in response to the tubercle bacillus, to fungi, and to many other organisms that cause chronic inflammation. It frequently happens therefore that in a tuberculoid reaction, in addition to epithelioid cells, a considerable number of giant cells are also present.

The reason why macrophages predominate in certain chronic inflammations and change to epithelioid cells under some circumstances is not well understood. Experimentally it has been found that macrophages develop into epithelioid cells when they have not undertaken phagocytosis, have completely digested phagocytosed material, or have successfully extruded phago-

Figure 8-2. Foreigh-body reaction, This is a section of an Etheron sponge that had been implanted for 40 days subcutaneously in a rat. The clear areas were occupied by fragments of sponge that had been dislodged during processing. They were surrounded by exuberant giant cells. Many of these have peripherally disposed nuclei and are of the Langhans type. Only a few have the nuclear arrangement of foreign-body giant cells. A similar type of chronic inflammatory reaction with giant-cell formation is seen around other foreign material, e.g., nylon or silk sutures (× 150).

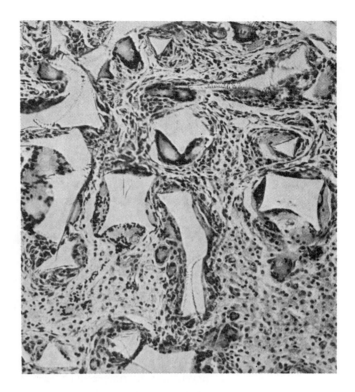

cytosed material by exocytosis. It follows that epithelioid cells contain few if any bacteria in an infection (*e.g.*, tuberculoid leprosy), whereas the undifferentiated macrophages in such an infection are stuffed with bacilli (see "Lepromatous Leprosy," Chapter 10).

The development of hypersensitivity is thought to be another factor in the development of a granulomatous reaction. Certainly, the hypersensitivity can lead to necrosis, which is often a feature of tuberculoid granulomatous inflammation. Indeed, three variants of this are recognized: (1) *noncaseating tuberculoid granuloma,* as seen in sarcoidosis, tuberculoid leprosy, and early lesions of tuberculosis (Fig. 10-3); (2) *caseating tuberculoid reaction,* as commonly seen in tuberculosis and also in some of the deep mycoses (Fig. 10-4); and (3) *suppurative tuberculoid reaction,* in which small abscesses filled with polymorphs are found and surrounded by a mantle of epithelioid cells. The commonest example of this is cat-scratch disease.*

Although the macrophage is traditionally regarded as a phagocytic scavenger cell, it has other important functions. As noted in Chapter 5, it acts as a *secretor cell,* and its products play a part in the production of fever as well as influencing the healing process that follows inflammation. Its role in the immune response is indicated later in this chapter and is described in more detail in Chapter 9.

Chronic Inflammation with Features of Healing. The formation of granulation tissue is a feature of many types of chronic inflammation. The tissue consists of endothelial cells forming blood vessels and lymphatics, fibroblasts forming collagen, and an infiltration by numerous lymphocytes and plasma cells. In hematoxylin and eosin sections it is often difficult to identify

---

*This curious disease is thought to be caused by a virus, although the agent has never been isolated. The appearance of an ulcerated nodule at the site of a cat scratch is followed by enlargement of the regional lymph nodes. These nodules suppurate, and the overlying skin may ulcerate so that the pus drains spontaneously. The pattern of infection and tissue response in the nodes closely resembles the changes seen in lymphogranuloma venereum (Chapter 11).

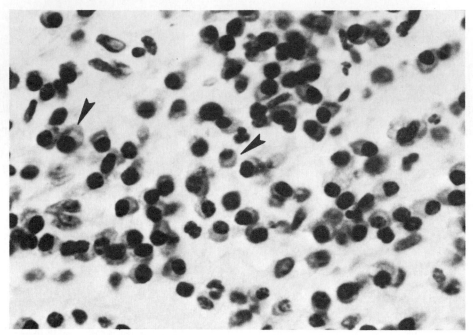

Figure 8–3.   Plasma cells. The section is of a chronically inflamed gum and shows numerous plasma cells. Note that the nuclei are placed eccentrically in the cells and that a clear zone is visible in the cytoplasm (arrows). This is the Golgi apparatus (×600).

each cell as either lymphocyte or plasma cell; therefore, the term *small round cell* is often used to encompass both groups. A heavy infiltration by such cells is a common finding in chronic inflammation.

Inflammatory granulation tissue is seen in the pyogenic membrane surrounding a chronic abscess and in the chronic inflammatory tissue in the base of an ulcer. Since the vascularity of the tissue can result in easy bleeding, chronic peptic ulcers are associated with intestinal bleeding. Likewise, chronic inflammation of the bronchial tubes leads to hemoptysis (coughing up of blood).

Fibroblasts are prominent in most chronic inflammation; since they lay down collagen, the end-result is fibrosis. This scar formation is characteristic of many chronic inflammatory lesions. It is seen in fibroid tuberculosis, in the base of a chronic peptic ulcer, and in the wall of an abscess. If fibrin is the hallmark of acute inflammation, fibrosis can be considered the salient feature of chronic inflammation. As scarring proceeds, the lumina of small arteries and arterioles are gradually obliterated by the thickening of the tunica intima; this process is called *endarteritis obliterans*. The end-result is a mass of dense avascular scar tissue. *Contracture* or *cicatrization* follows, and this leads to many important complications of chronic inflammation. Thus, chronic inflammation of the heart valves leads to stenosis and distortion of the valves; chronic gastric ulcers proceed to pyloric stenosis; and a chronic arthritis, such as rheumatoid arthritis, results in fibrous adhesions in the synovium and around joints.

Evidence of Regeneration.   In chronic inflammatory lesions involving specialized tissue, there is sometimes evidence of regeneration. This is usually seen in covering or lining epithelia; at times, the regeneration is followed by definite hyperplasia and even tumor formation. One of the best examples of this event is found in ulcerative colitis, which can proceed to polypoid overgrowth of epithelium and ultimately to cancer formation. In general, however, chronic inflammation in most organs is an infrequent precursor of cancer.

Chronic Inflammation with Evidence of an Immune Reaction. Although a few lymphocytes and plasma cells are found in uninflamed granulation tissue, many examples of chronic inflammation are characterized by a heavy infiltration of these cells (Fig. 8–3). Together with macrophages they are engaged in the processing of antigen and in the manufacture of either sensitized T cells or immunoglobulins. An infiltration by eosinophils is found in some examples of chronic inflammation in which hypersensitivity plays a part, *e.g.,* some parasitic infections.

The general effects of chronic inflammation depend on the nature and extent of the responsible agent. In a localized foreign body reaction or in a chronic ulcer of the leg, there is no noteworthy general response at all. On the other hand, in chronic infective diseases like tuberculosis there may be widespread changes in the reticuloendothelial system and in the blood stream.

Changes in the Reticuloendothelial System. Most chronic inflammatory reactions lead to hyperplasia of the reticuloendothelial (RE) system. The local accumulation of macrophages in some types has already been described; in addition, the lymph nodes draining a chronic inflammatory lesion generally show hyperplasia of the RE cells and sometimes of the germinal centers and medullary cords.

If organisms gain access to the blood stream, they are taken up by the other members of the RE system. These cells may destroy the organism or may themselves become parasitized. Overgrowth of the RE cells can lead to enlargement of the RE organs: of clinical importance is the enlargement of the spleen, since it can be detected readily. This RE hyperplasia is also a component of the immune response.

The Immune Response. Antibody production is a feature of most chronic inflammatory diseases, and the demonstration of specific antibodies is often a useful diagnostic procedure. Likewise, the detection of cell-mediated hypersensitivity is available as a diagnostic test.

The immune response is sometimes reflected in generalized enlargement of the reticuloendothelial system. Enlargement of lymph nodes, the spleen, and — at times — the liver is a manifestation of this response.

Finally, the long-continued stress on the antibody-producing mechanism may be associated with amyloid disease (see Chapter 25).

General Effects of Chronic Inflammation

Review Questions

1. Describe the role of the macrophage in chronic inflammation. Discuss its origin, functions, appearance, and the cells to which it may give rise.

2. It is sometimes stated that an infiltration by lymphocytes and plasma cells is typical of a chronic inflammatory reaction, and that a polymorph response is typical of acute inflammation. Elaborate on this statement.

Selected Reading

Walter, J. B., and Israel, M. S.: General Pathology. 5th ed. Edinburgh, Churchill Livingstone, 1979. Note, in particular, Chapter 11, which gives a detailed account of chronic inflammation as well as references to specific examples.

CHAPTER 9

The Immune Response

After studying this chapter the student should be able to:

- Define the terms antigen, epitope, hapten, active immunity, and passive immunity.
- Describe the development of the lymphoid tissues of the body and distinguish the B-cell system from the T-cell system.
- Describe the chemical nature of the immunoglobulins.
- Discuss how Ig produces (a) immunity to a toxic organism such as *Corynebacterium diphtheriae;* (b) immunity to an invasive organism such as the pneumococcus; and (c) hypersensitivity.
- Distinguish between type I, type II, and type III hypersensitivity reactions.
- Describe the symptoms, pathogenesis, and treatment of acute anaphylaxis in man.
- Give four examples of a type III reaction.
- List the lymphokines and relate their *in vitro* activity to (a) cell-mediated immunity; and (b) type IV hypersensitivity.
- Describe (a) transfer factor; (b) blast transformation of lymphocytes; (c) specific immunological tolerance; and (d) the Koch phenomenon.
- Define the following terms: autograft, homograft, allograft, syngeneic graft, and xenograft.
- Discuss the types of allograft rejection, the mechanisms involved, and the steps that can be taken to combat rejection.
- Classify the immunological deficiency diseases.
- Contrast the instructive theory of antibody formation with the selective theory.
- List the circumstances under which autoantibodies can be formed, and discuss the role of these antibodies in disease processes.

INTRODUCTION   A remarkable feature of the adult mammal is its ability to distinguish between its own constituents ("self") and those of external, or foreign, origin ("nonself"). Foreign material excites a reaction now called the *immune response*, and this results in the elimination of the alien matter. Since many of the foreign substances encountered are living organisms or their toxins, it follows that their elimination results in immunity to infection or limitation of its spread. In the first description of antibody formation in the last century, it was shown that animals injected with tetanus toxin produced substances that were present in the plasma and were capable of neutralizing the toxin. The antibodies, termed *antitoxins*, gave protection against the disease; the subject naturally grew around this central theme of immunity to infection. The immune response has presumably been evolved by animals during evolution as a means of self-preservation in a world teeming with microorganisms. Nevertheless, the immune response is not selective, and antibodies are formed against foreign substances regardless of whether they are bacterial products or not. Under certain circumstances these antibodies can react with foreign material, if it is reintroduced, and can produce severe damage to tissue components. The term *hypersensitivity* is applied to such a reaction. It is evident that the immune response is not concerned solely with immunity to infection, but that it plays a part in many disease processes and under some circumstances causes hypersensitivity.

Substances that are capable of eliciting an immune response are termed *antigens*; the antibodies that are formed are highly specific for the antigen evoking their formation. Antigens are high–molecular-weight substances, nearly always protein, and are recognized as foreign by special features of their chemical structure — probably by particular configurations of their external shape. The areas of the molecular surface that are involved are called *epitopes* or *determinant sites*. A single protein molecule has many such sites of either one or several distinct types. Hence, antibodies with separate specificities can be produced even with the injection of a single pure protein substance. Furthermore, it is possible to add a new epitope to a protein by the addition of a simple chemical substance called a *hapten*. Injection of a hapten alone will not lead to the formation of antibody. However, injection of a hapten-protein combination leads to the production of antibody that is specific for the hapten and will combine with it. Thus, *haptens are substances that are not antigenic in themselves but are capable of stimulating the formation of specific antibody when combined with a suitable carrier protein.* They are of great importance in human pathology, as a simple example will illustrate: Iodine and nickel are not antigenic but if applied to the skin of some individuals act as haptens. They combine with body proteins so that a new antigenic complex is formed. This stimulates an immune response that is specific for iodine or nickel. The next occasion on which the agent is applied to the skin a damaging antigen-antibody reaction occurs, and this produces an inflammatory response that manifests itself as allergic contact dermatitis (Chapter 41).

The immune response results in the formation of specific serum proteins termed *immunoglobulins*. These can be responsible for either immunity to infection or hypersensitivity. There is another arm to the immune response, and this leads to the formation of sensitized lymphocytes. This *cell-mediated immune response* can also lead to either immunity to infection or hypersensitivity.

To understand the two immune systems one must first appreciate the formation and structure of the antibody-forming tissues.

The Antibody-Forming Tissues

The cell most intimately concerned in the immune response is the small lymphocyte. This cell resides in the bone marrow, the thymus, the spleen, lymphoid aggregates such as the tonsils and the Peyer's patches of the small intestine, and the circulating blood. The development and functions of the lymphocyte have been subjected to intense investigation.

In the developing fetus, stem cells for the hematopoietic tissues (including lymphocytes) proliferate in the yolk sac, but later the liver and finally the bone marrow take over this function. Those stem cells destined to form lymphocytes migrate in one of two directions (Fig. 9–1). One group termed immature or early T cells migrate to the thymus and there develop into mature T cells. It is possible that some thymic hormone is necessary for this development. Having attained maturity, the cells leave the thymus via the blood stream and settle in the peripheral lymphoid tissues, predominantly in the paracortical zone of the lymph nodes (Fig. 9–2) and the equivalent area in the spleen. These T cells are mobile and long-lived. They enter the lymphatics, pass via the thoracic duct into the blood, and soon reach the lymphoid tissues again. T lymphocytes circulate in this way several times each day in the normal individual. Following the injection of an antigen, the T-cell system develops sensitized or *immune T cells*, which morphologically resemble small lymphocytes and are capable of reacting specifically with the antigen that elicited their formation.

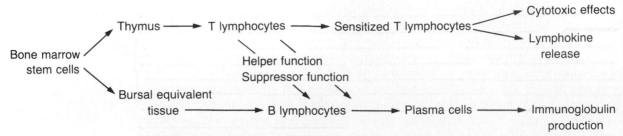

Figure 9–1. Diagram showing the postulated development of the peripheral lymphoid tissue. Stem cells that develop under the influence of the thymus become mature T cells. Contact with antigen causes them to become sensitized or committed. Further contact with antigen can lead to a cytotoxic effect by some direct action or there may be the release of lymphokines. B lymphocytes mature under the influence of the bursa or its equivalent. Contact with antigen causes them to mature into plasma cells and secrete immunoglobulins. T cells cooperate in this process and may act as either helper cells or suppressor cells.

The other group of lymphocytes from the bone marrow migrate to a structure that in birds is termed the *bursa of Fabricius,* an organ that is situated near the cloaca. Although no such structure is present in mammals, it has been suggested that there is an equivalent tissue that is more widely distributed and forms the lymphoid tissues of the appendix, colon, and Peyer's patches *(bursal equivalent lymphoid tissue).* It is now thought more likely that the bone marrow itself fulfills the function of the avian bursa. The bursa or its equivalent plays an essential part in the subsequent development of the lymphocytes, which when mature are termed *B lymphocytes.* They migrate into the blood stream and settle in various sites to populate the B cell areas of the peripheral lymphoid tissues such as lymph nodes and spleen. In the lymph nodes they are found in the medulla as well as the cortex. In the latter site they are aggregated into groups called follicles (Fig. 9–2), which when stimulated form central germinal centers. B cells tend to remain sessile in the lymphoid tissues, in contradistinction to the mobile, ever-wandering T cells. When stimulated in an immune response, the B lymphocytes develop an endoplasmic reticulum that leads to the formation of immunoglobulin. The fully developed cell is then known as a *plasma cell,* and in the lymph node it is found mainly in the medulla.

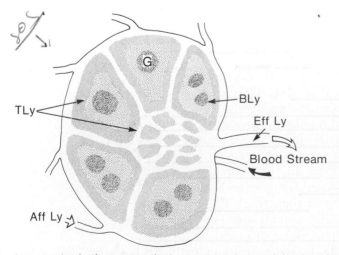

Figure 9–2. Diagram of a lymph node. Lymph enters the node through several afferent lymphatic vessels (Aff Ly) and percolates through a meshwork formed by reticulum cells and their reticulin fibers. In the medulla the fluid is collected into sinuses that are lined by phagocytic sinus-lining cells, which—like the reticulum cells—are members of the reticuloendothelial system. The cortex contains collections of B lymphocytes (B Ly), some of which have one or more germinal centers (G). Surrounding these areas, there is a mantle of T lymphocytes (T Ly); this is designated the *paracortical zone.* In the medulla there are groups, or cords, of B cells—both lymphocytes and cells that have differentiated into plasma cells. The B cells tend to remain in the node and are therefore described as being sessile. T cells, on the other hand, leave the node via the solitary efferent lymphatic vessel (Eff Ly), enter the blood via the thoracic duct, and finally return to a lymph node. They leave the blood stream by passing through the walls of the postcapillary venules in the paracortical zone. Lymph containing lymphocytes from tissues or other lymph nodes also enters the lymph node through one of the afferent lymphatics (Aff Ly). (Drawn by Margot Mackay, Department of Art as Applied to Medicine, University of Toronto.)

It is evident that the peripheral lymphoid tissue consists of two distinct types of lymphocytes — the T cells and the B cells — which, although morphologically almost identical, function quite differently. Indeed, the immune response can be regarded as having two distinct components: *(1) the T system of lymphocytes, which produces immune or sensitized lymphocytes, and (2) the B system of lymphocytes, which leads to the formation of immunoglobulins*. The immune response takes place in the peripheral lymphoid tissue. The thymus and bursal equivalent tissues play no direct part in this but are essential for the proper development of the immune system. This can be shown quite easily experimentally: If the thymus is removed from a developing embryo, the animal subsequently lacks T lymphocytes and never exhibits the cell-mediated component of the immune response.

Although it is convenient to describe the two components of the immune system as separate entities, it must be stated at the outset that this is an oversimplification of the situation. For most B-cell functions T cells are involved, either to help the response or to suppress it.

When an antigen such as diphtheria toxin is introduced into an animal for the first time, there is an interval of about two weeks before any specific immunoglobulin can be detected in the serum. Then follows a rise in antibody titer that reaches a plateau and subsequently declines (Fig. 9–3). This is termed a *primary response*.

When the same antigen is injected on a second occasion, there is a rapid rise in antibody titer that reaches a high level and subsequently falls again. This is a *secondary response*. Note that the time lag is shorter and there is a greater production of antibodies than at the first introduction of antigen. Evidently, the introduction of antigen in the first instance leads not only to the formation of antibodies but also to the formation of cells that have a "memory." On subsequent contact with the same antigen, consequently, there is rapid proliferation and formation of immunoglobulin. This *immunological memory* is an important aspect of the immune mechanism.

The plasma antibodies are globulins that mostly migrate in the γ fraction on electrophoresis; a few migrate in the α or β fraction. Nevertheless, antibodies have often been called γ-globulins, a term that is not strictly correct. Hence, they are now termed *immunoglobulins*, with the designation Ig regardless of their electrophoretic mobility. Each molecule consists of four polypeptide chains — two identical light chains and two identical heavy chains held together by disulfide bonds, as explained in Figure 9–4. The antibody-combining properties of the molecule reside in the Fab fragments, a

THE B-CELL SYSTEM — IMMUNO-GLOBULIN PRODUCTION

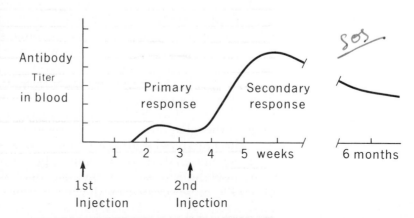

Figure 9–3. Diagram showing differences between a primary and a secondary response to an antigenic stimulus. (Drawn by Margot Mackay, Department of Art as Applied to Medicine, University of Toronto.)

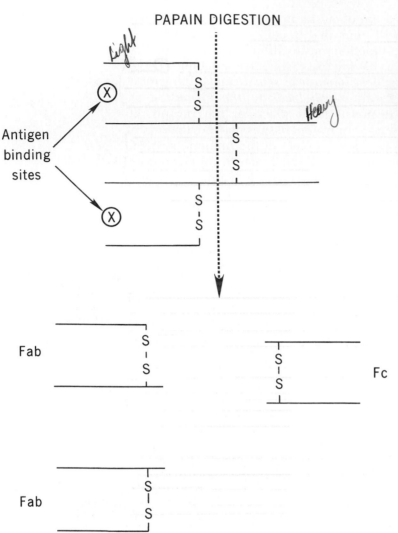

PAPAIN DIGESTION

Antigen binding sites

Fab

Fc

Fab

Figure 9–4. Degradation of the immunoglobulin molecule by papain. The immunoglobulin molecule is represented as two heavy long chains and two light chains joined together by disulfide groups. The antigen combining sites are indicated by ⊗ . Digestion with papain produces three fragments. Two are the Fab fragments, each with one antigen combining site and composed of a light chain and part of a heavy chain. The third fragment has no power to combine with antigen and is termed the Fc fragment (fragment crystallizable). The structure of the Fc fragment determines whether the antibody will fix complement or cross the placenta. (Drawing by Rasa Skudra, Department of Medical Photography and Art. Toronto General Hospital, Toronto.)

fact that harmonizes well with the divalent properties of most antibodies. The amino-terminal ends of the light chains and the associated ends of the heavy chains contain areas, called *domains,* that are *variable* because the amino acids that constitute them vary both in type and in sequence in each molecule. In some areas of these domains there are *hypervariable* regions displaying much more variation than others. Since antibody specificity is determined by amino-acid type and sequence, antibodies of different specificities occur, depending upon the exact structure of the variable domains (Fig. 9–5). The light chains and heavy chains also contain other areas or domains that are invariable or *constant.* These regions, particularly those on the Fc portion of the heavy chains, convey the biological activities of complement fixation, skin fixation, placental transfer, and opsonic activity. The last is due to the binding of antibody-coated organisms to macrophages and granulocytes via the phagocytes' Fc receptors. Killer cells also have Fc receptors, and this is described later in this chapter.

The immunoglobulins are themselves antigenic when injected into other species, and analysis of the antibodies produced has indicated that human immunoglobulins can be divided into *classes* according to the specific antigenic determinants on the heavy chains. There are five types of heavy chains that are named: γ, α, δ, ϵ, and μ. Each antibody molecule has a pair of

Figure 9–5. Representations of an antigen binding site. *A,* A two-dimensional representation of an antigen binding site formed by the apposition of peptide loops containing hypervariable regions depicted by shading. Three loops are shown belonging to the light chain and three belonging to the heavy chain. *B,* A simulated combining site formed by apposition of three middle fingers of each hand, each finger representing a hypervariable loop. It will be appreciated that variations in the amino acid sequence of the hypervariable areas will alter the shape of the antigen combining site such that its specificity is changed. (Drawing by Rasa Skudra, Department of Medical Photography and Art, Toronto General Hospital, Toronto. Modified from Figure 2–10 in Roitt, I. M.: Essential Immunology. 4th ed. Oxford, Blackwell Scientific Publications, 1980.)

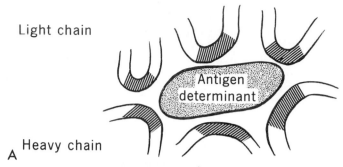

Light chain

Antigen determinant

A Heavy chain

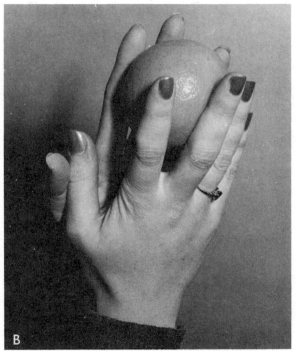

B

identical heavy chains, and therefore five *classes* are recognized — IgG, IgA, IgD, IgE, and IgM, respectively. Each class has been further subdivided into two groups, K and L, for Korngold and Lipari, the two workers who first recognized them. The difference lies in the light chains, which are termed κ (kappa) and λ (lambda). Each molecule, whether IgG, IgA, IgM, IgD, or IgE, has either two κ or two λ chains, but never one of each (Fig. 9–6).

The injection of a single antigen into an animal can lead to the production of any of the five classes of antibodies, so that in theory at least ten different chemical types of antibodies are formed, but they all have the same antigenic specificity. Furthermore, the antibodies are even more heterogeneous than that, since subdivisions are now recognized within each class; *e.g.,* IgG is known to be composed of at least four subtypes — IgG_1, IgG_2, IgG_3, and IgG_4.

Properties of the Five Classes of Immunoglobulins. IgG is the most abundant immunoglobulin present in the plasma. It is a 7S protein* with a molecular weight of about 150,000 daltons. It is the only immunoglobulin to cross the placenta.

---

*The sedimentation rate is measured in *Svedberg units* and is a measurement of the rapidity with which molecules move when subjected to centrifugal force in an ultracentrifuge. Larger molecules have higher Svedberg units. Thus, the 19S fragment contains those proteins of a molecular weight of about 10^6 daltons.

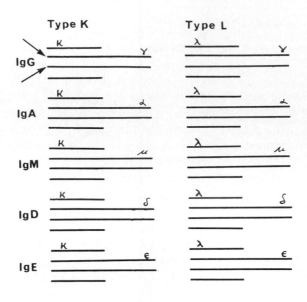

Figure 9–6. Structure of the immunoglobulins. Each immunoglobulin has two identical long, or heavy, chains and two identical short, or light, chains. There are five classes—IgG, IgA, IgM, IgD, and IgE —each differing in their heavy chains, which are γ, α, μ, δ, or ϵ, respectively. Of each class there are two types—type K and type L—the type depending on whether the light chain is κ (kappa) or λ (lambda). The specificity of each molecule is related to the two binding sites, which are indicated by the two arrows on the IgG type κ. Antibodies are therefore divalent. Note that following immunization by a single antigen, ten distinct types of immunoglobulin can be formed. They each have the same antibody specificity but differ in other respects, such as in chemical structure, physical properties, and in ability to sensitize, to fix complement, and to cross the placenta.

IgA is present in the plasma, but its highest concentration is found in secretions of mucous membranes, and its presence is an important factor in preventing infection of these membranes. IgA is manufactured locally in plasma cells and is secreted by epithelial cells as a dimer composed of two IgA molecules joined by a J chain. As the antibody is secreted by the epithelial cells an additional glycoprotein called a *secretory* or *transport component* is added. This serves to stabilize the IgA against proteolysis — *e.g.*, in the gut.

IgD has no known function, although it is possible that it is a component of B-cell membranes and serves as an antigenic receptor site.

IgE is a 7S fraction and is responsible for human anaphylaxis as well as for other type I hypersensitivity states. This is because it has an affinity for mast cells and renders them hypersensitive.

IgM is a 19S globulin with a molecular weight of 900,000 daltons; hence, it is also called a macroglobulin. It consists of five 7S monomers joined with a J chain to form a pentamer. Because of its size, IgM is largely restricted to the intravascular compartment. In an immune response it is often the first immunoglobulin to be produced. Later it is augmented by IgG in the secondary response.

Monoclonal Antibodies. It is evident that the injection of an antigen into an animal leads to a wide variety of antibodies. They vary not only in chemical nature and class but also in specificity, since one antigen may have several epitopic sites. The production of highly specific antiserum in animals is therefore difficult. A recent technique has revolutionized this subject. If an animal is injected with an antigen, the antibody-producing cells can be plated out and grown artificially. Individual cells producing a specific antibody can be selected and cloned. Since the cells are mature or maturing B cells that have a limited life span, they cannot be grown *in vitro* indefinitely. However, by fusing the selected cell with a malignant myeloma cell derived from a syngeneic animal a clone of cells can be grown that not only produces the specific antibody that has been selected but also has immortal life. Such antibody-producing clones are called *hybridomas,* and it is now possible to use them to produce highly specific antibodies. Their use to delineate the different types of T cells is described later in this chapter. Unfortunately, at the time of writing, these highly specific monoclonal antibodies are expensive, and their use is therefore limited by financial constraints.

Although the chemical nature of immunoglobulins is known in some detail, chemical analysis of plasma can determine only the total immunoglobulin content. Antibodies are highly specific, and a variety of techniques have been developed for measuring the amount of a particular antibody. If the antibodies produced after injection of a simple soluble protein, *e.g.*, egg albumin, are mixed with the appropriate antigen, a precipitate is formed when the antibody and antigen meet in approximately equivalent concentrations. An antibody that behaves in this way is termed a *precipitin* (Fig. 9–7). When the antigen is a particle, *e.g.*, a red cell or bacterium, antibodies produced to it can lead to the aggregation of the particles, thereby forming visible clumps. This reaction is termed *agglutination*, and antibodies that produce it are termed *agglutinins* (Fig. 9–8).

Soluble antigens can be attached to particles (*e.g.*, latex, bentonite, or prepared red cells) in the laboratory. The modified antigen so formed can then be used to detect antibodies by an agglutination reaction.

Antibodies can produce another important effect, for when combined with antigen the complex can activate the complement system.

The Complement System.   This system consists of a series of plasma proteins (termed C1 to C9) that, following activation, interact with each other in a sequential or cascadelike manner.* The system can be activated in two separate ways (Fig. 9–9).

The Classical Pathway of Complement Activation.   In the classical pathway antigen-antibody complexes activate C1q, and this is followed by the sequential activation of C1r and C1s. Then follows an action on C4 and C2 to form the important product C4b2a, often shortened to C42. This important

---

*A bar over the figure indicates an activated product. Thus, C$\overline{1}$ is the active form of C1.

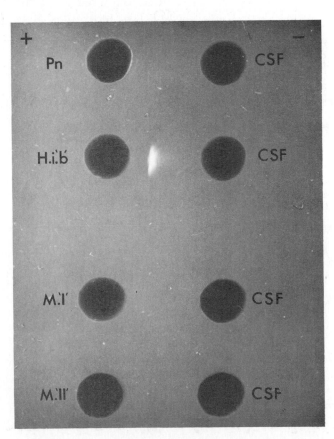

Figure 9–7. A precipitin reaction used to identify an antigen. A young child developed signs of meningitis and was admitted to a hospital after having received an antibiotic. A sample of cerebrospinal fluid (CSF) was obtained by lumbar puncture; although it contained many polymorphs, no bacteria could be cultured. Nevertheless, bacterial antigen was demonstrated by the technique of *countercurrent immunoelectrophoresis,* which is shown in the figure. The test is carried out in a sheet of agarose gel. CSF is placed in the four wells on the right, and specific antisera are placed in separate wells on the left. The meaning of each abbreviation is as follows: Pn, antipneumococcal serum. H.i.'b', antihaemophilus influenzae B serum; M'I', antimeningococcal type I serum. M'II', antimeningococcal type II serum. A current is passed through the gel, and bacterial antigen, which has a strong negative charge, is driven toward the anode (+). Under the conditions of the test, antibody moves toward the cathode (−). Hence, antigen and antibody move toward each other, and a precipitate is formed where specific antibody meets antigen in optimum proportions. The well-marked precipitin line that is shown indicates that the CSF contains *Haemophilus influenzae* antigen. This test is useful in demonstrating antigen when bacteria cannot be cultured because of previous antibiotic therapy. The test is also used in identifying bacterial antigens in sputum and blood.

Precipitin reactions can be obtained by allowing antigen and antibody to diffuse toward each other from separate wells in an agar sheet. However, the test is less sensitive, since diffusion occurs all around the periphery of the wells and the reagents are thereby diluted. Application of an electric field drives the two agents toward each other and thereby makes the test more sensitive. (Courtesy of Dr. C. Krishnan.)

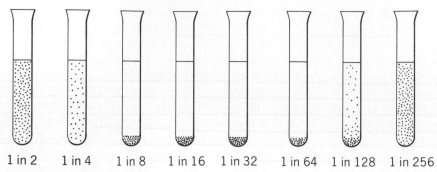

1 in 2   1 in 4   1 in 8   1 in 16   1 in 32   1 in 64   1 in 128   1 in 256

Figure 9–8. Agglutination test. A series of tubes is prepared, the first containing neat serum (left-hand tube), with each subsequent tube containing serum diluted with saline in proportions of $\frac{1}{2}$, $\frac{1}{4}$, $\frac{1}{8}$, etc. (*i.e.,* doubling the dilution). To each tube is added an equal volume of suspension of particles—bacteria, red cells, or latex particles coated with antigen. The tubes are incubated at 37°C for a suitable time. The final dilution of the serum in the last tube to show definite agglutination is described as the *titer of the antibody.* In this illustration the titer is 1 in 128. Sometimes the left-hand tube, which contains the highest concentration of antibody, fails to show agglutination. Such a situation is described as the *prozone phenomenon.* Examples of this type of agglutination test are the Widal (for typhoid fever), the Weil-Felix (for typhus fever), and the Paul-Bunnell (for infectious mononucleosis).

substance is also called C3 convertase, because it cleaves C3 to C3a and C3b. C3b combines with cell membrane sites, and when it is close to membrane-bound $C\overline{42}$, $C\overline{423b}$ or C5 convertase is formed. This cleaves C5 to C5a and C5b. C5b forms an active trimolecular complex with C6 and C7 to form $C\overline{5b67}$. This also binds to cell membrane sites. Finally, C8 and C9 are activated, and there is damage to the cell membrane that leads to lysis and destruction of cells.

The following points should be emphasized.

(1) Two molecules of IgG will activate complement, whereas IgM is a much more powerful complement activator since only one molecule is

CLASSICAL PATHWAY   ALTERNATE PATHWAY

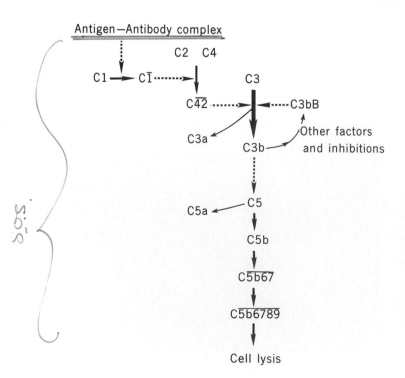

Figure 9–9. Pathways of the activation of complement. The complement system consists of nine proteins labelled C1, C2, etc., to C9. C1 in fact has three components, C1q, C1r, and C1s. In the classical pathway of activation, Ig$\underline{G}$ or IgM combines with antigen and activates C1 to C$\overline{1}$: This leads to the formation of C$\overline{42}$ or C3 convertase which cleaves C3 to C3a and C3b. C3b activates C5, and the subsequent activation of C6, C7, C8, and C9 leads to membrane damage and cell lysis. In the alternate pathway C3 is activated by an alternative activator depicted as C3bB. The details of this pathway are complex and may be triggered by nonimmunological mechanisms as well as by antigen-antibody interaction. (Drawing by Rasa Skudra, Department of Medical Photography and Art, Toronto General Hospital, Toronto.)

required. This is because IgM is a pentamer. IgA, IgD, and IgE will not activate complement.

2. The activation of complement consumes its components. When complement was first described it was considered to be a single substance, and it was therefore said to be "fixed" by antibody. Hence, the term "complement-fixing antibodies" is in common use, and tests designed to detect their presence are called antibody *complement fixation tests*.

3. When all components of complement are utilized, the effect is cell lysis. Hence, antibodies that cause this effect are termed lysins, *e.g.*, hemolysins lyse red cells and bacteriolysins lyse bacteria.

4. During the activation of complement the major components tend to be bound to cell membranes. In addition, low–molecular-weight substances are formed that are released into the fluid phase and have important actions. C3a and C5a are chemotactic to white cells and also cause mast cells to release their granules containing histamine, etc. (Chapter 5). These substances are called *anaphylatoxins*. The complex C567 also has chemotactic activity. Hence, the activation of complement augments the acute inflammatory reaction, and this can so alter the local environment that infecting agents are destroyed. In addition, however, lysosomal enzymes that cause cell damage can be released. These aspects are discussed later in this chapter under the headings "Immunity" and "Hypersensitivity."

5. C3b binds to cell membranes, and this can lead to the adherence (called *immune adhesion)* to cells with C3b receptors, *e.g.*, phagocytes. This is an important step in phagocytosis and is an example of an opsonizing effect.

The Alternate Pathway of Complement Activation.   C3 can be activated in this alternate pathway by an activator termed C3bB. This activator can be formed by the action of microbial polysaccharides (such as endotoxins) and aggregated IgA. The actual formation of C3bB is complex and poorly understood but involves a protein called properdin. Hence, the alternate pathway is sometimes called the properdin system. It is clearly a mechanism by which cells can be lysed and an inflammatory reaction augmented by a mechanism not involving the immune system itself.

Complement fixation tests are of great value in the diagnosis of many diseases, particularly viral infections, gonorrhea, and syphilis. The principle involved is described in Figure 9–10, which explains the Wassermann reaction for syphilitic antibody detection.

Some antibodies are capable of coating organisms (*e.g.*, pneumococci) and rendering them more readily susceptible to phagocytosis by polymorphs and macrophages. Such antibodies are termed *opsonins,* and their presence can be detected *in vitro* by incubating a suspension of organisms with polymorphs in a suitable medium. Opsonins are important *in vivo* in providing immunity to infection.

It should be noted that the globulin antibodies have been named according to the nature of the test used to detect them. It was at one time thought that each type of antibody was a distinct entity, but it is now known that a single type of antibody can perform several functions, depending upon the conditions under which it is examined. Thus, a substance may be capable of neutralizing toxin, *e.g.*, diphtheria toxin, in an *in vivo* experiment; it is therefore rightly called an "antitoxin." However, *in vitro* it can produce a precipitate with its antigen and may then be labelled a "precipitin." Some agglutinins, such as to red cells, produce agglutination only in the absence of complement. When this is present, complement is activated and the cell undergoes lysis.

FIRST REACTION	SECOND, OR DETECTOR, REACTION (HEMOLYTIC SYSTEM)
Patient's Serum Previously heated to 56° C for 30 min to inactivate complement; may or may not contain syphilitic antibody.	*Sheep Red Cells*
+	+
Antigen A standard quantity	*Hemolysin* Serum of a rabbit immunized against sheep red cells
+	+
Complement ⟶ A carefully measured amount	*Complement* If unused in the first reaction

Figure 9–10.   The Wassermann reaction for syphilitic antibody.   The test is carried out in two stages. In the first reaction, patient's serum (depleted of complement) is mixed with antigen and complement. If the patient's serum contains antibody, it combines with antigen and activates the complement, which is consumed or "fixed." Hence, no complement is available for the second reaction, and hemolysis does not occur. Conversely, if the patient's serum does not contain antibody, complement is available for the detector reaction (hemolytic system), and hemolysis occurs.

The antigen used in this test is an extract of heart muscle, which by chance has antigenic properties in common with *Treponema pallidum.* By the use of treponemal antigen the test can be made more specific. In practice, other tests are also employed (Chapter 10).

Effects of Immunoglobulin in the Body

Immunity

The exotoxins of the causative agents of diphtheria, tetanus, gas gangrene, and botulism are potent antigens, and their introduction into the body leads to the formation of antitoxins. These antibodies provide immunity to these diseases, since their presence in the blood leads to neutralization of toxin and to its subsequent elimination. An individual who has had diphtheria or even a subclinical infection is invariably immune for life, since immunological memory will lead to the rapid formation of antibody (secondary response) if the organism is ever encountered again. This immune state can be produced artificially by injecting *toxoid.* Toxoids are toxins that have been rendered less toxic by addition of formaldehyde but nevertheless are still highly antigenic. It is now a common practice to give a series of injections of tetanus toxoid and diphtheria toxoid so that active immunity is produced. *Active immunity* means that subjects are producing their own antibodies because of antigenic stimulations. In the case of patients suffering from these diseases, immunity can be provided by injecting specific immunoglobulin derived from an immune animal or another human being. This is *passive immunity.* It is a useful emergency procedure, because it provides immediate immunity. It is of a temporary nature, however, and as the antibodies are broken down (catabolized), immunity is lost.

In the case of most infective agents, the antibodies that are produced in response to infection are directed against antigenic components of the organism itself. These antibodies are therefore called *antibacterial, antiviral,* or *antifungal,* and because the organisms have many antigenic determinants, antibodies are produced that have different specificities. Some of these antibodies can lead to protection against subsequent infection, but others appear to have no protective activity; their detection in the blood, however, is useful in diagnosis.

Value of Antibody Detection in Diagnosis of Infective Disease.   The detection of a specific antibody to a particular organism in the serum of a patient is often of value in either making the diagnosis or confirming it.

Examples are the detection of agglutinins during the second and third week of typhoid fever (Chapter 6), and the VDRL in syphilis (Chapter 10). An isolated test is of limited value, since the presence of a specific antibody may merely indicate a past infection or previous immunization. A *rising titer* during the course of an illness is of much greater significance and may be taken as presumptive evidence in the diagnosis of a disease, provided it is associated with an illness that clinically is consistent with that diagnosis. The value of taking a sample of blood early in the course of a disease followed by a sample taken during convalescence is quite apparent. Antibody diagnosis is particularly useful in the detection of infections in which the organism cannot easily be isolated, *e.g., Legionella pneumophila,* or if the organism is plentiful only during the early, clinically nondiagnostic phase of the disease, *e.g.,* many virus infections.

The sharing of an antigen between different species is sometimes of value in diagnosis. For example, the Epstein-Barr virus shares an antigen with the red cells of sheep, and this forms the basis for the Paul-Bunnell test, (Chapter 26).

Immunization Against Invasive Organisms.   With invasive organisms, *active immunization* is carried out by injecting a suspension of the organism itself. Such a preparation, which is termed a *vaccine,* may contain either living or dead organisms. The precise preparation that is used is the one found in practice to produce the most effective immunity. Production of vaccines is very much a matter of trial and error. In the case of the staphylococcus, an effective vaccine has yet to be produced. Injecting a dead suspension of *Hemophilus pertussis,* on the other hand, has been found to be an effective means of preventing whooping cough. With tuberculosis, vaccines containing dead organisms are of no value, but those with living organisms are effective. The organism commonly used is a tubercle baccilus (used in the *bacillus Calmette-Guérin* vaccine, BCG), which has been grown in artificial media for so long that it has lost its virulence. A vaccine of this *attenuated* organism produces a very local infection, which leads to a reasonable (but not absolute) degree of immunity. Vaccinia virus* is used for "vaccination" against small-pox. Vaccines should not be confused with toxoids. A vaccine is a suspension of microorganisms, either alive or dead. A toxoid is a chemically altered preparation of bacterial toxin.

Passive antibacterial immunity can be provided by injecting human or animal sera containing specific antibodies. This has been used in the past (*e.g.,* antipneumococcal sera), but the discovery of potent antibiotics has made their use unnecessary. Passive immunization against viral infections still has a useful role; for example, antimeasles serum is used to prevent very young children from contracting this infection.

Mechanisms of Antibacterial Immunity.   In infection with invasive organisms the antibodies that appear are *antibacterial,* in the sense that they are directed against bacterial components or secretions. They are detected as agglutinins, precipitins, complement-fixing antibodies, antibacterial hemolysins, and so forth. The particular test employed to detect them in clinical practice is arbitrary — it is often the test that is most convenient or merely the one that was first discovered. The antibodies detected are not necessarily the ones that destroy the organisms *in vitro* or *in vivo.* Therefore, they do not necessarily provide immunity. A syphilitic patient with a strongly positive VDRL, far from being immune, is highly infectious.

---

*The precise origin of the vaccinia virus currently available is not known. It may be derived from an attenuated strain of smallpox virus or from cowpox virus. As noted elsewhere, vaccination against smallpox is not now recommended.

Invasive organisms are destroyed in the body by two major mechanisms. Either they are destroyed by cells, usually polymorphs or phagocytic cells of the reticuloendothelial system, or they are lysed by the activation of complement. Antibacterial antibodies can provide immunity, and they do this by aiding one of these mechanisms.

1. Opsonic Effect. Antibodies can neutralize the noxious surface antigens of certain virulent bacteria, for example, the capsular polysaccharide of pneumococci, which repel or kill phagocytes at close quarters. An opsonized bacterium is more easily phagocytosed. Polymorphs and macrophages have Fc receptors on their cell membranes, and the cells will therefore adhere to antibody-coated organisms. Likewise, if the antibody activates complement, C3b on bacterial membranes is also recognized by phagocytes' receptors, and this is a further mechanism by which the phagocytes are brought into close contact with bacteria and adhere to them. Adherence is an essential preliminary step to phagocytosis.

2. Antibody-Dependent Cell-Mediated Cytotoxicity. Target cells (*e.g.*, bacteria or larger organisms) coated with IgG can be killed by a mechanism not involving phagocytosis. Cells containing Fc receptors will adhere to such coated target cells and kill them by some direct cell-to-cell interaction, which is poorly understood. Cells that may be involved in this antibody-dependent cytotoxicity reaction include polymorphs, monocytes, and cells that resemble small lymphocytes and have Fc receptors. These have been called *killer cells (K cells)*, but their precise nature is not known. Some appear to have T-cell markers, whereas others are *null cells* having neither B- nor T-lymphocyte markers. It should be stressed that these lymphocytes are not sensitized and that the reaction appears to be nonspecific.

3. Activation of Complement. IgG and IgM can activate complement, which, if it proceeds to its final stages, leads to membrane damage and bacterial lysis.

4. Enhancement of the Inflammatory Reaction. Antibodies can enhance the acute inflammatory reaction in a variety of ways. By activating complement, C3a and C5a are formed. These are chemotactic to white cells and in addition act as anaphylatoxins, meaning that they cause mast cells to release histamine and other chemical mediators of acute inflammation. IgE has the property of adhering to mast cells, and when acted upon by a specific antigen, *e.g.*, that provided by a bacterium, will cause the mast cell to degranulate and again release mediators that will enhance the inflammatory reaction.

Hypersensitivity   Immunoglobulins can produce hypersensitivity in several distinct ways:

Type I Hypersensitivity — Anaphylaxis. This is best illustrated by a simple experiment. If a guinea pig is given an injection of a simple protein, such as egg albumin, it shows no obvious discomfort. About two weeks later, specific immunoglobulins (precipitins) appear in the plasma. A second injection of egg albumin is then given intravenously. Antigen reacts with a sensitizing antibody, and the animal rapidly develops difficulty in breathing. It becomes unconscious, convulses, and dies within a few minutes. The reaction, termed *generalized anaphylaxis* or *anaphylactic shock*, is highly specific; it is due to a damaging antigen-antibody reaction occurring on the surface of certain cells, which causes *histamine, slow-reacting substance of anaphylaxis* (SRS-A),* and other mediators to be liberated. The histamine

---

*SRS-A is so called because it produces a slow contraction of smooth muscle, in contrast to the rapid contraction induced by histamine.

produces vasodilatation (dilatation of blood vessels) and lowering of the blood pressure, and together with SRS-A it causes spasm of the bronchial muscle. In the guinea pig the second injection must be large and given intravenously. It first neutralizes the circulating plasma antibodies, and enough then remains to combine with sensitizing antibody that is fixed to cells. When anaphylaxis occurs in humans, the manifestations are the following:

1. *Bronchospasm,* which causes great difficulty in expiration. The sudden onset of wheezing dyspnea is characteristic.

2. *Edema* due to a generalized increase in vascular permeability. Sometimes edema of the larynx adds to the respiratory difficulty.

3. *Pallor.*

4. *Low blood pressure.*

In humans, the reaction is due to the formation of sensitizing IgE, which has a great affinity for mast cells, to which it becomes firmly attached. Very little need be present in the blood. Hence, unlike the situation of the guinea pig, very small doses of antigen can cause acute anaphylactic shock. Although rare, it is encountered under three circumstances:

(a) When horse gamma globulin is given to patients who are sensitized to horse protein, *e.g.,* in passive immunization against diphtheria and tetanus, whether prophylactic or therapeutic.

(b) When a drug that is capable of acting as a hapten is injected into a patient who is sensitive to it. Penicillin is such a drug; each year a number of people die of anaphylaxis from this therapy.

(c) Following the sting of a bee or wasp in highly sensitive individuals.

The danger of anaphylaxis should always be kept in mind by anyone administering animal sera or drugs by injection. At the first sign of anaphylaxis 0.5 to 1.0 ml of a 1:1000 solution of epinephrine should be given intramuscularly. The drug causes peripheral vasoconstriction and bronchodilatation. The dose should be repeated at 15-minute intervals until the crisis is over. A slow intravenous injection of an antihistamine should be given immediately after the adrenalin and repeated over the next 24 hours to prevent relapse. Edema of the larynx may necessitate emergency tracheostomy.

Dust and Food Hypersensitivity.   This group of hypersensitivity reactions occurs after the ingestion of certain foods and the inhalation of pollen or dust. The symptoms differ according to the route of absorption. The offending agent may be a complete antigen or a hapten.

Types. Inhalation of antigens like pollen, horse dander, and dust usually produces watering of the eyes or symptoms involving the respiratory tract: congestion of the nasal mucosa (allergic rhinitis or hay fever) and bronchial asthma. Mast cells sensitized by IgE release a number of agents when acted upon by specific antigen. In addition to histamine and SRS-A previously mentioned, there is a platelet-activating factor that causes platelets to undergo the release reaction, and an *eosinophil-chemotactic factor of anaphylaxis* (ECF-A). The nasal and bronchial secretions of patients with these atopic manifestations are therefore teeming with eosinophils.

Ingestion of certain foods produces either gastrointestinal symptoms or urticarial skin rashes. Some people are particularly sensitive to such foods as shellfish, mushrooms, strawberries, and milk. The lesions of this group of hypersensitivities are mostly exudative in type and are mediated by histamine. The antihistaminic drugs therefore have an ameliorative effect. Sensitive people can be detected by injecting into or pricking the skin with a minute dose of the offending antigen. Redness and a wheal appear *within a few minutes.* It will be noted that the phenomena of type I hypersensitivity appear within a minute or two of contact with antigen. For this reason the term *immediate hypersensitivity* is often applied to the group.

Patients with this type of hypersensitivity frequently give a family history of similar complaints. One member may have *hay fever,* another *extrinsic bronchial asthma,* and a third, *atopic dermatitis.* It seems that the capacity to react to certain antigens with the production of sensitizing IgE antibodies is related to genetic make-up. Individuals who have such a family background are termed *atopic* and are liable to suffer from *eczema in childhood.* They may later develop *allergic rhinitis* (hay fever), or *bronchial asthma* and are particularly liable to become susceptible to anaphylactic shock. It therefore follows that before any injection is given to a patient, any personal or familial liability to hypersensitivity should be determined.

Desensitization. Attempts to desensitize atopic patients are sometimes made by injecting small doses of the antigen (*e.g.,* pollen extract) at weekly intervals, but unfortunately the procedure is not uniformly successful. The dose is steadily increased, with an aim to produce an excess of blocking IgG in the blood so that antigen is intercepted before it reaches cells sensitized by IgE. Other explanations have been put forward. Repeated small doses of antigen could lead to the induction of tolerance, possibly by the action of suppressor T cells.

Type II Hypersensitivity — Antibody-Dependent Cytotoxic Hypersensitivity. Antibodies adherent to a surface antigen of a cell can cause destruction of that cell in a variety of ways. Activation of complement can cause lysis. Phagocytes, by becoming adherent because of their Fc or C3b receptors, can destroy the cells by phagocytosis. Nonphagocytic cells (*e.g.,* K cells) can cause destruction by the phenomenon of antibody-dependent cell-mediated cytotoxicity (see above). Most examples of type II reaction seen in human pathology concern the destruction of red cells. Occasionally during penicillin therapy the drug, by acting as a hapten, can become attached to a red-cell membrane and lead to the formation of destructive antibodies that cause hemolysis by complement activation. Similarly, autoimmune hemolytic reactions are examples of this type of hypersensitivity. Likewise, the hemolysis that occurs following a mismatched transfusion or in hemolytic disease of the newborn can be included under this heading. Whether type II hypersensitivity can cause destruction of cells other than red cells is less certain. Some aspects of the later changes in graft destruction suggest that this mechanism is operating. Also, the kidney damage seen in Goodpasture's syndrome may be mediated by this mechanism.

Type III Hypersensitivity — Immune-Complex Reactions. As noted previously, some types of antibodies have the property of combining with their respective antigen to form complexes that can activate complement. Chemotactic factors are liberated, and polymorphs, which are attracted to the complexes, release damaging lysosomal enzymes. The release of anaphylatoxins contributes to the inflammatory reaction so produced. Four examples in which damaging immune complexes produce disease will be described below.

The Arthus Phenomenon. Repeated weekly subcutaneous injections of antigen given to an animal lead to progressively more severe local reactions. Swelling and redness appear within one hour, and over the next few hours hemorrhage and necrosis develop. The pathogenesis is as follows: The injected antigen diffuses into vessel walls and encounters the specific IgG that is present in the blood. Antigen-antibody complexes activate complement in the vessel wall. Polymorphs accumulate and release their lysosomal

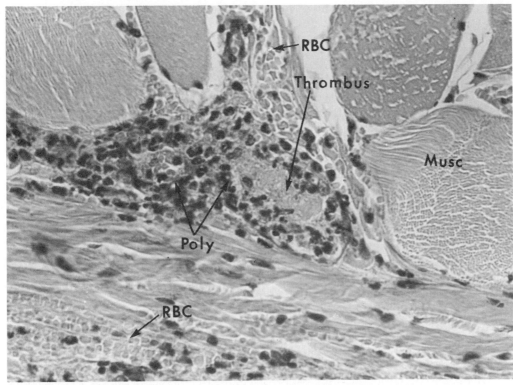

Figure 9–11. The Arthus reaction in a rabbit. This section is from the subcutaneous tissues and includes striated muscle (Musc). The blood vessel in the center is sectioned obliquely and shows occlusion of its lumen by a thrombus. Its walls are heavily infiltrated by polymorphs (Poly), many of which are degenerating. Free red cells (RBC) in the tissues bear witness to the severity of the vascular damage (× 550).

enzymes. The vessel wall is damaged, and thrombosis follows (Fig. 9–11). The Arthus reaction is thought to be the explanation of some types of vasculitis in man, such as that seen in gonococcal septicemia (Chapter 10). Farmer's lung provides another example (Chapter 30).

Serum Sickness. Serum sickness is a condition characterized by fever, joint pains, and urticarial eruptions that occur about 14 days after the administration of a large dose of foreign serum, such as horse immunoglobulin. The pathogenesis is explained in Figure 9–12.

Drug Hypersensitivity. Hypersensitivity to drugs is a common clinical event and is due to the drug or one of its degradation products acting as a hapten and stimulating the formation of sensitizing antibodies. Virtually any drug can produce a reaction, but common offenders are penicillin, sulfonamides, aspirin, barbiturates, and quinine. *Anaphylactic reactions* (type I reaction) can range from urticaria to severe anaphylactic shock. Sensitizing IgE antibodies are responsible. *Later drug reactions* begin several days after the administration of the drug and are much more common. Some of these have the features of immune-complex reactions. They are characterized by skin rashes that may be urticarial, papular, or petechial and are usually widespread, brightly erythematous, and intensely itchy. The rash is accompanied by fever and sometimes by pain in the joints, thereby showing some similarity to serum sickness. The antibodies concerned are IgG or IgM. Note that some later drug effects such as thrombocytopenia, hemolytic anemia, erythema multiforme, jaundice, and a syndrome resembling systemic lupus erythematosus are not clearly understood. Sometimes cytotoxic antibodies are

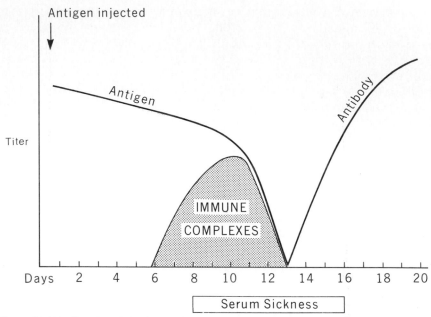

Figure 9–12.   Graph indicating changes in antigen and antibody titer during serum sickness. Following a single injection of a large dose of antigen, free antigen is present in the blood in higher titer. The titer drops rapidly with the onset of the immune response. As antibody enters the blood, antigen-antibody complexes form and are rapidly eliminated from the circulation by the activity of the reticuloendothelial system. It is during the period of circulating immune complexes that the illness of serum sickness occurs. The complexes are deposited in the kidney, skin, and joints. Complement is activated, polymorphs accumulate, lysosomal enzymes are released, and damage is done. It is not known why the lesions tend to be restricted to those three sites. As the immune complexes are catabolized, the symptoms of the illness subside, and free antibody appears in the blood. This illustrates how the immune response results in elimination of foreign protein from the body. (Drawn by Margot Mackay, Department of Art as Applied to Medicine, University of Toronto.)

produced (*e.g.*, as with penicillin), and sometimes immune complexes may be incriminated, but often the pathogenesis is quite obscure.

Chronic Immune-Complex Disease.   If daily injections of antigen are given to an animal in such quantity that antigen-antibody complexes are formed in the blood, a chronic glomerulonephritis develops. It is believed that some types of human glomerulonephritis have a similar pathogenesis, because granular deposits of immune complexes and complement are found in the glomeruli (Chapter 35). Likewise, the acute rheumatic fever that follows streptococcal sore throat is probably of similar nature.

Type IV Hypersensitivity.   This is also called *cell-mediated hypersensitivity* and is discussed later in this chapter.

Type V Hypersensitivity — Stimulatory Hypersensitivity.   This fifth type of hypersensitivity has been described to explain how an antibody can react with a hormone receptor and "switch on" the cell. Thyroid-stimulating immunoglobulin that is present in Graves' disease is the only well-documented example.

THE CELL-MEDIATED IMMUNE RESPONSE

Following contact with antigen, the body may develop a cell-mediated immune response. This is particularly prominent if the antigen is applied directly to the skin, is injected with Freund's adjuvant, or is in the form of a living organism, either a tissue graft or a bacterium or other parasite. The T-cell system responds by producing antigen-sensitive T cells (sensitized lymphocytes). These cells have various functions and properties, which can be detected *in vitro* when the cells come into contact with the appropriate antigen.

If the antigen is a virus, the T cells destroy the virus-infected cells by an ill-defined cell-to-cell interaction. The sensitized T cells do this first by *recognizing the surface HLA tissue antigens that have been modified by the multiplying virus* within the cell. In the rejection of foreign tissue grafts, sensitized lymphocytes again cause destruction of the cells following their recognition of the foreign HLA surface antigens. With bacterial infections, *e.g.*, tuberculosis, sensitized T cells probably do not directly kill the organisms, but they ultimately lead to their destruction by other cells — probably macrophages.

Cytotoxic Effect

Sensitized lymphocytes react specifically with antigen and release a number of low–molecular-weight substances termed *lymphokines*. These agents are at present ill-defined chemically but have been named according to specific demonstrable activity. They may be listed as follows:

Lymphokine Release

1. Migration-Inhibition Factor (MIF). This acts on macrophages and prevents their migration in a tissue culture system (Fig. 9–13). This agent is probably the same as the *macrophage-activating factor,* which makes cells more phagocytic and better able to kill organisms. It may be supposed that MIF is an important agent, which leads to the accumulation of macrophages during the demolition phase of acute inflammation and in many types of chronic inflammation in which granuloma formation is prominent.

2. Transfer Factor. This substance specifically transfers sensitization to previously uncommitted lymphocytes. Therefore, it probably recruits new cells to the site involved, *e.g.*, the site of infection, and is therefore important in multiplying the effect of immunity and also in multiplying the effect of hypersensitivity from the cell-mediated immune response.

3. Lymphotoxin. This agent has the property of destroying cells, an effect that can be demonstrated in fibroblast tissue cultures. Presumably, lymphotoxins can also destroy cells *in vivo*.

4. Skin Reactive Factor. This is presumed to be responsible for some of the phenomena of the Mantoux test, which is described later in this chapter.

5. Chemotactic Factor. Several types are produced and can attract neutrophils, monocytes, eosinophils, and lymphocytes.

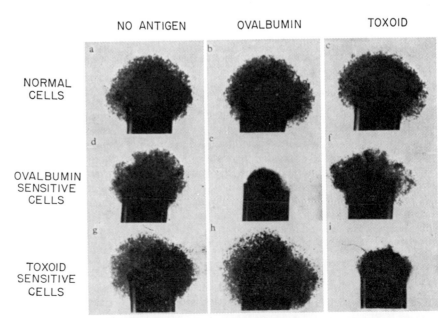

Figure 9–13. Specific inhibition by antigen of the migration of cells from sensitized animals. The cells, mostly macrophages and lymphocytes from a peritoneal exudate, are placed in capillary tubes and incubated in a microchamber. Normally, the macrophages migrate from the open end and produce a tufted appearance. The cells derived from animals with delayed hypersensitivity show no migration in the presence of specific antibody. (From David, J. R., al-Askari, S., Lawrence, H. S., and Thomas, L.: Delayed hypersensitivity in vitro. Journal of Immunology, *93*: 264–273, 1964.)

NO ANTIGEN   OVALBUMIN   TOXOID

NORMAL CELLS

OVALBUMIN SENSITIVE CELLS

TOXOID SENSITIVE CELLS

6. *Mitogenic Factor.* This agent causes blast transformation of lymphocytes and stimulates mitosis.

7. *Interferon.* This agent prevents intracellular viral replication and is described in detail in Chapter 12.

8. *Immunoglobulin.*

Helper Function

During the immune response to many antigens, T cells are necessary for the B-cell response that culminates in immunoglobulin formation. Hence, neonatal thymectomized mice lack these helper T cells and exhibit an impaired humoral response in addition to a defective cell-mediated immune response itself.

Suppressor Function

Some T cells have the reverse effect of the helper cells. They suppress not only T-cell response but also that of the B cells. As with the humoral immune response, the cell-mediated immune response can be associated with either immunity to infection or hypersensitivity. Immunoglobulins are not involved, and cell-mediated reactions cannot be passively transferred to another animal by transferring serum. Transfer can be effected only by lymphocytes. With animals the cells must be alive, but with humans extracts of lymphocytes are effective. The agent responsible is called *transfer factor*, and it acts on the recipient's lymphocytes to render them sensitized.

Cell-Mediated Immunity

Although it is relatively easy to assess humoral immunity by measuring the titer of specific immunoglobulins, there is no simple way of assessing cell-mediated immunity. Only the response to a challenging infection can reliably reveal its presence; in animals this is difficult, and in humans it is virtually impossible.

Cell-mediated immunity is probably a factor in immunity to all infections, but is particularly important in relationship to infections with viruses, fungi, and bacteria, especially those that are intracellular parasites, such as the mycobacteria that cause tuberculosis and leprosy.

Cell-mediated immunity has many aspects. Direct cytotoxicity by activated T cells is important in viral infections. The release of lymphokines augments the inflammatory reaction and recruits and activates phagocytic cells, particularly the macrophages.

Cell-Mediated Hypersensitivity

This is also known as *type IV* or *delayed hypersensitivity* and is exemplified by the Koch phenomenon.

The Koch Phenomenon. If tubercle bacilli are injected into a normal guinea pig, there is an incubation period of 10 to 14 days before the appearance of a nodule at the site of injection. Ulceration follows, bacilli spread to local lymph nodes, and finally they reach the blood stream. The animal dies of a generalized infection within 6 to 12 weeks. The injection of more tubercle bacilli into a different site in the same animal infected 4 to 6 weeks previously evokes a completely different type of response. A nodule appears within 1 to 2 days, ulcerates, and then heals. There is little tendency to spread to the local lymph nodes. This second type of response was first described by Robert Koch. It should be noted that the reaction of a tuberculous animal to the tubercle bacilli differs from that of a healthy one in three important respects: (1) the incubation is greatly shortened (this may be described as *hypersensitivity);* (2) the lesion heals quickly; and (3) there is little spread. These are the features of immunity.

The heightened tissue response of the tuberculous animal can be demonstrated not only with the living tubercle bacillus but also with a protein extract of the organism. Koch originally used a crude extract called *old tuberculin;* more recently, a purified protein derivative (PPD) has been introduced.

The injection of a small quantity of PPD into a normal animal results in a negligible inflammatory response. In the tuberculous animal, however, an indurated red lesion develops that appears within 12 to 24 hours and reaches a maximum by 48 to 72 hours. This is the *tuberculin,* or *Mantoux, test;* a positive result indicates the existence of hypersensitivity to tuberculoprotein.

This type of hypersensitivity differs in many important respects from the type I reactions described previously. Characteristics of the Koch phenomenon are as follows:

1. The reaction is delayed: *It takes at least 12 hours* to develop, as compared with only *a few minutes* in other types of hypersensitivity reactions.

2. Although there is a mild acute inflammatory reaction, the phenomenon is characterized by an accumulation of lymphocytes and macrophages rather than polymorphs.

3. The reaction is not mediated by histamine and is not blocked by antihistaminic drugs.

4. Immunoglobulins are not involved in the reaction. If plasma from a Mantoux-positive individual is injected into a Mantoux-negative person, there is no transfer of sensitivity.

5. Delayed hypersensitivity can be transferred to a normal animal by the transfer of T lymphocytes. Passive hypersensitivity persists for as long as the injected cells live in the new host. In some way, the transplanted cells alter the host's own lymphocytes so that these also take part in the delayed type of skin reaction that is subsequently elicited. In man, delayed hypersensitivity can be transferred not only by living cells but also by extracts of lymphocytes. First described by Lawrence in 1955, the action of the *transfer factor,* which is one of the lymphokines, is not known. However, it is evidently very potent, because a single injection of lymphocyte extract can render the recipient hypersensitive for many months.

Examples of Cell-Mediated Hypersensitivity

1. Following Infection.   A positive Mantoux reaction indicates past or present infection with the tubercle bacillus. The hypersensitivity reaction probably plays a major part in the production and persistence of tuberculous lesions. Delayed hypersensitivity is a feature of many other chronic infections — leprosy and histoplasmosis, for example. Much of the damage in these infections is produced not by the organism itself but by the host's own reaction.

2. Allergic Contact Dermatitis.   This follows the application of a sensitizing chemical to the skin. The reaction has been described previously.

3. The Graft Reaction.   See page 132.

4. Experimental.   Delayed hypersensitivity also follows the injection of antigen mixed with Freund's adjuvant. The latter consists of a water-in-oil emulsion mixed with killed tubercle bacilli or other mycobacteria. It is not known for certain how this curious concoction can potentiate the immune response, but it may be that it acts by leading to an accumulation of macrophages that can process the antigen (page 135) and also perhaps by activating helper T cells.

Blast Transformation.   One of the most remarkable observations of recent times is that the small lymphocytes of the blood can be stimulated *in vitro* to enlarge, develop basophilic cytoplasm, and undergo mitosis. Such cells are termed *immunoblasts* and are thought to be able to develop into plasma cells or lymphocytes. Agents that cause lymphocytic transformation are:

1. Phytohemagglutinin. This is an extract of the broad bean; the reason for its causing blast transformation is not understood.

2. Antigen if Added to the Lymphocytes of a Sensitized Individual. This occurs regardless of whether the sensitization is of the immediate or delayed type.

3. Contact with Foreign Cells.

4. Antigen-Antibody Complexes.

The precise role of blast transformation phenomenon in the intact animal is not known, but various suggestions have been made, as follows:

1. The proliferating cells form the germinal centers of lymph nodes, and in fact represent clones that produce antibody. The cells can develop endoplasmic reticulum and differentiate into plasma cells.

2. The blast cells can revert to a type of small lymphocyte, which could have several possible functions. It could act as a *memory cell,* so that when next simulated by antigen it could be transformed and produce antibody. It could also act as an *effector cell* in cell-mediated responses.

TISSUE GRAFTS*

In addition to its practical value in surgery, the transplantation of tissue has done much to extend our knowledge of the body's response to foreign tissue. To a considerable extent the fate of a graft depends upon its origin. The three types — autograft, homograft, and heterograft — will therefore be described separately.

Autografts

An autograft is a graft of tissue made from one site to another site in the same individual. Provided the graft obtains an adequate blood supply, it usually lives and functions normally.

Autografts have been used extensively in plastic surgery. Free grafts of skin may be applied to raw surfaces, *e.g.,* following a burn or wide excision of a tumor such as carcinoma of the breast. Whole-thickness flaps of skin may be used as pedicle grafts and swung from one part of the body to another area. With such a procedure, part of the original blood supply is maintained until the portion that has been moved acquires a new blood supply. When the latter is thought to be adequate, the original connection with the donor site is divided.

Homografts

A homograft is a transplant made from one individual to another of the same species. If the two individuals are of identical genetic structure, the graft is termed *syngeneic* or *isogeneic.* Such a graft is accepted as self, does not provoke an immune response, and behaves like an autograft.

An *allogeneic graft,* or *allograft,* is a graft made between individuals of the same species but of different genetic constitution. This is the common type of graft that is used in clinical practice.

As a general rule, allogeneic homografts are rejected, unless special steps are taken to avoid this. Three patterns of rejection are encountered:

Hyperacute Rejection. In hyperacute rejection, the graft never becomes vascularized and is rapidly destroyed. This type of rejection is mediated by preformed immunoglobulins. These may belong to the ABO system (Chapter 26) or may be directed against HLA antigens (page 134), owing to the fact that the patient has had a previous transfusion (containing leukocytes) or a previous tissue graft. The immunoglobulins induce platelet aggregation, and

---

*The terms *transplant* and *graft* are used interchangeably.

there is widespread vascular occlusion and necrosis. In clinical practice it is therefore important to test a person who is about to receive a graft for immunoglobulins that are specifically directed against the graft, particularly its major blood group antigens.

Acute Rejection.   Provided preformed immunoglobulins are not present most allogeneic grafts become vascularized. Ten to 14 days later, however, the graft may undergo necrosis and be rejected. This acute rejection is due to an infiltration by sensitized T lymphocytes that are directly cytotoxic to the graft cells.

The application of a second graft from the same donor, or from an animal that is syngeneic, results in an *accelerated graft rejection phenomenon.* The graft no longer becomes vascularized but is rejected in a few days. This action is also mediated by sensitized T lymphocytes. In patients who have had renal grafts and are treated with cytotoxic drugs, periodic phases of acute rejection may occur many months after the surgery. These phases of rejection are partially mediated by T lymphocytes, but humoral antibodies also play a part by causing vascular occlusion. Damage to antibody-coated cells through antibody-dependent cell-mediated cytotoxicity may also play a part.

Chronic Rejection.   This type of response occurs many months or years after the grafting. It has been studied most in renal grafts. Histologically, the reaction is characterized by gradual reduction in the size of the lumens of the vessels due to subendothelial thickening. The reaction is thought to be mediated by humoral mechanisms.

The vigor with which a graft is rejected is related to many factors, including the type of tissue and the amount of transplantation antigens present in the graft but not represented in the host. Some tissues, such as skin, are rapidly rejected and have no clinical application. Kidney grafts, however, have proved very successful. With the heart, the initial results were disappointing, but with the use of better techniques the outlook is far more promising. At Stanford the one year survival is reported to be 68 per cent, while 56 per cent of patients are alive at 5 years.

Various attempts have been made to prolong the life of allografts. These fall under three headings:

1. Tissue Matching.   Tissue matching of donor and recipient at the HLA loci is important. Matching is often only carried out at the HLA-A and HLA-B loci, whereas it is thought that the most important antigens are those related to the HLA-D locus. In practice this matching is more difficult. Hence, it follows that HLA matching between siblings produces good results with grafting, since they are likely to share one haplotype. HLA matching between unrelated subjects is less successful.

2. Immunosuppression.   A variety of immunosuppressive techniques have been used with considerable success, particularly with renal transplantation. Azathioprine (Imuran) and prednisone are the mainstays of therapy.

3. *Antigen-Specific Depression of Allograft Reactivity.*   If the recipient could be made tolerant of the graft's antigens, survival of the graft would be assured without the dangers of inducing generalized immunosuppression by drugs. Experimentally this has been achieved in various ways, but at the present time the techniques have not been applied to humans.

The function of the graft is dependent on the continued survival of its cells and is an example of a *homovital graft.* This contrasts with a *homostatic graft,* in which the cells die but the matrix persists and performs a useful function. The best example of this is a bone graft. The bone cells die, but the matrix remains and is gradually replaced by living bone tissue. The process is called *creeping substitution.* In the meantime, the bone provides valuable support. The cornea and heart valves have also been used as homostatic grafts.

Heterografts (Xenografts)

These are grafts from one individual to another of a different species. In general, vital grafts of this nature are invariably rejected and are not used in clinical practice. With homostatic xenografts the situation is more promising, and the replacement of damaged human heart valves with pig valves is widely used with success.

The Major Histocompatibility Complex in Man

The antigens concerned in the graft rejection are termed the *human leukocyte antigens* (HLA); they are determined by a group of closely linked genes that together constitute the *major histocompatibility complex* (MHC) on the short arm of chromosome 6. The following loci have been identified: HLA-A, HLA-B, HLA-C, HLA-D, and HLA-DR. For each locus there are many alternative alleles, *e.g.,* over 20 at locus HLA-A and over 33 at HLA-B. Since the genes are closely linked, they tend to be inherited as a group on chromosome 6, and an individual inherits one group (called a *haplotype*) from one parent and another haplotype from the other. Hence, a parent shares one haplotype with each of his offspring. With the large number of alternative alleles at so many loci, it is obvious that the chances of any one individual having exactly the same genetic make-up as any other are extremely remote, with the exception of identical twins.

Closely associated with the HLA-DR locus is another that is occupied by the *Ir* (immune response) genes. These code for the immune-associated (Ia) antigens. The immune response genes of an individual are of great importance because they determine to a large extent the way an individual reacts to a particular antigen. Thus, one person may react vigorously in an immunological sense to a particular antigen, whereas another may be a poor responder. The *Ir* genes are difficult to investigate, but since they are so closely associated with the other genes of the major histocompatibility complex, it follows that an individual's mode of immunological response is closely linked to HLA antigens. This is thought to be the explanation of the fact that some diseases tend to be associated with particular HLA antigens. The reason for this is that the pathogenesis of many diseases is so closely linked to the individual's immune response. Nowhere is this more applicable than in the group of autoimmune diseases to be described later in this chapter.

The HLA genes and their associated antigens are of great importance in transplantation medicine, but have probably been evolved for a completely different reason. They are thought to act as markers by which cells can be recognized as self by the individual. Modification of the surface antigens may be the way in which cells are recognized as being abnormal. Thus, virus-infected cells modify the surface HLA antigens and are ultimately destroyed by the T-cell system of the cell-mediated immune response. It is possible that alteration of self-markers is important in other diseases of a degenerate or neoplastic nature. However, it must be admitted that the precise significance of the HLA antigens is poorly understood. It would be convenient to regard them as important in the homeostatic mechanisms that control the development of cancer, but the evidence that cancer is due to a breakdown in immunological homeostasis is not convincing.

Immunological Deficiency Diseases

Primary immunological deficiency diseases are rare, but their existence has strengthened the view that the immune response has two separate components. In one group, the most common of which is congenital sex-linked agammaglobulinemia, there is a failure in the development of the B lymphocytes, and the subjects possess few plasma cells and manufacture little immunoglobulin. They are susceptible to repeated bacterial infections, which usually results in early death. In another group, there is failure of thymic development, and T lymphocytes are absent or abnormal. These individuals suffer from viral, fungal, and acid-fast bacterial infections. They also fail to develop delayed type hypersensitivity. In the most severe type of immunological deficiency disease there is complete failure of both T and B lymphocytes, and life is limited to a year or two.

Acquired immunological deficiency is of much greater practical importance and occurs in generalized lymphoma (particularly Hodgkin's disease), leukemia, and other related conditions. It is also a feature of therapy with cytotoxic drugs and glucocorticoids.

The following steps may be postulated as occurring after the introduction of an antigen: (1) *recognition* of antigen; (2) *processing* of antigen; and (3) *production* of immunoglobulins and immune lymphocytes.

Functional Steps in the Immune Response

Recognition.   A mechanism must exist for recognizing an antigen as foreign. There is good evidence that this recognition mechanism is under genetic control and is determined by genes at the Ir locus. It is believed that the cell that is capable of recognizing antigen and initiating an immune response is morphologically a small lymphocyte. It is evident that the cell must have a memory, because the response to a second injection of antigen is far in excess of that which follows a first encounter.

Processing of Antigen.   Once an antigen is recognized, it appears that its determinants are processed in such a way that the immune response is initiated. There is good evidence that the *macrophage* performs this function and that it processes antigen in such a way that the necessary determinants are presented to lymphocytes. In many instances these lymphocytes are helper T cells. Antigen that is not processed by macrophages appears to stimulate the formation of suppressor T cells. This explains why antigens in a particulate or aggregated form are much more immunogenic than are soluble antigens. As noted previously, T-cell function is not necessary for all types of immune response, and there are certain antigens that appear to act directly on B cells and lead to the formation of immunoglobulins. Such antigens are called T-cell independent.

Production of Antibodies and Reactive Cells.   This final process of the immune response has two components. In the T-cell system immune or sensitized lymphocytes are produced that are capable of reacting with antigen in a number of ways. The cells may be directly cytotoxic by some ill-defined cell-to-cell interaction, or they may produce chemicals described as lymphokines, which have a variety of actions that were described earlier in this chapter. It is not known how many cell types are involved in these various stages or how many functions a particular cell type can perform. It is known that some T cells act as helper cells and promote the immune response, whereas others have the reverse effect and are suppressor T cells.

The other arm of the immune response is responsible for the production of immunoglobulins by B cells, which mature into antibody-producing plasma cells. There is little doubt that in most immune responses T cells are also involved in this process. The helper T cells promote the response, whereas the suppressor T cells inhibit it.

It is evident that our understanding of the immune response is far from complete. Not only are there the various systems for the production of immune lymphocytes or antibodies, but there must be some mechanism for regulating the response, because when the antigenic stimulation is withdrawn, the immune response is turned off. Nevertheless, some memory remains that can be reactivated when next the antigen is encountered.

Lymphocytes play a key role in the immune response, and it is evident that many types exist. Morphologically they appear very similar and cannot be distinguished. It has been found that lymphocyte cell membranes contain markers that can be identified; thus, B cells contain immunoglobulins in their cell membranes. More recently, another series of cell markers has been identified and has been labelled OKT1, OKT2, OKT3, and so forth.* Specific antiserum against these cell markers can be prepared by using the hybridoma technique (page 118). It is now possible to identify the various stages in the development of B and T cells, and in the future the rather nondescript, small round-cell infiltrate of inflammation will no doubt be described in much more exact terms as to precisely which cell is involved. Another application is the typing of the various forms of lymphocytic leukemia and lymphoma.

Theories of Antibody Production

The Instructive Theory

It has been postulated that antigens play an instructive role in antibody production and that the extraordinary specificity of antibodies is related to the antigens acting as molds, or templates, during antibody synthesis. The theory, although superficially satisfying, has many drawbacks. It is believed that the specificity of immunoglobulins is related to their exact chemical structure, which by all current knowledge is determined by the genetic information in the antibody-producing cells. The possibility could be invoked that the complex immunoglobulin molecule could in some way fold itself around the antigen and thereby produce a specific binding site, but there is evidence against this. If specific antibody is so treated that its complex secondary structure is unwound, the antibody specificity is lost. If the molecule is then treated in such a way that its three-dimensional structure is re-formed in the absence of antigen, the specificity returns. It is therefore difficult to evade the conclusion that the specificity of antibodies is determined by their chemical structure, which is itself a reflection of genetic information. One must conclude that the body knows how to make antibodies against an antigen without ever having had prior contact with that antigen!

The Selective Theory

This theory postulates that in the adult there are cells capable of reacting to any nonself antigen that the individual is likely to meet. The antigen selects these cells and stimulates them to divide and mature into either immunoglobulin-producing cells or immune T lymphocytes. Hence, the antigen determines the quantity of antibody produced but not directly its specificity. Since the number of reactive cells increases, it may be assumed that many remain, so that on a second encounter with the same antigen there are more antigen-sensitive cells, and the immune response is correspondingly quicker and of greater magnitude.

This general theory, formulated by Jerne and elaborated by Burnet, provides one explanation of the phenomenon of the specific immunological tolerance that is described below. In its simplest form it is postulated that during the early stages of embryonic development many somatic mutations occur in the immunologically reactive cells. These mutations result in the formation of a whole range of cells that between them contain a number of cells capable of mounting an immune response specific for any antigen that the body may subsequently meet. In the adult, contact with antigen stimu-

---

*Named after the research worker Kung using T cells in the Ortho laboratories.

lates growth of these cells and in this way forms a body of cells, or clone.* As the clone increases in size, antibody production increases in intensity.

It is obvious that if somatic mutation occurs so frequently, cells will be formed that can produce antibodies against all possible antigens, and inevitably some mutations will result in cells capable of forming antibodies against the host's own developing tissues. For instance, as liver cells develop liver antigens, anti-liver antibodies should appear. Since this does not occur in the normal person, there must be some mechanism, activated *during embryonic life,* for the destruction of these harmful *forbidden clones.* Any antigen present in the developing embryo is recognized as self, and at birth there should be no cells present that could mount an immune response against it.

If the selective theory is accepted in principle, it is necessary to understand how the body could contain so many different types of cells, each capable of recognizing a different antigen and producing the appropriate antibody. It has been estimated that there should be 10^8 or more different types of antibody molecules. In the *germ line theory* it is assumed that we inherit all the necessary genetic information for manufacturing this vast number of different antibodies. The information is contained in genes that are separated by introns; each developed cell uses only particular parts of the genetic information, so that only one specific antibody is produced. The alternative theory is that the great diversity of genes is generated by somatic mutation. Possibly both mechanisms are involved, but the controversy remains unsettled.

Specific Immunological Tolerance

The administration of an antigen to an embryo results not in the formation of antibodies but in the acceptance of the foreign substance as "self." This phenomenon of specific immunological tolerance was first noticed by Medawar when embryo mice were injected with donor allogeneic cells, *i.e.,* from a mouse of a different genetic constitution. When the injected embryonic mice were born and reared, it was found that they would accept skin grafts from the same strain as the original donor but not from those of any other strain (Fig. 9–14). The tolerance was therefore specific and was not due to a generalized depression of the immune response.

Specific immunological tolerance to nonliving antigens can also be induced, but it persists only for as long as the antigen remains. Therefore, repeated injections are usually required. Tolerance can be induced in adult animals, but with difficulty. Usually *large doses of antigen* must be given (*high-zone tolerance*), and the lymphoreticular system must first be damaged either by the administration of cytotoxic drugs or by ionizing radiation. When antibody formation is temporarily in abeyance, it seems that the regeneration of the immunologically competent cells in the presence of antigen can lead to tolerance. Somewhat surprisingly, repeated administration of *small doses* of antigen can also lead to tolerance (*low-zone tolerance*). Tolerance is easier to induce with soluble antigens than with those in particulate form. This is probably because soluble antigens are less likely to be taken up by macrophages before being presented to the lymphocytes.

The precise explanation of tolerance is not known. The original theory of *clonal deletion* proposed by Burnett supposes that potentially reactive cells are physically eliminated. This may well be the explanation of tolerance that develops during embryonic life. A modification of this theory, *the clonal anergy theory,* supposes that the potentially reactive cells are not physically

---

*A clone is a group of cells of like hereditary constitution that has been produced asexually from a single cell. The word is derived from the Greek *klon,* meaning a cutting used for propagation.

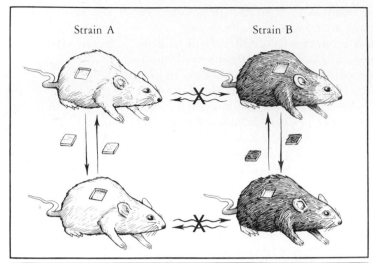

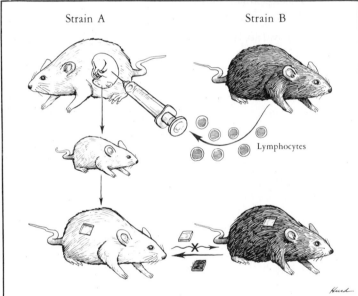

Figure 9–14. Representation of Medawar's experiment illustrating the fetal induction of tolerance in the mouse. Note that skin grafts can be exchanged between any two untreated mice of strain A or strain B but cannot be exchanged between mice of strain A and strain B. Injection of strain B cells into fetal strain A mice induces tolerance. If the cells consist of adult lymphocytes (immunologically competent cells), they may react against the host. This is called a *graft versus host* (GVH) reaction. If it is severe enough the baby mice are stunted and may die. Such a condition is called *runt disease.* The severity of the GVH reaction depends on the number and strength of tissue antigens present in the host (*i.e.,* strain A) and not present in the donor lymphocytes. (From Bellanti, J. A.: Immunology. Philadelphia, W. B. Saunders Company, 1971.)

destroyed but are in some way inactivated. Other mechanisms have also been proposed. Soluble antigen appears to lead to the formation of the suppressor T cells without stimulating helper T cells. In low-zone tolerance it is thought that the overproduction of suppressor cells leads to tolerance. With high-zone tolerance it is felt that helper T cell function is depressed. There seems little doubt that it is easier to suppress T function than B function, and in tolerant animals B cells may be present that are capable of reacting against a particular antigen if the necessary signal is given to them. Such a signal is not provided if T-cell function is defective.

It is evident that there are many possible mechanisms in the production of specific immunological tolerance, and probably each plays a part under particular circumstances. An understanding of tolerance is important because if there is a breakdown in the mechanism autoantibodies can be produced and disease may follow. This subject, autoimmunity, will be discussed in the next section.

AUTOIMMUNITY   Although it is evident that under normal conditions the body does not make antibodies against its own tissues, the mechanisms that prevent their formation may occasionally break down.

In theory, antibodies could be made against the individual's own tissues (*autoantibodies*) under three circumstances:

1. **Alteration in Antigenicity of Tissue Proteins.** This may be due to either of the following:

(a) Degenerative Lesions. Following necrosis of tissue, such as in skin burns, antibodies may be produced to a slightly altered skin protein. These antibodies are an effect of the disease and not its cause. It has been suggested that autoantibody formation plays a part in the normal elimination of damaged tissue or altered tissue proteins.

Autoantibodies could also be produced against a specific tissue haptenic grouping if the carrier protein is altered in some way — possibly by a degenerative process or owing to the effect of an infection. The antibodies would be specific for the tissue haptens and could in theory cause damage. Possibly, rheumatic heart disease is produced by this mechanism.

(b) Attachment of Hapten. With a condition such as allergic contact dermatitis, the antibodies are directed more specifically against the hapten than against the normal skin.

2. **Release of a Previously Isolated Antigen.** It is possible that some tissue antigens are anatomically isolated from the immunologically competent cells and are therefore not recognized as "self." When antigens are released into the tissues following injury or disease, autoantibodies are formed. It has been postulated that thyroglobulin in the thyroid acini is one such substance and that antibodies to it could damage the thyroid cells and lead to Hashimoto's disease (Chapter 39). The evidence is not convincing.

3. **Altered Reactivity of the Immune Mechanism.** If a disease process causes a *loss of tolerance,* self proteins would be regarded as foreign, and an immune response would be evoked. This occurs in some diseases of the lymphoreticular system. Autohemolysins are sometimes produced, causing a hemolytic anemia — a good example of a condition caused by an autoantibody.

The injection into an animal of normal syngeneic or allogeneic tissue mixed with Freund's adjuvant may result in a disease of the respective organ, which is presumed to be due to autoantibody production. If thyroid tissue is used, a condition resembling Hashimoto's disease is produced. If brain tissue is used, a cell-mediated allergic encephalomyelitis results. This bears considerable resemblance to the human disease that may follow administration of rabies vaccine, which itself contains rabbit spinal-cord tissue (Chapter 12).

It may be postulated that an autoimmune response may be cell-mediated or may result in the formation of immunoglobulins. The immunoglobulins might be of any class and of one of two types: (1) *Organ-specific immunoglobulins,* whose specificity is directed against a determinant present in one organ, *e.g.,* hemolysins and antithyroid antibodies; or (2) *non–organ-specific antibodies,* which are exemplified by those directed against DNA (in systemic lupus erythematosus), mitochondria, and immunoglobulin determinants (rheumatoid factor) (Fig. 9–15).

Antibodies may directly attack a tissue and cause damage. The immunoglobulins acquire destructive properties by activating complement, *e.g.,* hemolysins damage red cells, which results in acute hemolytic anemia. Antibody-dependent cell-mediated cytotoxicity is another possible mechanism. Immune T lymphocytes can also destroy cells, such as in allergic encephalomyelitis. Autoantibodies can also combine with antigen and form

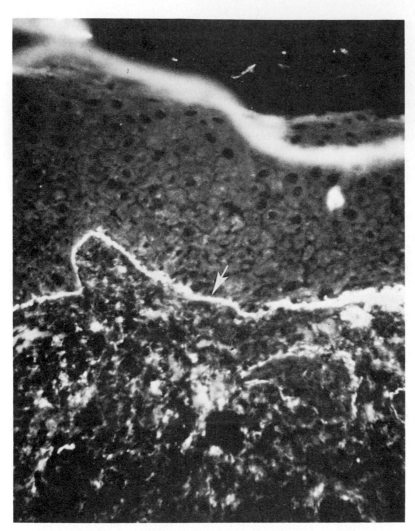

Figure 9–15. Deposition of IgG antibody in the basement membrane zone of skin in bullous pemphigoid. Bullous pemphigoid is a skin disease characterized by the formation of blisters, either vesicles or bullae (Chapter 41). IgG anti–basement membrane antibodies are present in the blood and are deposited in the basement membrane zone of skin and mucous membranes. A frozen section of skin from a patient with this disease was treated with fluorescein-labelled antihuman IgG and examined microscopically under ultraviolet light. The fluorescein glows brightly and acts as a stain for IgG. The linear staining of the basement membrane, indicated by the arrow, is characteristic of this disease and is useful as a diagnostic test. It is not known whether the skin lesions are caused by the deposition of antibody. Possibly, the skin is damaged by some other mechanism and the IgG deposition is a secondary incidental event.

The labelled antihuman IgG used in this test is obtained by immunizing an animal with human IgG. The animal is bled, and the antibody is purified. Attachment of fluorescein to the molecule is performed chemically.

damaging *antigen-antibody complexes.* The lesions of this immune-complex disease can resemble serum sickness if acute, but if the process is chronic, the kidney is the organ most often affected, and glomerulonephritis results. Diseases in which the major lesions are caused by an immune mechanism may justifiably be called autoimmune diseases. However, it must be stressed that the autoimmunity merely provides a mechanism in the pathogenesis of a disease. It does not explain the cause, which, as noted below, may be inherited or acquired.

Etiology of Immunologically Mediated Diseases

1. **Genetic Factors.** There is a definite tendency for some autoimmune diseases (*e.g.,* systemic lupus erythematosus and rheumatoid arthritis) to be familial.

2. **Acquired Factors.** Some extrinsic factors are known to precipitate an autoimmune process. Certain drugs and sunlight can precipitate the onset of lupus erythematosus. Mycoplasmal pneumonia is sometimes complicated by an autoimmune hemolytic anemia. When the cause of a disease is clearly established — as in smallpox — the immunologically mediated manifestations of the disease, such as the skin eruption, are readily accepted as part of the entire condition. It is when the cause of a disease is not known, such as with rheumatoid arthritis, that emphasis is given to the autoimmune component of the illness. The label "autoimmune disease" should not delude one

into thinking that one knows the cause of the disease; only part of the pathogenesis has been described.

SUMMARY

When antigen gains access to the tissues of the body, a complex series of events occurs. It is taken up by the phagocytic cells of the reticuloendothelial system, and changes occur in the lymphoid cells that result in a cell-mediated T-cell response or the formation of immunoglobulins by the B-cell system.

The relationship of this immune response to hypersensitivity and of immunity to infection is complex.

With simple protein antigens, or with haptens that combine with body proteins, immunoglobulins are produced. If the antigen is a bacterial toxin or a component of a bacterium, the antibody can afford immunity to infection. Sometimes the immunoglobulins are of such a type (IgE in humans) that they sensitize the cells of the body to the action of antigens, which in turn mediates hypersensitivity of the anaphylactic type. Sometimes antibodies form damaging complexes with antigen, leading to a nonspecific injury to various parts of the body, commonly the kidney and blood vessels. This is immune-complex disease, or type III hypersensitivity. Occasionally antibodies are specific for a particular tissue, as when hemolysins are formed. This is the type II reaction.

When the body is invaded by foreign living cells, the cell-mediated immune response is also stimulated. Immune or sensitized lymphocytes are formed, which, when confronted with the appropriate antigen, respond in a number of ways. They may have a direct cytotoxic effect or lead to the release of a variety of lymphokines. These have many effects; in particular, they recruit macrophages and enhance the inflammatory response. The cell-mediated immune response plays a big part in the rejection of foreign grafts and also causes damage to the skin in acute allergic contact dermatitis. Similarly, it plays a big part in the removal of invading bacteria, particularly those that multiply intracellularly. The role of type IV hypersensitivity is more difficult to understand, since it is a factor in prolonging the effect of some infections, which thereby become chronic. It must be admitted that the precise relationship between immunity and hypersensitivity in relation to infection is not clearly understood.

A response that eliminates foreign grafts is of no obvious evolutionary advantage. It has been suggested that the immune response, particularly the cell-mediated component, has evolved as a mechanism for eliminating abnormal cells that have been produced in the body as a result of either damage or genetic change. This scrutinizing or surveillant action of the lymphocytes may be an important homeostatic mechanism by which damaged or neoplastic cells are destroyed and eliminated (Chapter 17). It is becoming clear that the histocompatibility antigens play an important role in self-recognition and are involved in many ways in the immune response to foreign antigens. Closely associated with them are the genes that control the individual's immune response.

Review Questions

1. Describe what is meant by atopy. Under what circumstances is an atopic person liable to react adversely to medical treatment?

2. Describe the possible functions of a cell that morphologically resembles a small lymphocyte.

3. Compare type I hypersensitivity with type IV hypersensitivity with respect to the following:
   (a) antibodies involved
   (b) means of passive transfer to another individual
   (c) detection by skin testing

4. Describe the pathogenesis of the various hypersensitivity reactions that can follow the injection of penicillin.

5. A newborn infant is found to have no thymus. Predict what might happen if
     (a) he is given no treatment
     (b) he is injected with live syngeneic small lymphocytes from his identical twin
     (c) he is injected with live allogeneic small lymphocytes from a parent

6. Compare and contrast antitoxins with antibacterial antibodies with respect to their:
     (a) chemical properties
     (b) *in vitro* reactions with antigen
     (c) ability to prevent infection
     (d) ability to provide immunity to disease

Selected Readings

Austen, W. G.: Heart transplantation after ten years. New England Journal of Medicine, 298:682–684, 1978.

Bellanti, J. A.: Immunology II. Philadelphia, W. B. Saunders Company, 1978.

Benacerraf, B., and Katz, D. H.: The histocompatibility-linked immune response genes. Advances in Cancer Research, 21:121–173, 1975.

Bigley, N. J.: Immunological Fundamentals. Chicago, Year Book Medical Publishers, 1975. An elementary introduction to the subject in 225 pages.

Bloom, B. R.: In vitro methods in cell-mediated immunity in man. New England Journal of Medicine. 284:1212–1213, 1971.

Bodmer, W. F., Dick, M. H., Joysey, V. C., et al.: The HLA system. British Medical Bulletin, 34:213–316, 1978.

David, J. R.: Lymphocyte mediators and cellular hypersensitivity. New England Journal of Medicine, 288:143–149, 1973.

Good, R. A., and Fisher, D. W. (Eds.): Immunobiology. Stamford, Conn., Sinauer Associates, 1971. A multi-author textbook in 305 pages in which the fundamentals of immunology are presented by graphic style by many of the best-known immunologists.

Haurowitz, F.: The evolution of selective and instructive theories of antibody formation. Cold Spring Harbor Symposia on Quantitative Biology, 32:559–567, 1967.

Hayward, A. R.: Immunodeficiency. London, Arnold, 1977, 125 pages.

Hitzig, W. H.: Congenital immunodeficiency diseases: pathophysiology, clinical appearance and treatment. Pathobiology Annual, 6:163–201, 1976.

Humphrey, J. H., and White, R. G.: Immunology for Students of Medicine. 3rd ed. Oxford, Blackwell Scientific Publications Ltd. 1970, 757 pp.

Leading Article: Immunosuppression and malignancy. British Medical Journal, 3:713–714, 1972.

Leading Article: Lymphokines. Lancet, 1:1490–1491, 1973.

Leading Article: Transfer factor. Lancet, 2:79–81, 1973.

Leading Article: Immunological tolerance. Lancet, 1:555–556, 1975.

Leading Article: Lymphokines: an increasing repertoire. British Medical Journal, 1:62, 1978.

Leading Article: Cardiac transplantation. Lancet, 1:687–688, 1980.

Leading Article: Treatment of anaphylactic shock. British Medical Journal, 282:1011–1012, 1981.

Lepow, I. H., and Rosen, F. S.: Pathways to the complement system. New England Journal of Medicine, 286:942–943, 1972.

Ogra, P. L., and Karzon, D. T.: The role of immunoglobulins in the mechanism of mucosal immunity to virus infections. Pediatric Clinics of North America, 17:385–400, 1970.

Orange, R. P., and Austen, K. F.: Chemical mediators of immediate hypersensitivity. Hospital Practice, 6(1):79–89, 1971.

Patterson, R., Zeiss, C. R., and Kelly, J. F.: Classification of hypersensitivity reactions. New England Journal of Medicine, 295:277–279, 1976.

Roitt, I. M.: Essential Immunology. 4th ed. Oxford, Blackwell, 1980, 358 pp.

Rosenberg, L. E., and Kidd, K. K.: HLA and disease susceptibility: a primer. New England Journal of Medicine, 297:1060–1062, 1977.

Ruddy, S., Gigli, I., and Austen, K. F.: The complement system in man. New England Journal of Medicine, 287:489–495; 545–549; 592–596; 642–646, 1972.

Tomasi, T. B.: Secretory immunoglobulins. New England Journal of Medicine, 287:500, 1972.

Turk, J. L.: Delayed Hypersensitivity. 2nd ed. Amsterdam, North Holland, 1975.

Waldman, R. H.: Immune mechanisms on secretory surface. Postgraduate Medicine, 50:78–82, 1971.

Zuckerman, S. H., and Douglas, S. D.: The lymphocyte plasma membrane: markers, receptors, and determinants. Pathobiology Annual, 6:119–162, 1976.

Some Bacterial Infections — Pyogenic, Anaerobic, Mycobacterial, and Spirochetal

CHAPTER 10

After studying this chapter the student should be able to:

- Describe the characteristics of the following organisms and the common diseases caused by them: staphylococci, streptococci, pneumococci, gonococci, and meningococci.
- Classify the gram-negative intestinal bacilli and list the types of infection they produce.
- Describe the main features of diphtheria and compare them with a disease caused by an invasive organism.
- Compare and contrast gas gangrene with tetanus.
- Discuss the prophylaxis of tetanus in relation to the immune state of the patient.
- Describe the properties of *Mycobacterium tuberculosis* and the tissue reaction to the organism.
- Differentiate between the following types of tuberculosis: (a) infection caused by the bovine and the human strains; (b) childhood and adult types of infection.
- Describe the Koch phenomenon.
- List the factors that predispose to tuberculosis.
- Differentiate between lepromatous and tuberculoid leprosy with respect to: (a) tissue reaction, (b) the immune state, (c) the number of bacilli present in the lesions, and (d) clinical features.
- Describe three diseases caused by organisms of the genus *Borrelia*.
- Outline the sources of infection and the clinical features of human leptospirosis.
- Describe the three stages of syphilis and relate the gross findings to: (a) the pathogenesis of the disease, (b) the number of organisms present in the lesions, and (c) the diagnosis of the disease.

PYOGENIC INFECTIONS

Organisms that cause infection leading to suppurative inflammation are termed *pyogenic.* Important examples of such organisms are staphylococci, streptococci, pneumococci, gonococci, meningococci, and the coliform group of bacteria. The pathological effects of these bacteria are all similar. There is an acute inflammatory response culminating in a massive infiltration of polymorphs. If the inflammation succeeds in destroying the organism, the lesion abates. If the organisms gain the upper hand, the condition proceeds to tissue destruction and suppuration. The abscess so formed may burst spontaneously onto a free surface or may be drained surgically. The destroyed tissue is ultimately replaced by regeneration or repair. Sometimes, if the body's resistance is poor or if the organism is extremely virulent, there may be rapid local spread of infection and generalized dissemination. Fatal septicemia or pyemia is the result. Not infrequently, infection with pyogenic organisms results in chronic suppurative inflammation. Indeed, these organisms are responsible for much of the chronic bacterial inflammation that plays such an important role in everyday clinical practice.

Although the organisms termed pyogenic bacteria commonly produce suppurative inflammation, there are some circumstances in which infection leads to a different type of response. Hence, the lesions produced by each type of organism will be considered separately.

INFECTIONS PRODUCED BY INDIVIDUAL ORGANISMS

Staphylococcal Infections

Staphylococci are gram-positive cocci that tend to grow in clusters. They are common inhabitants of the skin and can be divided into two groups:

Staphylococcus albus.   This organism, which is so named because of the white appearance of its colonies, is almost nonpathogenic and a normal member of the skin's flora. It occasionally produces infection under unusual circumstances, such as with mainline drug abusers in whom it causes endocarditis (Chapter 28).

Staphylococcus aureus.   This organism is found on the skin of some normal people, particularly those who live in crowded communities such as those of hospitals. The reservoir of pathogenic staphylococci is in the anterior part of the nose. About 40 per cent of healthy adults are nasal carriers, but the figure may rise to over 70 per cent in a hospital population. From the nose, the organisms are readily transferred to the skin, particularly the hands. Here the organisms can multiply and spread to other objects and to other people.

Lesions Produced by Staphylococcus aureus

The typical staphylococcal lesion is a circumscribed area of inflammation with suppuration. Skin lesions are frequent and include stitch abscesses, boils, carbuncles, paronychia (inflammation of the nail fold), and impetigo (Fig. 10–1).

In *impetigo* the organisms invade the superficial layers of the skin and produce characteristic subcorneal bullae and pustules. This is common on the face in children. The blisters soon rupture and become covered by a honey-colored crust.

Infection of the hair follicles is common; the type of lesion produced depends upon how deeply the organisms penetrate. Since pus is produced, the term *pyoderma* is employed to describe this whole group of skin diseases. In *superficial folliculitis* numerous small pustules are seen at the openings of adjacent hair follicles. The face is a common site for this eruption to occur.

A more destructive and severe infection of the hair follicle is the *boil*, or *furuncle;* when pus is produced, it is discharged from a single opening. A *stye* is a particular type of boil in which an eyelash is implicated. Boils are particularly common in the axillae and on the back of the neck (Chapter 6).

In a *carbuncle* the staphylococcal infection extends to the underlying fatty subcutaneous tissue and spreads laterally. The subcutaneous tissue is divided into compartments by fibrous septa, which extend from the deep fascia to the dermis. It therefore follows that subcutaneous infections tend to be loculated, with each individual abscess bursting to the surface through its own hair follicle orifice. Thus, a carbuncle has multiple heads, and extensive areas of skin become undermined and are eventually sloughed off.

Staphylococci are the commonest cause of wound infection, usually the result of hospital cross-infection. Other important staphylococcal infections are bronchopneumonia, enterocolitis, and osteomyelitis, all of which are discussed elsewhere in this text. Staphylococcal infections sometimes involve veins (a condition called *phlebitis),* and this leads to thrombosis. If the

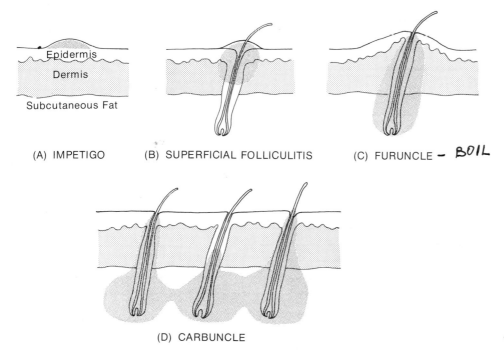

Epidermis
Dermis
Subcutaneous Fat

(A) IMPETIGO   (B) SUPERFICIAL FOLLICULITIS   (C) FURUNCLE – BOIL

(D) CARBUNCLE

Figure 10–1. Diagram illustrating some staphylococcal infections of the skin. *A, Impetigo.* The infection is very superficial, and a pustule forms beneath the stratum corneum of the epidermis. *B, Superficial folliculitis.* The suppurative inflammation involves the superficial part of a hair follicle. Clinically this appears as a small pustule; the condition is called impetigo of Bockhart. *C, Furuncle, or Boil.* The infection involves an entire hair follicle, and the inflammatory edema produces a considerable swelling, which can be 1 cm or more in diameter. Nevertheless, a boil has one head only. *D, Carbuncle.* The infection involves the subcutaneous tissues and loculated pockets of pus are present. These pockets are formed between fibrous septae, which are not shown in the diagram. Note the multiple heads through which pus can be discharged. (Drawing by Margot Mackay, Department of Art as Applied to Medicine, University of Toronto.)

thrombus is invaded by the organisms, it tends to soften and break off, forming septic emboli. This condition is called *pyemia* and is characterized by multiple pyemic abscesses and septic infarcts (Chapter 20).

Although staphylococci are typically invasive organisms, some strains produce toxins that have important effects. Three conditions should be noted:

Staphylococcal Toxins

Staphylococcal Food Poisoning. This is due to ingestion of preformed heat-stable enterotoxin formed by organisms growing in food products (Chapter 6).

The Scalded Skin Syndrome. Certain strains of staphylococci produce an epidermolytic toxin (exfoliatin), and when this organism affects young babies there is extensive shedding of the superficial layers of the skin so that the child appears to have been extensively scalded.

Toxic Shock Syndrome. Another epidermal toxin is produced by certain staphylococci. Infections by these organisms may be accompanied by a severe illness — high fever, generalized reddening of the skin, conjunctival hyperemia, watery diarrhea, hypovolemia, and renal failure. The syndrome was first described in children; in those who recover there is extensive desquamation of the affected skin and peeling of the palms and soles during convalescence. This toxic shock syndrome has recently been described in previously healthy young women who use particular types of tampons during menstruation. Characteristically there is a sudden onset of high fever, diarrhea, and other symptoms noted above. The pathogenesis is thought to be that the staphylococci multiply in the tampon and produce toxin, which after absorption causes the syndrome.

Streptococcal Infections

Streptococci are gram-positive organisms that tend to grow in chains, particularly in a fluid culture.

Types of Streptococci

The four major groups are recognized by the type of colony produced on blood agar:

1. *Alpha-hemolytic streptococci,* also called *Streptococcus viridans,* grow on a blood-agar plate as small colonies that produce a greenish pigmentation with an ill-defined surrounding narrow zone of partial hemolysis. Two important infections produced by this group of organisms are on the one hand the relatively trivial apical infections of teeth and on the other its lethal complication, subacute bacterial endocarditis (Chapter 28).

2. *Beta-hemolytic streptococci* produce a sharply demarcated zone of complete hemolysis on the agar plate. Many groups have been defined. Group A beta-hemolytic streptococcus is termed *Streptococcus pyogenes* and is the common human pathogen; it causes over 90 per cent of human streptococcal infections. Other groups produce disease in animals, such as bovine mastitis, in which the udder is infected. These organisms may be present in milk but are harmless to humans. Group B streptococcus is a common commensal in the female genitourinary tract and can cause *severe perinatal infections.* The manifestations are those of respiratory distress with shock, septicemia, and meningitis. Group C and Group G streptococci are occasional causes of *wound infection* and *puerperal sepsis.*

3. *Nonhemolytic streptococci* are also called *enterococci,* since they commonly occur in the gut.

4. *Anaerobic streptococci* are a separate group that is considered later.

Lesions Produced by Streptococcus pyogenes

The typical streptococcal lesion is a spreading infection of the connective tissues — a condition called *cellulitis.* Abscesses occur later than in staphylococcal infections, and the pus tends to be watery and often blood-stained. Streptococci are occasional causes of wound infection and are also responsible for a number of cases of *impetigo. Erysipelas* is a classic streptococcal lesion and consists of a spreading infection in the dermis. It affects the face and is seen as a raised, bright red plaque with a sharply defined edge that steadily advances.

Streptococci are important causes of *tonsillitis* and *pharyngitis.* Infection can spread to the middle ear to produce *otitis media* and down the tracheobronchial tree to lead to *bronchopneumonia.*

In days gone by, streptococcal infections of the uterus following labor were common *(puerperal sepsis).* Before the introduction of aseptic techniques and chemotherapy, this was one of the major causes of death following childbirth.

Some streptococci produce an *erythrogenic toxin,* which is absorbed into the blood and produces a punctate erythematous rash termed *scarlet fever.* The skin lesions are sterile, since they are produced entirely by this exotoxin. The usual streptococcal infection leading to scarlet fever is a sore throat.

Two other important diseases associated with streptococcal infections are *acute rheumatic fever* and *acute glomerulonephritis.* Both are thought to be related to the development of hypersensitivity and to be manifestations of immune-complex reactions (Chapter 9).

Pneumococcal Infections

Pneumococci closely resemble streptococci but have a well-defined capsule and tend to occur in pairs. The organism is a common commensal of the throat; about 80 different serotypes are known. A few of these types are highly virulent and can cause infection in healthy individuals. The organisms penetrate the defenses of the respiratory tract, invade the lung, and cause *lobar pneumonia*. This is accompanied by a septicemia that at times is complicated by metastatic lesions such as meningitis. The other category of pneumococci tends to be relatively avirulent but can act as secondary invaders causing *bronchopneumonia* either in elderly debilitated patients or in persons who have had a previous virus infection (Chapter 30).

The gonococcus is a gram-negative diplococcus whose only known host is man. The organism is generally transmitted by sexual intercourse and causes the important venereal disease *gonorrhea*. In the male, an *acute urethritis* appears 2 to 8 days after infection. A purulent penile discharge is the main symptom and is combined with difficulty and pain on passing urine. A smear of the pus on a glass slide when stained by Gram's method reveals typical *intracellular diplococci*. Diagnosis is confirmed by culture of the organism on special media. If treated correctly — usually with penicillin — the disease clears up rapidly. Untreated, the infection can spread to involve the seminal vesicles and epididymis. Chronic infection and its attendant fibrosis is a well-known cause of *urethral stricture*.

Gonococcal Infections

In the female, gonorrhea causes acute urethritis and cervicitis, but symptoms are frequently ignored or absent, and the infection goes unnoticed. These asymptomatic females are the main reservoir of gonorrhea in our society. Spread to involve the fallopian tubes leads to *acute salpingitis* and associated peritonitis. This event can present as an acute surgical abdominal emergency; the patient presents with abdominal pain and fever. Chronic gonococcal infection is a very common cause of *pelvic inflammatory disease (PID)* and may follow an acute attack or appear *de novo*. Salpingitis leads to fibrosis of the fallopian tube, which is an important cause of *sterility* in the female.

When the sulfonamides, and later the antibiotics, were introduced it was hoped that gonorrhea could be eliminated from our society, because the organism was very sensitive to these agents. Unfortunately, these hopes have not been fulfilled. Some cases are missed and continue to provide a source of infection. At the same time, drug-resistant strains of the gonococcus have evolved. The control of gonorrhea is an important public health function, and a vital aspect of this is the tracing of patient contacts. As with syphilis, the source of infection is another human being. There can never be an isolated case of either of these venereal diseases!

Two nonvenereal infections with the gonococcus are worthy of note:

Acute Vulvovaginitis.   This can occur in epidemic form in girls' schools and is transmitted by towels and communally used clothing. This infection does not occur after puberty, because the hormonal activity associated with sexual maturity leads to an acid pH in the vagina, and this acts as an efficient bactericidal chemical barrier.

Gonococcal Conjunctivitis and Ophthalmitis.   Infection of the baby's conjunctiva during delivery results in an acute purulent conjunctivitis. Corneal involvement with ulceration and even perforation is a dreaded complication, since it leads to blindness. This disease was said to be responsible for about 50 per cent of blindness in children before effective prophylaxis abolished it. As a routine, a drop of 1 per cent silver nitrate is placed in each conjunctival sac of a newborn child.

Gonococcal conjunctivitis is occasionally seen in adults when pus from a urethral discharge is transmitted to the eyes, generally by the patient's own hands.

The introduction of the gonococci usually leads to a local infection, but the invasive potential of the organisms should not be forgotten. Bacteremia can result in metastatic lesions, of which acute septic arthritis is the most common. Gonococcal septicemia has recently become an important complication. It usually affects young women, and its onset is triggered by a menstrual period. The fever, arthralgia (pain in the joints), and the development of skin lesions due to vasculitis are the outstanding symptoms of the condition (Fig. 10–2).

Meningococcal Infections

The meningococcus closely resembles the gonococcus morphologically and is a normal commensal of the nasopharynx. The first encounter with the organism causes an inconsequential infection in most individuals, but occasionally the organism spreads to produce a septicemia; finally, it settles in the subarachnoid space to cause *meningitis*. Septicemia is usually accompanied by a petechial skin rash, which gives the disease its alternative name of "spotted fever." Meningitis usually occurs in those individuals who lack immunity (usually children), but it also may appear in susceptible adults. The disease occasionally becomes epidemic when large numbers of adults are crowded together in confined quarters, such as in army barracks.

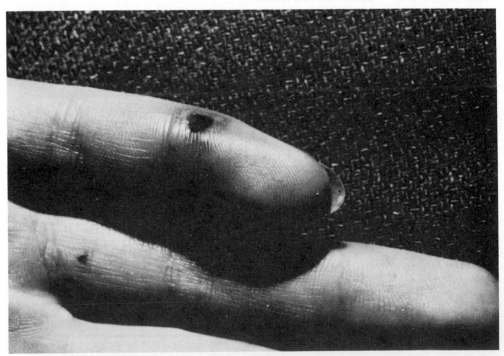

Figure 10–2. Gonococcal septicemia. The patient was a 24-year-old woman who complained of pain that flitted from one joint to another (polyarthralgia) and had been present for about five days. The pain dated from the onset of her last menstrual period. Pain and discomfort were particularly marked in the right knee; on examination, this joint was shown to be swollen and somewhat tender. A day or two after the onset of her arthralgia, she noted a rash that consisted of scattered lesions on the distal part of her arms and legs. Some of these lesions were small erythematous papules, but others were enlarged and developed hemorrhagic pustules in their centers. The figure shows one of these lesions on a finger. During the course of the disease the patient felt unwell, lost her appetite, and developed a mild fever every evening. A biopsy of one of the skin lesions showed an acute vasculitis. This finding, together with the history and clinical features, strongly suggested a diagnosis of gonococcal septicemia. A slight vaginal discharge was noted. A swab of the cervix subsequently grew gonococci. Penicillin therapy was started, and an uninterrupted recovery ensued.

The patient had been on a holiday two weeks before the onset of the illness. During that time she had had intercourse with a new acquaintance. Prior to that she was not aware of having had intercourse with anyone who had any discharge.

This is a large group of rod-shaped bacteria; the pus-producing members include *Escherichia coli*, *Proteus* species, and *Pseudomonas aeruginosa* (also called *Pseudomonas pyocyanea*). The organisms, commonly grouped as the "coliforms," are normal commensals of the lower small intestine and the colon, where, with the exception of certain enteropathic strains considered in Chapter 32, they cause no damage; indeed, their presence is beneficial. Once outside the confines of the gut, they cause infection with suppuration. They are always predominant in infective lesions derived from the bowel contents, *e.g.*, appendicitis and generalized peritonitis following perforation of the gut. Furthermore, the coliforms are the commonest agent in *urinary-tract infections*, reaching the kidney as part of a normal bacteremia from the colon, or else being introduced into the bladder by catheterization. The coliform organisms are sometimes troublesome causes of *wound infection* in hospitals. Not infrequently they cause *bronchopneumonia* and *middle-ear infection*. Septicemia may complicate any of these infections and is a potent factor in inducing shock (Chapter 21). The common pyogenic infections are summarized in Table 10–1.

Infections with Gram-negative Intestinal Bacilli

Salmonella and *Shigella* are important members of the gram-negative intestinal bacilli, and their pathogenic activity is largely confined to the intestinal tract. *Food poisoning* and *bacillary dysentery* are described in Chapter 32. *Typhoid fever* is considered in Chapter 6.

Diphtheria is an acute infectious disease caused by *Corynebacterium diphtheriae*. This organism is a gram-positive curved bacillus that produces characteristic colonies on special growth media. Spread is by inhalation of

Diphtheria

TABLE 10–1. COMMON PYOGENIC INFECTIONS

ORGANISM	SOURCE OF INFECTION	COMMON INFECTIONS
Staphylococcus *Staphylococcus aureus*	Skin of carrier or patient	Wound and skin infections; pyemia; pneumonia; osteomyelitis
Staphylococcus albus	Normal flora of skin	Mild wound infections; endocarditis
Streptococcus *Streptococcus pyogenes*	Throat of carrier or patient	Throat infections; wound infections; pneumonia
Streptococcus viridans	Normal flora of mouth	Apical tooth infection; endocarditis
Nonhemolytic streptococci (enterococci)	Normal flora of intestine	Wound infections; urinary tract infections; peritonitis
Pneumococcus	Normal flora of nose and throat; carriers	Pneumonia; meningitis
Gonococcus	Patients with chronic genital infection	Genital tract infections; gonococcal conjunctivitis; and ophthalmitis
Meningococcus	Normal flora of nose and throat; carriers	Meningitis

Gram-negative intestinal bacillus
  Escherichia coli
  Proteus species
  Pseudomonas aeruginosa
	Normal flora of intestine; fomites	Wound infections; urinary tract infections; peritonitis; pneumonia

droplets or airborne particles from an active case or a carrier. Generally the organism settles on the tonsils, adjacent soft palate, or nasopharynx; less commonly affected are the nose and larynx. The bacteria multiply on the surface, and after an incubation period of 1 to 7 days there are sufficient organisms present to produce enough of their powerful exotoxin to cause the epithelium to undergo necrosis. There is a severe underlying inflammatory reaction so that fibrin and neutrophils are added to the necrotic tissues to form the characteristic gray, tough, adherent *pseudomembrane*. Forcible attempts to remove this membrane lead to bleeding. This is in contradistinction to the exudate of acute streptococcal sore throat or of a *Candida* infection, which can easily be removed. Of interest is the origin of the term diphtheria—it is derived from a Greek word meaning skin or hide.

Clinically, the patient with diphtheria complains of a sore throat, and tender enlarged regional lymph nodes may be felt. If the larynx is involved there may be sufficient edema to cause respiratory difficulty; partial detachment of the diphtheritic membrane can add to this serious complication. Fever, malaise, and a neutrophil leukocytosis are present.

It must be stressed that the diphtheria bacilli do not invade the tissues, but their exotoxin produces damage not only locally but also to other tissues, which it reaches via the bloodstream. The toxin damages the myocardium and causes an acute toxic myocarditis. When clinically evident this has a poor prognosis. Damage to the nervous system becomes manifest at any time up to 8 weeks after the onset of the disease. Paralysis of the soft palate and eye muscles and a widespread peripheral neuritis are its usual manifestations.

After recovery from diphtheria the subject has sufficient antitoxic immunity to prevent reinfection (Chapter 9). Nevertheless, the throat (or other site) may still harbor *C. diphtheriae.* Such a person is immune to diphtheria but is a carrier of the organism and can infect other people.

Immunity to diphtheria can be assessed by performing the *Schick test,* in which a minute amount of diphtheria toxin is injected into the skin and the effect observed over the next week. If an acute inflammatory reaction ensues, it means that the subject has no antitoxins and is therefore susceptible to diphtheria. A negative reaction implies immunity.

Diphtheria was at one time common in Europe and North America, particularly in children, but since the introduction of mass immunization with toxoid it is now rare. However, the disease is not uncommon in the developing countries, and even in North America small outbreaks still occur. This emphasizes the necessity for continuing the immunization program.

ANAEROBIC INFECTIONS

The Clostridia comprise a group of organisms that are normal commensals of the intestine, form spores that are extremely resistant to destruction, and grow only in the absence of oxygen. The strict anaerobic requirement for growth makes laboratory isolation difficult and explains the curious circumstances under which these bacilli cause human disease. *Clostridium botulinum* has already been described in Chapter 6. This section deals with the clostridia that cause gas gangrene as well as *Clostridium tetani,* which causes tetanus.

Clostridial Infections

Gas Gangrene

Gas gangrene follows the contamination of a wound with spores of the pathogenic clostridia. Considering the ubiquitous presence of these spores and the rarity of gas gangrene, it is evident that a healthy wound that is contaminated does not develop infection. The essential factor necessary for spore germination is a reduced oxygen tension. This is present in a severely lacerated wound that contains dead tissue — particularly dead muscle that has lost its blood supply. The presence of soil in a wound is particularly dangerous, because the calcium salts in it may lead to considerable tissue necrosis. Any coincidental infection by one of the aerobic pyogenic organisms, such as staphylococci or streptococci, serves to augment the anaerobic conditions. Most examples of gas gangrene are exogenous in origin, and are due to the gross contamination of a severely lacerated dirty wound. Gas gangrene is frequent in battle casualties and in agricultural accidents. Indeed, it was during the First World War that this group of organisms was studied intensively and finally classified — so important was this type of infection in causing deaths. Occasionally, gas gangrene is endogenous and occurs when a wound is contaminated with the patient's own feces.

Pathogenesis and Lesions of Gas Gangrene.   Gas gangrene is never due to infection by a single type of clostridium; it is the result of a combined assault by several organisms working together. The true pathogens, best known of which is *Clostridium perfringens* (also called *Clostridium welchii*), produce powerful exotoxins that are liberated locally and produce tissue necrosis. Since muscle is usually involved, an extensive and progressive local muscle necrosis around the area of the original wound follows. At this stage the muscle appears red and is obviously dead, since it does not contract. The dead muscle excites an acute inflammatory response characterized by a tremendous outpouring of fluid with remarkably few polymorphs. The extensive inflammatory edema impairs the blood supply of the muscle, so that further growth of and invasion by the organism are favored. As noted above, many organisms are involved in the clinical condition of gas gangrene. The saprophytic group of clostridia, typified by *Clostridium sporogenes,* produce no potent toxins, but have the property of splitting protein. They attack the dead muscle and liberate hydrogen sulfide and other foul-smelling gases. The hydrogen sulfide combines with iron from hemoglobin, and the iron sulfide so formed gives the whole area a black color. The wound that is complicated by gas gangrene rapidly becomes black and discharges foul-smelling fluid in which there are bubbles of gas. Absorption of toxic substances, particularly the exotoxins of the pathogenic clostridia, leads to shock, and the patient dies unless the limb is expeditiously amputated.

Treatment of Gas Gangrene.   In the treatment of gas gangrene it is usual to give an antiserum prepared against the exotoxins of the main pathogens. Penicillin or other antibiotics are also useful, because they destroy the growing bacteria. For prophylaxis it is important that wounds be adequately treated surgically so that all dead tissue is removed and adequate drainage assured. This is as important as the administration of appropriate antibiotic therapy.

Tetanus

The spores of *Clostridium tetani* infrequently contaminate wounds, but as with gas gangrene organisms, a reduced oxygen tension is essential for their germination. The conditions conducive to tetanus infection are therefore similar to those described above. Nevertheless, quite often the degree of trauma may be mild, and an insignificant puncture wound, such as the prick of a thorn contaminated with manure, has quite commonly been the site of origin of a fatal tetanus infection.

Clinical Features.   The incubation period varies from a few days to several weeks; the shorter it is, the worse is the prognosis. Tetanus is clinically a disease of the central nervous system. The local lesion may be so mild that only a very careful search will reveal it, yet the exotoxin produced by the local infection may be sufficient to cause death.

After peripheral absorption, the toxin reaches the central nervous system — probably by passing along the motor nerve trunks to the spinal cord or medulla oblongata. At first, the toxin acts locally, which explains the early phenomenon known as local tetanus. This consists of spasm of those muscles controlled by the same spinal segment as that supplying the area infected. Stiffness of the muscles appears, and this is soon followed by an increase in muscular tone and painful spasms. After a while, the spasms become generalized; particularly striking is contraction of the jaw muscles, resulting in closure of the lower jaw or *trismus* (inability to open the mouth, or "lockjaw"). Finally, generalized convulsions occur, and death from asphyxia follows involvement of the respiratory muscles.

Prophylaxis of Tetanus. Since tetanus may complicate quite trivial wounds, by far the best method of prophylaxis is active immunization. This is carried out by giving a course of three injections of tetanus toxoid, thereby inducing a high blood level of specific antitoxin immunoglobulin.

In a patient who has sustained a deep wound — particularly if there is much ragged laceration of tissue, or if it has been contaminated with animal fecal material — the procedure used depends upon whether the patient has had previous active immunization or not. If previous injections of tetanus toxoid have been given, all that needs to be done is to give a further dose of toxoid. A rapid secondary immune response leads to a high level of antitoxin within one or two days. If, on the other hand, there has been no previous immunization, passive immunization with antitoxin must be considered. In the past, the administration of horse antitetanic serum (ATS) has been advised, but the danger of inducing anaphylactic shock or serum sickness is considerable. Furthermore, the duration of passive immunity is short, particularly if the subject has had previous injections of horse serum (see Fig. 9–12). Since the use of human antitetanic serum obviates these difficulties, it should be given whenever it is available. At the same time it is also advisable to give the first injection of tetanus toxoid. The patient should be instructed to return for further toxoid administrations. Tetanus is now an uncommon disease in the Western world, but the situation in the poorer countries is quite different. It has been estimated that over one million people die of tetanus each year, and that it is the leading cause of death in hospitals in many developing countries. Injecting quinine (for malaria), ear piercing, circumcising, and applying soil or even dung to the umbilicus of the newborn are all common modes of contamination that lead to infection in the unprotected population.

Other Clostridial Infections

Clostridium difficile is a minor normal inhabitant of the human bowel, but during the course of oral antibiotic therapy, particularly with clindamycin or lincomycin, bacterial overgrowth and accompanying toxin production can lead to a severe, sometimes fatal, pseudomembranous colitis (Chapter 32).

Ingestion of food (generally a meat or poultry stew) heavily contaminated with certain strains of *Clostridium perfringens* leads to acute food poisoning. Approximately one third of all outbreaks of food poisoning are due to this cause.

Gram-negative Anaerobic Intestinal Bacilli

The gram-negative intestinal bacilli of the genus *Bacteroides* form the bulk of organisms in the feces, and they are present also as part of the normal flora of the mouth and vagina. These organisms do not produce spores and are strictly anaerobic. They cause wound infection, pelvic abscesses, puerperal sepsis, and occasionally oral infection. But in these instances their role is probably secondary to infection with more pathogenic organisms. Their

TABLE 10–2. COMMON ANAEROBIC WOUND INFECTIONS

ORGANISM	SOURCE OF INFECTION	COMMON INFECTIONS
Clostridium welchii and others	Animal feces; normal flora of human intestine	Wound infection; myositis (gas gangrene); gangrenous lesion of intestinal tract
Clostridium tetani	Animal feces; occasional member of flora of human intestine	Mild wound infection with severe toxic effects (tetanus)
Anaerobic streptococci Bacteroides species	Normal flora of intestine, vagina, and the mouth, to a lesser extent	Wound infections; gangrenous lesions of intestinal tract: peritonitis; postpartum uterine infection (puerperal sepsis)

presence should be suspected in any infection associated with a foul odor. The organisms may on occasion invade the blood stream and cause septicemia with shock.

Anaerobic Streptococcal Infections

Anaerobic streptococci are normal inhabitants of the bowel and vagina. They were important causes of puerperal infection in the past and occasionally are associated with wound infection and gangrenous lesions.

The important anaerobic infections of wounds are summarized in Table 10–2.

MYCOBACTERIAL INFECTIONS

The mycobacteria or acid-fast bacilli have features that distinguish them from other bacteria. They are difficult to stain (see Ziehl-Neelsen stain, below), and the two important human pathogens *Mycobacterium tuberculosis* and *Mycobacterium leprae* grow slowly *in vivo*. They have some affinity with fungi and were so named on this account (*mykes* is Greek for "fungus").

Tuberculosis

The importance of tuberculosis cannot be judged by its present incidence in the Western world. In the past it was a common and dreaded disease, but the sanitoria and hospitals for "consumption" (as the disease was once called) either have shut down or have changed their names and directed their attention to other diseases. In part, this has been effected by early diagnosis and better treatment; in the main, however, improvement in social conditions, removal of slums, and the pasteurization of milk have played the major role. In areas of the world where poverty and overcrowding are rife, so also is tuberculosis.

The Causative Organism. Tuberculosis is caused by *Mycobacterium tuberculosis*, of which there are several strains, the most important being the *human* and the *bovine* varieties. The organisms contain a waxy material in their cell walls that is responsible for their special properties. Since stains cannot easily penetrate the organism, a smear receiving the ordinary Gram stain will show no bacteria. A special stain must be employed: heating a smear with strong carbolfuchsin. Once this stain has penetrated the organism, it cannot easily be removed by acid or alcohol. This forms the basis of the Ziehl-Neelsen (ZN) stain. Mycobacterium tuberculosis is therefore spoken of as being "acid-alcohol-fast." The organism is demanding in its cultural requirements and takes several weeks to produce visible colonies. It follows that tuberculous specimens treated in a routine way will be reported as sterile. Special methods must be employed, and the laboratory technologists must be aware of the necessity for this. The organisms also grow slowly *in vivo*, and tuberculous infections tend to develop slowly and to be chronic.

The Tissue Reaction to Tuberculous Infection. When tubercle bacilli are introduced into a tissue, there is a rapid acute inflammatory response with a polymorph infiltration. This tends to be quite mild and fleeting. It is soon followed by massive accumulation of macrophages, which ingest the bacilli and then become modified to form *epithelioid cells*. These have more cytoplasm than the typical macrophage and lose their ability to ingest material. The accumulation of epithelioid cells tends to be focal, and small nodules or *tubercles* are formed (Fig. 10–3). These are about 0.5 to 1.0 mm in diameter and are just visible to the naked eye. Some macrophages, instead of becoming epithelioid cells, form giant cells that are of the Langhans type. Surrounding the mass of epithelioid cells, there is a diffuse zone of lymphocytes with a few plasma cells and fibrocytes. Within two weeks necrosis begins in the mass of tissue containing not only the epithelioid cells but also those cells peculiar to the part involved. The necrosis is called *caseation*, and the dead tissue forms a dry, firm, coagulated mass, which has fancifully been likened to cheese. Caseation is probably caused by the development of hypersensitivity to the products of the bacilli, as explained in Chapter 9.

The end-result is a fully formed tubercle follicle (Fig. 10–4). It consists of a central mass of caseation surrounded by epithelioid cells and occasional giant cells. This, in turn, is surrounded by a wide zone of small round cells. The appearance is highly characteristic of tuberculosis, but a similar reaction can be seen in other infections, particularly those caused by fungi. Adjacent tubercles tend to fuse, and as the caseous process extends, wide areas of tissue are destroyed. The lesion can now be seen with the naked eye, and the caseation can extend for many centimeters. Progressive caseation is the hallmark of spread of tuberculosis. In some instances, the firm caseous tissue undergoes liquefaction. The precise reason for this is not known, but

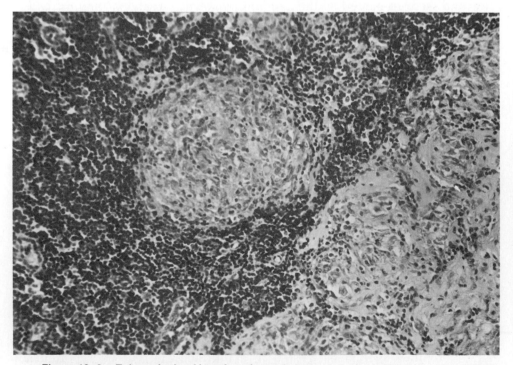

Figure 10–3.   Tuberculosis of lymph node; early lesion. In the center of the picture there is a circumscribed collection of epithelioid cells forming a follicle that stands out clearly against the dark background provided by the closely packed small lymphocytes. On the right-hand side several follicles have fused together.

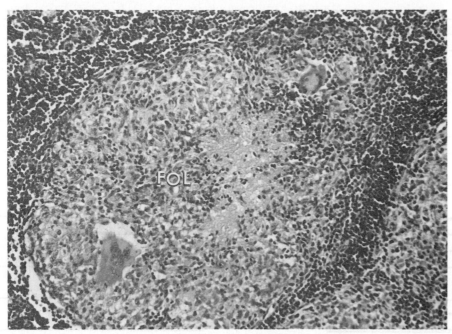

Figure 10–4. Tuberculosis of lymph node; follicle with caseation. Compared with the lesion shown in Figure 10–3, this tuberculous follicle (Fol) has enlarged, and its center has become caseous. Two giant cells are shown. The one with many nuclei arranged around its periphery has the characteristic features of a Langhans giant cell. Although this is an active tuberculous lesion, bacilli are scanty and would be very difficult to find in a section stained with Ziehl-Neelsen's carbolfuchsin. Culture in a suitable medium or guinea-pig inoculation is used to isolate the organism.

increased hypersensitivity is generally incriminated. A cavity is then formed containing liquefied caseous material that is teeming with bacilli. Conventionally, this is called pus, although technically this term in inaccurate, since few polymorphs are present. The tuberculous pus tends to track in the line of least resistance, providing for one means by which a tuberculous lesion can extend.

Tubercle bacilli are typically intracellular parasites and can be spread locally in the tissues by the migration of macrophages. Satellite lesions are therefore formed, and their eventual fusion with the original focus is the means by which the lesion enlarges. Tubercle bacilli also spread via the lymphatic vessels, causing the regional lymph nodes to contain typical tubercles. In susceptible individuals this spread continues to the blood stream, and widespread dissemination occurs. The subject becomes severely ill, having numerous tubercles, particularly in those organs with a high reticuloendothelial content such as the spleen, bone marrow, and liver. The meninges are also affected, and *meningitis* frequently accompanies this condition, which is called *generalized miliary tuberculosis*. The name is derived from the numerous small tubercles that at one time were likened to millet seeds.

Tuberculosis causes mastitis in cows, and the organism is therefore present in milk. On ingestion of the milk by man, a local infection occurs either in the tonsils or in the small intestine. This local lesion is small and clinically silent, but the organism spreads to involve regional lymph nodes in a massive way. The situation is similar to that of tuberculosis in the guinea pig. Bovine tuberculosis was once common in children in whom large masses of caseous cervical or mesenteric lymph nodes were characteristic. Human

Tuberculosis Due to the Bovine Strain of Tubercle Bacillus

beings have considerable innate immunity to tuberculosis, and the disease usually stopped its spread at this point. Occasionally, continued spread resulted in miliary tuberculosis and death.

The eradication of tuberculosis from our herds and the almost universal pasteurization of milk have made bovine tuberculosis so rare that this form of the disease has virtually ceased to exist in the Western world.

Tuberculosis Due to the Human Tubercle Bacillus

The mode of infection is by the inhalation of organisms present in fresh droplets or in the dust of dried sputum expectorated by a person having an open case of pulmonary tuberculosis.

It has been recognized for a long time that tuberculous infection manifests itself differently in children and adults. At all ages the lung is the principal organ involved.

Childhood Tuberculosis. In childhood the primary focus (the Ghon focus) is a small lesion situated at the periphery of the lung field. This subpleural focus may heal and produce no clinical illness, while the infection may spread to the hilar lymph nodes, which become greatly enlarged and caseous and eventually form a conspicuous primary complex (Fig. 10–5A). Either it heals and calcifies (Fig. 10–6), or the infection spreads and the child dies of miliary tuberculosis with meningitis.

Adult Tuberculosis. In adult life a pulmonary focus is almost always either atypical or subapical. The lesion either heals or progresses slowly with softening and liquefaction. In this way a cavity is formed (Figs. 10–5B and 10–7). The destruction of lung tissue leads to bleeding, which often leads to hemoptysis. This is accompanied by a chronic cough, low-grade fever, weight loss, and a raised erythrocyte sedimentation rate (ESR). The patient feels unwell and lacks energy. Depending upon the resistance of the patient, there is a tendency for either healing with fibrosis or extension of the cavitating process. In severe cases there can be great destruction of lung tissue. At any time, caseous debris may be inhaled into other bronchi to produce areas of tuberculous bronchopneumonia. This may occur on a small scale and result in extension of the disease, but if it is widespread in a highly sensitized person, it can lead to massive consolidation of lung tissue. This is quite uncommon nowadays.

In summary, adult tuberculosis is a chronic disease in which phases of spread alternate with phases of healing and fibrosis.

Precisely why the morphology of adult tuberculosis of the lung is so different from that seen in childhood is not known. One explanation is that the adult type is a reinfection. The previous infection induces immunity, so that with a reinfection the disease does not spread but remains localized to the

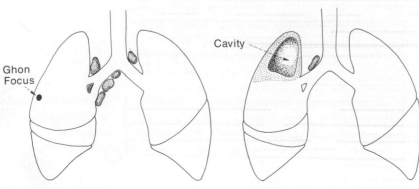

Figure 10–5. Pulmonary tuberculosis. In childhood tuberculosis, the lung lesion is small, but the spread to hilar and mediastinal lymph nodes is extensive. In adult tuberculosis, there is a destructive lung lesion (often apical and with cavitation), and the lymphatic spread to the hilum is minimal. (Drawing by Margot Mackay, Department of Art as Applied to Medicine, University of Toronto.)

Cavity

Ghon Focus

(A) CHILDHOOD TUBERCULOSIS   (B) ADULT TUBERCULOSIS

Figure 10–6. Tuberculosis of lung. This section of lung shows a circumscribed, partly calcified lesion called a *Ghon focus* (see also Fig. 10–5A), which is indicated by the upper right arrow. This is thought to be the primary focus of a previous tuberculous infection. The adjacent pleura is thickened, and the overlying pleural space is obliterated by fibrous adhesions. In Europe this type of lesion is usually due to a previous tuberculous infection; however, it is often difficult to prove this by finding organisms in the focus itself. In North America histoplasmosis can produce a lesion that has an identical appearance.

The specimen was from a patient who had died of miliary tuberculosis. The Ghon focus had evidently become reactivated, and bacilli had spread throughout the body via the blood stream. Two miliary tubercles are indicated by arrows. (Specimen courtesy of the Boyd Museum, University of Toronto.)

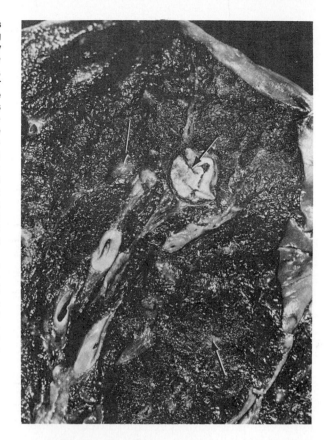

Figure 10–7. Chronic pulmonary tuberculosis in an adult. This radiograph shows a typical chronic destructive tuberculous infection in the right upper lobe. Two areas of cavitation are evident. The large one is indicated by the two arrows; below and slightly to the right there is a smaller cavity. The infection has now spread to the lower lobe, where extensive areas of tuberculous bronchopneumonia are evident. (Photograph courtesy of Dr. D. E. Sanders.)

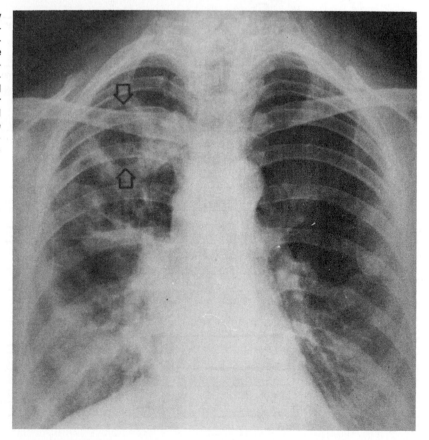

lung. Unfortunately, hypersensitivity leads to extensive destruction of lung tissue. Undoubtedly, there is some truth in this explanation, but although the situation is similar to that seen in the Koch phenomenon, it is not exactly the same. In the Koch phenomenon the lesion of reinfection heals because immunity develops (Chapter 9), whereas in human pulmonary adult tuberculosis, the lesion tends to heal slowly, and the disease remains chronic and progressive.

Metastatic Tuberculosis.   At any stage in the development of a tuberculous lesion, a transient bacteremia can occur. This can result in small metastatic tuberculous lesions being produced in virtually any organ of the body. These usually remain quiescent, but years later they may become active and produce active tuberculous lesions at that site. Bone, kidney, brain, epididymis, fallopian tube, and joints are areas where this response is particularly frequent. The lesions are typically those of a chronic inflammation with progressive destruction of parenchyma and its replacement by fibrous tissue. Caseation is usually an obvious feature; if there is liquefaction, the pus can spread in the line of least resistance. With renal tuberculosis, the pus ruptures into the pelvis of the kidney and is passed in the urine. Large cavitated areas extend from the pelvis of such a kidney. When tuberculous pus is formed adjacent to tuberculosis of the spinal column, the pus enters the psoas sheath, tracks down to below the inguinal ligament, and finally opens onto the skin surface.

Factors Determining the Response of Tissues to Tuberculous Infection.   It is evident that a tuberculous infection may be followed by a minimal reaction that heals rapidly or may lead to a progressive disease with rapid spread culminating in death. The factors determining tissue response are the following:

1. *The Dose and Virulence of the Organism.*
2. *Innate Immunity.*   For the most part, human beings have considerable immunity to tuberculosis, but it does seem that certain races (*e.g.,* the Eskimos and the Irish) are especially susceptible. Nevertheless, it is difficult to separate the effects of environment from those of innate immunity, because poverty, starvation, and ignorance are the forerunners of tuberculosis in any race.
3. *Age and Sex.*   In days gone by, tuberculosis was particularly common in early adulthood, especially in females. With the improvement in social conditions and the great decline in the incidence of tuberculosis, this trend is no longer apparent. In old age, immunity to tuberculosis diminishes, and the disease even now is not infrequent in our senior citizens.
4. *General Health of the Individual.*   Malnutrition and chronic debilitating disease, particularly diabetes mellitus, are notorious predisposing factors to tuberculosis. For example, an attack of measles can activate a previously quiescent tuberculous focus.
5. *Occupational Factors.*   Those whose work carries the hazard of atmospheric pollution by particles of silica (*e.g.,* tunnelers, miners, and quarrymen) are liable to develop pulmonary tuberculosis. To a lesser extent the same hazard applies to those who manufacture asbestos products.
6. *Acquired Immunity and Sensitivity.*   This has been described previously (Chapter 9). It is generally held that the immunity to tuberculosis is T cell–dependent. It follows that in diseases where T cell function is impaired, tuberculosis is particularly liable to occur; if infection has already been acquired, it is likely to spread. Patients with Hodgkin's disease and other lymphomas treated with immunosuppressant drugs are extremely susceptible to terminal fulminating tuberculosis infection.

Leprosy is caused by *Mycobacterium leprae,* which was one of the first bacteria to be incriminated as a cause of human disease and will probably be the last to be cultured in an artificial medium. Investigation of the disease, in particular the sensitivity of the organism to antibiotics, has been greatly hindered by our inability to grow the organism and the great difficulty encountered in infecting laboratory animals. So far, the organism has only been grown in the foot pads of mice and in the nine-banded armadillo. In practice, pathological diagnosis depends on demonstrating the organism by ZN staining of smears or sections.

Introduction

Although the disease is of great antiquity, it is uncertain whether the accounts in the Old Testament in fact describe leprosy. There seems little doubt that the disease was present in the Middle East before the birth of Christ, and during the Middle Ages it was common in Europe, having been introduced there by the returning Crusaders. The disease has now retreated from Europe and is endemic in the Far East, India, the Middle East, Africa, and Central and South America, where overcrowding and poverty are still rife. To those who live in the affluent parts of the world it may come as a surprise to learn that there are over 12 million cases of leprosy in the world. The disease was probably introduced into the continental United States by the Negro slaves, and is still endemic in some southern states and Hawaii.

The terms leper and leprosy conjure up such distasteful images in most people's minds that the disease is best called *Hansen's disease* — named after Gerhard Hansen, the Norwegian physician who described the causative bacillus.

The mode of infection is unknown, but the disease is probably spread by contaminated nasal secretions. It has been estimated that over 90 per cent of humans have such high innate immunity to the lepra bacillus that they are very unlikely to develop infection even if exposed to the disease. The remaining 5 to 10 per cent are susceptible. The disease is generally acquired in childhood, and the first lesion is an insignificant scaly skin patch. This *indeterminate lesion* may heal spontaneously or progress to one of the two major forms of the disease.

Mode of Infection

Tuberculoid Leprosy. This type of leprosy occurs in individuals with a relatively high state of natural immunity. The skin lesions consist of one or several *well-demarcated* papules or plaques, which are associated with local nerve involvement, causing the skin of the area to become hypoesthetic. Microscopically the skin and involved nerves show a noncaseating tuberculoid reaction similar to that seen in early tuberculosis. Lepra bacilli are extremely sparse. The lepromin reaction (Fernandez reaction)* which is similar to the Mantoux, is positive and indicates a high state of cell-mediated immunity.

Types of Leprosy

Lepromatous Leprosy. In lepromatous leprosy the lesions consist of multiple macules, papules, and plaques, which are of *widespread distribution* and tend to be *symmetrical.* The lesions are *poorly delineated,* and often there is a diffuse infiltration of the skin. Microscopically the dermis is

---

*The lepromin test is performed by injecting a preparation of human lepromatous tissue into the skin. An inflammatory reaction at 48 to 72 hours is comparable to a positive Mantoux test. It is termed the *Fernandez reaction* and is positive in tuberculoid leprosy. A reaction that develops at 3 weeks or more (*Mitsuda reaction*) indicates that the individual can react to the lepra bacillus with a granulomatous reaction. *The test is positive in many uninfected normal people* and indicates that their innate immunity is very high and that they are unlikely to develop leprosy. A negative Mitsuda reaction, on the other hand, indicates a low resistance to infection, and should such an individual become infected, the lepromatous form of the disease will probably ensue.

diffusely packed with macrophages, which are themselves stuffed with lepra bacilli. Since the lesions tend to occur in the cold parts of the body, the hands and face are particularly affected. The diffuse thickening of the skin of the face leads to a lionlike appearance (leonine facies). There is diffuse involvement of nerves, so that a symmetrical peripheral neuritis is characteristic.

In lepromatous leprosy, the nasal mucosa is also infiltrated by bacteria-laden macrophages, and the destruction of the nasal bones leads to the characteristic appearance (Fig. 10–8). Because the nasal secretions contain a large number of bacilli, it is probable that this is the manner by which the disease is disseminated.

In lepromatous leprosy there is defective T-cell immunity, causing the lepromin reaction to be negative. As if to compensate for this, there is an overproduction of immunoglobulins, and the hyperimmunoglobulinemia is associated with *acute reactional phases* that are a great hazard in leprosy. Exacerbation of the skin lesions, iridocyclitis, orchitis, nerve damage, fever, prostration, and death can occur during these acute phases, which may either develop spontaneously or be precipitated by ill-advised vigorous treatment. The damage is probably mediated by the deposition of immune complexes with antigen excess (Chapter 9). The large number of bacilli present in the lesions provides the antigen for the formation of these complexes.

Leprosy provides a fascinating example of the effects that an immune response has on the pattern of an infection. In the tuberculoid type, T-cell immunity is well developed, the lepromin test is positive, few bacilli are present in the lesions, and the inflammatory response is characterized by a tuberculoid reaction with plentiful Langhans giant cells. The pattern of reaction is similar to that encountered in the common type of tuberculous infection. In lepromatous leprosy on the other hand, T-cell function is in abeyance and vast numbers of bacilli are present in the lesions, which are

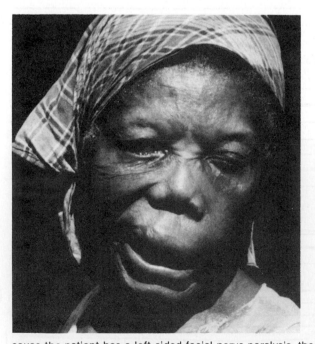

Figure 10–8. Leprosy. This patient is a voluntary resident of a leper colony in the Caribbean. Years before this picture was taken she was found to be suffering from lepromatous leprosy, and has been taking a sulfone or other antileprous drug ever since. Her condition is not now infectious; indeed, she may be completely free of the lepra bacillus, although this is difficult to prove. Nevertheless, she exhibits some of the devastating effects of the disease. Inflammation of the nasal mucosa (rhinitis) accompanied by destruction of the nasal bones has resulted in collapse of the bridge of the nose. Repeated attacks of iritis have led to glaucoma and cataract so that the sight of both eyes has been gravely affected. The left eye is completely blind, but the right is able to detect movement and the difference between light and dark. Because the patient has a left-sided facial nerve paralysis, the muscles of the left side of the face do not move. This can be detected by the drooping of the left eyelid, and the failure of the left side of the mouth to move backwards when the patient smiles or talks.

characterized by a diffuse infiltration by macrophages ("lepra cells"). Occasionally an analogous situation is encountered in tuberculosis. In the terminal stages of miliary tuberculosis, the tuberculin test becomes negative, and the lesions teem with bacilli.

2. **Borderline or Dimorphous Leprosy.** Cases occur in which the clinical and pathological features are between the two polar types of tuberculoid and lepromatous leprosy. In these borderline cases, acute reactional states are particularly common, and the disease tends to terminate in one of the two major forms, often the lepromatous type.

Leprosy is a chronic disease that is now amenable to treatment with a number of chemotherapeutic drugs. The sulfones are the mainstay of these drugs, because they are not only effective but also readily available and cheap. Also, when treated with sulfones the disease soon becomes noninfectious, so that there is no need for patients with Hansen's disease to be isolated.

SPIROCHETAL DISEASES

Spirochetes are long, slender, spiral filamentous organisms. The human pathogens are classified according to three genera: *Borrelia, Leptospira,* and *Treponema.*

Borrelia

Two species of *Borrelia* cause *relapsing fever.* The European type is spread by lice, whereas the African variety is tickborne. Relapsing fever has an incubation period of three to four days and is characterized by an abrupt onset, a high fever, and the appearance of spirochetes in the blood stream. After three to five days, circulating immunoglobulin antibodies appear, the blood is cleared of organisms, and the fever abates. Some days later, organisms return to the blood, and another attack of fever ensues. Up to ten similar attacks may occur, thereby giving the disease its descriptive name.

The pathogenesis of this remarkable relapsing disease is that the organisms are able to mutate with extreme rapidity. No sooner does the immune response develop and kill off the organism than a new immunological variant emerges, followed by a relapse of fever until the host has had time to develop new specific antibodies. A similar type of relapsing fever is also seen in trypanosomiasis; this, too, is due to the high mutability of the organism.

Borrelia vincentii is another large spirochete; it is a naturally occurring contaminant of the mouth. When local resistance is impaired, *e.g.,* in agranulocytosis and leukemia, the organism in association with *Bacteroides* causes ulcerative oral lesions. It is also an important member of the bacteria that are incriminated in gingivitis. During the First World War the condition of acute ulcerative gingivitis was so common in soldiers that it was known as "trench mouth." This was due to poor nutrition and poor dental hygiene.

Leptospirosis

Many strains of leptospira are known and are normally carried in the kidneys of many species of animals such as rodents, dogs, cattle, birds, and amphibians. The organisms rarely cause harm in their usual host, but if transmitted accidentally to another animal species or to human beings they give rise to a clinical infection called leptospirosis. Leptospirosis is transmitted to man in water contaminated by the urine of carrier animals, usually rats or dogs. It is therefore an occupational hazard of such persons as sewer workers, military personnel, and veterinarians.

Leptospirosis can vary from a mild influenzalike disease to a severe illness with renal and hepatic damage. The latter type is known as Weil's disease. Occasionally meningitis is a dominant feature of the clinical presentation.

Syphilis   The causative organism of syphilis, *Treponema pallidum*, is a delicate spiral filament or spirochete which is difficult to stain and has never been cultivated in a synthetic medium. It is difficult to infect animals with this organism; rabbits, however, develop an acute orchitis after intratesticular inoculation. This method is used to obtain a supply of spirochetes for use in some diagnostic tests.

During the course of infection, the patient develops immunoglobulins that are of great diagnostic importance. The best known is the Wassermann antibody, which fixes complement in the presence of a phosphatide extract of heart muscle (cardiolipin) or produces a precipitate in the presence of a similar type of antigen (Kahn reaction, the Venereal Disease Research Laboratory [VDRL] test, and other modifications). Since the antigen used is not a specific component of the spirochete, it is not surprising that these *standard tests for syphilis* (STS) are also sometimes positive in nonspirochetal diseases — for example, leprosy, malaria, and systemic lupus erythematosus. Pregnancy, too, is occasionally associated with a false positive reaction.

In recent years it has been found that syphilitics also develop a specific treponemal antibody in their sera. When mixed with a suspension of live organisms it leads to their immobilization, and this forms the basis for the *treponemal immobilization (TPI) test.* Specific treponemal antibody will adhere to the organism, and this can be detected by a fluorescent technique (*fluorescent treponemal antibody test* [FTA]). Dead organisms adherent to a slide are used in this test, in contrast to the living, and therefore infectious, organisms required for the TPI test. If nonspecific antibodies are first absorbed by mixing the patient's serum with a nonpathogenic strain of treponema (the Reiter strain), the test is made more specific for syphilis. This is the *FTA-ABS* test and is the one most commonly performed. These *treponemal tests* are not performed routinely but are of great value in verifying ambiguous results and eliminating false positive reactions. It is unfortunate that even the specific tests cannot distinguish between syphilis and yaws.*

The Disease. Apart from congenital syphilis, the infection is nearly always acquired venereally. Unlike the tubercle bacillus, *Treponema pallidum* is very rapidly destroyed both in water and by drying. Intimate direct contact is therefore necessary for infection to occur. The spirochete is one of the most invasive organisms known, for once having penetrated the surface, it spreads along the lymphatics to the regional nodes and reaches the blood stream in a matter of hours. Therefore, systemic dissemination occurs long before any local manifestations appear.

The disease is divisible into three active stages, described below.

Primary Syphilis   The primary lesion of syphilis is the *chancre*, which usually appears on the genital area three to four weeks after infection. It commences as an indurated nodule, which breaks down to form an ulcer that characteristically is painless and is accompanied by enlargement of the regional lymph nodes (Fig. 10–9). Extragenital chancres are not uncommon (*e.g.*, around the anus, and on the lips, tip of tongue, tonsil, or other part of the oral cavity). The chancre heals even without treatment and leaves an inconspicuous atrophic

---

*Yaws is a disease that has much in common with syphilis and is caused by *Treponema pertenue*. It is frequent in some tropical countries and is not of venereal origin. The primary lesion is extragenital; secondary and tertiary stages follow. Significant cardiovascular and nervous system involvement is rare as compared with syphilis. It is possible that *Treponema pallidum* developed as a variant of *Treponema pertenue*, which became adapted to venereal transmission.

scar. Its occurrence can easily be missed, particularly in women, in whom the lesion can be on the cervix or vaginal vault. In passive homosexual males an anal lesion may likewise evade detection. In passing it may be noted that syphilis is common in homosexual males, partly because the chancres can be missed, and partly because these people tend to be more promiscuous than most heterosexuals.

CASE HISTORY I. (See Figure 10–9.) The patient, who had been consorting with a number of sexual partners, had noticed a small ulcer on the penis about a week before this picture was taken. This ulcer had steadily enlarged. Although it was not painful, he was persuaded to seek medical advice when he noticed swelling of his left inguinal region. On examination an oval ulcer with a firm base on the penis was noted, and this was associated with large inguinal lymph nodes on the left side. Characteristically, the ulcer was not painful. The ulcer was firmly squeezed, and its base gently rubbed with a bacteriological loop. The drop of fluid that was obtained was examined by dark-field illumination and showed numerous active spirochetes. A blood sample taken at this time showed a negative VDRL. Following the administration of penicillin, the ulcer healed and the lymphadenopathy subsided. The patient's sexual partners were traced, and only two were found to have had intercourse with him during the last three months. Both were found to have a positive VDRL and were treated for syphilis. This cases illustrates three important points: (1) A VDRL can be negative during the early stages of primary syphilis. (2) The response to penicillin is dramatic. (3) Contacts must be traced in an effort to prevent the further spread of the disease. Tracing the contacts is an important public health function.

The fact that the spirochetes become disseminated long before there is any local lesion suggests that hypersensitivity plays an important part in the pathogenesis of the lesion. The chancre is not comparable with a boil, for it is not a local inflammatory reaction tending to limit the infection. A possible explanation is that sensitizing antibodies are first formed at the site of infection and in the regional lymph nodes. During the incubation period, the organisms multiply; as sensitizing antibodies are produced, a damaging antigen-antibody reaction occurs to produce the primary lesion and its associated lymphadenitis.

A definite diagnosis of primary syphilis rests entirely upon finding the

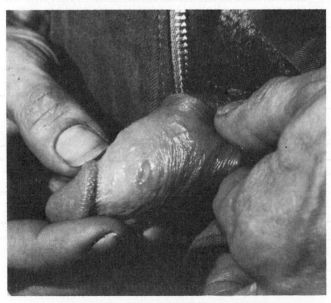

Figure 10–9. Primary chancre of syphilis. For a more complete description, see Case History I.

organisms in the lesion by direct microscopic examination using the dark-field method (Chapter 1). Soon after the appearance of the chancre, antibodies appear in the blood and the serological tests for syphilis become positive.

Secondary Syphilis   Within two to three months of exposure, the disease becomes clinically generalized. Tradition has it that syphilis, or at least a virulent form of the disease, was introduced into Europe by the returning sailors of Columbus in 1493. The disease was sometimes fatal and indeed sufficiently severe to warrant naming it the "Great Pox." The disease spread rapidly like a plague throughout Europe, reaching as far as Scotland by 1497. Even to this day *lues* (from the Latin for pestilence) is used as an alternative name for the disease. Nowadays, secondary syphilis is much milder and is characterized by the appearance of a generalized macular or papulosquamous erythematous rash.* Characteristically, this does not itch and affects the whole body, including the palms and soles (Fig. 10–10).

Papules* affecting moist areas such as the genital, axillary, and submammary regions can enlarge to produce flat, warty lesions (*condylomata lata*). The primary chancre may still be present or may have healed by the time the secondary lesions appear.

CASE HISTORY II. (See Figure 10–10.) The patient had developed a generalized nonitching rash composed of red palpable lesions (0.2 to 1.0 cm in diameter) covered by loose, keratin scales (this constitutes a generalized, nonpruritic, erythematous, papulosquamous eruption; see Chapter 41). Lesions were most obvious on the trunk, but they were also present on the limbs, including the palms and soles. Because the patient was in the habit of taking a barbiturate sleeping pill each night, the possibility of the rash being due to an adverse drug reaction was also considered. However, drug rashes generally itch, and the presence of a nonitching rash, particularly if it affects the palms and soles, is very suggestive of secondary syphilis. The patient denied ever having had an ulcer on his penis but admitted to having had homosexual encounters. Blood was taken for a VDRL test. The patient was treated with penicillin. Within eight hours he had developed a fever, and the rash had become more obvious before it faded. The VDRL was subsequently reported as being strongly positive.

This case illustrates the following points:

1. Any generalized nonpruritic papulosquamous rash, particularly one affecting the palms and soles, should be diagnosed as syphilis until proved otherwise.
2. The VDRL test is always positive in secondary syphilis.
3. No history of a primary lesion is obtainable in some patients — particularly in females and in male homosexuals.
4. Successful treatment with penicillin often causes an immediate accentuation of the lesions. This response is known as the Herxheimer reaction and is presumed to be due to the massive release of bacterial antigen as the organisms are killed.
5. The patients should be treated before laboratory confirmation is obtained. This helps to prevent the spread of the infection.

A low-grade fever, headaches, joint pain, anemia, generalized lymph node enlargement, iritis, and many other symptoms may be noted at this stage. Shallow ulcers may occur on the mucous membranes; these, like other secondary lesions, particularly the condylomata, are teeming with organisms and are highly infectious. Diagnosis at this stage depends either on identification of the organism by microscopy or on confirmation by serological means. The serological tests are always positive in secondary syphilis. If a negative result is reported, the prozone phenomenon should be suspected (Chapter 9).

---

*See Chapter 41 for definition of these terms.

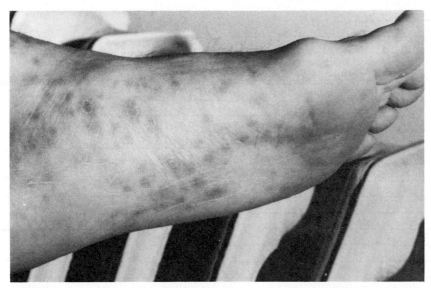

Figure 10–10. Lesions of secondary syphilis. For a more complete description, see Case History II.

Even without treatment the lesions of secondary syphilis heal and the patient enters into a latent phase.

This is an asymptomatic state that can be diagnosed only on history or by obtaining a positive serological test for syphilis. During the first two years after infection *(early latent syphilis)* the patient is still considered infectious and may develop recurrent secondary lesions, *e.g.*, skin lesions, and these are not as symmetrical as are the early rashes. Indeed, they may easily be misdiagnosed by the unwary. After two years *(late latent syphilis)* the patient is probably not infectious, although a female may still give birth to a syphilitic child. At any time one of the tertiary lesions may appear, but even in cases of untreated syphilis, they occur in approximately only one third of patients. The remaining two thirds remain asymptomatic for life, although about half of them still have a positive serological test for syphilis.

Latent Syphilis

Local destructive lesions may appear two to three years after infection and continue to erupt sporadically for many years. The lesions are presumably due to marked hypersensitivity, since spirochetes are few and the reaction to them is excessive. Two types of lesions can be recognized: localized gummas and diffuse inflammatory lesions characterized by parenchymatous destruction.

Tertiary Syphilis

Localized Gummas. The gumma is the classic lesion of tertiary syphilis. It is usually a solitary tumorlike mass and consists of a central large area of coagulative necrosis that has a slimy, stringy, gumlike mass from which the name gumma is derived. The necrotic tissue is surrounded by a granulomatous inflammatory reaction. Gummas are described as being most frequent in the liver, testes, subcutaneous tissues, and bones — including the nasal and palatal bones. In the latter situations the destruction produced by the gummas leads to perforation of the hard palate. With the introduction of penicillin and other antibiotic treatment of syphilis, *gummas are now extremely uncommon.*

Diffuse Lesions.   The really severe effects of tertiary syphilis fall on the cardiovascular and the nervous systems.

In *syphilitic aortitis* the elastic aortic wall is steadily destroyed by a chronic inflammatory reaction and is replaced by fibrous tissue. The weakening of the aorta results in aneurysmal dilatation; ultimately, the vessel may rupture. The disease tends to affect the thoracic aorta, causing widening of the aortic ring, which can lead to incompetence of the aortic valve.

Neurosyphilis may be meningovascular or parenchymatous. In the former type there is focal meningitis and vascular occlusion of small vessels. Isolated cranial nerve paralyses are produced.

Parenchymatous neurosyphilis includes the two well-known conditions of general paralysis of the insane and tabes dorsalis. *General paralysis of the insane* (GPI) is a chronic syphilitic meningoencephalitis in which the frontal lobes are particularly affected. This results in progressive dementia and paralysis. *Tabes dorsalis* is a degenerative condition of the posterior columns of the spinal cord and the posterior roots of the spinal nerves. The loss in sensation leads to loss of postural sense and a typical staggering gait.

The diagnosis of tertiary syphilis is primarily clinical, but it may often be substantiated by serological examination of the blood and cerebrospinal fluid. In most cases of overt syphilis the serological reactions are positive. Gummas are usually diagnosed by biopsy or following excision. It has frequently been stressed that syphilis is the great mimic in medicine and that virtually any lesion or disease can be faithfully copied by syphilis. Hence, a routine VDRL test is a common clinical procedure. Note, however, that the serological tests for syphilis frequently remain positive during the latent periods and that a syphilitic patient can suffer from other diseases. Thus, a mass present in the lung in a patient with a positive VDRL is more likely to be a carcinoma, which is common, than a gumma, which is rare.

Congenital Syphilis   During the first two years of infection, an untreated syphilitic mother is very liable to transmit the disease to her fetus, particularly in the later months of pregnancy. Abortion may result, or a severely affected infant may be born alive but die soon after birth.

More frequently, the child survives and may then exhibit early stigmata of the infection: skin eruptions, nasal infection (snuffles), and involvement of bones. Destruction of the nasal bones leads to a saddle-shaped deformity of the nose. Sometimes stigmata appear only in later childhood. The notched,

ORGANISM	SOURCE OF INFECTION	DISEASE PRODUCED
Borrelia		
Borrelia recurrentis	Body louse	European relapsing fever
Borrelia duttonii	Ticks	African relapsing fever
Borrelia vincentii	Normal flora of mouth	Gingivitis, gangrenous lesions of mouth
Leptospira		
Leptospira icterohaemor-rhagiae and others	Urine of rodents, dogs, and many other species	Leptospirosis (Weil's disease)
Treponema		
Treponema pallidum	Human case of syphilis	Syphilis
Treponema pertenue	Human case of yaws	Yaws

deformed upper incisor teeth, inflammation of the cornea (interstitial keratitis), periostitis, and nerve deafness are all well-known features. In effect, the early lesions of congenital syphilis are comparable to those of the secondary stage, whereas the later manifestations have the destructive features of tertiary syphilis as encountered in the adults.

The spirochetal diseases described in this section are summarized in Table 10–3.

1. Compare and contrast infections with *Staphylococcus aureus* with those produced by *Streptococcus pyogenes* in terms of the following:
   (a) site of infection
   (b) type of local lesion produced
   (c) spread of infection
   (d) lesions produced by exotoxin
   (e) sterile lesions produced by immune mechanisms

2. List the lesions produced by the gonococcus. Indicate how the organism reaches each of the sites mentioned.

3. A patient has driven a fork through his foot while digging in the garden. What measures should be taken to prevent the development of tetanus under these conditions:
   (a) if he has had tetanus toxoid injections previously
   (b) if he has never had tetanus toxoid or does not know whether he was ever given toxoid

4. A soldier sustains a gunshot wound of the thigh. The lacerated wound is contaminated by soil, and he is unable to receive medical attention for 24 hours. Describe the signs and symptoms that indicate the development of:
   (a) infection with a pyogenic organism, such as a gram-negative intestinal bacillus
   (b) tetanus
   (c) gas gangrene

5. Compare a chronic staphylococcal lung abscess with a cavitated tuberculous lesion with respect to:
   (a) the tissue reaction
   (b) the contents of the cavity
   (c) the methods of demonstrating the causative organism

6. Compare and contrast leprosy with tuberculosis in terms of the following:
   (a) properties of the organisms
   (b) methods of diagnosis
   (c) tissue response to infection
   (d) immune response to infection
   (e) organs or tissues affected

7. Syphilis is an excellent example of a disease in which the lesions are produced, not by the organism acting alone, but by an interplay between the organism and the host reacting to it. Discuss this response in relation to the three active stages of the disease.

Review Questions

Browne, S. G.: Mycobacterial diseases: leprosy. *In:* Fitzpatrick, T. B., et al. (Eds.): Dermatology in General Medicine. 2nd ed. New York, McGraw-Hill Book Company, 1979, pp. 1492–1505.

Christie, A. B.: Infectious Diseases. 2nd ed. Edinburgh, Churchill Livingstone, 1974. See, in particular, Chapter 22, "Tetanus," and Chapter 28, "Leptospiral Infections."

Cruickshank, R., Duguid, J. P., Marmion, B. P., and Swain, R. H. A.: Medical Microbiology. 12th ed. Vol. 1. Edinburgh, Churchill Livingstone, 1973. An excellent account of medical microbiology, with the accent on laboratory findings and the properties of bacteria and viruses.

Glasgow, L. A.: Staphylococcal infection in the toxic-shock syndrome. New England Journal of Medicine, *303*:1473–1475, 1980.

Leading Article: Clostridia as intestinal pathogens. Lancet, *2*:1113–1114, 1977.

Leading Article. Toxic shock and tampons. British Medical Journal, *281*:1161–1162, 1980.

Selected Readings

Moschella, S. L., Pillsbury, D. M., and Hurley, H. J., Dermatology. Philadelphia, W. B. Saunders Company, 1975. See pp. 808–825 for a well-illustrated, detailed account of leprosy.

Robbins, S. L., and Cotran, R. S.: Pathologic Basis of Disease. 2nd ed. Philadelphia, W. B. Saunders Company, 1979. See Chapter 10, "Infectious Diseases," which provides a useful reference to the pyogenic infections and tuberculosis.

Scofield, C. B. S.: Sexually Transmitted Diseases. 2nd ed. Edinburgh, Churchill Livingstone, 1975.

Woodruff, A. W. (Ed.): Medicine in the Tropics. Edinburgh, Churchill Livingstone, 1974. See Chapter 24, "Leptospirosis."

Wroblewski, S. S.: Toxic shock syndrome. American Journal of Nursing, 81:82–85, 1981.

Youmans, G. P., Paterson, P. Y., and Sommers, H. M.: The Biological and Clinical Basis of Infectious Diseases. Philadelphia, W. B. Saunders Company, 1975. An excellent account of medical microbiology and infectious disease, with particular emphasis on the clinical features.

Mycoplasmal, Chlamydial, and Rickettsial Infections

CHAPTER 11

After studying this chapter the student should be able to:

- Outline the main features of mycoplasmal pneumonia and the organism that causes it.
- Compare chlamydia with mycoplasma and describe the important human diseases caused by members of the chlamydial group of organisms.
- List the four types of typhus fever and describe the main features of one of them.
- Describe the main features of Q fever.

This chapter describes infection with members of three groups of organisms. The microorganisms are all much smaller than the true bacteria; many of them are obligatory intracellular parasites, and some of them in the past have been confused with viruses. Nevertheless, unlike viruses they are capable of simple division and do not exhibit the complex intracellular mode of reproduction that is so characteristic of viruses.

Mycoplasmal Infections

Mycoplasma are the smallest organisms (150 to 250 nm) that are capable of growth in a cell-free medium. They lack a cell wall and therefore tend to be very pleomorphic; coccobacillary, filamentous, and branching forms are common. The only known human pathogen is *Mycoplasma pneumoniae*, an organism causing a type of pneumonia that tends to occur in small epidemics. The onset is insidious, and the x-ray changes of patchy consolidation are often more extensive than the clinical picture would suggest (Fig. 11–1). Recovery is invariable and can be hastened by tetracycline therapy. Before the nature of the causative organism was understood, the disease was labeled "primary atypical pneumonia" or "viral pneumonia" (see Case History 13–I). Two curious features of the disease are the development of cold autohemagglutinins (Chapter 26) and a positive standard test for syphilis. A complement fixation test is available and is the most widely used method of diagnosis.

CASE HISTORY I. (See Figure 11–1.) The patient was a 36-year-old female who had developed an upper respiratory infection that persisted for two weeks and was accompanied by a dry, hacking cough. Although she was treated with penicillin, she showed no improvement. At the end of the third week the patient still felt ill and was troubled by a persistent cough, shortness of breath, and an evening fever. She was diagnosed to have mycoplasmal pneumonia.

Since the patient was found to be three months pregnant, she was not administered tetracycline, the usual drug of choice. Tetracycline is contraindicated in pregnancy, particularly during the last three months, because it impairs fetal tooth development. The patient was given erythromycin and made a slow recovery.

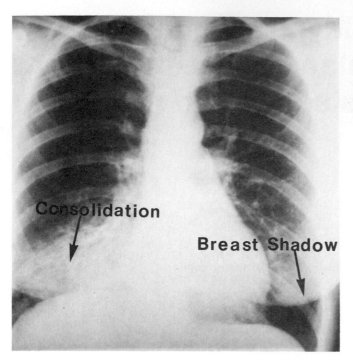

Consolidation

Breast Shadow

Figure 11–1. Chest radiograph of patient with mycoplasmal pneumonia. Note bilateral, patchy consolidation, most marked in the lower lung fields, particularly on the right side. A diagnosis of mycoplasmal pneumonia was confirmed by the finding of specific antibodies of a titer of 1 in 3000. (Photograph courtesy of Dr. D. E. Sanders.) For a more complete description, see Case History I.

Chlamydial Infections   The chlamydia, previously called *Bedsonia* after Samuel Bedson, who was a pioneer in the field, are small, obligatory intracellular parasites about 300 nm in diameter. Several are pathogenic to human beings. Since growth in tissue cultures is difficult, the organisms are generally isolated by injecting the yolk sac of the chick embryo. Chlamydia contain both DNA and RNA and have been divided into two subgroups: *Subgroup A* includes the chlamydia of trachoma-inclusion conjunctivitis and lymphogranuloma venereum. *Subgroup B* contains the organisms causing psittacosis and ornithosis.

Trachoma. This is an infection of the conjunctiva that becomes chronic, tends to spread to the cornea, and causes scarring. The disease is uncommon in the Western world but is a very important cause of *blindness* in the Middle East and other areas of poverty and overcrowding. Diagnosis is confirmed by isolating the organism or demonstrating the inclusion bodies in a smear from the conjunctiva.

Inclusion Conjunctivitis. This disease is so named because inclusion bodies can be seen in infected cells. It affects newborn babies (in whom it forms a type of ophthalmia neonatorum) as well as adults (causing "swimming pool conjunctivitis"). The organism is transmitted venereally and causes urethritis in the male ("nongonococcal urethritis") and cervicitis in the female. Indeed, the genital area is the reservoir of infection. Transfer to the eyes of babies occurs during labor; transfer in adults occurs via the hands or imperfectly chlorinated pool water. The TRachoma-Inclusion Conjunctivitis chlamydia are often grouped as the TRIC organisms. Why the organisms cause the severe disease trachoma in some parts of the world and the much milder conjunctivitis or genital infection in other areas is not known.

Lymphogranuloma Venereum. This is an uncommon venereal disease characterized by the appearance of a local genital ulcer and regional lymph node enlargement.

Psittacosis (Ornithosis). Psittacosis is a disease of birds of the parrot family (psittacine birds). Ducks, chickens, turkeys, pigeons, gulls, and other birds may also have the disease, in which case it is termed ornithosis.

Diagnosis is confirmed by a complement fixation test. Infection in humans is caused by inhalation of dust containing contaminated bird excreta, and it usually presents as a type of pneumonia. The regulations relating to the importation of psittacine birds have made this an uncommon disease. Occasional outbreaks still occur, however, because native birds, such as poultry and pigeons, can harbor the organism.

Rickettsial Infections

The rickettsial organisms are obligatory intracellular parasites that are widely distributed in nature, infecting many species of mammals that form their natural reservoir. Infection is transferred by lice, fleas, ticks, and mites. Humans are infected when they accidentally intercept the life cycle of infection from insect vector to animal reservoir. The only exception to this mode of transfer is with epidemic typhus, in which humans, themselves, are the only known reservoir.

Typhus

The typhus group of fevers is currently of little day-to-day importance; in the past, however, it has been responsible for epidemics of ferocious intensity. These have occurred in time of war when humans, rats, fleas, and lice have shared a common habitation. No doubt, future catastrophes will once again highlight the virulence of the rickettsiae, and it is for this reason that some knowledge of this group of diseases is important.

Mode of Infection. Some rickettsiae are injected by the bite of an infected tick or mite. On the other hand, lice and fleas pass contaminated feces as they feed on their animal host, causing rickettsial organisms to be introduced when the site of the bite is scratched.

Types. The typhus fevers have an incubation period of 7 to 10 days, and their onset is of dramatic suddenness with rigors, fever, and severe headaches accompanied by prostration. The organisms multiply in the endothelial cells of blood vessels and the far-reaching vascular damage accounts for the widespread nature of the lesions seen in the disease. A skin rash appears in most cases about the fourth day of clinical illness. The following types of typhus are important:

*1. Epidemic, Louse-borne Typhus.** Caused by *Rickettsia prowazeki*, this disease is associated with a high mortality and was responsible for the typhus epidemics of the two World Wars. DDT, with its lousicidal activity, proved to be an effective weapon in controlling this disease. Unlike the case in all other forms of typhus, with this disease man is the only mammal host. Since infected lice soon die, one would expect the disease to die out. A parasite that often kills its only hosts should not be successful. The explanation of the paradox is that following an attack of the disease humans can harbor the organism for many years. A recrudescence of the disease (Brill-Zinssler disease) can occur; the illness is mild but of great importance, because the victim constitutes a potential source of infection. If he happens to harbor lice, and lives in overcrowded squalor, he can initiate the next epidemic.

2. Endemic, Flea-borne Typhus. This disease is endemic in many parts of the world, including the U.S.A. It is caused by *Rickettsia mooseri* and is transmitted by the *rat flea*.

3. Rocky Mountain Spotted Fever. This disease, endemic throughout North America, is caused by *Rickettsia rickettsii* and is a severe form of

---

*In addition to rickettsiae, the body louse also transmits one type of relapsing fever (Chapter 10). Infestation can generally be recognized by the presence of itchy papules and numerous scratch marks ("vagabond's disease"). It is important to note that the parasite lives in clothing and not on the skin. Hence, when infestation is suspected, the underclothing —particularly its seams — should be carefully examined.

typhus transmitted by the bite of a tick. A widespread hemorrhagic rash is an outstanding feature. Similar types of tick-borne diseases occur in other parts of the world.

4. Scrub Typhus.   This was the mite-borne type of typhus that constituted a problem in the Pacific area in World War II.

Laboratory Diagnosis.   Patients with typhus develop antibodies that by chance agglutinate certain strains of proteus organisms. This reaction has been utilized in a diagnostic test, which is called the *Weil-Felix reaction* and is analogous to the Widal reaction for typhoid. A rising titer during the course of a febrile illness helps to confirm the diagnosis. Specific antirickettsial complement-fixing antibodies can also be demonstrated. Isolation of the organism is performed by inoculating a suitable laboratory animal.

Treatment.   Treatment of typhus has been revolutionized by the introduction of chloramphenicol and tetracycline. Typhus now has a low mortality, unless the patient is already the victim of other disease or starvation.

One other form of rickettsial disease is of interest:

Q Fever.   Q (for *query*) fever, caused by *Coxiella burneti,** is transmitted from animal to animal by the bite of a tick. Sheep, goats, and cows are naturally infected, and human disease is caused either by drinking contaminated milk or by inhaling dust contaminated by animal material. Q fever in humans is characterized by a long incubation period (about 19 days), and the disease resembles other forms of typhus, except that although a rash is very uncommon, evidence of pneumonia or hepatitis is frequently found.

Review Questions

1. Describe the antibodies that are formed during the course of an infection with mycoplasmal and rickettsial organisms. How may these aid in diagnosis? How may their presence cause confusion with other diseases?

2. How does infection with *Rickettsia prowazeki* in humans differ from infection with other rickettsial organisms?

3. Write brief notes on the infections caused by the TRIC group of organisms.

4. List the diseases that are spread by the body louse. Where would one expect to find this parasite in a verminous person?

Selected Readings

Castleman, B. (Ed.): Case records of the Massachusetts General Hospital. A case of Rocky Mountain spotted fever. New England Journal of Medicine, 288:1400–1404, 1973.
Cruickshank, R., Duguid, J. P., Marmion, B. P., and Swain, R. H. A.: Medical Microbiology. 12th ed. Edinburgh, Churchill Livingstone, 1973, Chapters 50–52.

---

*Named after Burnet, the Australian virologist, who is better known for his concepts in immunology (Chapter 9). The genus *Coxiella* is closely related to the genus *Rickettsia*.

Viral Infections CHAPTER 12

After studying this chapter the student should be able to:

- Compare and contrast viruses with higher organisms with respect to the following:
  - (a) size
  - (b) structure
  - (c) chemical composition
- Describe how viruses enter a cell, how new viral material is produced, and how new particles are released.
- Describe the range of effects that a viral infection can have on a cell.
- Describe the immunity that a viral infection can evoke, particularly in relation to the following:
  - (a) immunoglobulin formation
  - (b) T-cell immunity
  - (c) interferon production
- List the nine groups of viruses described in this chapter and give examples of the common members within each group.
- Distinguish among the following: the incubation period, the prodromal stage, enanthem, and exanthem. Use measles and smallpox as examples.
- Describe the pathogenesis of poliomyelitis as well as the means available for preventing this disease.
- Describe the hazards of vaccination against smallpox.
- Discuss the relationship between varicella and zoster. Outline the clinical features of each.
- Compare hepatitis A with hepatitis B in regard to these factors:
  - (a) incubation period
  - (b) mode of transmission
  - (c) clinical features and complications
  - (d) etiology
- Describe the three particles that have been found in the blood of patients with hepatitis B. Indicate their antigenic interrelationship.

Introduction

Viral infections are common and are of many types. At times, some have reached epidemic proportions and have been so severe that through the ages man has made strenuous attempts at preventing them; by chance, some attempts have been successful. Thus, Jenner, who knew nothing of virology, found a way to prevent smallpox. Pasteur postulated that the cause of rabies was an infinitesimally small microorganism, and without ever isolating it, he devised a means of protecting against rabies. The theory that disease could be caused by organisms smaller than bacteria was finally confirmed by Iwanowsky in 1892, when he showed that tobacco mosaic disease was due to an agent so small that it could pass through the pores of a filter that would retain all known bacteria. It was at the turn of the century that the first human disease, yellow fever, was proved to be caused by a similar ultramicroscopic, filterable virus. Until the advent of electron microscopy, the structure of viruses was poorly understood. We now have a wealth of knowledge concerning their structure and chemical composition, and this can best be understood in relation to the properties of bacteria.

GENERAL PROPERTIES OF VIRUSES

Bacteria are all within the range of the light microscope and are complete cells surrounded by a cell membrane and often by a cell wall.* They contain both DNA and RNA together with many chemicals, such as enzymes, for their own maintenance and reproduction. They multiply by simple division. Since bacteria are complete cells, the majority of them can be grown by the bacteriologist on an artificial medium; the causative organisms of leprosy and syphilis are the two notable exceptions. Viruses, on the other hand, are much smaller, although the large poxviruses are just within the range of the conventional light microscope. *Viruses contain either RNA or DNA, but never both.* They have no mitochondria and cannot produce high-energy adenosine triphosphate (ATP). They possess no ribosomes. Indeed, viruses consist of little more than structural protein and nucleic acid. They can multiply only in the protoplasm of a cell, and they do this by utilizing the structures and chemicals of the infected cell and perverting them for their own purposes. Indeed, the essential differences between viruses and all other organisms is that the synthetic processes that attend multiplication take place within the protoplasm of the infected cell in viruses but in the body of the organism itself in all other infective agents.

Structure of Viruses

A complete infective virus particle that can exist outside a cell is called a *virion,* and it consists of a core of either DNA or RNA, which is surrounded by a protein coat, or *capsid.* Some viruses, e.g., herpes simplex virus, have an outer *envelope* derived from the nuclear membrane or the plasma membrane of the cell from which the virus was released.

Electron microscopy has shown the coat to consist of subunits, or *capsomeres,* each of which is made of protein and consists of a hollow tube pointing outwards. The capsomeres are closely packed and so arranged with their neighbors that the virion has a definite geometric shape. Three major types of viruses can be recognized: (a) *viruses with cubic symmetry,* which have the form of an icosahedron, a solid, roughly spherical structure having 20 facets, each consisting of an equilateral triangle and meeting at 12 corners (Fig. 12–1); (b) *viruses with helical symmetry,* which consist of a filament

---

*Animal cells do not possess a cell wall. Penicillin acts by inhibiting the formation of cell-wall material. After division, penicillin-treated bacteria have a defective cell wall, are fragile, and are easily killed.

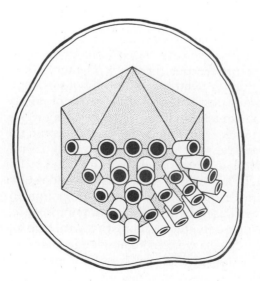

Figure 12–1. Diagrammatic representation of a typical virus showing cubical symmetry. The core of the virus has the form of an icosahedron having 20 facets. It is covered by symmetrically arranged capsomeres, each consisting of a hollow tube. The covering of capsomeres constitutes the viral capsid. The virion (consisting of the genetic material and the capsid) has an outer membrane that is derived from the altered host plasma or nuclear membrane. (Drawing by Frederick Lammerich, Department of Art as Applied to Medicine, University of Toronto.)

Figure 12–2. Helical arrangement of capsomeres. The covering envelope of a paramyxovirus has been ruptured; its RNA content has been released. The photograph shows the long thread of nucleoprotein surrounded by the capsomeres arranged in a helical fashion (× 117,450). (Photograph courtesy of Micheline Fauvel, Department of Medical Microbiology, Faculty of Medicine, University of Toronto.)

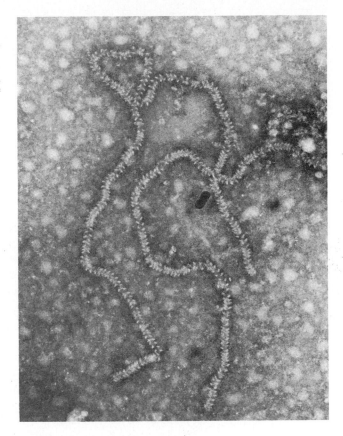

with capsomeres arranged around the nucleic acid as a *helix* (Fig. 12–2); and (c) *complex viruses*, in which the virus particle does not conform to either cubic or helical symmetry, *e.g.*, bacteriophages and poxviruses (Figs. 12–3 and 12–9). Bacteriophage is a virus that infects bacteria and is commonly called "phage" for short; it has a head attached to a central core from which arise six tail filaments (Fig. 12–3).

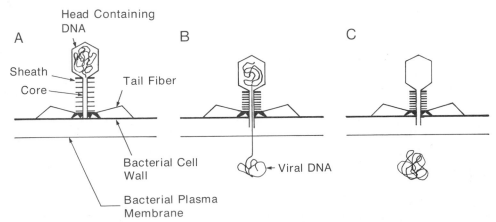

Figure 12–3. Diagrammatic representation of the entry of bacteriophage into a bacterial cell. The bacteriophage consists of a head containing DNA, a rigid core surrounded by a sheath to which is attached a tail piece, and tail fibers. *A*, The first event in the entry of the phage is the attachment of the tail fibers to the receptors of the bacterial cell wall. *B*, Contraction of the sheath results in the injection of viral DNA into the bacterial cell substance. *C*, The protein component of the phage shown attached to the cell wall is subsequently lost, leaving the viral DNA within the substance of the bacterium. Here, it can replicate and lead to lysis of the bacterial cell, or it can remain latent as prophage. (Drawn by Sue Reynolds.)

Growth of Viruses

Viruses will grow only in living cells. In the early days of virology, whole live animals were used for growth of these structures, but the animal's immune response was a complicating factor and the method was ethically undesirable as well as expensive. Also, the animals often harbored their own viruses, and these sometimes served as contaminants. Embryonated hen's eggs were next used, but apart from the absence of an immune response they had similar disadvantages. Cell culture has now largely replaced these methods.

Animal cells (*e.g.*, kidney cells or fibroblasts) will grow as a single monolayer on a glass surface if this is covered by a suitable culture medium. Subcultures can be obtained from such a growth; unfortunately, after repeated subculture, however, the cells cease to multiply and die off. Apparently normal animal cells cannot live forever. Occasionally, the cells undergo an alteration and continued subculture is possible. The process is called *transformation,* and the cells are malignant (Chapter 17). Established cell lines of this type can be kept growing indefinitely and are used for virus culture. The best known of these is the HeLa cell.

Mechanism of Viral Growth.   The first stage of virus-cell interaction is *attachment* of the virion to the cell surface. This is believed to be the result of an affinity of the virus for some specific cell receptors. With the relatively simple bacteriophage, the protein capsid of the organism remains on the outside of the cell, but the phage acts as a type of microsyringe, its DNA content being squirted into the cell substance (Fig. 12–3). With animal viruses the process is less simple, because the stage following attachment is *penetration* of the virus particle into the cell by a process of *endocytosis*. To begin with, the virus is contained within a phagosome; then, by means that are not clearly understood, it escapes from the phagosome and enters the cytoplasm proper. The next stage is one of *uncoating* of the virus so that the free nucleic acid is released. The virus now ceases to exist as a particle and may not even be infective. Nevertheless, its component parts can still be detected. This stage in viral multiplication is known as the *eclipse phase* and is a feature of the reproductive cycle of all true viruses.

The information in the viral nucleic acid is transcribed and diverts the host's cell activity into synthesizing viral coded enzymes, regulating protein synthesis and ultimately leading to the production of more viral nucleic acid and viral structural proteins. The precise way in which this occurs varies considerably from one virus to another.

DNA Viruses.   The viral DNA encodes for specific mRNA, and this is translated on host ribosomes. This leads to the formation of enzymes that are needed later for the subsequent synthesis of new viral DNA and structural proteins that form the viral coat.

RNA Viruses.   Viruses in this group vary considerably in how they replicate within cells. With some viruses (*e.g.*, poliovirus), the viral RNA acts as messenger RNA that encodes for enzymes and viral proteins and as a complementary RNA that is used as a template for the formation of new viral RNA. With other viruses, especially those that are enveloped, such as the myxoviruses, the viral RNA leads to the formation first of a complementary strand of RNA, which then acts as mRNA for the production of new enzymes, viral protein, and new viral RNA. The replication of tumor RNA viruses is quite different from either of the two previous methods. Virus-specific DNA is formed by reverse transcriptase and becomes incorporated in the host cell's genome. Virus RNA is transcribed from this virus-specific DNA.

It is evident that the replication of viruses is a complex affair. The result is that the specific nucleic acid, either RNA or DNA, is manufactured together

Figure 12–4. A myxovirus. An electron micrograph of influenza A/2, England 4272, which is demonstrated by negative staining. The irregular shape of the virus is clearly seen, and the well-marked covering membrane from which numerous prickles project is also observable. These projections contain hemagglutinin; it is to these structures that red cells become adherent. The RNA within the virion is not apparent in this photograph (× 120,000). (Photograph courtesy of Micheline Fauvel, Department of Medical Microbiology, Faculty of Medicine, University of Toronto.)

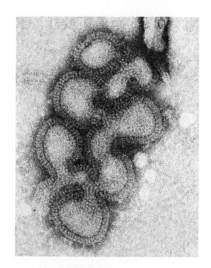

with the protein component of the capsomeres. The final result is assembly of mature virus particles, and this may occur either in the cytoplasm or in the nucleus. Finally, the particles are released from the cell.

Release of Virus Particles. The virus-infected cell may be so damaged that it disintegrates, and mature virus particles are released in a burstlike fashion. Under other circumstances, the cell is not destroyed, and virus particles are released slowly. In the latter type of infection, the virus frequently receives an additional coat, termed an *envelope*, from a cell membrane. Thus, the orthomyxoviruses receive an envelope of cell membrane (Fig. 12–4). This membrane is not a completely normal cell membrane, but one that has been modified by the effect of virus and contains viral type antigens. Herpesvirus, a DNA virus that is assembled in the nucleus, acquires an envelope of modified nuclear membrane from the host cell (Fig. 12–5).

As noted above, viruses sometimes kill the cells that they infect. In tissue culture this is termed a *cytopathic effect* and is useful in diagnostic virology. If known specific antiserum is added to a culture, inhibition of the cytopathic effect helps to identify an unknown virus (Figs. 12–6 and 12–7).

Sometimes an infecting virus alters the cell, but it does not kill it. A common effect is the formation of a mass of homogeneous material, called an *inclusion body*, either in the nucleus or in the cytoplasm of the infected cell. Inclusion bodies consist of maturing viral material and can be used as markers in the identification of a viral disease. Thus, the finding of characteristic inclusion bodies (Negri bodies) in the neurons of a dog is diagnostic of rabies.

Viral nucleic acid can sometimes enter the nucleic acid pool (genome) of the host cell and become incorporated into the host's genetic material. The viral nucleic acid then replicates when the cell divides; in fact, it behaves like a gene. This symbiotic relationship can result in the cell showing no evidence of infection. The virus is *latent*.

Under certain circumstances the nucleic acid of a latent virus can replicate and behave once more as an infective agent. The cell may then be damaged. Some examples illustrating the implications of this remarkable relationship are as follows:

1. Some bacteria contain a latent bacteriophage. This can suddenly lead to lysis of a whole culture. Such a strain of bacteria is termed *lysogenic*.

Effect of Viruses on Cells

2. Herpes simplex virus can remain latent for many months or years in human beings. The development of fever from any cause, exposure to sunlight, or the onset of menstruation can upset the balance between the person and the virus, and then herpes blisters, or *coldsores*, appear on the skin.

3. The cell containing a latent infection may show altered function. Thus, production of toxin by the diphtheria bacillus is determined by the presence of a phage.

4. Some viruses can cause normal animal cells to be transformed into cancer cells. Since such cells are stimulated to grow, this response has very important implications when one considers the possible causes of cancer (Chapter 17).

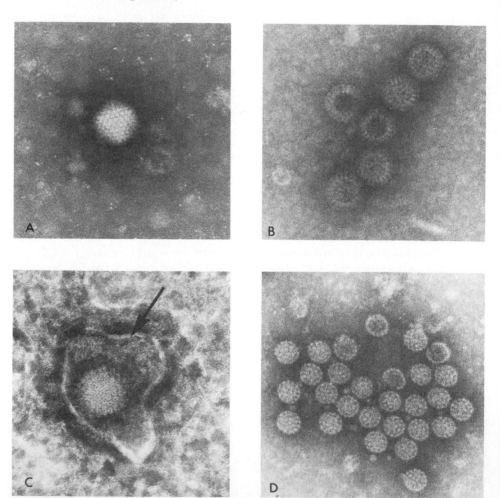

Figure 12–5. *A, Adenovirus.* This virus, which is demonstrated by negative staining, has the typical icosahedral form and has no outer envelope (× 167,760). *B, Rotavirus.* This virus has not yet been grown in tissue cultures. It can be found by electron microscopy in the stools of some infants with acute gastroenteritis. This disease is a major cause of illness during childhood and is particularly common in infants under the age of two years; it often occurs in winter. Some cases are due to bacterial infection (e.g., *Salmonella, E. coli*), but most cases appear to be due to viruses (× 136,300). *C, Herpes simplex virus.* The envelope, which is clearly shown (arrow), is derived from the modified nuclear membrane of an infected cell. The hollow capsomeres of the virion are clearly visible (× 139,800). (Compare this with Figure 12–1.) *D, Papovavirus, S.V. 40.* This organism was found as a contaminant in a culture of African Green Monkey kidney cells. Another important member of this group of viruses is the polyoma virus. In tissue culture, the cells show characteristic vacuolation. The name "papova" is derived from *PA*pilloma, *PO*lyoma, *VA*cuolating agent (× 136,300). (Photographs courtesy of Micheline Fauvel, Department of Medical Microbiology, Faculty of Medicine, University of Toronto.)

Figure 12–6. Normal HeLa cells in tissue culture. The confluent sheet is composed of plump polygonal cells derived from a malignant epithelial cell line that originated from a carcinoma in a patient named *Helen Lane*—hence, the name "HeLa." A giant cell form is conspicuous in this field. This photograph was obtained by using phase contrast microscopy (× 200).

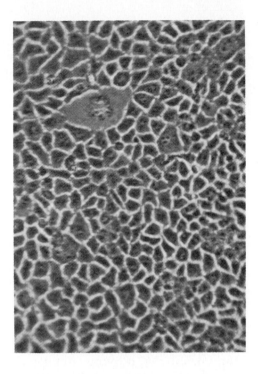

It was once fashionable to classify viruses according to the tissue they affected. Thus, a *derma*totropic virus affects the skin, whereas a *neuro*tropic one involves the nervous system. This classification is quite unsatisfactory, because many viruses can affect different tissues. Thus, the dermatotropic virus, herpes simplex, which causes coldsores, in fact lies latent in the nerve cells of the ganglion that is related to the sensory nerve supply of the part affected. Herpes simplex virus can cause pneumonia and encephalitis. It is therefore quite unreasonable to classify it as a dermatotropic virus. The

Classification of Viruses

Figure 12–7. HeLa cells in culture infected with adenovirus. The sheet of cells is broken up, and the swollen, refractile cells have fused to form irregular masses. This response is called the *cytopathic effect of the virus.* Specific antisera will inhibit this effect. Using known antisera, one can identify a particular virus. Likewise, if cultures of a known virus are used, the ability of a serum to inhibit the cytopathic effect can be used to estimate the titer and specificity of antibody (× 200).

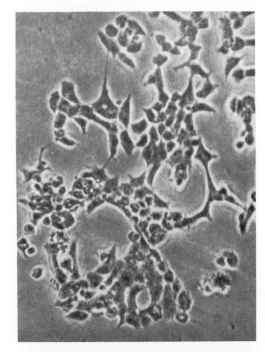

modern classification of viruses is under constant review, but major groups are now being separated with reference to the following criteria:

1. The type of nucleic acid present — whether it is DNA or RNA.
2. The symmetry of the virus — whether cubic, helical, or complex.
3. The size of the virion and the number of its capsomeres.
4. The presence or absence of an envelope.
5. The antigenic structure of the virus. Some viruses share common antigens with others, and these are then included in one group; for example, the adenoviruses all possess a common group antigen.

Mechanism of Immunity to Viral Infections

The mechanism of immunity to viral infection is complex and has several components.

Protection by Immunoglobulins.   Plasma antibodies play an important part, especially in the disseminated infections. Most viruses possess several antigens, some associated with the protein envelope and others with the nucleoprotein. The antibodies reacting with the protein coat are those that are of importance in immunity; they prevent the virus from attaching itself to the cell receptor. The virus is invulnerable to antibody when it is intracellular. These plasma, virus-neutralizing immunoglobulins belong mostly to the IgG class.

Note that after recovery from an attack of poliomyelitis, or following immunization with living attenuated virus administered orally, a subsequent dose of poliovirus does not flourish in the cells of the small bowel. This is due to the action of IgA antibodies produced locally in the intestine and present in the secretions. People who have been immunized with a killed suspension of poliovirus administered parenterally (Salk vaccine) usually exhibit unhindered multiplication of viruses in the small bowel despite a considerable antibody response in the blood.

It should be stressed that no live viral vaccine should be given to any patient with an immunological defect. Likewise, a live vaccine should not be given to pregnant women for fear of infecting the fetus.

Cell-mediated Immunity.   There is also a T-cell–mediated immunity independent of circulating antibodies. Children with congenital immunoglobulin deficiency can resist viral infections, but if they have a T-cell defect, death is often due to widespread viral disease. T cells can kill viruses and the cells that harbor them in a variety of ways. There may be a direct cytotoxic effect of sensitized T cells, or lymphokines may be released (Chapter 9). These agents have many effects. They can recruit inflammatory cells, particularly macrophages. One of the lymphokines is interferon (see below).

Antibody-dependent cell-mediated cytotoxicity (Chapter 9) is a mechanism whereby non-sensitized cells — neutrophils, lymphocytes, and macrophages — can acquire cytotoxic activity in the presence of specific immunoglobulins. Cellular immunity is particularly important in herpesvirus and poxvirus infections.

Interferon.   The infection of a cell with one virus sometimes prevents a second infection by another virus. This phenomenon is termed "viral interference," and an important mechanism is the production of a protein called *interferon* by the cell. Interferon is a protein of low molecular weight, which readily diffuses from the cell and causes other cells to produce agents called *translation-inhibiting proteins* (TIP), which are thought to prevent translation of viral mRNA. Interferon has no effect on the cell's protein synthesis, but by being able to distinguish between viral and cellular mRNA, it can prevent viral replication in the cell. The production of interferon does not save an infected cell, but by affecting neighboring cells, the interferon probably prevents the spread of a viral infection within the body. Interferon does not produce lasting immunity to viral infection but is probably a major factor in recovery from an acute attack.

Various attempts have been made to use interferon as a prophylactic agent; unfortunately, it is species specific and only human interferon is effective in the treatment or prophylaxis of human disease. This has posed severe technical difficulties, but nevertheless, interferon is now being manufactured from human white cells, lymphoblastoid cells (Chapter 1), and fibroblasts. The compound is not generally available, but in the future it is likely that the techniques of recombinant DNA will be used to insert the appropriate genetic information into bacteria so that interferon can be made on a large scale (Chapter 3).

Viral Chemotherapy

The very close relationship between the virus and its host cell at one time made it appear unlikely that specific chemotherapeutic agents could be developed for viral diseases. If a virus utilized cell ribosomes and other enzymes, then it seemed unlikely that a specific blocking agent could be found. This initial pessimism was not justified. Viruses have very specific actions, starting with their attachment to the cell, their penetration, their uncoating, their production of viral material, and their assembly and release. These are highly specific events, each of which is a point of attack. Already a number of compounds are known that will act as chemotherapeutic agents, but unfortunately most of them are toxic and have not come into general use. *Amantadine* specifically blocks the penetration of influenza A virus into cells and has been used as a prophylactic drug. It could be used in the event of a widespread epidemic. 5-Iodo-2-deoxyuridine (idoxuridine or 5-IDU) inhibits the growth of vaccinia and herpes simplex viruses. This has been used as a local application at two hourly intervals to treat herpes keratitis. Its use for the common herpes infection (coldsores) of the skin is disappointing. *Cytosine arabinoside* and *adenine arabinoside* have been used in the treatment of herpetic encephalitis and severe varicella-zoster infections. Like 5-IDU they are too toxic to be useful agents except in desperate situations. It is to be hoped that in the future better, less toxic agents will be available for the treatment and prophylaxis of viral disease.

These will be described under nine headings; (1) The Enteroviruses; (2) The Poxviruses; (3) Viruses Affecting the Respiratory Tract; (4) The Arthropod-borne Viruses; (5) The Herpesviruses; (6) Infectious Warts and Other Papovavirus Infections; (7) Viral Hepatitis; (8) Rabies; and (9) The Slow Viruses.

EXAMPLES OF VIRAL INFECTIONS

The enteroviruses are a group of small, spherical, single-stranded RNA–containing viruses found particularly in the intestine. They are members of a large group called the picornaviruses (pico = small + RNA), to which the rhinoviruses, the cause of the common cold, belong. Three main groups of enteroviruses will be described.

The Enteroviruses

1. The Coxsackie Viruses.   This group was so named because they were first isolated in the town of Coxsackie in New York State. There are a large number of viruses in this group, and they cause a variety of illnesses ranging from an upper respiratory infection resembling a cold to meningitis and myocarditis.

*2. The ECHO Viruses.** There are many types, causing a variety of infections, as do the Coxsackie viruses.

---

*ECHO = Enteric, cytopathic, human, orphan viruses. These viruses were first noted in children's feces and could not at first be linked with any disease.

3. *Poliovirus.* Poliomyelitis is an important disease and will be discussed in some detail.

Poliomyelitis. Poliomyelitis (infantile paralysis) is the most important of the enterovirus infections. There are three separate strains of the organism, and the disease is acquired by ingesting material that has been contaminated by virus-containing feces. The virus proliferates in the cells of the bowel, and if the infection is not arrested at this stage, the virus enters the blood stream via the lymphatics. It multiplies in various extraneuronal sites, and after 7 to 14 days (the incubation period of the disease) virus particles re-enter the blood stream and fever commences. Even at this stage of viremia, the disease may be arrested without severe effect.

If the condition proceeds, the virus finally settles in the central nervous system and localizes in the motor nerve cells of the medulla and spinal cord. Some of the infected cells are destroyed, and paralysis ensues. It should be stressed that although many people are infected with poliomyelitis, only a few develop a clinical disease, and of these only some develop paralysis. A number of factors are known which appear to precipitate paralytic poliomyelitis. One of these is local trauma. If a patient who is already infected with poliomyelitis has his tonsils removed, paralysis of the pharynx can occur. This is known as the bulbar type of disease. Likewise, an injection at any site can precipitate paralysis. It is therefore important that during an epidemic of poliomyelitis, no one should be subjected to unnecessary surgical trauma nor should injections for immunization against other disease, such as diphtheria, be given.

Active Immunization. The first effective vaccine was devised by Salk, who used poliovirus grown in monkey kidney cells and subsequently inactivated by formaldehyde. The Salk vaccine is administered by intramuscular injection, and three or four doses are given to ensure adequate antigenic stimulation. The vaccine stimulates the production of immunoglobulins. This does not prevent infection of the intestine with poliovirus, but it does prevent subsequent spread of the virus to involve the central nervous system. The vaccine can advantageously be combined with other vaccines and toxoids.

The vaccine developed by Sabin is a live attenuated virus and is given by mouth. The attenuated virus causes an intestinal infection that, like the Salk vaccine, stimulates the formation of immunoglobulin antibodies. However, there is one important difference between the vaccines: the Sabin vaccine also produces intestinal immunity because of the local formation of IgA. Thus, the Sabin vaccine prevents the subsequent infection with poliovirus, and it may be presumed that if large populations are immunized with Sabin vaccine, virulent strains of the virus will eventually die out. Because the Sabin vaccine is easier to administer and more effective, it has become the more popular of the two methods of immunization. It is usual to give the three separate strains of poliovirus. As noted previously, the infection of a cell with one virus sometimes prevents infection with other viruses. To overcome this interference, three separate doses of the trivalent vaccine are administered.

Rotaviruses. Although not strictly enteroviruses, the rotaviruses are considered here since they are also found in the intestinal tract. They have recently attained importance as a possible cause of *acute infantile gastroenteritis.*

The Poxviruses   The poxviruses are a group of large, brick-shaped, DNA-containing viruses that produce vesicular and pustular lesions of the skin. Many animals have their own variety of pox disease, *e.g.,* cowpox and mousepox. The human disease is *smallpox,* or *variola.* The virus that causes the common skin disease molluscum contagiosum is included among the poxviruses (Fig. 12–8).

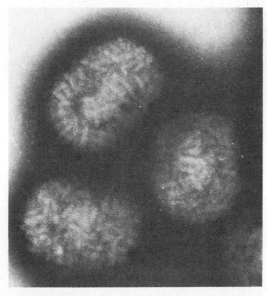

Figure 12–8. Poxvirus from molluscum contagiosum. Molluscum contagiosum is a viral disease of the skin that is characterized by the formation of small umbilicated papules. It is common in children and is a self-limiting disease. A suspension of material from a human lesion was mixed with a solution of 2 per cent phosphotungstic acid and allowed to dry on a suitably prepared copper grid coated with a film of carbon. Under the electron microscope, the electron-dense background produced by the phosphotungstic acid allows the viral particles to stand out quite clearly. This technique, which is known as "negative staining," is frequently used to demonstrate viral particles. Poxviruses are large, square, and structurally complex. The outer protein layer consisting of strands is shown here. Because vaccinia and smallpox viruses have a similar morphology, the identification of particles of this type in a case of suspected smallpox would lead to a provisional diagnosis of this disease. Confirmation by culture and serological means would be required ($\times$ 105,850). (Photograph courtesy of Micheline Fauvel, Department of Medical Microbiology, Faculty of Medicine, University of Toronto.)

Smallpox

The disease is acquired by inhalation of virus either directly from a patient or indirectly from fomites. The bedding is particularly dangerous as a fomite, and there are many instances on record where laundry workers have acquired the disease. It is believed that the primary site of infection is in the nasopharynx and that following local multiplication of virus, the organism spreads via the lymphatics; following a transient primary viremia, it spreads to involve the reticuloendothelial system. Viral multiplication is followed by a second phase of viremia about 10 days later, and this coincides with the onset of symptoms. The initial illness, before the development of the rash, is called the *prodromal stage* and lasts for about four days. The rash starts first on the mucous membranes (the *enanthem*) and then on the skin (the *exanthem*). Skin lesions are at first erythematous but rapidly become vesicular and pustular. Characteristically all the lesions are at the same stage of development, and they tend to be more frequent on the face and distal parts of the body. The trunk, particularly the front of the chest and abdomen, is relatively spared. Smallpox is highly infectious, and in the past has been responsible for devastating epidemics having a mortality of up to 50 per cent. In those who survive, the skin lesions heal with scarring, which leaves the typical "pockmarks" on the face.

Active Immunization. The first really effective attempt at smallpox immunization was performed by Edward Jenner, who discovered that the natural pox infection of bovine animals, cowpox, could produce a similar but localized lesion in human beings and that this would lead to protection against subsequent smallpox infection.

Since then a third virus has emerged: vaccinia virus. Its origin is obscure. It is believed to be a mutant of either variola or cowpox viruses; probably most strains used at the present time originated from cowpox.

Until recently, vaccination has been a recommended procedure for protection against infection with smallpox. However, it has certain dangers:

1. Eczema Vaccinatum. Patients with pre-existing skin disease, particularly atopic dermatitis, can develop a generalized rash that somewhat

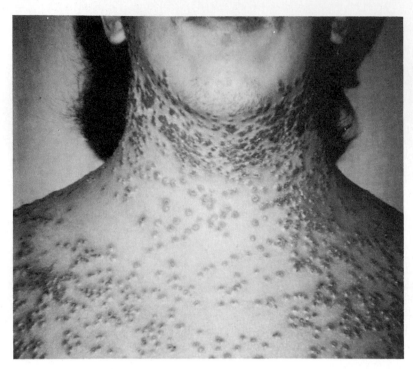

Figure 12–9. Kaposi's varicelliform eruption. The patient is a young man who was eager to travel; he was vaccinated at his own request by his physician. As a child he had suffered from infantile eczema and periodically had developed areas of atopic dermatitis. At the time of vaccination he appeared normal; nevertheless, shortly afterward he developed a widespread eruption that was particularly severe on the chest, neck, and back. Each lesion consisted of a pustule, the center of which was somewhat depressed and umbilicated in appearance. (Note: Any patient with a widespread skin eruption —particularly atopic dermatitis—should not be vaccinated against smallpox.) Accidental inoculation of the lesions with the virus produces Kaposi's varicelliform eruption; if widespread, this can be fatal. A similar widespread infection can occur in patients with burns. Herpes simplex can also produce a similar clinical picture. Electron microscopy of the fluid from one of the pustules is an easy means of distinguishing between the two types of infection.

resembles smallpox itself. This is known as *Kaposi's varicelliform eruption* (Fig. 12–9). It appears to be due to generalized spread of the vaccinia virus in those patients who are particularly susceptible. Occasionally a similar type of generalized eruption is seen from herpes simplex virus infection.

2. Generalized Vaccinia.   This condition occurs as a blood-borne spread from the local vaccination site. It is a self-limiting, relatively benign condition.

3. Progressive Vaccinia.   In this condition the local lesion continues to spread and the outcome is generally fatal. This disease occurs in patients who have T-lymphocyte deficiency.

4. Postvaccinal Encephalomyelitis.   About two weeks after vaccination an encephalitis occurs that has a 50 per cent mortality. It appears to be due to some type of autoimmune reaction, but its precise pathogenesis is not understood.

In view of these unpleasant, though admittedly rare, complications of vaccination, the wholesale use of vaccination became less widely used as the incidence of smallpox declined. The last known case of smallpox in the world occurred in September 1978 in Birmingham, England, where a woman died of the disease acquired from a research laboratory. Prior to that unfortunate event, the last case of confirmed smallpox occurred in Somalia in October 1977. Since no known carrier state exists, smallpox is now regarded as having become extinct. The only possible way of acquiring the disease is from a strain of virus kept in a reference laboratory. Vaccination against the disease is a thing of the past, and Jenner's true claim to fame must be the eradication of a disease rather than the development of a vaccine to prevent it.

Viruses Affecting the Respiratory Tract

Orthomyxoviruses

This is a group of spherical or irregularly shaped viruses having a characteristic envelope that has the property of adhering to red cells (Fig. 12–4). Within the envelope there is a strand of ribonucleoprotein having helical symmetry (Fig. 12–2). The orthomyxoviruses cause influenza — an illness characterized by an acute tracheobronchitis of abrupt onset. The severity of the illness varies from a mild upper respiratory infection with fever and chest pains (the flu) to a rapidly fatal illness with extensive pneumonia. The pneumonia may be due to the virus itself or to a coexistent bacterial infection — generally streptococcal or staphylococcal. Three types of influenza virus are known. *Influenza virus type A* is the most important and causes epidemics or pandemics of varying severity. In some, such as the pandemic of 1918, tens of millions of people died. Influenza virus type A readily mutates, so that new strains are continually appearing. Occasionally a virulent strain emerges, and an epidemic ensues because the population has no immunity to it. *Influenza virus type B* causes endemic cases and occasional epidemics, although these tend to affect a localized area. Type B virus shows less antigenic variation than type A. *Influenza virus type C* appears to exist as one single type and causes a subclinical or very mild upper respiratory infection.

These viruses resemble the orthoviruses in morphology but are larger and more pleomorphic. The group includes the viruses described below: **Paramyxoviruses**

Parainfluenza Viruses.   These cause respiratory infections similar to influenza. In infants parainfluenza viruses cause *croup* or *acute laryngo-tracheobronchitis*. This is characterized by hoarseness and cough and may lead to severe respiratory distress. Bronchiolitis and pneumonia may occur.

Respiratory Syncytial Virus (RSV).   This virus produces a cytopathic effect in tissue culture, and the virus-infected cells tend to fuse together to form giant cells or a syncytium, from which the virus acquires its name. Infection may occur at any age to produce a common cold–like illness, but the importance of this virus is that it is a common cause of *bronchiolitis and pneumonia in infants* under 1 year of age and is indeed the most common cause in those under 6 months.

Mumps Virus.   Mumps is a disease that has a long incubation period (18 to 21 days) and is characterized by fever and enlargement of one or both parotid glands (acute parotitis). In adult males this may be complicated by involvement of one or both testes (acute orchitis). Infection of the ovaries may also occur, and in both sexes meningoencephalitis and pancreatitis are well-recognized complications.

Measles (Morbilli).   This is the most infectious of the common fevers. A 10-day incubation period is followed by a 4-day illness with fever, tracheobronchitis, and conjunctivitis. The characteristic enanthem appears on the buccal mucosa as grains of salt on a red background; these "Koplik's spots" are diagnostic of the disease during this early catarrhal infectious phase. On the fourteenth day after exposure, the characteristic maculopapular exanthem appears. *German measles* (rubella) resembles measles clinically but has a longer incubation period (16 to 18 days), and the prodromal stage is mild or absent. This otherwise trivial disease is of importance because it causes malformations and other abnormalities in the unborn children of pregnant women who contract the disease (Chapter 16). The virus of German measles is probably not a paramyxovirus, and as yet it remains unclassified. It is included here for convenience.

The adenoviruses are DNA-containing viruses that are common commensals of the upper respiratory tract. They cause a variety of mild upper respiratory infections and conjunctivitis (Fig. 12–5).   **Adenoviruses**

These are small RNA-containing viruses that cause the common cold, by far the most frequent form of respiratory viral infection. The incubation period   **Rhinoviruses** is 2 to 4 days, and the disease is characterized by nasal discharge, sore throat, cough, and fever. There are a large number of different subtypes, and repeated attacks can occur since neutralizing antibodies merely have a protective effect against reinfection with the particular serotype responsible.

The Arthropod-borne Viruses

The arthropod-borne viruses contain RNA and have been grouped together as *arboviruses*. In fact they consist of several distinct families. Two main types of disease can be recognized:

Arbovirus Encephalitis

Many types are known and tend to be restricted to particular parts of the world. Some (*e.g.,* Western equine encephalitis of North America and Venezuelan equine encephalitis) are mild, while others (*e.g.,* Eastern equine encephalitis of North America and Japanese B encephalitis) are severe.

Arbovirus Fevers and Hemorrhagic Fevers

One of the most severe diseases of this group is *yellow fever,* which is caused by a flavivirus and is spread by a mosquito. The disease is endemic in West Africa and Central America. The virus causes a severe illness characterized by hepatic necrosis resulting in jaundice, renal failure, and a high mortality.

Dengue is a major health problem in Southeast Asia, India, and the Pacific Islands. The disease is characterized by a severe febrile illness with a rash and severe pains in the limbs. It is rarely fatal, except in young children, in whom it may cause the *dengue hemorrhagic shock syndrome.* This resembles a number of other distinct viral infections that are collectively known as the *hemorrhagic fevers* and have a high mortality.

The Herpesviruses

Although the well-known clinical features of varicella (chickenpox) and zoster are poles apart, there is good evidence that they are both caused by the same virus.

Varicella and Zoster

Chickenpox. This disease has a pathogenesis similar to that of smallpox. It exhibits an enanthem with vesicles on the oral mucosa followed by an exanthem of vesicles on the skin, which subsequently become pustular. Clinically, the disease bears some resemblance to smallpox, but the prodromal stage is much less severe; the skin eruption tends to occur in crops, so that lesions at a different stage of development are present at the same time, and the distribution of the rash is different. In chickenpox the lesions are not clustered in areas of pressure and tend to be most profuse on the trunk. In smallpox the limbs, face, and back are most severely affected.

Zoster (Shingles).   Following an attack of chickenpox the virus may lie latent in the posterior root ganglia of the spinal, trigeminal, or facial nerves. In later life the virus can be reactivated, and can spread down the nerve fibers to the skin, producing the lesions of herpes zoster (Fig. 12–11).

The onset of an attack is characterized by discomfort or pain in the area affected. Next erythema (redness) and swelling appear, followed by crops of papules and vesicles, which often become hemorrhagic before maturing to form pustules (see Chapter 41 for definitions of these terms). These dry, and the crusts finally fall off to leave areas of scarring and irregular pigmentation (Fig. 12–10). Shingles commonly involves one or more of the branches of the fifth cranial nerve, and if the eye is affected, special care is needed to prevent permanent damage to the cornea (Fig. 12–11). Pain is a feature of shingles and is often severe when the face is involved. The pain can persist for many months after the skin lesions have healed (*post-herpetic neuralgia*). This emphasizes the fact that shingles is primarily an infection involving nerves.

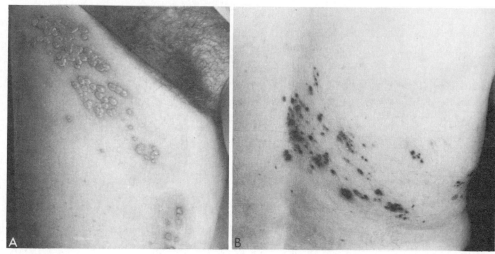

Figure 12–10. Shingles (zoster). *A,* The photograph shows the right thigh of a patient with early zoster. Skin lesions consist of grouped, tender water blisters (vesicles), each surrounded by a zone of redness (erythema). The lesions are distributed along the second lumbar nerve. As the disease progresses, the lesions dry up and become encrusted. *B,* This print shows a typical case of zoster at the stage of crusting. Note how the lesions follow the line of the cutaneous nerves that parallel the ribs. The lesions do not cross the midline; this is an important sign that helps to distinguish zoster from other localized blistering diseases, such as a contact dermatitis. The lesions of zoster heal with scarring and are often painful, particularly in elderly patients.

Figure 12–11. Shingles (zoster). This patient has well-advanced lesions of zoster involving the ophthalmic and maxillary divisions of the right fifth cranial nerve (trigeminal nerve). Although the eyelids are swollen and show vesicles with crusting, the conjunctiva and cornea were spared. The branch that supplies the cornea also supplies the tip of the nose, which in this patient is also uninvolved.

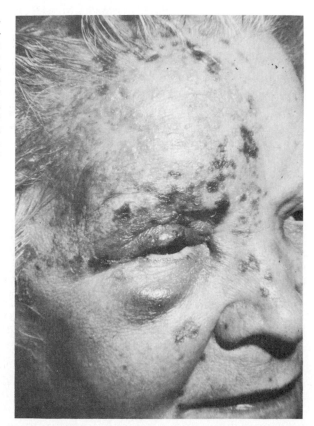

Children exposed to a patient with zoster can develop chickenpox if they are susceptible.

Herpes Simplex

The virus of herpes simplex is one of the most widely distributed viruses in human beings (Fig. 12–5C). It has been estimated that about 60 per cent of the population is affected. Of these, only 10 per cent exhibit primary childhood lesions, such as gingivostomatitis, keratoconjunctivitis, and vulvovaginitis. Two antigenically distinct types of virus are known. Type I commonly affects the mouth and skin, whereas Type II affects the genitalia. It should be noted that the acute primary gingivostomatitis is characterized by numerous painful ulcers in the mouth. It is associated with malaise and fever. Following recovery the subject does not develop recurrent mouth ulcers but may be liable to recurrent cold sores on the skin, particularly that adjacent to the lips.

Abrasions of the skin sometimes lead to primary herpetic infection (traumatic, or inoculation, herpes simplex). A good example of this is the painful *herpetic whitlow*, which is seen in nursing attendants working in neurosurgical wards. These people acquire their infection while inserting endotracheal tubes into the mouths of unconscious patients.

Usually, however, the primary infection remains subclinical, and the virus remains latent in the cells of the host. This symbiosis tends to be disturbed by intercurrent infections, such as the common cold, pneumonia, and malaria, and in very susceptible victims even by menstruation, emotional strain, and exposure to sunlight. There then develop typical *herpetic blisters* (coldsores), especially around the mucocutaneous junction of the lips. Occasionally lesions recur in the conjunctiva and cornea. The remarkable feature of herpes simplex is the tendency for lesions to recur at the same site. Thus, one patient complained of developing lesions on the left knee every spring for six consecutive years. The tendency for herpes simplex to recur at the same site as well as its continued chronicity has led to the belief that the virus resides in the sensory root ganglia and that the pathogenesis is therefore similar to that of zoster.

Type I herpes simplex virus occasionally disseminates and leads to an *acute necrotizing encephalitis.*

Type II herpes simplex virus usually affects the genitalia and leads to recurrent lesions. Vesicles develop on an erythematous base and quickly evolve into shallow painful ulcers that last 1 to 2 weeks. In the male the lesions are usually on the glans or shaft of the penis while in women there is recurrent ulceration of the vulva, vaginal wall, or cervix. Infection is acquired by intercourse, and herpes genitalis is now one of the common venereal diseases. It causes great emotional and physical upset and is particularly serious during pregnancy. If active lesions are present at the time of labor, the infant may be infected during its passage through the birth canal. *Neonatal infection* is a severe generalized disease associated with liver damage and a high mortality. The infection can be averted by cesarean section.

Epstein-Barr (EB) Virus

This herpesvirus causes classical *infectious mononucleosis* with a positive Paul-Bunnell test. It is also associated with nasopharyngeal carcinoma and Burkitt's lymphoma (Chapter 17).

Infectious Warts and Other Papovavirus Infections

The common wart is due to a small DNA-containing virus that belongs to a group of organisms that also cause papillomas in other animals (Fig. 12–6D). They have been labeled the *papovaviruses*. Included in this group is a passenger virus quite commonly found in monkey kidney cells — the *SV-40* virus, which under some circumstances is capable of inducing tumor formation. It has not been proved to be harmful to humans.

There are two distinct diseases that come into this category. They are **Viral Hepatitis** traditionally called infective hepatitis and serum hepatitis, but the terms *hepatitis A* and *hepatitis B* are now used since the causative agents have been isolated and the adjectives "serum" and "infective" are not accurately descriptive of the diseases.

Hepatitis A has an incubation period of about *1 month* and tends to occur **Hepatitis A** in epidemics in places where young adults are crowded together, such as in military and academic institutions. This disease is caused by a small (25 to 28 nm) RNA virus with cubic symmetry. It can be transmitted to chimpanzees and has recently been grown in tissue culture. The virus can be demonstrated in the blood and feces during the acute illness and persists in the feces for 3 to 4 weeks during convalescence. The disease is spread from case to case via the fecal-oral route or is acquired by the ingestion of food or water contaminated by feces containing hepatitis A virus (HAV).

The onset of the disease is usually insidious and is accompanied by malaise and mild gastrointestinal upset. Aversion to cigarette smoking is a curious early symptom, and sometimes urticaria and joint pains are prominent, suggesting that immune complexes play a part in the pathogenesis of this stage of the disease. After a few days, jaundice and other evidence of liver cell damage appear. Following a prolonged course of several weeks, recovery occurs. The disease has a low mortality.

This disease has an incubation period of about *3 months* and tends to be **Hepatitis B** more severe than hepatitis A, although an absolute distinction between the two is not possible on clinical grounds. The disease has an appreciable mortality, and there is a tendency for it to be followed by progressive liver damage and cirrhosis. Hepatitis B is nearly always contracted by the injection of blood or serum from a person carrying the infective agent. Minute quantities are capable of transferring infection. In the past the disease has occurred in venereal disease clinics where patients were lined up and therapeutic agents were injected with a common needle. Likewise, it is a major hazard among drug addicts. The disease is also rife in those who handle human blood or work in hemodialysis units.

In spite of the fact that hepatitis B is due to an infective agent (termed *virus B*), it has proved to be incredibly difficult to isolate the agent. The virus is clearly no ordinary virus! Indeed, the first clues as to its nature came from a most unlikely source: an abnormal antigen of lipoprotein constitution was noted in the serum of an Australian aborigine, and this was at first believed to be a plasma protein of unusual type determined by an abnormal gene. The antigen was subsequently found in cases of leukemia, lepromatous leprosy, and finally in patients who had a history of having had hepatitis. The antigen was called the *Australia antigen*, and its presence in the blood was found to be associated with the ability of the blood to transmit serum hepatitis. Electron microscopy of Australia antigen–positive serum revealed two types of particles, marked "a" and "b" and shown in Figure 12–12. At first it seemed that these must be the infective agents of hepatitis B, but the discovery that neither of them contained nucleic acid proved to be a stumbling block. Surely no infective agent could exist without nucleic acid! The search for Australia antigen–positive individuals was greatly aided by the observation that patients who had received many blood transfusions (*e.g.*, hemophiliacs) and also those who had recovered from serum hepatitis had a variable titer of

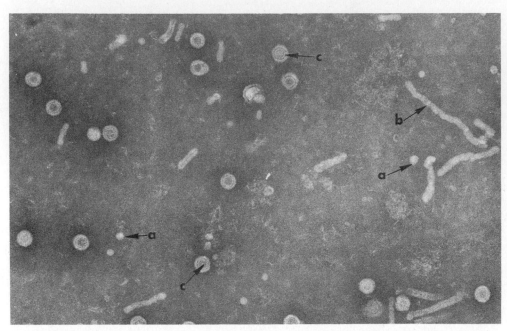

Figure 12–12. Hepatitis B; negative-stained preparation of Australia-antigen positive serum. Three types of particles can be seen: spherical particles 20 nm in diameter (a); elongated tubular filaments up to 230 nm in length, 20 nm in diameter (b); and Dane particles, 42 nm in diameter and having a double shell (c) ($\times$ 119,700). (Photograph courtesy of Micheline Fauvel, Department of Medical Microbiology, Faculty of Medicine, University of Toronto.)

antibodies against this particular antigen. Further investigations of patients with hepatitis B revealed a third type of particle now known as the *Dane particle* (Fig. 12–12). This consists of a central core that is surrounded by a double-shelled structure. The shell and the other two particles share a common surface antigen, and this is now termed the HB_SAg. This is the original Australia antigen. It is not infective and cannot be the cause of hepatitis B. The core of the Dane particle, on the other hand, has another antigen, which is now labeled HB_CAg (Fig. 12–13). The core contains some RNA and also a DNA polymerase. This indeed appears to be the essential agent in hepatitis B, and the Dane particle is currently regarded as the virion responsible for this disease. Identification of the core antigen is at present difficult, owing to the lack of suitable antisera. For the time being, detection of HB_SAg is used to screen blood for its likely infectivity in transfusion work. It seems that the two particles depicted in Figure 12–12 (*a* and *b*) as well as the outer coat of the Dane particle are protein components of the virus, and that these are produced in excess during an infection of hepatitis B.

Although hepatitis B is commonly transmitted by the transference of infected serum, there must be some other means of transmission. Ingestion of contaminated material (*i.e.*, feces) is one possibility, but two other alternatives have recently been investigated. Infection could occur during sexual intercourse when the male acquires infection from the menstrual blood of the female. Secondly, infection could be congenital, since it has been shown that antigen-positive mothers give birth to antigen-positive babies. The investigation has indeed come almost full circle, for in the first instance it was believed that the Australia antigen was a genetically determined factor passed from the parent to the child! This perhaps reiterates the close similarity between the genetic material contained within viruses and the genetic material contained within chromosomes.

The subject of hepatitis has been dealt with at some length, partly because the disease is of current interest and tends to affect young healthy

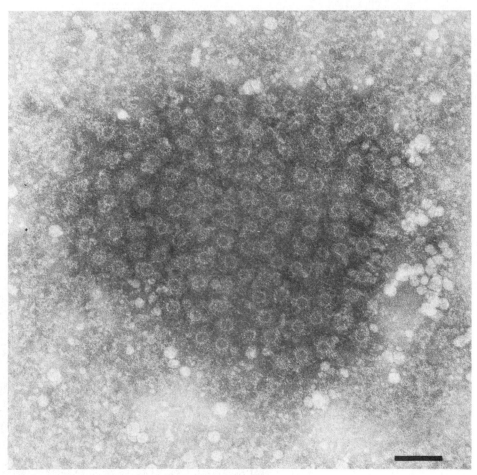

Figure 12–13. Immune electron microscopy test with Dane core antigen incubated with human serum. A concentrated sample of Dane particles was treated with a detergent (polysorbate 80) in order to disrupt the outer coat and to release the internal component. This Dane core measures 27 nm in diameter. The suspension of particles was incubated with serum from a patient who had recovered from an attack of virus B hepatitis. An anticore antibody causes the core particles to adhere to each other and to form immune complexes. This method can be used to detect anti-HB$_c$Ag (see text; bar represents 100 nm) ($\times$119,700). (From Fauvel, M., Babiuk, L., Sheaff, E. T., and Spence, L.: Preparation of a Dane core (hepatitis B) antigen from human plasma. Canadian Journal of Microbiology, *21*(6):905–910, 1975.)

adults, and partly because it illustrates the fact that the pathogenesis of viral diseases is by no means simple. The relationship is not as straightforward as that between the staphylococcus and a boil.

Prophylaxis of hepatitis is possible. Immune serum administered after infection will largely prevent type A hepatitis. With type B or serum hepatitis, the position is less certain, perhaps because the antibody titer of globulin used has been so low that it is virtually ineffective.

A vaccine for hepatitis B has now been prepared from HB$_S$Ag obtained from human serum. Its value is under investigation, but preliminary results suggest that it gives a good degree of protection.

Non A, Non B Hepatitis

Sensitive methods are now available for the detection of HB$_S$Ag, and all prospective blood donors who give a history of jaundice or whose blood contains HB$_S$Ag are rejected. Hence, hepatitis B is no longer a major hazard of blood transfusion. Nevertheless, post-transfusional hepatitis continues to occur. In the U.S.A. about 10 per cent of cases are due to hepatitis B infection, indicating that the tests used are not capable of detecting small amounts of infectious hepatitis B virus. The majority of cases are not due to hepatitis B virus, hepatitis A virus, or any other known virus. Such cases are thought to be due to another virus or group of viruses, which have provisionally been labelled non A, non B. The disease is not clinically distinguishable from other types of viral hepatitis but is generally milder. There is some evidence that the disease is liable to progress to chronic liver disease. Non A, non B hepatitis is spread mainly by the parenteral route (*i.e.*, by injecting infective material), but contact spread in families has been reported.

Rabies   Rabies is caused by a bullet-shaped virus belonging to the group of rhabdoviruses, which normally infect certain species of animals. The disease is rare in human beings, but it is of intense interest for two reasons. With one possible exception, there has never been recorded a human case of rabies in which the patient survived. Although many diseases are fatal, the mode of death in rabies is particularly unpleasant. An initial phase of excitement with spasms and convulsions is characteristic. Particularly common are painful contractions of the pharyngeal muscles initiated by attempts to swallow water. Hence the term *hydrophobia*, meaning that the patients fear water. The stage of excitement is followed by one of generalized paralysis, and death usually occurs within a few days of its onset. Treatment is entirely supportive; the only hope is that the diagnosis is wrong. The second reason for considering rabies important is that the infection is always a threat in North America and in continental Europe. Only in England is the disease virtually unknown and likely to remain so, owing to the strict quarantine regulations that are enforced.

Rabies is endemic in the fox population in Europe, whereas in North America it affects many species of animals, particularly the skunk. Following the bite of an infected animal the virus spreads to the nervous system via the nerve fibers. Rabies in dogs is invariably fatal within 10 days, and if a person is bitten by a dog, it is important to keep the dog under surveillance for this period. If the dog dies or is killed, examination of the brain for Negri bodies is an important investigation.

If the person is bitten by a rabid animal or by an animal that escapes, the question of immunization is of paramount importance. It has been estimated that about 30,000 persons in the U.S.A. are given treatment each year for rabies immunization.

The original method of immunization against rabies was devised by Pasteur. He noted that rabbits infected with rabies developed a virus of fixed virulence. When the spinal cords of infected rabbits were removed and dried for varying periods, it seemed that the virus lost its pathogenicity. Thus, material derived from a rabbit spinal cord that had been dried for some time failed to produce rabies on injection into a human being. A series of 14 injections, each given at daily intervals, was administered — each one being from a rabbit cord preparation dried for a lesser period of time. Unfortunately, the injections are painful and produce ever-increasing local inflammatory reactions. The repeated injection of foreign spinal cord tissue can on occasion lead to an autoimmune encephalomyelitis (Chapter 9). The problem with rabies prophylaxis is whether the risk of inducing a disabling encephalomyelitis outweighs the risk of developing rabies. Antiserum prepared in horses is now available, and vaccines prepared in duck eggs have been developed. The latter are used for immunizing animals, but whether they are sufficiently potent for human use, or indeed whether they are safe, has yet to be determined.

The Slow   *Scrapie* is a disease of sheep that is characterized by itching and by
Viruses   degeneration of the brain. It can be transmitted to sheep, goats, and mice, but

the incubation period is long — rarely less than four months. The infective agent has unusual properties: it can withstand boiling, x-irradiation, and treatment with formalin. It contains little, if any, nucleic acid. Its nature is not understood, but it is grouped with other similar agents as a *slow virus*.

Kuru is a slowly progressive degenerative nervous disease of the Fore people of New Guinea and was originally thought to be inherited. It usually affected women and children of either sex, but not men. A tribal ritual was for women and children to eat the brains of deceased relatives, including those who had suffered from kuru, and it is believed that the disease is caused by a slow virus acquired by this quaint tribute to the dead.

These rare and curious diseases have been mentioned not because they are ever likely to be encountered by a medical practitioner but because they reveal the existence of patterns of infective disease quite different from those previously recognized. Two other human "degenerative" nervous diseases are known to be caused by viruses. One is Creutzfeldt-Jakob disease and the other subacute sclerosing panencephalitis. The latter is caused by the measles virus acting in an obscure way that is quite different from that seen in ordinary measles. The hope is that other diseases will be found to be of similar nature and that ways will be found to combat them.

Review Questions

1. Compare and contrast the methods available for the production of immunity against the following:
    (a) smallpox (variola)
    (b) poliomyelitis (infantile paralysis)

2. It was once fashionable to classify viruses according to the tissues that they affected. Describe why this is now considered an unsatisfactory approach to classification. In particular, use the following viruses to illustrate your answer: the poliovirus, the mumps virus, herpes simplex virus, and the influenza virus.

3. How does the immunity to a virus infection differ from that produced against a bacterial infection? Illustrate your answer with reference to diphtheria, influenza, poliomyelitis, and smallpox.

4. Under what circumstances would you consider it inadvisable to vaccinate a person against smallpox? What are the possible complications of vaccination?

5. List the viruses that cause an upper respiratory infection.

6. Compare hepatitis A with hepatitis B. What is the most common viral cause of post-transfusional hepatitis in North America?

Selected Readings

Cruickshank, R., Duguid, J. P., Marmion, B. P., and Swain, R. H. A.: Medical Microbiology. 12th ed. Vol. 1. Edinburgh, Churchill Livingstone, 1973. Chapters 12, 13, and 14 give a good account of the general properties of viruses. All of Part III is devoted to a detailed account of viral diseases.

Dale, S.: Early events in cell-animal virus interactions. Bacteriological Reviews, 37:13–135, 1973.

Holland, J. J.: Slow, inapparent, and recurrent viruses. Scientific American. 230:32–40, 1974.

Keck, J., and Swerhun, P.: Hepatitis B: an occupational risk. The Canadian Nurse, 76:33–35, 1980.

Leading Article: Diagnosis and management of human rabies. British Medical Journal, 3:721–722, 1975.

Leading Article: Post-transfusion hepatitis, British Medical Journal, 283:1–2, 1981.

Middleton, P. J., Szymanski, M. T., Abbott, G. D., Bortolussi, R., and Hamilton, J. R.: Orbivirus acute gastroenteritis of infancy. Lancet, 1:1241–1244, 1974.

Temin, H., and Baltimore, D.: RNA-directed DNA synthesis and RNA tumor viruses. Advances in Virus Research, 17:129–186, 1972.

Timbury, M. C.: Notes on Medical Virology. 6th ed. Edinburgh, Churchill Livingstone, 1978. A very concise account of medical virology.

Youmans, G. P., Paterson, P. Y., and Sommers, H. M.: The Biologic and Clinical Basis of Infectious Diseases. 2nd ed. Philadelphia, W. B. Saunders Company, 1980. Chpaters 5 to 8 describe the general properties of viruses. Individual infections are discussed in other parts of the book in terms of regional or clinical findings.

CHAPTER 13 Fungal Infections

After studying this chapter the student should be able to:

- Classify the fungi into four groups on the basis of their morphology.
- List the various regional types of ringworm.
- Describe the forms of *Candida* infection and relate them to the types of people who are liable to be affected.
- Describe cryptococcosis, histoplasmosis, candidiasis, North American blastomycosis, and South American blastomycosis with respect to:
  - (a) geographic distribution
  - (b) primary site of infection
  - (c) organs affected in the disseminated forms.

Classification of Fungi

In the past, fungi have been regarded as plants without roots, stems, and leaves and as being incapable of photosynthesis because they lack chlorophyll. They are now regarded as neither plants nor animals; they are placed in a separate group. Although their classification is complex and unsatisfactory, for practical purposes four varieties can be recognized:

1. *Molds,* which grow as long filaments *(hyphae),* which branch and interlace to form a meshwork or *mycelium.*

2. *Yeasts,* which are unicellular and grow by budding only.

3. *Yeastlike fungi,* which grow partly as yeasts and partly as long filamentous forms called *pseudohyphae.*

4. *Dimorphic fungi,* which can grow either as hyphae or as yeasts, according to the cultural conditions.

The great majority of fungi are saprophytic and play an important part in nature by breaking down organic material. They have been of great service to man in the production of bread, cheese, and alcoholic beverages. In the last several decades, they have attracted interest because they produce antibiotic agents.

Diseases Caused by Fungi

Fungal infections *(the mycoses)* may be divided into two groups. The *superficial mycoses* are very common and affect skin only (tinea). The *deep* or *systemic mycoses,* on the other hand, are uncommon causes of clinical illness, but they have recently come to the fore because they complicate illnesses in which there is impairment of the T-cell component of the immune response. In this classification *Candida* occupies an intermediate position, since the common infection is superficial but on occasion the organism disseminates widely.

The Superficial Mycoses

Ringworm or Tinea. Ringworm is caused by a group of fungi that are termed the *dermatophytes* and have the property of digesting the keratin of skin or hair. The dermatophytes are molds that grow as a mycelium and reproduce by the formation of various types of spores.

Ringworm, which is due to invasion of keratin by one of the dermatophytes, can affect the scalp (causing *tinea capitis* in which involvement of hair shafts causes a bald patch), the body skin (causing *tinea corporis* with its variant *tinea cruris* affecting the inguinal region), the foot (causing athlete's foot, or *tinea pedis*), the hands (causing *tinea manuum*), and sometimes the nails (causing *tinea unguium*). Clinically, each type of ringworm has its own particular characteristics, but in general the lesions are erythematous, scaly, sometimes vesicular, and tend to have a sharp red spreading border that gives the lesions a ringlike shape from which the disease acquires its name. Diagnosis is easy: Scrapings of keratin can be examined by direct microscopy for hyphae, and from the culture one can readily identify the particular strain of mold responsible. Local treatment with antifungal agents is effective, except in the case of ringworm of the nails, for which the only effective treatment is prolonged oral administration of griseofulvin, one of the few antibiotics that are effective against these fungi.

Not all ringlike lesions are ringworm. Psoriasis and nummular eczema can mislead the unwary; vigorous, ill-advised treatment can lead to contact dermatitis. Most patients who complain of "ringworm" and "athlete's foot" do not have a fungal infection.

Infection with *Candida* species is one of the most frequent fungal infections in man. The organism most commonly involved is *Candida albicans* (previously called *Monilia albicans*), a yeastlike fungus that reproduces by budding but sometimes elongates to form pseudohyphae. The yeast form is characteristic of superficial candidal infections, whereas the pseudomycelial growth is found when the organism invades deeper tissues. *Candida albicans* is a common commensal in the *oral cavity, alimentary tract*, and *vagina*. Infection occurs when general or local conditions become suitable. Superficial infections of the mucous membrane appear as white patches called *thrush*. In the mouth this is very common in infants — especially premature ones — and it may be accompanied by perianal lesions. Oral candidiasis can occur at any age during the course of any debilitating disease. Vaginal thrush is common during pregnancy, in women using the birth control pill, and in patients with diabetes mellitus. Cutaneous candidiasis can occur in moist intertriginous areas, such as in the groin, under the breasts, and in the nail folds (chronic paronychia) of those whose occupations bring their hands repeatedly into water. Candidiasis constitutes one type of *diaper rash*, while at the other extreme of age *Candida* may cause *angular stomatitis*. This occurs because elderly subjects with dentures suffer from loss of vertical height between the mandible and the maxilla secondary to atrophy of the alveolar bone following the extraction of teeth. The moist folds at the corners of the mouth form a ready site for a troublesome *Candida* infection.

Generalized infection with *Candida albicans* is occurring more frequently and is a serious and often fatal opportunistic infection (see Chapter 6). Steroid therapy, the presence of lymphomas, the administration of cytotoxic drugs, and indeed any disease in which cell-mediated immunity is impaired are predisposing factors for widespread invasion by the organism. Disseminated lesions affect many internal organs.

Less extensive candidal infections are seen under particular circumstances. Endocarditis occurs in addicts who inject themselves intravenously with narcotics. Mouth lesions can spread to produce extensive gastrointestinal infections following the prolonged oral administration of a broad-spectrum antibiotic that upsets the balance of the local bacterial flora. Finally, there is an inherited type of immunological T-cell deficiency, in which there is a selective susceptibility to *Candida* infection. These patients have persistent widespread skin and mucous-membrane infections with *Candida* that defy all

Candidiasis (Moniliasis)

treatment. Nevertheless, despite the distressing skin lesions, dissemination to the internal organs does not occur.

Deep Mycoses   In certain parts of the world fungal infections are of considerable importance. In general, the organisms are found as saprophytes in the soil, and infection is acquired by inhalation. A primary lesion may occur in the lungs, but in the majority of people it is asymptomatic and is followed by healing. Occasionally, however, the organisms produce more severe local damage and spread to involve other organs. In their pathogenesis the diseases therefore resemble tuberculosis to a considerable extent. Indeed, the tissue reaction to these organisms sometimes also closely resembles that seen in tuberculosis.

Cryptococcosis. The causative organism, *Cryptococcus neoformans* (previously called *Torula histolytica*), is a yeast of worldwide distribution. The primary lung lesion is usually small, heals by fibrosis, and passes unnoticed. Occasionally, the organism spreads widely and has an affinity for the central nervous system, where it causes *meningitis*. This widespread dissemination is particularly common in patients with T-cell deficiency.

Histoplasmosis. The causative organism, a dimorphic fungus named *Histoplasma capsulatum*, has a worldwide distribution; infection, however, is particularly common in the Mississippi valley of the U.S.A., and skin tests indicate that up to 90 per cent of the population have been infected. The organism is found in the soil and is particularly abundant in soil contaminated with bird droppings, *e.g.*, in chicken houses. Once again, the primary lesion is in the lung and the disease closely resembles tuberculosis. Unless the initial infection has been heavy, the disease is generally asymptomatic. Healing usually occurs with calcification. Occasionally the lung lesion cavitates, and metastatic lesions occur elsewhere. Even more rarely, the fungi invade the blood stream in a massive way and cause a generalized infection. An extract of the organism is used in the *histoplasmin test* (analogous to the tuberculin reaction) and is positive in infected individuals.

CASE HISTORY I.   In 1953, at the age of 25 years, the patient, an Englishwoman, developed a flulike illness that was accompanied by pain in the chest on taking a deep breath. Pleurisy complicating "virus pneumonia" was diagnosed initially, but markedly enlarged hilar lymph nodes and normal lung fields were revealed by a chest radiograph. The diagnosis was changed to primary tuberculosis, but since the patient produced no sputum, the diagnosis was never proved; nevertheless, her tuberculin test was initially negative and became strongly positive. This Mantoux conversion was taken as good evidence of a tuberculous infection. Three months of rest in a sanatorium was ordered. The patient made a rapid recovery, married, and had two children without recurrence of the lung infection. She emigrated to North America in 1965.

In 1971 at the age of 43, the patient developed another "flulike" illness (see radiograph, Fig. 13–1). A "coin lesion" was noted in the right lung field *(A)*, and a tomogram *(B)* revealed the shadow with greater definition. Although the patient was a nonsmoker, a diagnosis of lung cancer was considered. However, a radiograph taken two years previously showed a lesion of similar size to be present. A cancerous lesion probably would have enlarged during this period. Nevertheless, it was decided that this was insufficient evidence on which to exclude such a serious disease. A needle biopsy was performed under local anesthesia, and necrotic tissue was obtained. Neither organisms nor tumor cells could be identified in this. A histoplasmin test proved to be strongly positive. Histoplasmosis is much more common in North America than in England, and the presence of a lung lesion with a strongly positive histoplasmin test in a recent immigrant was regarded as presumptive evidence of primary histoplasmosis. No treatment was given, and the patient remains well to this day.

This case illustrates four points:

1. Persistent lung infections in young people should always raise the possibility of tuberculous infection.

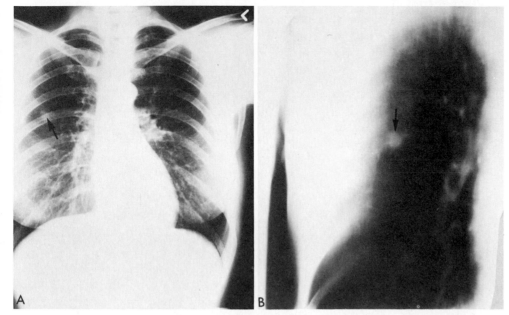

Figure 13–1. Chest radiograph of a 43-year-old female patient with histoplasmosis. *A,* Note "coin lesion" in the right lung field. *B,* Tomogram reveals the shadow with greater definition. (Radiographs courtesy of Dr. D. E. Sanders.)

2. The development of hypersensitivity to an organism or its products during the course of a disease is good evidence of infection by that organism, provided the clinical features are consistent with such a diagnosis.

3. A lung lesion in a person over the age of 40 should be regarded as cancerous until proved otherwise.

4. A knowledge of the geographic incidence of disease can help in arriving at a correct diagnosis.

Coccidioidomycosis. This disease is caused by *Coccidioides immitis,* a dimorphic fungus that is common in the dry desert regions of California, Arizona, and Argentina. In these places the majority of the inhabitants acquire a primary infection of the lung, but as with other diseases of this type, the lesion soon heals and is either asymptomatic or else causes a mild influenza-like illness known locally as "valley fever" or "desert fever." Occasionally, the disease is progressive, and the destructive lung lesions closely resemble tuberculosis. Rarely, the organism invades the blood, and infection of many organs may subsequently occur.

North American Blastomycosis. This is caused by infection with the yeast *Blastomyces dermatitidis.* The primary lesion is usually in the lung (Fig. 13–2) but may be cutaneous. Widespread dissemination occasionally occurs and tends to involve the bones, skin, and lung.

South American Blastomycosis (Paracoccidioidal Granuloma). The causative organism, *Paracoccidioides brasiliensis,* is a yeast that usually produces a primary infection in the region of the nasopharynx. Destructive local lesions and regional lymphadenopathy ensue. Untreated, the disease runs a prolonged course, and ultimately death occurs as a result of spread to lung, skin, and other organs. It is a more serious infection than the other deep-seated mycoses mentioned; unless treated, it is frequently fatal.

Over 100,000 species of fungi are known, and of these about 100 are pathogens. Apart from those previously described, there are others that occasionally produce infection under particular circumstances. For the most part they act as secondary invaders in the course of other diseases, or they

Other Fungal Infections

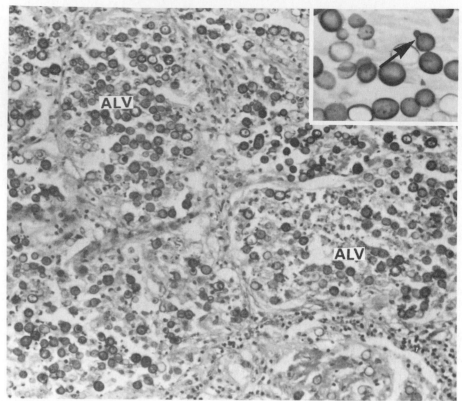

Figure 13–2. Blastomycosis of the lung. The alveolar walls are intact, but the alveoli themselves (ALV) are *consolidated,* being completely airless and filled with inflammatory exudate (compare with Figs. 5–7*A* and 30–2). This condition is called *consolidation.* The exudate contains amorphous fibrinous material, disintegrating polymorphs, and large numbers of fungi (× 250). The inset is from the same case, but it shows a section that has been stained by a silver impregnation method. The budding form ot the fungus, marked by the arrow, is typical (× 600).

occur as opportunistic infections when immunity is weakened. One of the best known examples of the latter is the *Aspergillus* species, which sometimes affects the lung. The organism has a great propensity to invade blood vessels, so that the tissue reaction is complicated by extensive necrosis due to infarction. Mucormycosis (caused by *Mucor* and other genera) is another opportunistic infection. It tends to affect diabetic subjects as well as those with immune deficiencies. Infection may involve the nasal sinuses, lungs, or gastrointestinal tract.

In India, injuries to the feet are sometimes infected with fungi, leading to chronic suppurative lesions involving the skin, subcutaneous tissues, and bone; such a condition is known as *maduromycosis* or *Madura foot.* This is caused not only by various species of fungi, but also by certain higher bacteria.

In conclusion, it can be appreciated that although serious infections due to fungi are not common, fungal disease can assume considerable importance under specific conditions. These circumstances include climate and treatment of patients in specialized units with cytotoxic or immunosuppressive drugs.

Treatment of Fungal Infections

Few drugs are available for the treatment of the deep fungal infections. Amphotericin B offers some hope in the treatment of systemic fungal infections, but unfortunately the drug causes renal damage. Topical nystatin is effective for superficial candidal infections, but nystatin cannot be administered systemically.

1. A coin lesion, similar to that shown in Figure 13–1, is found in a radiograph taken as part of a routine health inspection. List the possible causes. Modify this list after reading Chapters 16, 17, and 30.

2. Classify the fungi into four groups and give at least one example of each group.

3. A patient has several red, scaly skin lesions, ranging from 1 to 3 cm in diameter, each having a raised border. How would you attempt to arrive at a diagnosis?

Cruickshank, R., Duguid, J. P., Marmion, B. P., and Swain, R. H. A.: Medical Microbiology. 12th ed. Volume 1. Edinburgh, Churchill Livingstone, 1973. Chapter 53 gives a good review of the pathogenic fungi.

Reese, P. L., and Dixon, D. M.: Opportunistic mycoses. American Journal of Nursing, *81*:1160–1165, 1981.

Youmans, G. P., Paterson, P. Y., and Sommers, H. M.: The Biologic and Clinical Basis of Infectious Diseases. 2nd ed. Philadelphia, W. B. Saunders Company, 1980. Chapter 32 gives a detailed account of histoplasmosis, coccidioidomycosis, and blastomycosis.

Helminthic Infections

After studying this chapter the student should be able to:

- Distinguish between the definitive and the intermediate host of a parasite.
- Describe the major differences between the tapeworms, the flukes, and the roundworms.
- Describe the life cycles of the helminths listed in Table 14–1 and outline the effects on human beings of infection with these parasites.

The worms, or helminths, that plague mankind are classified as belonging within two phyla of the animal kingdom (Table 14–1).

The phylum *Platyhelminthes*, or flatworms, is further subdivided into two classes (1) *Trematoda*, and (2) *Cestoda*. The *Trematoda*, or *flukes*, are flat, leaflike creatures that live in the *intestine, liver,* or *lung* (the distomes) or in the *blood stream* (the schistosomes). The *Cestoda,* or *tapeworms,* are segmented and possess a head or scolex, a neck, and a varying number (often hundreds) of proglottides. Both cestodes and trematodes are hermaphroditic.

The phylum *Nemathelminthes* contains the roundworms, which are never segmented, possess an alimentary canal, and in general have separate sexes.

The helminths of medical importance form a very small fraction of the total number known, and their study and recognition is a very specialized field.* Only some common examples will be described in this chapter.

The life cycle of many worms is complex. The *definitive host* is the one in which the parasite reaches maturity and produces gametes. The *intermediate host* is one in which the parasite passes through its larval stage or stages; in some instances, several intermediate hosts are required. Most parasites are extremely exacting in their demands, and knowledge of their host requirements is a valuable weapon in designing methods of eliminating them.

In general, the spread of parasites is encouraged by unsanitary conditions, overcrowding, and a warm climate. The Arctic is less hospitable for harboring these organisms than the Nile region. It follows that helminthic infections are much more common in the tropics. Nevertheless, a worm can travel by air as easily as its host; even in temperate climates, therefore, it is important to be aware of common "tropical diseases."

The Trematodes or Flukes

The life cycle of the flukes involves one or two intermediate hosts (Fig. 14–1). Man is the definitive host and acquires the infection by ingestion of infected fish, crayfish, or vegetation (causing the disease distomiasis) or by penetration of the skin by the parasite (schistosomiasis).

---

*The diagnosis of parasitic infections generally depends on identification of the worm itself or its ova. In some instances, specific antibodies demonstrated by complement fixation or the presence of delayed hypersensitivity is useful in diagnosis.

TABLE 14–1. CLASSIFICATION OF WORMS DESCRIBED IN THIS CHAPTER

PHYLUM	CLASS	EXAMPLES
Platyhelminthes (Flatworms)	Trematoda (Flukes)	Distomes *Fasciola hepatica* *Clonorchis sinensis* *Fasciolopsis buski* *Paragonimus westermani*
		Schistosomes *Schistosoma hematobium* *Schistosoma mansoni* *Schistosoma japonicum*
	Cestoda (Tapeworms)	*Taenia saginata* *Taenia solium* *Diphyllobothrium latum* *Echinococcus granulosus*
Nemathelminthes (Roundworms)	Nematoda (Roundworms)	*Ascaris lumbricoides* Ancylostomes *Ancylostoma duodenale* *Necator americanus*
		Strongyloides stercoralis *Enterobius vermicularis* (pin- or threadworm) *Trichuris trichiura* (whipworm) *Trichinella spiralis*
		Filariae *Wuchereria bancrofti* *Onchocerca volvulus* *Loa loa* *Dracunculus medinensis*

The Liver Flukes. *Fasciola hepatica* is a common parasite of sheep and is occasionally acquired by human beings following the ingestion of watercress containing metacercariae (the resting stage of a trematode parasite). The parasite reaches the intestine, penetrates the wall, crosses the peritoneum, and reaches the liver, where it matures to form an adult fluke.

Clonorchis sinensis, or Chinese liver fluke, has a similar life cycle, but the metacercariae are found beneath the scales of a freshwater fish. Eating raw fish is the mode of infection. The flukes can obstruct the bile ducts, cause inflammation, and ultimately lead to hepatic fibrosis and cirrhosis.

Intestinal Flukes. Infection with *Fasciolopsis buski* is limited to the Far East. Adult worms live in the upper small intestine.

Lung Flukes. *Paragonimus westermani* resides in the lungs, where it causes recurrent hemoptysis and, ultimately, chronic lung inflammation with fibrosis. Infection results from eating raw crayfish in which the metacercariae reside.

The Distomes

Schistosomiasis (also called bilharziasis after Bilharz [1852], who discovered the worm) is the most important disease caused by flukes, because of its worldwide distribution and the severity of its lesions. It is caused by three closely related flukes, described below.

Schistosoma hematobium. The adult flukes live in the portal venous system; after copulation they migrate against the blood flow to the venous plexus around the bladder, where the female lays eggs. As these mature, they secrete a lytic substance that destroys the surrounding tissues. Some ova die and become calcified. A chronic cystitis with hematuria ensues, and the

The Blood Flukes or Schistosomes

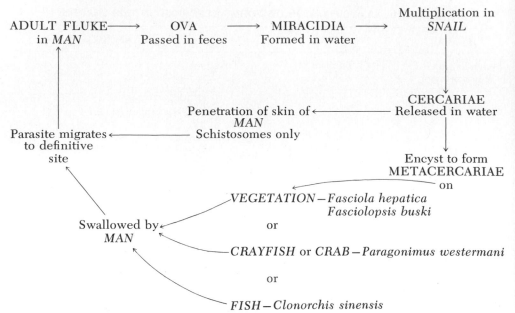

Figure 14–1. Life cycle of the common flukes. Note that the schistosomes have only one intermediate host: a snail. The other parasites shown have a second intermediate host: freshwater *vegetation,* a *crab* or other *crustacean,* or a *fish.* The parasites are shown in capital letters, Roman type, whereas the hosts are in capital letters, italic type.

epithelial hyperplasia that is a component of this process sometimes progresses to carcinoma. Viable ova that penetrate the mucosa are passed in the urine. On contact with fresh water, the ova hatch and liberate ciliated forms — the *miracidia.* These have about eight hours in which to search for the intermediate host, a specific snail. If the search is successful, the parasite proliferates in the snail, and one to two months later thousands of infective larvae, called *cercariae,* are liberated into the water. Cercariae are able to penetrate the skin of an unsuspecting bather, then enter venules, and finally pass through the lungs and heart, reaching the portal vein to start their remarkable life cycle once again. This type of schistosomiasis is common in the African continent, particularly in the Nile Valley.

Schistosoma mansoni. This type of schistosome has a life cycle similar to that of *Schistosoma hematobium* and is found in South America, the Caribbean, and Africa. The adult worm resides in the intrahepatic portal veins, from which the ova are distributed to the venules of the colon, rectum, liver, and lung. An initial phlebitis with surrounding inflammation is eventually followed by fibrosis. Intestinal involvement causes diarrhea, pain, and melena. The liver becomes fibrosed, and portal hypertension leads to esophageal varices and splenomegaly. Pulmonary fibrosis is less common. Ova are passed in the feces, contaminate fresh water, and develop into cercariae. The cycle starts once again.

Schistosoma japonicum. This fluke causes schistosomiasis in the Orient and is similar to the mansoni type but is more severe. The colon, the liver, the lungs, and other organs — including the spinal cord — are involved, and death usually occurs within five years of onset unless effective treatment is given (Fig. 14–2).

The continued existence of schistosomiasis is related to poor sewage disposal as well as to the popular habit of passing urine and feces into water channels that are used for bathing. The reversal of such habits is difficult, and education is all-important.

Figure 14-2. Schistosome ova in pancreas. The ova are probably dead, since they are calcified and stain deeply with the hematoxylin owing to their calcium content. In spite of their being dead, they can still excite a chronic inflammatory reaction (× 250).

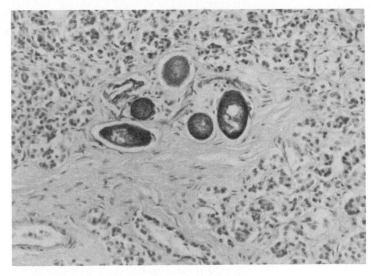

Villages can be located away from known contaminated streams. Mass treatment of patients and snail control are other methods of checking this disease. Nevertheless, schistosomiasis is a disease of great antiquity, and it gives no evidence of decreasing in frequency. Indeed, estimates suggest that the disease is spreading and is increasing in prevalence. Schistosome eggs have been identified in the Egyptian mummies of the twentieth dynasty (1200 to 1190 B.C.). Present estimates of 180 million infected persons bear witness to the continued success of this parasite.

Tapeworms possess a head (scolex) and a neck followed by a chain of segments or proglottides arranged in a ribbon, often many feet long (Fig. 14-3). Two hosts are necessary; man is the definitive host of three common tapeworms and the intermediate host of one other (hydatid disease).

The Cestodes or Tapeworms

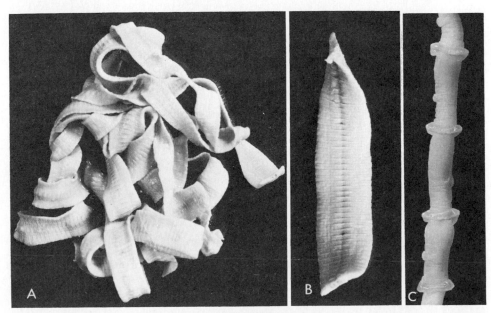

Figure 14-3. Tapeworms. *A,* Part of the tapeworm *Diphyllobothrium latum.* The total length of the worm is over 30 feet. The head is about 1 mm in diameter, and the immature segments are much smaller than the mature segments shown above (× 1.5). *B,* Part of the worm shown in *A.* It is made up of many proglottides or segments, each of which is wider than it is long. *C,* Part of the tapeworm *Taenia saginata.* Each segment is longer than it is wide.

Taenia saginata.   The beef tapeworm grows only in the human intestine. It has up to 2000 segments and can be 30 feet long. The mature terminal segments contain vast numbers of eggs, which are passed in the feces. As mature segments are cast off at one end, new ones are formed in the neck region. The worms are very long-lived — some have reportedly lived over 40 years.

When cattle eat the mature proglottides or isolated eggs, the embryos hatch out, penetrate the intestine, and migrate to the skeletal muscle, where they form the next larval stage, which is cystic (this stage of the tapeworm is called the *cysticercus*). Man becomes infected by eating undercooked infected beef. Symptoms consist of vague abdominal pains or skin eruptions (*e.g.*, urticaria) due to hypersensitivity.

Taenia solium.   This is the pork tapeworm. It has up to 1000 segments and can extend to 20 feet in length. The intermediate host is the pig. Humans acquire intestinal infection by eating undercooked pork containing cysticerci.

Occasionally man eats the eggs of *Taenia solium,* and cysticerci develop in muscles, heart, brain, skin, and other organs. The human being then becomes the intermediate host. Symptoms of the condition known as cysticercosis are mainly neurological.

Diphyllobothrium latum.   This is the largest of the tapeworms, measuring up to 33 feet in length, and has over 3000 proglottides. The intermediate host is a fish, and the disease is most prevalent among the inhabitants of the fish-eating countries: Scandinavia, parts of Russia, and Asia.

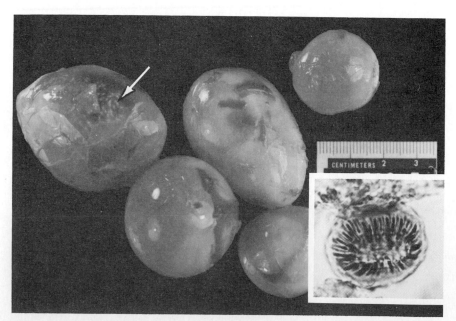

Figure 14–4. Hydatid cysts. The patient had emigrated to North America at 21 years of age after having previously lived and worked on a sheep farm in Yugoslavia. Nine years later he developed a rapidly expanding mass in the upper abdomen. Laparotomy was performed, and multiple hydatid cysts were found in the liver. The largest of these were drained, but unfortunately some of the cysts' contents were spilled into the peritoneal cavity. The parasite was thus disseminated. During the next 10 years, four further operations were necessary for removal or drainage of cysts in the peritoneal cavity, spleen, mediastinum, and pleural cavities.

The figure shows five separate hydatid cysts. These have an epithelial lining from which small cysts or brood capsules develop. These are pinhead sized (see arrow), and within them scoleces of the head of the worm project. The inset shows one scolex with its characteristic hooklets. On being ingested by a dog or wolf this structure will form the head of a new tapeworm.

Hydatid Disease. *Echinococcus granulosus* is a small tapeworm found in the intestine of dogs, wolves, and other carnivorous animals. Ova are ingested by sheep, which constitute the usual intermediate host. The cysticercal forms, called *hydatid cysts*, develop in the liver, the lungs, and elsewhere (Fig. 14–4). Dogs become infected by eating infected sheep carcasses. Occasionally, humans ingest eggs and also develop hydatid cysts. These are commonest in the liver and lungs, but they may occur in any part of the body. The disease is particularly prevalent in the sheep-raising areas of Australia.

The Nematodes or Roundworms

Ascaris lumbricoides. The adult ascarides are 15 to 35 cm in length and live in the small intestine, where they usually cause no trouble except in those instances of a heavy infection, when their bulk causes obstruction (Fig. 14–5). Ova are passed in the stools and develop in soil into embryonated ova. When these are ingested, they hatch into larvae, which penetrate the gut wall and reach the lungs via the blood stream. They enter the alveoli, ascend the bronchi and trachea, and finally pass down the esophagus to reach the intestine. Why this parasite pursues this remarkable course is quite unknown. Perhaps its ancestors had a different life cycle (*i.e.*, like that of *Ancylostoma duodenale*, described below), and the migrating habit has been retained by the worm for no more useful purpose than as a reminder of its heritage. During the migratory phase, the patient may experience asthmatic attacks and develop patchy pneumonic consolidation. Blood eosinophilia is common, as it is in many helminthic infections, particularly when the parasites are migrating through the tissues.

Ancylostomiasis (Hookworm Disease). This disease, which is of worldwide distribution, is caused by *Ancylostoma duodenale* in the Old World and *Necator americanus* in the New World. The worms attach themselves to the wall of the small intestine and cause bleeding. With a heavy infection, the blood loss may lead to a severe chronic iron deficiency anemia, which, when combined with undernutrition, is an important cause of chronic ill health in underdeveloped countries. Elsewhere, it is rare.

Eggs are passed in the feces and hatch in the soil into larvae that have the ability to penetrate the skin of a barefooted passerby. They migrate via the blood to the lungs, penetrate the alveoli, ascend the trachea, and finally reach the gut to develop into adult worms.

Enterobius vermicularis (Pinworm or Threadworm). This nematode is very common in all parts of the world and lives in the lower gut. The females deposit their fully infective eggs around the anus, particularly at night, when their host is asleep. In so doing they cause severe itching (*pruritus ani*); pinworm infection should always be suspected as a cause of this condition,

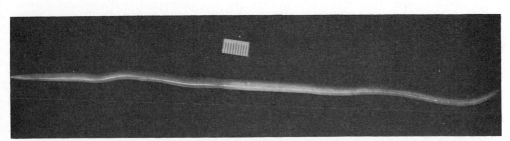

Figure 14–5. *Ascaris lumbricoides.* This worm is the largest roundworm parasite of humans and superficially resembles an earthworm (from the Latin *lumbricus*, an "earthworm"). It ranges in length from 15 to 35 cm. The specimen above was approximately 20 cm (8 inches) in length. Other common roundworms are considerably smaller: *Trichuris trichiura,* 3 to 5 cm: *Enterobius vermicularis,* 8 to 13 mm; and *Ancylostoma duodenale,* up to 1.0 cm. (The scale above the roundworm shown is 1 cm.)

particularly in children. Infection is acquired by swallowing the eggs, which develop into adult forms in the intestine. The worms have a short life span (one to two months), but continuous reinfection will maintain the infection unless strict personal hygiene is enforced. One cannot but admire the ingenuity of this worm: the severe anal itching demands scratching and results in deposition of eggs under the nails. How many small children can refrain from sucking their fingers at some stage during the day?

Diagnosis is most easily accomplished by pressing a piece of adhesive tape (*e.g.*, Scotch tape or a specially prepared material) against the child's perianal skin in the morning just after wakening. Ova will be found adherent to the tape.

Trichuris trichiura (Whipworm).   Infection with the whipworm is extremely common, but it rarely causes any symptoms. The life cycle of the whipworm is similar to that of the pinworm, except that ova are passed in the feces, and infection is acquired by ingesting the ova in contaminated food or in water.

Trichinella spiralis.   The ban on eating pork imposed by some religious groups and the tradition of eating only well-cooked meat by others probably originated with some understanding of the life cycle of this worm.

Trichinella spiralis is primarily a parasite of rats. In the intestine the adult male worm dies after copulation — a fate that is not uncommon in the world of worms. The pregnant female burrows into the intestinal wall and discharges hundreds of larvae into the blood stream. When these reach skeletal muscle, they curl up and form small cysts. Those larvae that reach other tissues are less fortunate — they die. When rats eat infected rat muscle, the dormant, encysted parasites awaken and develop into adult worms. Pigs and bears become infected by eating the carcasses of diseased rats, and human beings acquire infection (trichinosis) by eating undercooked pork or bear.

The symptoms of trichinosis vary. Minor infection is common, and there are no symptoms. With heavy infection the early symptoms are gastrointestinal; these are followed by systemic symptoms such as fever, generalized edema, and muscle pains. Involvement of the respiratory muscles or heart can, on occasion, cause death. In Canada this is an occasional sequel to an otherwise successful bear party.

The diagnosis is suggested by the clinical features (particularly muscle pains) combined with a marked blood eosinophil leukocytosis. The diagnosis is confirmed by one of the serological tests (complement fixation or precipitin reaction). Finding the parasite in a muscle biopsy provides the most convincing proof.

Strongyloidiasis.   Strongyloidiasis is an intestinal infection of human beings by *Strongyloides stercoralis,* a tiny (2 mm) roundworm that resides in the mucosa of the upper jejunum. Generally, the infection is asymptomatic. The common life cycle of the parasite is similar to that of the hookworm, and infective larvae, which develop in the soil, enter the skin and return to the intestine via the lungs.

The organism is, however, remarkable for having several alternative life cycles. In one of these, the ova in the intestine develop into infective larvae that penetrate either the intestinal wall or the perianal skin. Autoinfection can thus occur. In the immunologically suppressed patient, massive infection can result in a severe illness characterized by colitis, pneumonitis, and meningitis as well as a complicating gram-negative bacteremia. Strongyloidiasis, when diagnosed, should therefore be treated even if asymptomatic because of this potential lethal complication.

Filariasis is caused by a type of nematode that invades the subcutaneous tissues and lymphatics of man (Fig. 14–6). The female produces vast numbers of larvae, or *microfilariae,* which pass through the one intermediate host that transmits the infection to the human host.

Bancroft's Filariasis.   This disease, commonly referred to as "filariasis," is caused by *Wuchereria bancrofti,* which is a worm about 10 cm in length that resides in lymphatics. The females produce large numbers of microfilariae, which are liberated at night into the blood stream, where they can be sought for diagnosis. If an infected individual is bitten by a mosquito (also nocturnal), the mosquito becomes a carrier of the disease and infects persons it subsequently bites.

The adult forms of *Wuchereria bancrofti* produce little damage to lymphatics until they die. There then follows a severe chronic inflammatory reaction that results in lymphatic obstruction. The lymphatics most commonly affected are those of the groin; the leg consequently develops severe lymphatic edema. Marked overgrowth of the skin and subcutaneous tissues produces enormous swelling of the limb and sometimes the scrotum. The condition is called *elephantiasis* and occurs in many tropical and subtropical countries.

Three other filarial diseases are worthy of note:

Onchocerciasis.   This is caused by *Onchocerca volvulus,* which in man usually resides in the skin and causes an inflammatory reaction that leads to subcutaneous nodule formation. The microfilariae produced by the females migrate into the adjacent tissues; the most serious complication of this migratory phase of the disease is produced when the eye is invaded. Involvement of the cornea, the vitreous humor, and the ciliary body can result in blindness. The disease is seen in Africa, Mexico, and Guatemala.

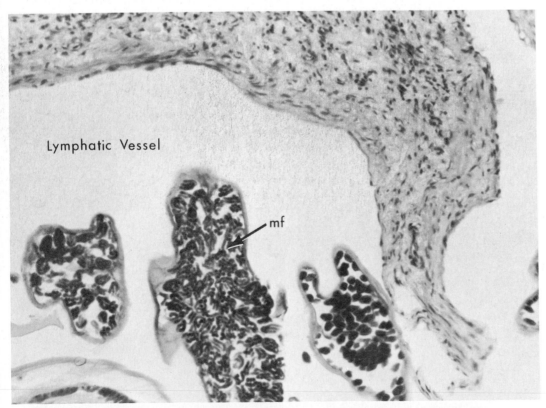

Lymphatic Vessel

mf

Figure 14–6. Filariasis.   Section of a nodule from a patient with onchocerciasis. The lymphatic vessel contains adult worms shown in cross section. Numerous microfilariae (mf) are present in the body of the gravid female ($\times$ 250).

Loiasis.   This is a form of filariasis restricted to tropical West Africa. The causative organism, *Loa loa,* is also known as the eyeworm. The adult worm occurs in the skin and at times invades the eye. In contrast to Bancroft's filariasis, the microfilariae of loiasis appear in the peripheral blood during the day. The disease is transmitted by a fly that bites during the daytime.

Dracunculiasis.   This type of filariasis occurs in the Middle East, India, and parts of Africa. The parasite is known as *Dracunculus medinensis,* or the guinea worm. The adult male is small and dies after copulation. The female worm is about 1 meter in length and wanders about the subcutaneous tissues, particularly of the legs. The worm burrows through the skin to produce a small papule, which finally develops into an ulcer through which its embryos are discharged. The embryos are taken up by a freshwater crustacean of the genus *Cyclops,* and after a period of maturation, the larvae are infective. Infection is acquired by swallowing the larvae.

The guinea worm is of interest, not because it is common, but because of its history. It is believed to be the oldest known parasite. The account of the fiery serpents sent by the Lord among the Israelites is believed to be an early description of dracunculiasis.*

The traditional treatment is to apply water to the area of ulceration of the leg so that the worm can be grasped and wound onto a stick. Steady pressure day by day results in extraction of the entire worm. Tradition has it that this is the origin of the serpent wound around the staff which is the emblem of the medical profession.

This account of human helminthic diseases has included only some examples of worms that affect persons in widespread areas of the world. Many other examples are known, some restricted to particular geographic areas. Thus, a localized outbreak of infection by *Capillaria philippinensis* has been described in the Philippine Islands and is manifested as a type of enteritis with a high mortality. It is caused by a minute whipworm and is acquired by eating infected fish and crustaceans. The latter are often eaten alive in a form of "jumping salads"!

Review Questions

1. Describe two tapeworm infections in which man is the intermediate host.

2. Compare the life cycle of *Ancylostoma duodenale* with that of *Enterobius vermicularis.*

3. List the helminthic infections that can be acquired in the following ways:
   (a) going barefooted
   (b) eating undercooked or raw pork
   (c) eating raw fish

4. What helminthic infections would you suspect as a cause of the following conditions:
   (a) pruritus ani
   (b) muscle pains
   (c) jaundice
   (d) chronic lung damage with hemoptysis
   (e) chronic iron-deficiency anemia
   (f) elephantiasis
   (g) hematuria

Selected Readings

Isselbacher, K. J., et al. (Eds.): Harrison's Principles of Internal Medicine. 9th ed. New York, McGraw-Hill Book Company, 1979. See pp. 890–918, "Diseases Caused by Worms."
Jeffrey, H. C., and Leach, R. M.: Atlas of Medical Helminthology and Protozoology. 2nd ed. Edinburgh, Churchill Livingstone, 1975. An atlas giving the morphology, life cycle, and major effects of common parasites. Useful for parasite identification.
Robbins, S. L., and Cotran, R. S.: Pathologic Basis of Disease. 2nd ed. Philadelphia, W. B. Saunders Company, 1979. See pp. 466–476 for a description of the pathological features of helminthic infections.

---

*Numbers, 21:6.

Protozoal Infections CHAPTER 15

After studying this chapter the student should be able to:

- Describe the clinical features of amebiasis, the nature of the causative organism, its mode of transmission, and the importance of carriers.
- Describe the effects of infection with *Giardia lamblia.*
- Explain the worldwide importance of malaria, the life cycle of the organism, and the features of the disease in man.
- Discuss how malaria is diagnosed and the approaches available for its control.
- Describe the manifestations of toxoplasmosis in the adult and in the newborn.
- Discuss the mode of transmission of trypanosomiasis and the main features of the three forms of the disease in man.
- Compare and contrast the three types of leishmaniasis in man.
- Describe the importance of *Trichomonas vaginalis* as a pathogen.
- Discuss the importance of *Pneumocystis carinii* as a human pathogen.

Protozoa are unicellular motile animals that have a well-defined nucleus. Some travel by ameboid movement, while others are ciliated or have a single flagellum. They are widely distributed in nature, but few species are pathogenic to man. Yet one of these causes malaria, which is currently the major human infectious disease problem. Worldwide, approximately 125 million people are believed to be infected.

AMEBIASIS

It has been estimated that about 10 per cent of the world's population harbor *Entamoeba histolytica,* the incidence ranging from under 5 per cent in the United States to over 40 per cent in the tropics. The majority of these people are asymptomatic and act as carriers.

Entamoeba histolytica exists in two forms: an active amebic trophozoite, which is present in active lesions of the disease, and a cyst, which develops when the organism is confronted by adverse conditions. It is by the swallowing of cysts that the disease is acquired. Cysts can withstand the acidity of the gastric juice and develop into active trophozoites, which by invading the mucosa of the large intestine cause catarrhal inflammation and ulceration. Following infection, symptoms are absent (in *asymptomatic carriers*), or they consist of intermittent diarrhea with the passage of blood and mucus (*chronic amebic dysentery),* or sometimes the colitis is severe and has an abrupt onset. Fever, severe abdominal pain, and the passage of profuse blood-stained stools are the features of this *acute amebic dysentery.* Cases of the acute form occur sporadically, and almost always in the tropics. Why the ameba is so aggressive in some people but causes a symptomless state in the majority of patients is not known. The existence of virulent strains of *Entamoeba histolytica* has been postulated, but it seems more likely that a synergistic action exists between the ameba and the intestinal flora in certain individuals.

Entamoeba histolytica occasionally penetrates the portal venous circulation, and this leads to *amebic hepatic abscess* formation. A diagnosis of this condition is often difficult because the complication is seen more commonly in cases of asymptomatic infection of the colon than in patients with overt dysentery. The diagnosis of active amebic colitis depends on identification of the active trophozoites by microscopic examination of fresh warm stool.* Serological tests are also available. In the absence of diarrhea, the trophozoites encyst before leaving the gut. The feces of asymptomatic carriers contain cysts only and are the chief source of infection. Food is the common vehicle of transmission, being contaminated by infected food handlers or by flies. The use of human feces as fertilizer may directly contaminate vegetables. Outbreaks of amebic dysentery are generally waterborne and are never as explosive as are those of bacillary dysentery (Chapter 32).

GIARDIASIS   Giardiasis is a protozoal infection of the small intestine that has come into prominence during the last decade because of an increased awareness that it can cause significant disease. The causative organism, *Giardia lamblia,* exists in two forms — a *trophozoite* that is found attached to the mucosa of the jejunum, and a *cyst* that is the infective form, since on being swallowed it can resist the acid contents of the stomach. Both forms of the parasite are present in the feces during active stages of the disease when diarrhea is present.

Giardiasis can be asymptomatic, but it may also cause acute attacks of diarrhea. The infection can also be responsible for chronic diarrhea, and this may be associated with malnutrition, steatorrhea (excess fat in the stools), and a condition resembling celiac disease (Chapter 32). Outbreaks of giardiasis have recently been held responsible for attacks of diarrhea in infant day care centers, among male homosexuals, and in travellers with "traveller's diarrhea" (Chapter 32).

As with amebiasis, it is not known whether the virulence of giardia varies from one strain to another, or whether host factors determine whether infection causes an acute disease or a chronic one or merely persists as a symptomless carrier state.

MALARIA   Malaria is a protozoal disease caused by infection by a member of the genus *Plasmodium.* It is characterized by paroxysms of fever, each lasting 2 to 4 hours and initiated by a severe rigor. The paroxysm passes through the classic cold, hot, and sweating stages (Chapter 22). The infection is acquired from the bite of a female anopheline mosquito whose injected saliva contains sporozoites that travel via the blood stream to reach the liver cells, where they multiply (Fig. 15–1). This *exoerythrocytic stage* occurs during the incubation period of the disease. Finally, infective forms return to the blood stream, invade the red cells, and divide asexually to produce sporozoites, each of which breaks up into numerous merozoites. These are liberated as the red cell ruptures, and each merozoite invades another red cell. This asexual cycle (schizogony) takes 48 hours with *Plasmodium falciparum.* It is a remarkable fact that the maturation cycle of each parasite soon becomes synchronized. The release of merozoites is accompanied by the onset of a paroxysm — each third day with tertian malaria (due to *Plasmodium vivax* and *Plasmodium ovale*) and each fourth day with quartan malaria (*Plasmodium malariae*). Paroxysms are more erratic with malignant malaria (due to *Plasmodium falciparum*). The last type of malaria is so named because it is the most severe and is accompanied by two serious complications.

Cerebral Malaria.   A complication of malignant malaria, cerebral malaria is characterized by the rapid development of a high fever (hyperpyrexia), coma, and death. (See Fig. 22–2).

---

*Both trophozoites and cysts of *Entamoeba histolytica* must be distinguished from those of *Entamoeba coli,* which are part of the normal flora of the colon.

Bite by Infective Mosquito

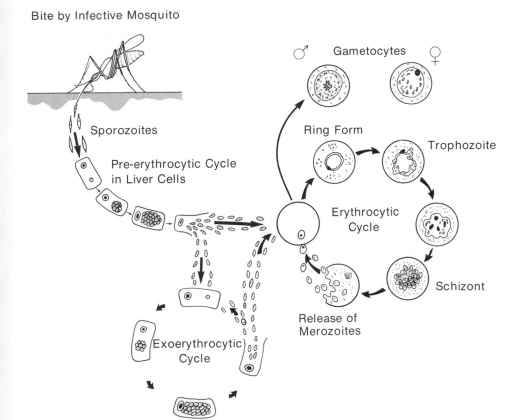

Figure 15–1. Development of malaria parasites in humans. Infection begins with the bite of an infective mosquito. The injected sporozoites travel in the blood stream and enter the liver cells, where they develop. Infective forms are released into the blood, and the majority of these enter red cells, develop into ring forms, and mature to form trophozoites. The erythrocytic cycle is completed by the development of a schizont; with the subsequent destruction of the red cell, infective merozoites are released. Except in the case of *Plasmodium falciparum* some malaria parasites continue to multiply within liver cells and constitute the exoerythrocytic cycle that is responsible for the persistence of the malarial infection. The male and female gametocytes, which are formed by some parasites, do not develop further in the human host but must await the bite of another mosquito. The precise shape and form of the malarial parasites vary according to the species. In the diagram the forms approximate those of *Plasmodium vivax.* (After H. C. Jeffrey and R. M. Leach: Atlas of Medical Helminthology and Protozoology. 2nd ed. Edinburgh, Churchill Livingstone, Medical Division of Longman Group Ltd., 1975. Reproduced by permission. Drawing by Margot Mackay, Department of Art as Applied to Medicine, University of Toronto.)

Blackwater Fever.   In blackwater fever, a malarial paroxysm is followed by massive intravascular hemolysis, hemoglobinuria, cessation of urine formation (anuria), and frequently death. The pathogenesis is not understood, but this complication is usually seen in chronic falciparum malignant malaria treated episodically with quinine. An autoimmune type of anemia probably plays an important part.

Course of Malaria.   The first attacks of malaria are often severe, but as time goes by the episodes become more mild. Persistence of infection is due to the persistence of the exoerythrocytic forms in the liver. In endemic areas, reinfection constantly occurs, and a state of chronic infection ensues. This state is characterized by anemia, enlargement of the spleen (splenomegaly), debility, and cachexia, leaving the patient open to other infections. Tuberculosis, cholera, bacillary dysentery, and bronchopneumonia all take their toll in patients with chronic malaria.

Control of Malaria.   The malarial parasites divide asexually in man, who is therefore the *intermediate host.* Gametocytes are formed in some infected red cells, but their maturation to form gametes and subsequent union to form zygotes occurs only in the female mosquito (Fig. 15–2). The anopheline mosquito is therefore the *definitive host*. The control of malaria involves mosquito control and the treatment of patients, who serve as the reservoir for the disease. Neither of these has proved to be easy, and eradication of the disease has not proved to be possible. Mosquitoes have developed immunity to insecticides, and drug-resistant strains of plasmodia have emerged. Evolution, which designed the complex life cycle of the plasmodia, is not easily relinquishing such a prize.

Diagnosis of Malaria. The diagnosis of malaria rests on finding the parasite in a suitably stained blood film. (See Figs. 15–2 and 22–2.)

TOXOPLASMOSIS

Toxoplasmosis is caused by an infection with *Toxoplasma gondii,* a parasite that primarily affects members of the cat family, which are the definitive hosts. The organisms multiply in the cells of the small intestine and develop into oocysts that are passed in the feces and subsequently mature into infective forms that remain viable for months. Humans and other animals acquire the disease by eating these mature oocysts. In the intestine the cysts develop into sporozoites that penetrate the bowel wall and migrate to lymph nodes, brain, and other tissues, where they encyst. When such cysts (*e.g.*, in a mouse) are eaten by a cat, the life cycle is completed.

It has been estimated (as judged by the presence of antibodies) that up to 70 per cent of humans are infected by *T. gondii* but that in the vast majority of people the infection is subclinical. A very few individuals develop a severe illness with brain involvement, while others have a mild febrile illness that resembles infectious mononucleosis because its symptoms include lymphadenopathy and a skin rash.

The tragedy of toxoplasmosis lies in its tendency to be transmitted transplacentally to the fetus. The mother, though infected, is symptomless. The effects on the fetus vary. A very severe infection may precipitate abortion. More often, the child survives but develops a severe generalized disease a

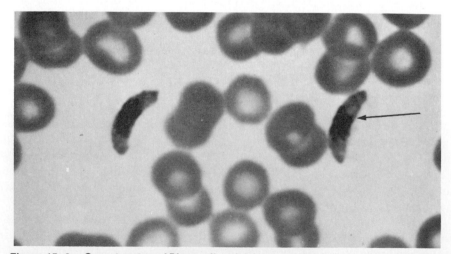

Figure 15–2. Gametocytes of *Plasmodium falciparum*. The two gametocytes shown were found in a routine blood film of a Malayan soldier. He was asymptomatic at the time. The crescentic shape of the organism is characteristic of this species of malaria parasite. One gametocyte (arrow), which has a more pointed end, is male; the other is female. The patient had a history of previous attacks of malaria, but he evidently had developed sufficient immunity to remain as an asymptomatic carrier. After a host has been bitten by a mosquito, gametocytes develop into gametes, which fuse to form a zygote. This zygote develops further and ultimately produces vast numbers of sporozoites that are ready to be injected when the mosquito bites her next victim.

few weeks after birth. In other cases, the disease appears later, and there is severe involvement of the central nervous system and the eye.

The trypanosomes are protozoa with a terminal flagellum and an undulating membrane. They cause infections of many animal species and pose a great economic problem in many parts of the world. Millions of acres in Africa are sparsely populated because of the impossibility of keeping domestic animals free of trypanosomiasis. Two types of infection occur in man (Table 15–1).

TRYPANOSO-MIASIS

African trypanosomiasis is caused by infection with *Trypanosoma brucei*, of which there are two strains. Humans are the only known victims of the Gambian strain *(T. brucei gambiense)*, while the Rhodesian strain *(T. brucei rhodiensis)* is primarily a parasite of wild game, with man acting as an occasional and accidental host. Man is infected by the bite of a fly of the genus *Glossina* (the tsetse fly), which injects infective forms with its saliva. A local skin lesion, which may pass unnoticed, is followed by a generalized infection that is characterized by fever, skin rashes, lymphadenopathy, and splenomegaly. After about one year infection can involve the central nervous system, and the patient becomes lethargic and lapses into a coma. It is this latter feature that has given the disease its other name — *sleeping sickness*.

African Trypanosomiasis

Trypanosoma cruzi is transmitted by a reduviid (kissing) bug, which tends to bite the face of the victim around the mouth, a habit that has earned it its name. After feeding, the bug defecates and passes infective forms of the trypanosome that enter the bite wound. A local nodule appears and is followed by evidence of generalized parasitemia, with fever and involvement of many organs — skin, mucous membrane, lymph nodes, and the central nervous system.

Chagas' Disease, or South American Trypanosomiasis

Chronic Chagas' disease is characterized by parasitization of the heart muscle. This accounts for many cases of heart failure in some parts of South America. There is no treatment for it.

The leishmania are protozoa that are transmitted by species of sandflies (genus *Phlebotomus*). In the fly the organism has a flagellum, but in the lesions of man and other animal hosts, the organism is nonmotile (forming Leishman-Donovan bodies) and parasitizes macrophages (Fig. 15–3). Dogs, jackals, rodents, and other animals form the natural reservoir of infection of most of the leishmania that cause human disease. In some areas man is the only known host. Three main types of leishmaniasis are known (Table 15–2).

LEISHMANIASIS

CASE HISTORY I. (See Figure 15–3). The patient was a 25-year-old Maltese male who was serving in the British Army in London. He had been complaining of general malaise for several weeks and was noted to be running a low-grade fever. His spleen was markedly enlarged and could be felt about four fingers' breadth below the left

TABLE 15–1. TYPES OF TRYPANOSOMIASIS

TYPE	ORGANISM	VECTOR	LESIONS
African	*T. brucei*	Tsetse fly	Localized skin ulcer Generalized infection Brain
South American	*T. cruzi*	Reduviid (kissing) bug	Skin nodule Generalized infection Encephalitis Myocarditis

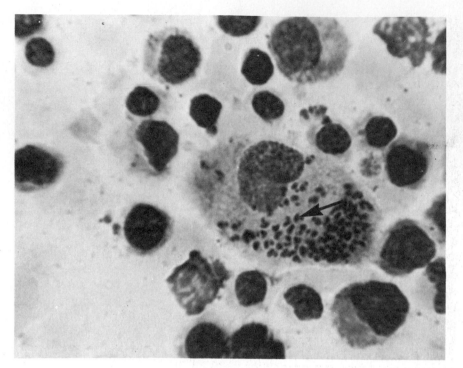

Figure 15–3. Photomicrograph of stained bone marrow of patient with leishmaniasis. The specimen illustrated here was taken from a sternal puncture. In the center is a large macrophage stuffed with parasites. Each organism has one large nucleus and a smaller rod-shaped structure called a *kinetoplast*. The arrow points to a typical organism showing these two structures. The membrane surrounding each individual organism is not clearly seen in this photograph. For more information on the patient with leishmaniasis, see Case History I.

costal margin. There was also some enlargement of the liver. Lymph nodes in both axillae were enlarged. A blood count showed a mild anemia, reduction in platelet count, and a white count of 3.5×10^9/L (3500/μL). The leukopenia was due to a reduction in the number of polymorphs (see Fig. 15–3 for a stained section of bone marrow).

The patient was treated with a pentavalent antimony compound and consequently made an uninterrupted recovery.

Visceral leishmaniasis, or kala-azar, in addition to being found in the Mediterranean, is found in China, Russia, India, Africa, and Central and South America.

Kala-Azar, or Visceral Leishmaniasis

Kala-azar is widely distributed, affecting the Far and Middle East, the area around the Mediterranean, particularly Malta and Greece, Africa, and to a lesser extent Central and South America.

TABLE 15–2. TYPES OF LEISHMANIASIS

TYPE	ORGANISM	VECTOR	LESIONS
Kala-azar (visceral leishmaniasis)	*L. donovani*	Sandfly (*Phlebotomus*)	Local skin ulcer in some types only
			Generalized infection of reticuloendothelial system
Cutaneous leishmaniasis of the Old World (oriental sore, Aleppo button, Baghdad boil, Delhi boil, and others)	*L. tropica*	Sandfly	Skin only
Cutaneous leishmaniasis of the New World	*L. braziliensis, L. mexicana,* and others	Sandfly	Skin and sometimes mucous membranes of mouth and nose

Kala-azar is caused by *Leishmania donovani,* of which there are probably several species, since the disease shows considerable geographical variations. Generally there is no local lesion at the site of the sandfly bite, and the organism proliferates in the reticuloendothelial cells of the spleen, lymph nodes, liver, and bone marrow. Compensatory reticuloendothelial hyperplasia leads to enormous splenomegaly and hepatomegaly. Involvement of the marrow leads to anemia and a low granulocyte count.

The mortality rate in untreated kala-azar is about 90 per cent, but the disease responds to treatment with antimony compounds.

Cutaneous Leishmaniasis of the Old World, or Oriental Sore

Oriental sore, which is the least serious form of leishmaniasis, occurs in countries bordering the Eastern Mediterranean, in Asia Minor, and in India. The causative organism, *Leishmania tropica,* produces a local infection of the skin at the site of the sandfly bite. A chronic ulcer is formed, and this heals spontaneously after a protracted course.

Cutaneous Leishmaniasis of the New World

The best-known variant of this type of leishmaniasis is American mucocutaneous leishmaniasis, or espundia, due to *Leishmania braziliensis.* One or more cutaneous lesions first appear and resemble oriental sore. However, the organisms spread to involve the mucosa of the mouth and nose. Here, even after the skin lesions have been treated, the disease progresses and leads to great tissue destruction, secondary bacterial infection, and death. Infections with other organisms (*e.g., Leishmania mexicana*) tend to be less severe than espundia and often involve the skin only.

TRICHOMO-NIASIS

Trichomonas vaginalis is the cause of a common vaginal infection that produces itching and a profuse, watery, yellow, frothy, vaginal discharge. The diagnosis is made by examining a fresh specimen of the discharge under the microscope and identifying the motile trichomonads. On the fixed smear stained by the Papanicolaou method the organisms can be seen, but often with difficulty.

In the male, a mild urethritis is the only evidence of infection. Usually the male carrier is symptomless. Transmission is by sexual contact, and both patient and sexual partners should be treated simultaneously.

PNEUMOCYS-TOSIS

Until recently, infection with *Pneumocystis carinii* was an uncommon cause of pneumonia in malnourished or premature infants. However, it also infects immunologically deficient subjects of any age and is being recognized with increasing frequency as a cause of terminal pneumonia in patients who have an immunological defect, either of congenital origin or due to malignant disease, administration of glucocorticoids, or therapy with antimetabolites (Chapter 9).

Pneumocystis carinii is probably a widely distributed organism and present in many apparently healthy people. It is a protozoan, but its life cycle has not yet been determined. The pneumonia it causes is an example of an opportunistic infection (Chapter 6).

Diagnosis of pneumocystis pneumonia often presents difficulty. The organism is best demonstrated by a special silver stain (methenamine silver nitrate stain). It may be found in the sputum, but often recourse has to be made to lung biopsy. This may be transbronchial, although an open lung biopsy is often performed. The latter has the advantage that tissue is obtained for histopathological examination as well as for culture for other possible opportunistic infecting organisms, such as cytomegalovirus and *Aspergillus* species.

Review Questions

1. A patient with kala-azar develops an acute gingivitis and an ulcerative pharyngitis. Can you suggest why?

2. Why is a polyclonal hypergammaglobulinemia, together with enlargement of the lymph nodes, liver, and especially spleen, so common in kala-azar?

3. Describe the possible aftereffects of eating a salad that has been washed in water contaminated by fecal material containing:
   (a) *Entamoeba histolytica*
   (b) *Giardia lamblia*

4. Outline the steps that can be taken in an attempt to control malaria in a community.

5. Enumerate the organisms that might be responsible for a vaginal discharge. How could the diagnoses be confirmed?

Selected Readings

Baker, J. R.: Parasitic Protozoa. London, Hutchinson University Library, 1970.

Belding, D. L.: Textbook of Parasitology. 3rd ed. New York, Appleton-Century-Crofts, 1965.

Bruce-Chwatt, L. J.: Malaria eradication at the crossroads. Bulletin of the New York Academy of Medicine, 45:999–1012, 1969.

Dyer, R., and Keystone, J.: Malaria, a Canadian problem. The Canadian Nurse, 77:20–23, 1981.

Elsden, R.: Amebiasis as a world problem. Bulletin of the New York Academy of Medicine, 47:438, 1971.

Faust, E. C., Russell, P. F., and Jung, R. C.: Clinical Parasitology. Philadelphia, Lea & Febiger, 1970.

Garnham, P. C. C.: Malaria Parasites and Other Haemosporidia. Oxford, Blackwell Scientific Publications, 1966.

Juniper, K.: Amebiasis in the United States. Bulletin of the New York Academy of Medicine, 47:448, 1971.

Koberle, F.: Chagas' disease and Chagas' syndromes: The pathology of American trypanosomiasis. Advances in Parasitology, 6:63–116, 1968.

Stagno, S.: Toxoplasmosis. American Journal of Nursing, 80:720–721, 1980.

World Health Organization: Amoebiasis. World Health Organization Technical Report Series, 421, 1969.

World Health Organization: Parasitology of malaria. World Health Organization Technical Report Series, 433, 1969.

Disorders of Growth
CHAPTER 16

After studying this chapter the student should be able to:

- Describe the causes of developmental anomalies.
- List 10 types of malformation and give an example of each.
- Describe the lessons learned from the thalidomide tragedy.
- Describe the fetal alcohol syndrome.
- Compare and contrast hypertrophy with hyperplasia.
- Define the following terms: atrophy, hypoplasia, aplasia, metaplasia, dyscrasia, and dysplasia.
- Classify the causes of atrophy and give examples of each.
- Discuss the use of the term dysplasia as applied to diseases of the skin, cervix uteri, and breast.

Introduction

Disorders of growth and differentiation most commonly occur during the period of embryonic development. This is hardly surprising, since a single fertilized ovum can transform itself into an entire animal in a short space of time — 21 days in the case of the mouse and 9 months in the case of human beings. Errors that occur during this period of marked change can result in gross defects. Postnatal development, on the other hand, is a relatively sedate affair, and the likelihood of an error occurring is correspondingly less.

Minor variations in development are so common that the resulting changes are regarded as normal. More serious errors in development result in the production of malformations that are usually present at birth but may not become evident until during the growing periods of childhood and adolescence. Gross abnormalities are often incompatible with life and result in abortion, stillbirth, or neonatal death.

The changes that are described in this chapter concern the abnormalities of cell growth: too much, too little, or the wrong sort. Such changes form a heterogeneous group; they often appear to bear little relationship to each other. Nevertheless, the changes are worthy of study, for they form cellular or functional entities that are commonly encountered in many disease processes.

It is convenient to divide the abnormalities of cell growth into two groups:

Developmental Anomalies. These arise before the affected part has reached its mature, adult form.

Acquired Anomalies. These arise in an organ or tissue after the mature configuration has been attained.

Inevitably, there is some overlap between these two groups, because it is sometimes difficult to decide at what point in time a particular organ does attain maturity. Nevertheless, the classification has some merit. A "developmental anomaly" is found in an organ that has never been normal. In contrast, an "acquired anomaly" occurs in an organ that has previously attained normal adult stature.

DEVELOPMENTAL ANOMALIES

Causes

Genetic Errors.   Inherited conditions, such as achondroplasia, and gross chromosomal anomalies (Chapter 3) are well-known causes of malformations. When one encounters a patient with a developmental anomaly, it is wise to carry out a chromosomal analysis and to investigate the family for a history of similar anomalies. Genetic counseling is a practical way of avoiding future abnormalities.

Environmental Factors.   It is becoming increasingly obvious that many external agents are capable of causing serious developmental anomalies if they act *in utero*. Such agents are termed *teratogens*. Infection transmitted from the mother to the fetus can cause serious damage, particularly if the transmission occurs during the first three months of pregnancy when the development of important organs, such as the heart, is proceeding rapidly. German measles has acquired a particularly evil reputation in this respect. Deformities occur in as many as 25 per cent of babies born to mothers who have had this infection during pregnancy. Congenital heart disease frequently occurs in children of women exposed to German measles. The first month of pregnancy is the most dangerous period to be exposed.

The fetal abnormalities that result from hemolytic disease of the newborn are described in Chapter 26.

The tragedy that followed the administration of the sedative drug thalidomide has highlighted the selective toxic effects that some drugs have on the developing embryo. The most common anomalies found in the "thalidomide babies" were absence of limbs or parts of limbs, angiomatous malformations (see *hamartomas*, discussed later) of lips and nose, as well as other malformations of the heart, alimentary tract, and genitourinary system. Since the deleterious (teratogenic) effects of a particular drug on the human fetus can be established only by testing the substance on pregnant women, it is current policy to avoid administration of any drug during pregnancy unless it is absolutely vital (see the following section).

Thalidomide: A Teratogenic Drug.   Thalidomide was first introduced in 1956 as a pleasant and safe hypnotic. During 1960 and 1961 an outbreak of *phocomelia*, or "seal extremity," occurred in West Germany. With this type of deformity the long bones of the limbs are defective, and rudimentary hands and feet arise from the trunk like the flippers of a seal. Viruses, radioactive fallout, food preservatives, and contraceptives were among the agents considered as possible causes, but thalidomide was finally incriminated. Similar outbreaks were reported from other parts of the world; by the end of 1961 the drug had been withdrawn from the market. By that time, tragically, many thousands of babies had been affected. Approval for the drug was delayed by the Food and Drug Administration of the U.S. because of other side effects (*e.g.*, peripheral neuritis). Fortunately, its effects on the fetus became known and general distribution in the U.S.A. was avoided. Nevertheless, some thalidomide babies were born as a result of premarketing clinical trials. The tragedy has taught us some lessons:

1. New drugs must be tested on pregnant laboratory animals.

2. Pregnant women should avoid all unnecessary drugs, particularly during early pregnancy. The use of thalidomide is dangerous during the crucial period from 37 to 54 days after the first day of the last menstrual period.

3. All adverse drug reactions should be reported to a central bureau for evaluation. It took five years to associate the striking birth deformities with thalidomide. Minor or subtle defects may never be recognized unless information is gathered and expertly analyzed.

4. New drugs are not necessarily the best drugs.

The Fetal Alcohol Syndrome.   Expectant mothers who consume large quantities of alcohol tend to give birth to infants that are short and below average weight. There is often underdevelopment of the maxilla with prominence of the forehead and lower jaw, a small head (microcephaly), and mental retardation. The failure of growth and mental development persists even if the child is later cared for by foster parents. It is evident that alcohol in the fetal blood presents a very real teratogenic hazard.

Malformations can affect any part of the body, and a large number have been described. It is convenient to group them under the following ten headings:

Types of Malformations

1. Failure of Development. There may be a complete failure of a part to develop *(agenesis)*, or the part may remain rudimentary and never attain a full mature size *(hypoplasia)*. An example of this lack of or incomplete development has already been mentioned in the case of the thalidomide babies' limbs. Likewise, one or both kidneys can show either agenesis or hypoplasia. The possibility of this anomaly is important to the surgeon who is considering the removal of one kidney. It is essential to check that the other kidney is present and normal.

2. Failure of Fusion. During development many structures normally fuse together, and a failure to do so can result in abnormality. A harelip or cleft palate is a common example of this failure to fuse.

3. Failure of Separation. A good example of this malformation is the webbing that may persist between the fingers or toes (Fig. 16–1).

4. Failure of Canalization. Many channels in the body originate as solid cords and subsequently canalize. A failure in this process leads to a congenital obstruction, which is frequently termed *atresia*. Examples of this are esophageal atresia and imperforate anus (anal atresia).

5. Ectopia. Sometimes organs and tissues are found at abnormal sites. This is termed *ectopia, heterotopia,* or *aberrance*. An interesting example of this is the ectopic thyroid that develops at the base of the tongue. In such a case, no thyroid tissue is found in the normal location, *i.e.,* in the neck. Aberrant blood vessels are quite common. They may even be noticed by a patient and cause anxiety, such as when the radial artery runs a superficial course at the wrist and its pulsation can be seen. Aberrant renal arteries can be damaged by a careless surgeon who relies on the normality of the patient's anatomy.

6. Heteroplasia. Sometimes there is an anomalous differentiation of a particular tissue in an organ. For instance, tissue identical to gastric mucosa

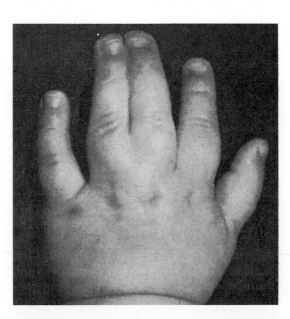

Figure 16–1. Syndactyly. The third and fourth fingers of the hand are joined together. This abnormality can easily pass unnoticed in a young baby. (Photograph courtesy of V. S. Brookes.)

may be found in the esophagus. Sebaceous-gland formation may occur in the oral mucosa; the small white dots that this produces can be seen in the buccal mucosa of many otherwise normal individuals.

7. *Local Gigantism.* Occasionally, there is a simple overgrowth of an organ or tissue. Thus, there may be an enlarged limb in neurofibromatosis. Likewise, there may be enormous overdevelopment of the female breast or breasts at puberty.

8. *Supernumerary Organs.* Additional or supernumerary organs are not uncommon. A good example is hands or feet that exhibit six digits (polydactyly). Supernumerary nipples are not uncommon, and infrequently these are associated with breast tissue.

9. *Hamartomas.* *A hamartoma is a tumorlike malformation in which the tissues of the particular part of the body are arranged haphazardly, usually with an excess of one or more components.* The term was coined by Albrecht and is derived from the Greek word *hamartanein*, meaning "to err." The concept of the hamartoma is of great importance, because a large number of common lesions fall into this general category.

The best-known example of a hamartoma is a simple mole or melanotic nevus of the skin. The lesion is composed of an excess of melanocytes that subsequently change into nevus cells. This lesion is described in detail in Chapter 41.

Some hamartomas (both of the skin and elsewhere) are composed of vascular spaces. Like many other hamartomas, these vascular lesions are given a name resembling that given to a tumor (hemangioma), even though, strictly speaking, this is incorrect, since they are not tumors. Hemangiomas of the skin may produce a noticeable mass (Fig. 16–2), or a flat lesion that cannot be felt but is obvious because of its bright red color. This type is called a "port-wine" stain (Fig. 16–3).

An uncommon but important hamartoma is found in the lung. This consists of a nodule of cartilage and a few spaces lined by a respiratory type of epithelium (Fig. 16–4). The lesion appears on a radiograph as a circumscribed opacity, commonly called a "coin lesion"; its discovery can lead to the mistaken diagnosis of cancer. Radical surgery for such a lesion is a medical catastrophe.

Some hamartomas tend to be multiple: Hemangiomas of the face can be associated with similar hemangiomas of the retina or brain. The skin lesions are thus pointers to the more serious underlying condition. Another well-known but distinctly uncommon example is neurofibromatosis (von Recklinghausen's disease). This inherited autosomal dominant trait results in widespread hamartomatous overgrowths of nerve-sheath tissue. These lesions closely resemble tumors and are generally loosely described as "neurofi-

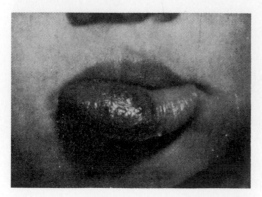

Figure 16–2. Hemangioma of the lower lip. (Photograph courtesy of Mr. G. S. Hoggins.)

Figure 16–3. Hemangioma affecting the skin of the right side of the face in the region of the maxilla.

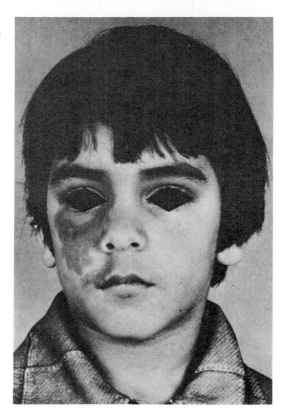

Figure 16–4. Hamartoma of the lung. In the center of the upper lobe there is a circumscribed, pearly-white, hard, round mass. It consists predominantly of mature cartilage, and there is no obvious capsule around it. (Specimen ER 22.1. Reproduced by permission of the President and Council of the R.C.S. Eng.)

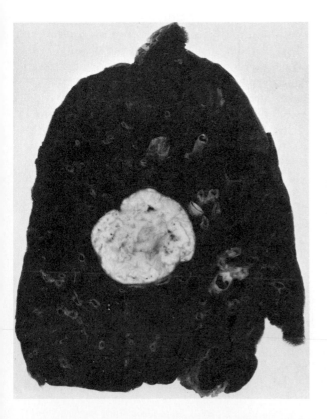

bromas." There is sometimes localized regional overgrowth, and gross deformity can result.

10. Persistence of Normally Vestigial Structures. During the course of development, many structures are formed that are of immediate importance to the developing embryo but that ultimately disappear and become obliterated by the time of birth or shortly thereafter. Occasionally, such structures persist and lead to trouble. The two most important complications are neoplasia and cyst formation. These tumors are considered in the next chapter. Patent ductus arteriosus is described in Chapter 28.

A good example of a *developmental cyst* is the dermoid cyst. This is due to the sequestration and growth of a piece of skin beneath the surface and occurs when folds of skin fuse together during development. During the complex development of the face, various folds are formed and fuse. Dermoid cysts tend to occur along the lines of these fusions, such as at the angles of the eye or mouth. Another example is persistence of a segment of the thyroglossal duct, which results in a midline cystic swelling in the neck, known as a *thyroglossal cyst*.

ACQUIRED DISORDERS OF GROWTH

In the mature individual, all organs and tissues (with the notable exceptions of muscle fibers and neurons) show a steady turnover, with mitosis compensating for cell death. In some organs, such as the liver, the turnover is slow; in others, such as the lymphoid tissue, it is fast. The mechanism controlling this turnover is not understood, but the end-result is that most organs remain at a constant normal size. Furthermore, there is a considerable reserve of tissue that can be drawn upon whenever additional work is demanded of it. Therefore, under normal conditions, no structural adjustment is necessary other than that of regulating the blood flow through the organ. Thus, tissues at rest are maintained by an intermittent blood flow through their supplying capillaries. This mechanism results in an economical use of the circulation, and it explains why noxious substances spread by the blood stream may nevertheless produce patchy effects. When more work has to be performed, the shut-down vessels dilate, and the organ shows an increased blood flow (active hyperemia). This is well illustrated by the tremendous increase in blood flow that occurs in skeletal muscle during periods of activity and in the salivary glands during eating.

Under abnormal circumstances, organs and tissues may show a change in size that is due either to an increase or a decrease in the bulk of parenchymal cells. Abnormalities of cellular growth are found in virtually all tissues, and only a few examples will be given here.

Quantitative Abnormalities of Cellular Growth: Hyperplasia

An increase in the number of cells of a tissue or organ that results in enlargement is called *hyperplasia*. The cause is generally related to the overaction of a tangible stimulus, which is often a basically physiological one acting to excess. Hyperplasia is therefore often the result of an increased demand for function. Following blood loss, there is consequently an increased demand for red-cell production, and hyperplasia of the bone marrow ensues. Likewise, in chronic infection the draining lymph nodes are stimulated so that there is hyperplasia of their component reticuloendothelial and lymphoid cells. In bacteremia there is also reticuloendothelial hyperplasia of the spleen, causing this organ to become enlarged.

In passing, it should be noted that enlargement of an organ is commonly denoted by the use of the suffix -*megaly*. Thus, enlargement of the spleen is described as "splenomegaly." The term gives no indication of the cause of the enlargement; for example, it might be due to hyperplasia of the spleen's constituent cells, or it could equally well be caused by an abscess or a tumor. As always, since there are exceptions to any rule, enlargement of the lymph nodes is spoken of as "lymphadenopathy."

Hyperplasia is generally regarded as an adaptive mechanism by which an increased number of cells is produced as a useful response to a stimulus. Thus, chronic physical irritation of the skin results in thickening of the epidermis; calloused hands are well suited to manual work. When the physical irritation is removed, the epidermis returns to normal. This response is different from that seen in neoplasia, in which withdrawal of the stimulus does not lead to a return to normal (see Chapter 17 for further discussion). Nevertheless, there are examples of cellular overgrowth in human disease that, although classified as hyperplasia, are neither produced by any known stimulus nor necessarily self-limiting or useful. An example of this is the hyperplasia of the thyroid gland in Graves' disease. The precise stimulus for this hyperplasia is not known, but the gland shows enlargement with massive production of new cells and considerable overactivity, so that there is excessive production of thyroid hormones and the patient suffers from hyperthyroidism. Other examples of hyperplasias in which the cause is not known are the epithelial and connective tissue hyperplasias seen in mammary dysplasia in women (Chapter 38) and in the extremely common condition of benign prostatic enlargement encountered in elderly men (Chapter 36).

Hypertrophy is defined as the increase in size of an organ or tissue due solely to an increase in the size of its constituent specialized cells. In practice, this phenomenon applies only to muscle, and the stimulus for this enlargement is almost always a mechanical one.

Any muscle that is continually stimulated by overwork tends to show enlargement. This is commonly seen in skeletal muscle, in which the bulging muscles of the athlete contrast with the slender ones of the sedentary worker. Cardiac muscle, likewise, shows enlargement if the heart is constantly forced to overwork. This is seen when the heart has to force blood through a stenosed orifice (*e.g.*, when there is left ventricular hypertrophy in aortic stenosis; Fig. 16–5) or when it has to contract against a high blood pressure (*e.g.*, in patients with left ventricular hypertrophy in systemic hypertension).

It is noteworthy that the human heart at birth weighs approximately 30 gm, and thereafter no new cells are formed. The heart muscle cells steadily increase in size; by maturity, therefore, there has been a tenfold increase in weight and a tenfold increase in size of muscle fibers. Any further enlargement is due to additional increase in muscle size. Although these large fibers are initially capable of vigorous contraction, it is unfortunate that they ultimately fail. This appears to be due to an inadequate blood supply, since enlargement of muscle-fiber size is not accompanied by an increase in number of blood vessels. It follows that an enlarged heart (cardiomegaly) due to hypertrophy is a diseased heart, and one that will ultimately fail to function efficiently.

Hypertrophy of smooth muscle cells is seen in the muscular coats of hollow organs, which are forced to expel their contents against resistance. The muscular urinary bladder wall hypertrophies when the prostate gland enlarges and causes urethral obstruction. The intestinal muscular wall undergoes hypertrophy proximal to any stenosis (*e.g.*, the stomach wall thickens in pyloric stenosis).

Nomenclature. A small organ or tissue is often spoken of as *atrophic*   **Atrophy**
when its diminution in size is due to a decrease in either the size or number of

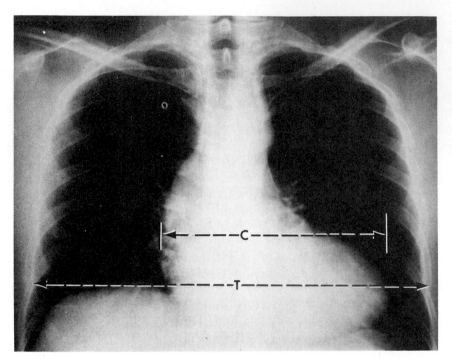

Figure 16–5. Hypertrophy of the left ventricle. This patient had aortic stenosis with enlargement of the heart (*cardiomegaly*) due to hypertrophy of the muscle of the left ventricle. It is convenient to assess the size of the heart by comparing the maximum width of the heart shadow (C) with the width of the chest cavity at the level of the highest point of the right side of the diaphragm (T). The cardiothoracic ratio, C/T, is normally less than 0.5. Here, of course, the ratio is greater than 0.5. (Photograph courtesy of Dr. D. E. Sanders.)

its constituent specialized cells. Only in muscle is the decrease in size of cells a major factor. In all other instances the number of cells is also reduced. Atrophy of the bone marrow is commonly called *hypoplasia* whereas extreme atrophy is known as *aplasia*. This is unfortunate, because the term hypoplasia is also used by some pathologists in a different connotation indicating an imperfect development of an organ or tissue.

Physiological Atrophy. There are many examples of structures that are well developed at a certain time of life but subsequently undergo atrophy. Many fetal structures, such as the thyroglossal duct and the hyaloid artery, which supplies the developing lens, completely disappear before birth. Other structures, such as the ductus arteriosus, atrophy early in postuterine life. From adolescence the lymphoid tissues of the body undergo steady atrophy; after parturition the uterus undergoes atrophy (commonly called *involution*); in old age most tissues (particularly the sexual organs) sustain a generalized process of atrophy.

Pathological Atrophy. Generalized atrophy occurs in starvation and is also a feature of the cachexia of malignant disease. Hypopituitarism, for example, results in atrophy of most of the endocrine glands. The widespread atrophy of bone, termed *osteoporosis*, is described in Chapter 40.

Local Atrophy. Local atrophy is usually the result of impaired blood supply (ischemia). As the blood vessels supplying the brain steadily become obstructed in many persons past middle age, the brain undergoes atrophy. This results in the rigidity of mind and loss of intellect that all too frequently accompany old age.

A particular variant of ischemic atrophy is that which is produced by local pressure. A steadily enlarging cyst or an expanding tumor produces pressure on adjacent tissues and leads to atrophy of the parenchyma. The fibrous tissue stroma tends to be more resistant; it persists and forms a capsule round the lesion.

Disuse Atrophy. It has been tritely stated that what a patient does not use, he loses. A striking example of this is the effects of immobilization of a limb. There is marked atrophy of bone, ligaments, and muscle following joint

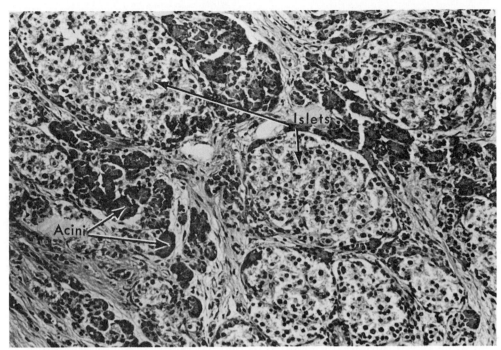

Figure 16–6. Atrophy of the pancreas. This patient had chronic pancreatitis, which caused the formation of a hard mass in the head of the organ. The mass had obstructed the main pancreatic duct. The section illustrated was taken from the body of the organ and shows atrophy of the exocrine component of the gland. Many acini have disappeared; those that remain are small. The shrinkage of the exocrine portion of the gland has resulted in condensation of the islets of Langerhans, which are themselves unaffected. At least seven are present in the field illustrated. Compare this with Figure 2–3. There is some increase in the amount of fibrous tissue and a sparse infiltration by small round cells, indicating a mild degree of chronic inflammation. This case illustrates the principle that if the duct of a secreting gland is obstructed, its parenchyma undergoes atrophy. It is of historical interest that Banting and Best ligated the pancreatic duct to remove the exocrine portion of the pancreas so that insulin could be extracted from the endocrine component without the complicating action of trypsin on their tissue extracts.

immobilization; it is the task of the physical therapist to prevent this. Similar atrophy occurs when a joint is fused *(ankylosed)* or when movement is prevented by pain. Thus, atrophy of muscles and ligaments is common around rheumatoid and tuberculous arthritic joints. Disuse atrophy of a gland following obstruction of its duct is illustrated in Figure 16–6.

There are a number of conditions in which tissues undergo atrophy for no obvious reason. Sometimes there appears to be a genetic defect; sometimes there appears to be an autoimmune mechanism; in most instances, however, there is no apparent cause. A distressing example of this is the atrophy of the brain that occurs prematurely in some people and leads to severe mental deterioration (dementia). Various types of this presenile dementia are known and are categorized under different names, *e.g.*, Alzheimer's disease. Idiopathic endocrine atrophy is seen in some cases of Addison's disease (Chapter 39) and in hypothyroidism and cretinism.

Metaplasia is a condition in which there is a change in one type of differentiated tissue such that it takes on the characteristics of another differentiated tissue. Two forms of this condition are described below.

Abnormalities of Cellular Differentiation

Metaplasia

Epithelial Metaplasia. It is quite common for the pseudostratified columnar ciliated epithelium of the trachea and bronchi to be replaced by a stratified squamous type of epithelium that may even undergo keratinization and resemble epidermis. This *squamous metaplasia* generally seems to be the result of chronic irritation. This condition is also found in the urinary tract, particularly in association with urinary stones and infection. Sometimes metaplasia can be more subtle. The bronchial lining can be replaced by a columnar epithelium in which simple mucus-secreting goblet cells predominate. This is extremely common in chronic bronchitis and is one of the factors that results in the excessive production of mucus that is continually coughed up (expectorated). The concept of metaplasia is important, because it helps to explain why tumors of the lung can resemble those normally arising in the skin (squamous-cell carcinoma) or in a mucus-secreting gland (adenocarcinoma).

Connective Tissue Metaplasia.   The fibroblasts of connective tissue and scar tissue can sometimes take on the characteristics of osteoblasts and lead to the laying down of bone. Spicules of bone are often found in chronically inflamed tonsils, in old scars, and in the fibrous elements of goiters. Since these areas of bone formation are visible in radiographs, they are of importance in diagnostic radiography.

Other Cellular Abnormalities

The term *dystrophy* is commonly used, but it is difficult to define. It is generally applied to any condition in which there is an alteration in the structure or function of an organ or tissue that does not readily fit into the other categories (*i.e.,* agenesis, atrophy, hypertrophy, or metaplasia). For example, in *corneal dystrophy* the cornea becomes opaque at about the time of puberty and ultimately results in blindness. Some varieties are inherited, and these appear to be degenerative. Dystrophy is also used to describe the crumbly, deformed nails affected by fungal infection or psoriasis. It is evident that the term dystrophy has no precise definition and is used in many specialties to describe diseases of widely differing nature.

The term *dyscrasia* is now used only by hematologists to describe some blood disorders of unknown cause and undetermined pathogenesis. The term serves no useful function and should be abandoned.

Dysplasia has been used to describe an abnormal development of tissue; like dystrophy, however, the term is also used by specialists in many fields to describe conditions of widely divergent nature. Thus, when applied to the breast (mammary dysplasia), dysplasia denotes a complex condition of unknown origin in which there is irregular hyperplasia and metaplasia of breast substance. In the cervix uteri, dysplasia has acquired a completely separate meaning. It is used to describe a type of epithelial overgrowth that is thought to progress steadily to *carcinoma-in-situ*, and ultimately to invasive cancer. In the skin, dysplasia is used in a similar context to describe the atypicality and irregular maturation seen in the epidermis in actinic keratoses and in Bowen's disease (see Figs. 17–15, 17–16, and 17–17). In these organs, therefore, the term "dysplasia" denotes a change that is thought to precede the onset of cancer.

From this short account, it is evident that the terms *dystrophy, dysplasia,* and *dyscrasia* are used quite arbitrarily to denote various types of conditions, the nature of which is poorly understood.

In this chapter many different perversions of cell growth have been described. The one factor they all have in common is that they are self-limiting and reversible if the stimulus is removed. In the following chapter, *neoplasia* is discussed. With this condition the perversion of cell growth persists even when the stimulus that produced it is eliminated.

Review Questions

1. At what stage of gestation is a drug most likely to produce severe fetal abnormalities? Describe the steps that can be taken to protect the fetus against potentially harmful drug action.

2. Define *hamartoma* and give three examples of those affecting the skin.

3. Describe how metaplasia differs from heteroplasia and dysplasia.

4. Differentiate between regeneration and hyperplasia.

5. Describe the changes that might occur when a leg is encased in a plaster cast for three months.

Clarren, S. K., and Smith, D. W.: The fetal alcohol syndrome. New England Journal of Medicine, *298*:1063–1067, 1978.

Editorial: Thalidomide's long shadow. British Medical Journal, *4*:1155, 1976.

Gillis, L.: Thalidomide babies: management of limb defects. British Medical Journal, *2*:647–651, 1962. See this article for pictures of thalidomide deformities.

Lawrence, D. R., and Bennett, P. N.: Clinical Pharmacology. 5th, ed. Edinburgh, Churchill Livingstone, 1980, pp. 94–98. Provides a fascinating account of the thalidomide disaster.

Marymont, J. H., and Herrmann, K. L.: Rubella in pregnancy: review of current problems. Postgraduate Medicine, *56*(4):167–172, 1974.

Taussig, H. B.: A study of the German outbreak of phocomelia. Journal of the American Medical Association, *180*:1106–1114, 1962. See this article for pictures of the thalidomide deformities.

Willis, R. A.: Some unusual developmental heterotopias. British Medical Journal, *3*:267–272, 1968.

Selected Readings

CHAPTER 17 Neoplasia

After studying this chapter the student should be able to:

- Define a neoplasm.
- Give a classification of tumors in tabular form.
- Define the following terms: adenoma, papilloma, cystadenoma, fibroma, and leiomyoma.
- Define carcinoma, sarcoma, adenocarcinoma, squamous-cell carcinoma, anaplasia, teratoma, dormant cancer, carcinoma-in-situ, and metastasis.
- Describe the microscopic features of malignant neoplasms and compare them with those of a benign neoplasm.
- Discuss the effects of a malignant neoplasm and contrast them with those of a benign neoplasm.
- List the malignant tumors that commonly metastasize to bone.
- Describe what is meant by staging of a tumor and indicate the value of the procedure.
- Give an account of the important features of
    - (a) squamous-cell carcinoma
    - (b) carcinoma arising from a glandular epithelium
    - (c) fibrosarcoma
- Subdivide the lymphomas into two groups and describe their salient features.
- Illustrate the structure and behavior of an intermediate tumor, using basal-cell carcinoma as an example.
- Discuss the difficulties in classifying neoplasms in relation to tumors of melanocytes, placenta, and embryonic rests.
- Give examples of carcinogenic chemicals that cause tumors in human beings.
- Outline the steps involved in the evolution of a malignant tumor following the application of a chemical carcinogen.
- Give examples of physical carcinogenic agents that affect humans.
- List the human tumors in which there is a hereditary predisposition.
- Discuss the relationship between hormones and cancer.
- Give examples of viruses that have been incriminated as a cause of cancer in animals. Indicate the relevance to human disease.
- Describe the development of cancer through the stages of dysplasia and carcinoma-in-situ.
- Discuss the evidence indicating that cancer starts in one cell rather than in many cells simultaneously.
- Describe the genetic and epigenetic theories of cancer.

Introduction   The presence of a lump or mass is a common clinical finding, and the term "tumor" was applied at one time to such a lesion; the suffix -*oma* was used to denote it. The practice of classifying all swellings as tumors became established long before the nature of the lesions was understood, and even today this relic of medical history persists in the use of names like "hematoma," "hamartoma," "tuberculoma," and "granuloma." In due course, the swellings of known origin, especially the infective ones, were excluded from the category of tumors, and a large group of swellings of unknown cause, which apparently had arisen as a result of the unrestrained growth of the individual's own cells, was left. In all other pathological processes the growth of cells appears to be coordinated and under strict control. A tumor is regarded as resulting from a breakdown in this mechanism and has been defined by Willis as *an abnormal mass of tissue, the growth of which exceeds and is uncoordinated with that of the normal tissues and persists in the same excessive manner after cessation of the stimulus that evoked the change.* This definition is unsatisfactory in several respects. First, it implies that the stimulus producing a tumor need act only for a short time. Second, it implies that the regulating mechanism governing cell growth is abolished. Unfortunately, we do not know the nature of this regulating mechanism, and we are consequently not able to prove or disprove that it is nonfunctional.

Although the excessive growth of cells is often manifested by the production of a tumor mass, this does not always occur. Sometimes the migration of newly formed cells from the site of formation outweighs the bulk of abnormal proliferation and no swelling as such exists. One excellent example of this is the diffuse infiltrating carcinoma of the stomach; another is leukemia. *Neoplasia,* which literally means "new formation or new growth," is a more suitable term. It implies that there is an abnormal type of growth that may be evident not only in the intact animal but also in cells grown in culture. Nevertheless, the terms "tumor" and "neoplasm" are commonly used synonymously and in this book will be used in this manner.

A neoplasm is regarded as resulting from an unrestrained growth of cells, and it follows that one possible classification can be based on the cell of origin. Since the tissues of the body have been divided into either epithelium or connective tissue, tumors can likewise be placed into one of two groups. Furthermore, each group can be subdivided. Thus, epithelial tumors can be grouped into those arising from stratified squamous epithelium, those from columnar epithelium, etc. This delineation, based on the cell type of origin, is an important component of our present-day classification. In itself, it is quite inadequate, since the effects of a tumor are determined not only by the tissue of origin but also by its biological behavior. In some tumors the dividing cells adhere to each other, and the neoplastic mass remains as a circumscribed lesion. Such a lesion is termed a *benign tumor,* and its behavior can be contrasted with that of tumors in which the cells do not adhere to one another and are thereby enabled to invade the surrounding tissues. These are the *malignant tumors,* or *cancers.* Cancer cells often enter natural channels such as lymphatics or blood vessels, and groups of tumor cells are carried as emboli to other parts of the body, where they grow and set up *secondary growths,* or *metastases.* Local invasion and embolic spread are the two characteristics of malignant tumors. The term "malignant" is particularly suitable, for, with the very few exceptions of spontaneous regression, this type of tumor inevitably causes death unless effective treatment is instituted. Nevertheless, the rate of progression varies markedly from one tumor to another, as will be seen from some examples studied later.

In addition to the typical benign and malignant tumors, there are other types that show patterns of behavior not fitting into either group. Most important are the *intermediate tumors,* in which tumor cells invade locally but do not metastasize. These are best called "locally malignant" tumors. *Carcinoma-in-situ* and the phenomena of *spontaneous regression* and *dormant cancer* are considered later.

The neoplastic cells are supported and nourished by a network of host connective tissue that consists predominantly of blood vessels, lymphatics, fibroblasts, and a varying amount of collagen. This network is called the stroma and, although an intimate part of the tumor, is not considered to be involved in the neoplastic change. Both benign and malignant tumors

Classification of Neoplasms

produce a number of factors that seem to promote stroma formation. One of these factors is called *angiogenic factor,* since it encourages the ingrowth of blood vessels.

When the patient is first seen clinically, the organ of origin is the most striking feature of many tumors. If the cell type of origin and biological behavior of the tumor can be determined, a satisfactory diagnosis may be obtained. In practice, however, it is not possible to assess behavior by leaving the tumor alone and awaiting development. It has been found that behavior can frequently be related to the microscopic appearance of the tumor. The ultimate classification of a particular tumor is therefore attained by establishing its site of origin, its tissue of origin, its behavior, and its microscopic appearance. An outline of the classification in current use is shown in Table 17–1.

Cancer is often regarded as a single disease, and one frequently hears references to its cause and treatment. It should be evident from this short discussion on classification, however, that "cancer" does not constitute a single entity but rather encompasses a large number of separate diseases. At the present time, it would seem to be as futile to search for the cause or cure of cancer as it would be to look for the cause and cure of "infection."

BENIGN NEOPLASMS

These are of two main types. Benign neoplasia of a surface or lining epithelium produces a warty tumor called a *papilloma* (Fig. 17–1). In a compact gland, such as the breast or the thyroid, the tumor is embedded in the tissue and is called an *adenoma.*

Benign Epithelial Tumors

Papillomas. Papillomas may occur on any epithelial surface. Some have a broad base and are described as *sessile,* whereas others become pedunculated and are called *polyps,* a morphological term applied to any pedunculated mass attached to a surface and not necessarily neoplastic. Papillomas are supplied by a core of connective tissue stroma containing blood vessels, lymphatics, and nerves. This is covered by a folded neoplastic epithelium composed of stratified squamous, transitional, or columnar cells, according to the type from which it has arisen. The cells show an orderly arrangement, and the epithelial basement membrane is intact unless there is distortion due to inflammation. The epithelial cells are entirely restricted to the surface and do not show invasion.

Stratified squamous-cell papillomas are common on the skin and are seen as warts (Fig. 17–2) and seborrheic keratoses (Chapter 41). Since the common wart (verruca vulgaris) is a squamous-cell papilloma, the term *verrucous* is commonly used to describe any papillary or wartlike lesion, whether it be on the skin or elsewhere, benign or malignant.

Adenomas. An adenoma is composed of a mass of glandular tissue that closely resembles the structure of the parent tissue. Adenomas are quite common in the colon, where they arise from the glands in the mucosa. As with papillomas, they frequently become polypoid (see Fig. 32–10).

In some adenomas the glandular spaces enlarge to form cysts (causing a *cystadenoma*), and papillomas can grow into these cysts (causing a *papillary cystadenoma*). Such a tumor is common in the ovary.

Benign Connective Tissue Neoplasms

A benign neoplasm, which can arise from any connective tissue, is composed of a mass of cells whose structure closely resembles that of the parent tissue. Common tumors in this group are lipomas derived from fat, leiomyomas derived from the smooth muscle (Fig. 17–3), neurofibromas (schwannomas) derived from the Schwann cells of the nerve sheaths, and fibromas derived from fibroblasts. These tumors are generally well circumscribed.

TABLE 17–1.　CLASSIFICATION OF TUMORS

TISSUE OF ORIGIN	BEHAVIOR		
	Benign	*Intermediate*	*Malignant*°
EPITHELIUM			
Types			
1. Covering and protective			
(a) Squamous	Squamous-cell papilloma		Squamous-cell carcinoma
(b) Transitional	Transitional-cell papilloma		Transitional-cell carcinoma
(c) Columnar	Columnar-cell papilloma		Adenocarcinoma
2. Compact and secreting	Adenoma; if cystic, cystadenoma or papillary cystadenoma		Adenocarcinoma; if cystic, cystadeno-carcinoma
3. Others	Adenoma	Basal-cell carcinoma Pleomorphic salivary gland tumors Carcinoid tumor (argentaffinoma)	Carcinoma
CONNECTIVE TISSUE			
Fibrous	Fibroma		Fibrosarcoma
Nerve sheath	Neurofibroma		Neurofibrosarcoma
Adipose	Lipoma		Liposarcoma
Smooth muscle	Leiomyoma		Leiomyosarcoma
Striated muscle	Rhabdomyoma		Rhabdomyosarcoma
Synovial	Synovioma		Malignant synovioma
Cartilaginous	Chondroma		Chondrosarcoma
Bone osteoblast	Osteoma	Giant-cell tumor	Osteosarcoma
Blood vessels and lymphatics	Benign hemangioma and lymphangioma		Angiosarcoma
Neuroglia		Astrocytoma, Oligodendroglioma, and Ependymoma†	
FETAL TROPHOBLAST	Hydatidiform mole		Choriocarcinoma
GERM CELLS	Benign teratoma		Malignant teratoma
EMBRYONIC TISSUE			
Pluripotential cell			
Kidney			Nephroblastoma
Unipotential cell			
Retina			Retinoblastoma
Hindbrain			Medulloblastoma
Sympathetic ganglia and adrenal medulla	Ganglioneuroma		Neuroblastoma
HAMARTOMA			
Melanotic nevus			Malignant melanoma
Neurofibromatosis	Neurofibroma		Neurofibrosarcoma

°Any malignant tumor may be so undifferentiated that it must be classified on a histological basis, *e.g.*, carcinoma simplex, spindle-cell sarcoma. The lymphomas and many rare tumors are not included in this table.

†These tumors are difficult to classify. The common types are locally malignant, but some also metastasize within the central nervous system. Rarely, they appear to be benign in children.

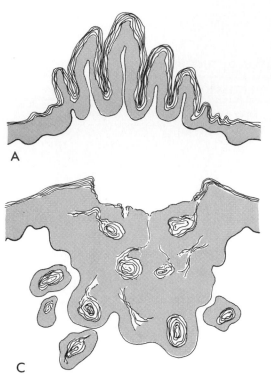

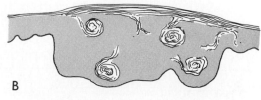

Figure 17–1. Tumors of the epidermis. Three types of neoplasia of a keratinizing stratified squamous epithelium (*e.g.*, epidermis) are shown. *A,* Benign neoplasia results in an excessive production of regular epithelium, which is thrown into a complicated folded structure in order to be accommodated. This formation is called a *papilloma.* The epidermal cells mature in an orderly way from the basal cells to the superficial squames. *B,* In *carcinoma-in-situ* there is excessive growth of epidermis, which thereby becomes thickened (acanthosis). Maturation of the cells is disorderly; foci of keratinization are found within the epidermis instead of being present only on the surface (dyskeratosis). *C,* In *carcinoma* the atypical epidermal cells break through the basement membrane and invade the underlying tissues. (Drawings by Margot Mackay, Department of Art as Applied to Medicine, University of Toronto.)

General Considerations of the Effects of Benign Neoplasms

The cells of a benign neoplasm show no tendency to invade the surrounding tissues but do produce an expanding mass that has two local effects:

Pressure Atrophy. The adjacent specialized parenchymatous tissue undergoes atrophy, while the more resistant connective tissue survives to form a capsule. *Benign tumors are therefore usually well encapsulated* and are not intimately connected with the surrounding tissues except at points of entry of the supplying blood vessels (see Fig. 37–2). Benign tumors can therefore be excised with relative ease; if local removal is complete, they do not recur. Nevertheless, a benign tumor cannot be dismissed as inconsequential. One

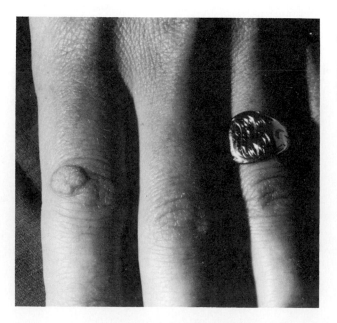

Figure 17–2. Verruca vulgaris. This patient has a common wart overlying the proximal interphalangeal joint of the left index finger. The lesion is a squamous-cell papilloma, which is caused by a papovavirus.

Figure 17–3. Leiomyoma of the uterus. The tumor consists of spindle-shaped smooth muscle cells arranged in sheaves, some of which are cut longitudinally, while others are seen in transverse section. No mitoses can be seen in this benign tumor (× 250).

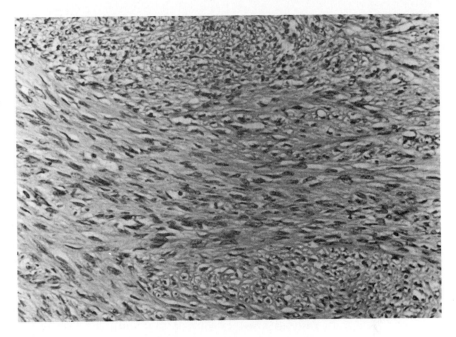

within the skull or vertebral column can produce serious pressure effects and even death. The shape of a benign tumor is generally spherical, but it may be modified by firm local structures.

Obstruction. A benign tumor may obstruct a natural passage, causing extensive damage. Thus, blockage of a bronchus can lead to bronchiectasis and bronchopneumonia (see Fig. 30–13). A tumor of the intestine can produce obstruction. Benign tumors generally grow slowly and rarely ulcerate on the surface. Hence, bleeding is uncommon as a symptom, except for certain vascular surface papillomatous growths such as those of the colon or bladder. Benign tumors of endocrine tissue occasionally produce an excess quantity of the associated hormone; this oversecretion of hormone can lead to serious and sometimes fatal effects. A good example of this is the adenoma of the islets of Langerhans, which can lead to fatal hypoglycemia as a result of the overproduction of insulin. It is therefore not true that benign tumors cannot cause death.

Microscopically, the cells of a benign tumor closely resemble those of the parent tissue. They are therefore described as being "well differentiated." The cells tend to be regular in size and uniform in staining and shape; mitoses are scanty and when present are of normal type.

MALIGNANT NEOPLASMS

General Considerations

The cells of a malignant tumor infiltrate surrounding tissues, normal cells are enveloped and destroyed, and the edge of the tumor is poorly defined. Microscopic spread occurs beyond the naked-eye edge of the tumor, and complete excision by surgery is therefore difficult. Even if much surrounding, apparently normal, tissue is included in the excision, malignant cells can often remain behind; their continued growth results in a *local recurrence*. The invading malignant cells spread in the planes of least resistance: fingerlike processes extend outward from the main tumor mass, and the growth has a fanciful resemblance to the silhouette of a crab. It is from this mode of spread that the term "cancer," from the Latin word meaning *crab*, is derived. In lay language it is generally applied to all malignant tumors. In medical terminology it is often used as being synonymous with *carcinoma, which is defined as a malignant tumor of the epithelial cells. A sarcoma is a malignant neoplasm derived from connective tissue cells.*

Embolic spread of tumor cells is responsible for the production of distant metastases. Local invasion and embolic spread are the two characteristics of malignant tumors. Both are related to the reduced cell adhesiveness that appears to be a fundamental characteristic of malignant cells, for this property is evident not only *in vivo* but also in tissue culture. The cells do not resist mechanical separation as well as do those of normal tissue (see cell transformation, page 251). The power to invade and spread, combined with the capacity for progressive growth, makes the term "malignant" particularly apt for this type of tumor. Death is inevitable in untreated cases, except for those very rare — though well-documented — cases of *spontaneous regression*, in which proven cancers have disappeared either with no treatment or with very limited palliative treatment.

Gross Characteristics

Malignant tumors do not possess a limiting capsule, although with some very rapidly proliferating growths, such as secondary tumors in the liver, they may appear circumscribed. Microscopy, however, shows tumor extension beyond the apparent edge of the growth. Malignant tumors tend to be irregular in shape and are usually larger than their benign counterparts. As would be expected from their destructive properties, they tend to ulcerate along a free surface. Hence, any area of ulceration that fails to heal within a reasonable time should be regarded as malignant until proved otherwise. Since tumors invade and destroy blood vessels, bleeding is a frequent symptom. *Bleeding and ulceration are thus features of malignant tumors.*

Microscopic Features

Several important microscopic features should be noted. Tumor tissue may resemble the parent tissue to a considerable extent, but the similarity is not as great as with benign tumors. Differentiation is not so well developed, and recognition of the tissue of origin is often difficult or even impossible. Tumors showing little or no differentiation are called *undifferentiated*.

Malignant tumors usually show much mitotic activity. The synthesis of DNA prior to division results in nuclear enlargement and hyperchromatism. This synthesis, together with the formation of polyploid cells, accounts for the irregularity in size and shape (*pleomorphism*) and the mode of staining that is so characteristic of malignant tumors. Mitoses are not only numerous but also abnormal (Fig. 17–4). A number of cells may deviate from the normal complement of 46 chromosomes, and occasionally cells are seen to divide into three instead of two (*triradiate mitosis*).

Anaplasia is a term that at first was introduced to describe new cells deviating from normal and resembling those of embryonic origin. It was at one time thought that tumors were derived from rests of embryonic cells. This concept has been abandoned, but the term anaplasia is still used to describe those cellular changes that are found in malignant tumors. Therefore, a tumor said to show a high degree of anaplasia has cells that are pleomorphic, poorly differentiated (scarcely reproducing the parent tissue), and exhibiting frequent and bizarre mitoses.

Effects

Malignant tumors produce their ill effects in a number of ways, which are described below:

Mechanical Pressure and Obstruction. Like benign tumors, malignant tumors cause obstruction to natural passages and lead to serious consequences. Thus, a tumor of the colon produces intestinal obstruction; a tumor of the bronchus leads to collapse and bronchopneumonia in the lung beyond it (see Fig. 30–18).

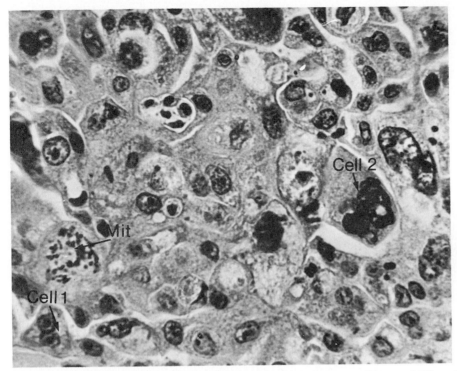

Figure 17–4. Anaplastic carcinoma of lung. The tumor shows no evidence of differentiation, and its cells exhibit marked pleomorphism. One cell possesses two nuclei, each with a prominent nucleolus (Cell 1), whereas another has many hyperchromatic nuclei (Cell 2). In an atypical mitosis scattered chromosomes can be identified (Mit) (× 550).

Destruction of Tissue. Both primary and secondary tumors infiltrate and destroy tissue. This is most obvious with cancer of the skin (Fig. 17–5) and is also well illustrated by tumors in bone, in which destruction may be so marked that minimal trauma produces a fracture. This is known as a *pathological fracture* and may sometimes be the first symptom of a previously missed tumor.

Hemorrhage. Malignant tumors that involve any surface usually ulcerate and bleed. Repeated bleeding can cause anemia; occasionally, a fatal sudden hemorrhage can occur where a large vessel is eroded. *Clinically unexplained bleeding from any site should be treated seriously, since it is a common symptom of cancer.*

Infection. All ulcerating cancers are bound to become secondarily infected with bacteria. Infection often follows in the wake of obstruction, such as bronchopneumonia with cancer of the lung and urinary tract infection with cancer of the bladder. *Repeated bouts of infection in an organ should always lead to a suspicion of an underlying malignant tumor.*

Starvation. Cancer of the mouth, pharynx, esophagus, and stomach can so obstruct the passage of food that direct starvation occurs.

Anemia. Anemia is common and is due to a variety of causes. There may be direct blood loss from an ulcerating tumor, malabsorption of essential dietary components, or bone-marrow replacement if there are multiple bony metastases.

Cachexia. The emaciated appearance of patients with advanced cancer is characteristic, but it is nevertheless not uncommon for some patients to remain obese. The cause of the weight loss and the generalized body atrophy in many patients with cancer has given rise to much speculation. At one time,

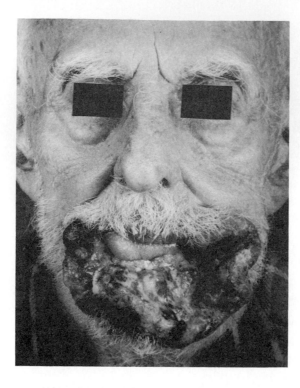

Figure 17–5. Squamous-cell carcinoma of the lower lip. This patient was a recluse and neglected himself. The carcinoma has destroyed the whole of the lower lip and part of the jaw. Cervical lymph nodes were invaded by metastatic growth. Histologically the tumor was a keratinizing squamous-cell carcinoma similar to that depicted in Figure 17–9.

a toxic product from the tumor was postulated, but this has never been substantiated. The present tendency is to attribute cachexia to secondary factors such as starvation, hemorrhage, infection, and liver damage.

In advanced malignancy there is usually fever, a raised erythrocyte sedimentation rate (E.S.R.), and a neutrophil leukocytosis. In part, these are effects of infection and in part they are due to the pressure of necrotic tissue both in the tumor and in the surrounding tissues.

Hormonal Effects.   Malignant tumors of the endocrine glands can sometimes produce effects by overproduction of the relevant hormone. This is less common than with benign tumors, as would be expected, since malignant tumors are less differentiated both in structure and in function.

Carcinomatous Syndromes.   A variety of syndromes have been reported in association with tumors that are not explicable in terms of infiltration by either a primary tumor or its metastases. Muscle weakness, skin eruptions, signs of an intracranial tumor, and venous thrombosis are some examples of this. At necropsy no local tumor is found to explain these features. A possible explanation is the deposition of immune complexes containing tumor antigen. For the most part, however, these strange manifestations of cancer have not been explained.

Another curious phenomenon is the hormonal effect produced by tumors of nonendocrine origin, which are particularly common in cancer of the lung. The tumor appears to be able to secrete hormonelike substances, and symptoms of hypercorticalism (Cushing's syndrome), hyperinsulinism, and hyperparathyroidism may occur. It is apparent that the atypical cells of malignant tumors can produce and secrete hormones or hormonelike substances into the circulation. This is an instance of abnormal differentiation of a malignant tumor.

Spread of Malignant Neoplasms

Direct Spread.   Tumor cells spread into the surrounding tissues, particularly along tissue planes and natural spaces. This is a feature that is used by the pathologist as an aid to the microscopic diagnosis of malignancy. Clinically, local invasion is often evident by the way in which the tumor becomes attached to adjacent structures. Thus, a carcinoma of the breast eventually becomes attached to the skin and the underlying pectoral muscles.

Invasion of Lymphatics. Carcinoma, but not sarcoma, shows a particular tendency to invade lymphatic vessels at an early stage, and the cells may grow as a long, ever-extending cord. The process is called *lymphatic permeation,* and the lymphatic obstruction it produces can cause lymphatic edema (Fig. 17–6).

Invasion of the Arteries and Veins. This is a common event and may lead to thrombosis and obstruction.

Spread by Metastasis. Groups of malignant cells may become detached, travel in some natural passage to a distant site, become implanted, and finally grow to produce secondary deposits, or metastases. The lymphatics, blood vessels, and serous cavities are the most important pathways.

Lymphatic Spread. Detached groups of tumor cells that have invaded lymphatic channels travel to the regional draining lymph nodes (Fig. 17–7). If the cells survive and grow, they replace the lymph node with tumor; the cells then move on to the next group of nodes. This is a common event with carcinoma and melanoma, but it is rare with sarcoma.

Blood Spread. The occurrence of blood-borne metastases is the feature of malignant disease that is responsible for death in most cases. It is the factor that limits the surgical and radiotherapeutic treatment of cancer. At first sight,

Figure 17–6. Spread of carcinoma by lymphatic permeation. Section of skin showing dilated lymphatic vessels filled with carcinoma. The specimen was taken from the skin of a woman with advanced carcinoma of the breast. Although the tumor is derived from a glandular structure, it shows no evidence of differentiation. The tumor may therefore be labeled an undifferentiated carcinoma, a polygonal-cell carcinoma, a spheroidal-cell carcinoma, or a carcinoma simplex (× 250).

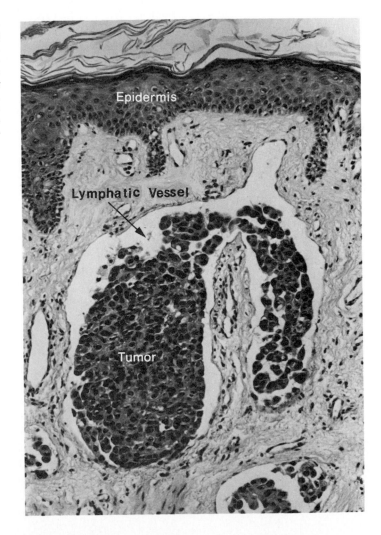

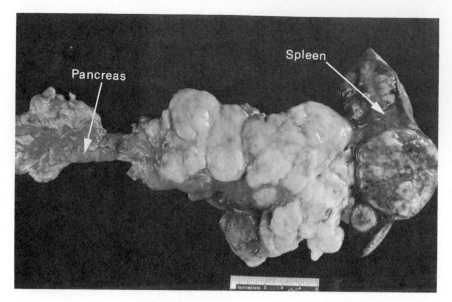

Figure 17–7. Lymph node metastases. The specimen shows a group of peripancreatic lymph nodes that are greatly enlarged by metastatic carcinoma. Several nodules of tumor are also present in the spleen. The primary growth was a small-cell (oat-cell) carcinoma of the lung. This tumor is highly malignant and metastasizes early and widely. In general, secondary deposits are infrequent in the spleen, but they are often found in patients with widespread metastases from oat-cell carcinoma of the lung or malignant melanoma.

The growths seen in these enlarged lymph nodes are not diagnostic of secondary carcinoma. An identical picture, including the splenic involvement, could be seen in a lymphoma such as Hodgkin's disease.

the mode of production of secondary tumors is easy to understand. Malignant cells invade small venules, become detached, and are then carried in the blood stream until they become impacted in the next capillary network that they encounter. There the emboli take root, and the cells proliferate and develop into secondary tumors. A second route of blood-borne metastases is via the lymphatics, for all the lymph eventually drains into the venous circulation.

As would be expected, the lung is one of the commonest sites of metastasis for all tumors. Primary tumors arising in an area drained by the portal vein regularly metastasize to the liver. Purely mechanical factors seem to account for this distribution, but such an explanation seems untenable upon a closer examination of the facts.

Many tumors, *e.g.*, of the breast and the kidney, give rise not only to lung metastases but also to secondary growths in the liver, bones, and other organs; such systemic metastases sometimes occur without apparent deposits in the lung. It is possible that such deposits are, in fact, present but are missed at an inadequate necropsy examination. Alternatively, one can postulate that the cells pass through the lung capillaries and travel to the systemic circulation, where they lead to secondary deposit formation.

One might expect that the distribution of metastases would be related to the blood supply of each organ. Such is not the case. Cardiac and skeletal muscle have an abundant blood supply, and yet it is rare to find metastases in muscle. The spleen also has a very large blood supply, yet splenic metastases are also quite uncommon. *Selective metastasis* is the term used to describe this distribution of metastases.

There is considerable evidence that malignant cells often reach the blood stream where most of them die. Only a selected few are able to take root and grow into secondary deposits. In part this depends on the nature of the tumor, as experimental work on the mouse will illustrate. Isolated cells of a transplantable malignant mouse melanoma can be cloned by growth in tissue culture. When these cells are injected intravenously into other mice of the same strain, metastases predominate in one organ (lung or brain) according to the nature of the clone that has been selected.

Some examples of selective metastasis should be noted:

Liver. The commonest organ in which blood-borne metastases are found is the liver, regardless of whether the primary tumor is in an area drained by the portal vein or not. Although massive enlargement of the liver is common, it is rare for liver failure to occur (Fig. 17–8).

Lung.   This is the next most common site of metastases.

Bone.   Carcinomas of the breast, lung, and prostate commonly metastasize to bone. Such spread is less frequently seen with other tumors. *Pain* is a common presenting symptom, particularly when the spine is involved and nerves are compressed.

Brain.   Cancer of the lung is notorious for the frequency with which it metastasizes to brain. Indeed, secondary lung cancer is a common type of tumor to be found in the brain.

Adrenal Glands.   This is a frequent site for secondary lung and breast cancer, an infrequent site for other primary growths.

Transcelomic Spread.   When a malignant tumor invades the serosal layer of a viscus, it causes a local acute inflammatory response. This results in the formation of a serous inflammatory exudate in the cavity, and bleeding usually occurs. It follows that the presence of a blood-stained effusion into any serous cavity, such as that of the pleura or peritoneum, should always arouse suspicion of malignancy. Withdrawal of some fluid and an examination for malignant cells will sometimes lead to a positive diagnosis. Cells that travel in the effusion can form the basis of numerous secondary seedling growths.

Grading and Staging of Malignant Tumors

In order to compare the results of various forms of treatment and to assess the likely outcome of a tumor (*i.e.,* to give a *prognosis*), efforts have been made to classify individual types of tumor.

Grading is an attempt to assess the biological malignancy of a tumor by examining its microscopic appearance, taking into consideration its degree of differentiation, its number of mitoses, and other factors. A grade I tumor is well differentiated, has few mitoses, and tends to have a good prognosis. A grade III tumor is poorly differentiated, has many mitoses, and tends to have a poor prognosis. Sometimes four grades are used. Unfortunately, the correlation between grade and prognosis is not good. Tumors may vary greatly from one area to another, and the assessment of the grade is very subjective.

Staging is more satisfactory and is based on the size of the primary tumor

Figure 17–8. Liver with metastatic carcinoma.   The liver contains numerous white nodules of metastatic carcinoma from a primary tumor in the nasopharynx. The nodules are of varying size; one of them is 13 cm in diameter.

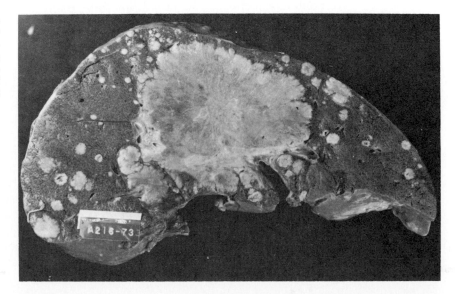

and its known extent of spread. The most widely used today is the *TNM system*. T1 to T4 describe the size of the tumor. N indicates the presence and extent of lymph node involvement; thus N0 indicates no nodal involvement. M indicates the presence and extent of distant metastases. The details of the classification vary with each specific tumor.

Dormancy   One difficulty with staging is the tendency for some metastases to appear many years after the primary tumor has apparently been treated successfully. Patients may remain well for 10, 20, or even 30 years after removal of a primary tumor and then suddenly develop multiple secondary deposits despite the absence of any local recurrence. It is assumed that tumor cells were present in the body during the entire period, but for reasons unknown they remained dormant. This is one of the most mystifying aspects of malignant disease, and were we to know the factors responsible for keeping cancer cells dormant, we might well have an adequate treatment for the disease. Carcinoma of the breast and kidney and melanoma of the eye are tumors that are notorious for this tendency toward metastases developing after a period of dormancy.

Malignant Epithelial Neoplasms   Malignant epithelial neoplasms are the *carcinomas*, the most common of all malignant tumors. Three types may be recognized:
    (1) Squamous-cell carcinoma
    (2) Glandular epithelial carcinoma
    (3) Transitional-cell carcinoma
Squamous-Cell Carcinoma.   This histological type of tumor arises at any site normally covered by stratified squamous epithelium — skin, mouth, esophagus, and other similar regions. Squamous-cell carcinoma arises via the invasion of the underlying connective tissues by the germinal cells situated in the basal layer of the epithelium. Malignant cells may infiltrate separately, but more usually they form clumps and columns as they proceed into the connective tissue. The cells tend to differentiate into prickle cells and form keratin, so that in a well-differentiated tumor, clumps of cells are seen with a central whorl of keratin (Fig. 17–9). This is called an *epithelial pearl* and is in effect an attempt by the malignant cells to reproduce the stratum corneum of the normal skin. Tumors that are less well differentiated form no keratin, but they do contain prickle cells. Poorly differentiated tumors show few recognizable structures and are difficult to distinguish from poorly differentiated tumors of other types. Purely descriptive terms are used to name such tumors: giant-cell carcinoma, spindle-cell carcinoma, and large-cell carcinoma.

Squamous-cell carcinoma can also arise from columnar or transitional epithelium. This can occur in one of two ways. The normal epithelium can undergo metaplasia to squamous epithelium, and tumor growth subsequently occurs in this. A second, and more likely, explanation is that the tumor arises in the epithelium first, and then the tumor cells show squamous differentiation. One of the most common tumors of lung, arising from the bronchial mucosa, is a squamous-cell carcinoma. Likewise, squamous-cell carcinoma is also found in the urinary bladder and less frequently in the gallbladder. It should be noted that the term "squamous-cell carcinoma" is used to describe a particular microscopic appearance of a tumor showing differentiation into a keratinizing squamous type of cell. It does not always mean a tumor arising from a squamous epithelium.

Glandular Epithelial Carcinoma.   This type of carcinoma may arise from a surface secreting epithelium, such as that which lines the stomach, or from a solid gland, such as liver or breast. The pattern of invasion of neoplastic

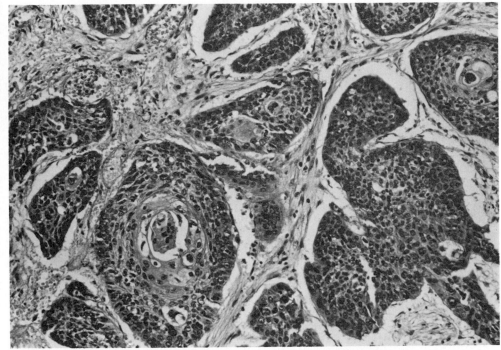

Figure 17–9. Squamous-cell carcinoma of skin. The dermis has been invaded by malignant cells that have grown to form clumps. In some areas the central tumor cells have differentiated into keratin and have formed cell nests or epithelial pearls. This is characteristic of a well-differentiated squamous-cell carcinoma. Note that the groups of tumor cells are sharply separated from the stroma (compare this with Figure 17–3).

epithelial cells is similar to that already described with squamous-cell carcinoma. In the case of the tumors arising from glandular epithelium, groups of cancer cells, instead of producing keratin, tend to arrange themselves into acinar structures containing a central lumen into which some secretion is poured (Figs. 17–10 and 17–11). The well-differentiated cancers showing excellent acinus formation can closely mimic the original glandular structure. If differentiation is poor, the tumor is composed of masses of cells with only occasional tubule formation. A tumor derived from glandular epithelium and showing glandular differentiation is called an *adenocarcinoma*.

In poorly differentiated tumors there are merely clumps of cells surrounded by a stroma and no evidence of central cavitation to produce an acinus. The names *carcinoma simplex, spheroidal-cell carcinoma* and *polygonal-cell carcinoma* are applied in this type of cancer (Fig. 17–6). Such tumors are particularly common in the breast and stomach.

Mucoid Cancer. Occasionally a carcinoma derived from glandular epithelium shows such excessive production of mucus that to the naked eye the tumor appears as a gelatinous mass and microscopically there are pools of mucus in which are floating malignant cells. Sometimes the cells contain one large droplet of mucus with the nucleus pushed to one side, giving the appearance of a signet ring. This type of tumor occurs in the stomach or large intestine.

Transitional-Cell Carcinoma. This type of tumor occurs in the urinary tract and often shows areas of squamous differentiation.

Stromal Reaction to Carcinoma. The reaction of the invaded tissue to carcinoma cells varies; its growth may be so stimulated that a hard fibrotic or *scirrhous* type of tumor is produced. Most breast cancers are of this type. As

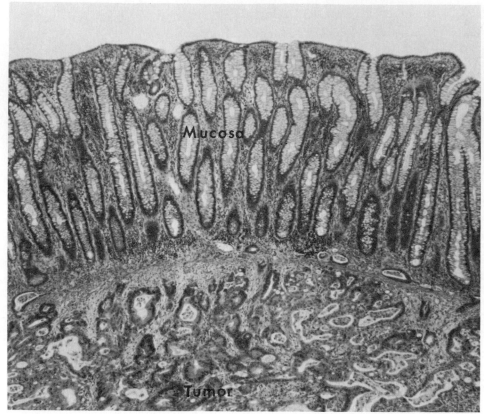

Figure 17–10.   Adenocarcinoma of the colon.   At this magnification the mucosa appears normal. The section was taken from an area adjacent to a carcinoma; tumor has invaded the submucosa. Normally this layer consists of loose connective tissue similar to that seen in the small intestine (Chapter 2) (× 60).

with wounds, the dense fibrosis appears to be associated with a contracting tendency that is poorly understood. It is this effect that leads to obstruction with many carcinomas of the colon. The contraction causes a purse-string deformity.

When a tumor has little stroma in relation to the cell bulk, it is soft or brainlike and is described as *medullary*, or *encephaloid*. It should be noted that carcinoma cells, like normal epithelial cells, tend to grow in solid sheets or clusters with close cell-to-cell apposition. Only with very anaplastic tumors do the cells separate, and their growth then resembles that of a sarcoma (see below).

Malignant Connective Tissue Neoplasms

These malignant tumors are called *sarcomas* and are much less common than carcinomas; like carcinomas, they occur at all ages. On the whole, sarcomas spread more rapidly than carcinomas, and the prognosis is correspondingly more grave. The cells of a sarcoma tend to separate after mitosis and to be intimately associated with the stroma and its blood vessels. This helps to explain why blood-borne metastases appear early: the lungs are often riddled with secondary deposits. Lymphatic involvement is very much less common than with carcinoma.

Fibrosarcoma.   Fibrosarcomas can arise in any fibrous connective tissue and can vary in their degree of differentiation. A well-differentiated tumor shows some cellular irregularity and good collagen formation; distinction from a fibroma can be extremely difficult. Poorly differentiated tumors show

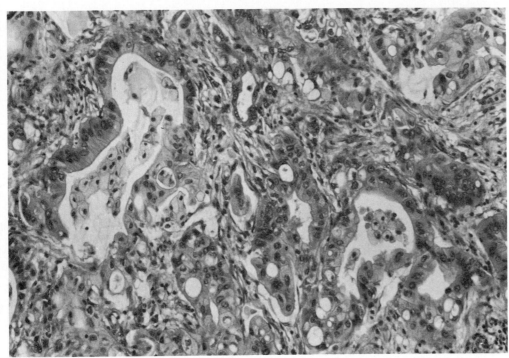

Figure 17–11. Adenocarcinoma of colon. This section is from a lymph node metastasis of the tumor shown in Figure 17–10. Although the growth is well differentiated, the pattern of glandular formation is quite different from the normal. Some malignant cells line large spaces, whereas others form solid clumps (× 250).

little or no collagen formation and are then termed *spindle-cell sarcomas.* A distinction from anaplastic carcinomas is sometimes difficult.

Osteosarcoma.   This is one of the commonest forms of sarcoma and is further described in Chapter 40. Other types of sarcoma are known. They arise from blood vessels (*angiosarcoma*), fat cells (*liposarcoma*), and smooth muscle cells (*leiomyosarcoma*) and are all uncommon.

The neoplastic lesions of these cells are the *lymphomas* and tumors of the *hematopoietic tissues.*

Lymphoma.   The lymphomas are all malignant tumors and arise from the cellular elements of the lymph nodes, bone marrow, and occasionally other organs having a reticuloendothelial content. They are the second most common malignant tumors; carcinomas occur most often. They generally start at one site — usually a lymph node — but spread to other lymph nodes and eventually become disseminated, with deposits being found in the spleen, liver, bone marrow, lungs, and elsewhere. Whether this represents metastasis or multicentric origin is debatable. Unlike many types of sarcoma, they are generally extremely radiosensitive. Sometimes a local lesion can be cured by radiotherapy, but unfortunately recurrence and spread throughout the body are the rule. Two major types of lymphoma can be recognized:

Hodgkin's Disease.   This is the commonest of the lymphomas and affects young and middle-aged adults predominantly. Lymph nodes are first affected and are replaced by tumor tissue that consists of atypical histiocytes together with lymphocytes, eosinophils, plasma cells, and often much fibrous tissue. In the past there has been much argument as to whether the disease represents an infective granulomatous process or a neoplastic disease. The consensus is that it is a neoplasm and therefore a type of lymphoma. The essential neoplastic element is believed to be the histiocytes. In particular, Reed-

Tumors of the Stem Cell and Its Derivatives

Sternberg cells must be identified in order to substantiate the diagnosis. These cells usually have two nuclei, each with a prominent nucleolus, and the nuclei are so arranged that the one appears to be the mirror image of the other. If the disease is treated while it is still localized, the prognosis is quite good, but when the disease has become systemic, the outlook is poor. The prognosis also depends on the histological appearance of the tumor present. Various classifications are in vogue that relate histological appearance to prognosis.

Non-Hodgkin's Lymphoma.   Many classifications of this group of lymphomas have been proposed, but none has attained international recognition. The subject is under constant review. These lymphomas lack the diagnostic atypical histiocytes of Hodgkin's disease and tend to be monomorphic, *i.e.,* they consist of one type of cell. At one time two main groups were recognized:

1. *Lymphosarcoma,* in which the cell type is either a small or a large lymphocyte. Lymphocytic leukemia is sometimes associated with this type.

2. *Reticulum cell sarcoma,* in which the tumor is composed of large cells thought to be neoplastic reticulum cells.

It was later realized that the large-celled lymphomas were derived not from reticulum or reticular cells but from histiocytes. These are the fixed cells of the reticuloendothelial system. These tumors were therefore renamed *histiocytic lymphomas.* The tumors of lymphocyte origin became the *lymphocytic lymphomas.* This classification is still in common use, but Lukes and his colleagues have pointed out that the neoplastic "histiocytes" are in fact transformed lymphocytes! Thus, it is now realized that the majority of non-Hodgkin's lymphomas are derived from lymphocytes. The use of cell markers has shown that the majority are of B-cell origin. T-cell lymphomas are uncommon, the best known example being mycosis fungoides, which is a disease that primarily attacks the skin. A few lymphomas have neither T- nor B-cell markers, while others appear to be derived from histiocytes. The name histiocytic lymphoma is still retained for the latter group. The various subdivisions of the B- and T-cell lymphomas are complex and will not be discussed further, except to mention one particular variant. This is Burkitt's lymphoma, a tumor that occurs extensively and almost exclusively in the low-lying moist region of Central and West Africa. It is almost entirely confined to children between the ages of 2 and 14 years and affects the jaws, ovaries, lymph nodes, and kidneys. The usual mode of presentation is an enormous facial swelling with loosening of the affected teeth. The fascination of this tumor is that it is thought to be caused by the Epstein-Barr virus.

Malignant Conditions of the Hematopoietic Tissue.   The most important of these are the *leukemias,* in which the malignant cells are found circulating in the peripheral blood, and *multiple myeloma,* in which the bone marrow is replaced by plasma-cell tumors. Both conditions are considered in detail in later chapters.

INTERMEDIATE NEOPLASMS

In their behavior, intermediate tumors are between the benign and the malignant groups. Since local invasion occurs, the tumors cannot be regarded as benign. Nevertheless, they do not show the steady, inexorable growth pattern of true malignant tumors. The victims do not inevitably die of the disease if left untreated. The most common tumor in this group is the *rodent ulcer,* or *basal-cell carcinoma.* This invades locally, but almost never metastasizes (Figs. 17–12 and 17–13).

Another tumor in this group is the pleomorphic salivary gland tumor. Histologically, this is an adenomatous growth and is unusual in that the stroma appears to consist of cartilage (see Fig. 31–7). The tumors often appear encapsulated, but the capsule is infiltrated by lateral extensions of growth.

Figure 17–12. Basal-cell carcinoma. This badly neglected tumor involves a large area of the face and has invaded the orbit and nasal cavity. Tumor invasion has combined with infection to cause considerable tissue destruction. The basal-cell carcinoma almost never metastasizes. This particular tumor was cured by radiotherapy together with excision of the left eye. This picture should be remembered when one considers the effects of any invasive tumor that is not readily visible. From this picture one can appreciate how an ulcerated carcinoma of the stomach, colon, or bladder could be accompanied by tissue destruction, infection, and bleeding. (Photograph courtesy of Professor D. D. Smithers.)

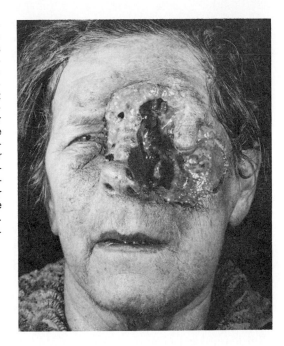

Simple enucleation is therefore followed by recurrence. Blood-borne metastases may develop, but this is a rare event.

In this group of tumors with erratic behavior are the carcinoid tumors of the lung (Chapter 30) and of the intestine (Chapter 32).

Although it might seem that all malignant tumors could be classified as either carcinoma or sarcoma, there are certain instances in which this cannot be done.

Difficulties in Tumor Classification

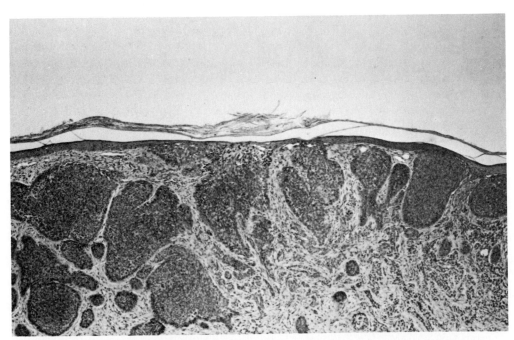

Figure 17–13. Basal-cell carcinoma of the skin. Masses of tumor cells are seen to be arising from the basal layer of the epidermis. Some still maintain their attachment to the epidermis, while others have become detached and are spreading deep into the dermis. This is a typical basal-cell carcinoma and shows no tendency to form keratin (× 60).

Neoplasms of Indeterminate Origin

The best example of such tumors is the melanoma of the skin (Chapter 41). Some authorities have called the melanocyte an epithelial cell, and its tumors have been called *nevocarcinomas*. Others regard them as of connective-tissue origin and label the tumors *melanotic sarcomas*. In practice, the term *malignant melanoma* is used to avoid this problem.

Placental and Embryonic Neoplasms

Tumors can arise from cells that are not normally present in the adult body. Two examples can be recognized:

(a) tumors of placental origin — hydatidiform mole and choriocarcinoma (Chapter 37).

(b) tumors of embryonic origin.

These tumors arise from cells that, although present in the developing embryo, should normally have disappeared by the time of birth. Such tumors generally arise in children; the best-known examples are the following:

1. The *retinoblastoma*, which arises in the eye generally before the age of four.

2. The *neuroblastoma*, which is a malignant tumor derived from primitive neuroblasts. Note that the stable nerve cells cannot divide and therefore cannot give rise to tumors. Primitive neuroblasts, on the other hand, can divide and subsequently differentiate into nerve cells. Neoplastic neuroblasts may behave similarly, thereby explaining the occasional occurrence of a tumor that appears to be forming nerve cells. A well-differentiated tumor of this type is benign and is called a *ganglioneuroma*.

3. The *nephroblastoma*, which is one of the common malignant tumors of childhood, involves the kidney. The tumor, which is derived from a primitive kidney cell, shows differentiation not only into renal tubules but also into connective tissue elements such as fibroblasts and striated muscle cells; even structures resembling glomeruli can be formed.

Teratomas

The commonest tumor of the ovary in young women is a benign teratoma or "dermoid cyst." The lining consists of epidermis together with normal skin appendages, including hair. Thus, the cyst contains sebaceous material and matted hair. In its wall other structures can be found, including thyroid tissue, teeth, bone, brain, and spaces lined by a variety of different types of epithelia (Fig. 17–14). This tumor clearly contains derivatives of all three embryonic germinal layers and could have arisen only from a totipotent cell that was capable of differentiating into virtually any of the normal tissues of the body. Such a tumor is called a *teratoma*. The tumor is thought to be of germ cell origin. A similar type of tumor occurs in the testis, but here the various tissues are poorly formed, and the tumor is nearly always malignant.

THE INCIDENCE AND CAUSE OF TUMORS

Observations on the incidence of tumors both in individuals and in ethnic and geographic groups have led to the unraveling of many factors that are involved in the production of tumors. These will be considered under the following headings:

1. Chemical Carcinogenesis.
2. External Carcinogenic Physical Agents.
3. Hereditary Predisposition.
4. Hormonal Factors.
5. Viral Infections.
6. Cancer Following Chronic Disease.

Figure 17–14. Teratoma of ovary.
For five years, the patient had had occasional episodes of abdominal pain. At the age of 32 she experienced a particularly severe attack, which led to her being admitted to a hospital. A rounded swelling was palpated in the abdomen above the pubis. A cystic ovarian tumor was removed at laparotomy.

The specimen shows the opened cyst. It is lined by skin, and on one side a hard mass projects into the cavity. This is covered by spongy skin containing numerous sebaceous glands and from it is growing a tuft of hair. The mass contains bone in which a number of teeth are partially embedded. One of these is clearly shown in the photograph. The mass of tissue (Seb) contains hair but is otherwise lying free in the cyst cavity. It consists largely of sebaceous material and desquamated keratin. (Photograph of specimen courtesy of the Boyd Museum, University of Toronto.)

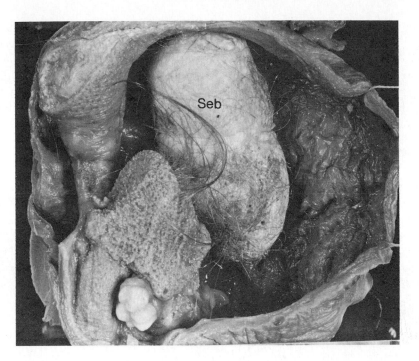

Chemical Carcinogenesis

The observation by Percivall Pott in 1775 that cancer of the scrotum was common in chimney sweeps led to the conclusion that soot and its derivatives cause cancer of the skin. It has been amply confirmed both in humans and in animals that certain chemicals, termed *carcinogens,* can lead to the formation of tumors. As would be expected, the first group of chemicals to be discovered were those derived from coal tar, and of these 1,2:5,6 dibenzanthracene and 3:4-benzpyrene are among the best known. When applied to the skin of animals, they cause squamous-cell carcinoma, and when injected into deeper tissues, they cause a variety of other tumors, including sarcomas. It has been found that when skin is painted with relatively small doses of carcinogen, no obvious change may be apparent. Nevertheless, if the skin is subsequently irritated by relatively nonspecific agents, such as croton oil, tumors can arise upon it. The supposition is that the carcinogen produced a change called *initiation,* such that relatively nonspecific stimuli can subsequently *promote* the formation of a malignant tumor.

The initiation process is thought to begin by the binding of the active carcinogen to some part of the cell, either DNA, RNA, protein, or other component. The biochemical damage so caused may be repaired enzymatically, and the cell can return to its normal state. Alternatively, the change may become fixed if cellular proliferation occurs. Thus, it is difficult to initiate tissues in which mitotic activity is normally low, *e.g.,* liver and kidney. On the other hand, it is easy to understand how hormonal stimulation or regeneration following injury (*e.g.,* viral hepatitis in the case of liver) can aid initiation. Likewise, epidermis can be initiated with ease because it normally exhibits considerable mitotic activity. The state of initiation appears to be long-lasting. By contrast, the effects of a promoting agent are of brief duration. All complete carcinogens are both initiators and promoters, but the relative potency of each activity varies. Thus, saccharin in large doses in animals is a weak initiator but a more powerful promoter in the bladder epithelium. Asbestos fibers act as a promoter in human lung previously initiated by cigarette smoking.

The simple two-stage development of cancer described by Berenblum (initiation and promotion) has now been extended to envisage a *multi-step process*. There is selective growth of the initiated cells to form focal areas of proliferation — some showing atypical hyperplasia, others dysplasia, adenomas, or papillomas. There seems to be progressive evolution of clones through the stages of hyperplasia, dysplasia, and carcinoma-in-situ to carcinoma of low malignancy and finally carcinoma of high malignancy. The whole process takes many months in the case of animals and many years in humans. The process may stop at any point, and indeed some of the stages are reversible. The probability of regression decreases as the lesions become more malignant, but even highly malignant tumors with metastases do on occasion regress — sometimes by differentiation into normal type cells. Possibly keratoacanthoma (Chapter 41) can be explained in this way. It is unfortunate that we know very little of the factors that govern the evolution of tumors.

Many hundreds of carcinogenic compounds have now been identified. Some are positively charged compounds (called *electrophilic reactants* because they react with sites on molecules that are rich in electrons). These agents (*direct acting carcinogens*) act directly on cells to induce cancer. The majority of carcinogens (*procarcinogens*), however, must be activated to form an electrophilic *ultimate carcinogen*. This activation is often accomplished within cells by enzymatic action (Chapter 4). The ultimate carcinogen may act on the cell where it is formed, or it may affect a susceptible tissue that it reaches through the blood stream, or via the urine, bile, or other secretion.

The appreciation that chemicals can cause cancer has been of great significance in industry, and it is convenient at this point to mention the carcinogens of importance.

Polycyclic Aromatic Hydrocarbons. These are formed whenever organic material is heated. Hence, they are ubiquitous, being present in food, car exhaust fumes, cigarette smoke, and coal tar derivatives.

Aromatic Amines. Naphthylamine and benzidine used in the chemical and rubber industries are converted in the liver into an ultimate carcinogen that is excreted in the urine and causes *bladder cancer*.

Nitrosamines and Nitrosamides. Nitrites (used to preserve meat) and nitrates (present in food and water) can be converted into carcinogenic nitrosamines and nitrosamides in the stomach and colon. Bacterial action plays a part in this conversion. These carcinogens may well be responsible for cancer of the stomach and colon. The increasing use of refrigeration as a means of preserving meat could be a factor in the declining incidence of stomach cancer.

Naturally Occurring Carcinogens. The mold *Aspergillus flavus*, which contaminates ground-nut meal, produces a toxin *(aflatoxin)* that is a powerful liver carcinogen. This may explain why liver cancer is so prevalent in Africa. *Betel nuts* commonly chewed in India are a factor in the development of mouth cancer.

Other Compounds. Many other chemicals have been incriminated as possible human carcinogens. Saccharin and cyclamates have been linked to bladder cancer; vinyl chloride, the monomer of polyvinyl chloride, to hemangiosarcoma of the liver; diethylstilbestrol (DES) given to pregnant women, to carcinoma of the vagina in their female offspring; and chromium, nickel, and asbestos, to cancer of the lung. Indeed, the list is never-ending and other examples will be cited when the causes of individual tumors are discussed.

Carcinogenic substances may be formed within the body from its own constituents. Bile salts may be modified in the gut to produce carcinogenic chemicals.

The testing of new compounds for carcinogenic activity is an important public health undertaking. Administration to animals is expensive, time-consuming, esthetically unpleasing, and above all unreliable since the activity of a particular carcinogen shows great species variation. An alternative is the *Ames test,* in which the compound is tested for its ability to cause mutations in bacteria. Since 90 per cent of carcinogens prove to be mutagenic, this procedure, or some variant of it, is used as a quick, easily performed screening test. The ultimate proof of safety remains as before — the use of the chemical on human beings.

Inhibition of Chemical Carcinogenesis.   Many compounds are known to inhibit the tumor-producing ability of chemical carcinogens. They include anti-oxidants, derivatives of vitamin A (retinoids), anti-inflammatory steroids, and perhaps vitamin C. These agents may have their effect by preventing the activation of procarcinogens (see above), or they could block the processes of initiation or promotion.

Some authorities believe that up to 80 per cent of human cancers are caused by the activity of some chemical carcinogen. Hence, there is hope that some of these carcinogens may be avoided and that the incidence of cancer will decline. Nevertheless, it is evident that the evolution of cancer is a complex process and that drastic changes in living style might have unexpected effects, for not only may carcinogens be removed from our environment but so also may protective anti-carcinogens be eliminated.

External Carcinogenic Physical Agents

The discovery of ionizing radiations was soon followed by an appreciation that these rays can cause cancer. Cancer of the skin occurred in the early radium workers and in those exposed to x-rays. The ingestion of radioactive compounds can lead to more widespread damage. The most famous example of this was recorded in female workers who painted luminous watch dials. They sucked their brushes to point them and thus ingested radioactive compounds used in the luminous paint; these compounds were deposited in the bones. The patients developed sarcoma of the bones as well as leukemia. The most recent demonstration of the carcinogenic activity of ionizing radiation has been the increased incidence of malignant disease in the survivors of the Hiroshima and Nagasaki bomb explosions. It is now appreciated that even diagnostic radiology carries a minor risk; consequently, all efforts are made to minimize the dosage received for essential radiographic procedures. Since it is believed that the embryo is particularly susceptible, the radiation of pregnant women is now carried out only for vital reasons.

Ultraviolet light is another carcinogenic agent. The common lesions it produces are solar keratoses and basal-cell carcinomas.

The damage caused by both ionizing radiation and ultraviolet light can be repaired by the cell. Cancer is therefore liable to develop only if radiation is received at a rate that exceeds the cells' ability to repair the damage. Hence, individuals with little protective melanin pigment in their skin, such as those of North European stock, are particularly liable to develop malignancies of the exposed skin if they live in a sunny climate, such as that of Australia.

There is a rare inherited disorder (xeroderma pigmentosum) in which there is a defective DNA repair mechanism. The unfortunate sufferers are destined to develop multiple skin cancers and to die early unless they are adequately protected from damaging sunshine.

Hereditary Predisposition

It is possible to breed a strain of animals in which virtually all members of the strain will die of a particular cancer if they live long enough. It seems likely, therefore, that some hereditary predisposition is a factor in the development of tumors. Nevertheless, it is doubtful whether this is of any great importance in human pathology, since statistical surveys among relatives of cancer patients have not yielded convincing evidence of an increased incidence of tumors. Cancer of the breast is possibly more common in the relatives of affected women than in the population at large.

There are, however, a number of very uncommon neoplastic diseases that are inherited. The condition *polyposis coli* is transmitted as an autosomal dominant trait; sooner or later one of the lesions becomes malignant, and the patient dies of carcinoma of the colon, usually before the age of 40 years. The very uncommon tumor *retinoblastoma* (Chapter 42) is also inherited as a mendelian dominant trait. With these and a few other extremely rare exceptions, there is little evidence that the tendency to develop cancer is inherited.

Hormonal Factors

The early observations that the administration of estrogens to mice led to an increased incidence of cancer of the breast was at first thought to indicate that hormonal imbalance could cause cancer in humans. However, it was soon appreciated that in mice cancer of the breast is related to a viral infection by the Bittner virus, and that the major effect of the estrogens was to allow the male mice to develop breasts in which cancer could develop. There have been similar instances in human pathology. Some men who have been deliberately castrated and undergone "sex change operations," and who have been administered estrogens for developing breasts, have subsequently developed cancer of the breast and have died of this disease. There is indeed little evidence that hormones play a major part in the cause of most human tumors. Nevertheless, hormones are related to tumors in various subtle ways. Some teenage girls whose mothers were given the synthetic estrogen *diethylstilbestrol* during pregnancy have subsequently developed *carcinoma of the vagina*. This disease is extremely rare under normal conditions. It seems that the effect of estrogens on the developing fetus is to allow certain vestigial structures to remain; these subsequently develop into tumors during the offspring's adolescence.

Hormone-Dependent Tumors. If hormones can seldom be directly incriminated in the cause of human cancer, they are undoubtedly of great importance in maintaining the growth of some tumors, which are called *hormone-dependent tumors*. The best example is carcinoma of the prostate.

Both the normal prostatic epithelium and the carcinoma derived from it are dependent for their integrity upon a supply of testosterone. If patients with cancer of the prostate are castrated, there is often a dramatic relief of symptoms and regression of both the primary tumor and its metastases. Both castration and the administration of estrogens are now used in the treatment of carcinoma of the prostate. Unfortunately, although there is some initial response, the patients ultimately die of the tumor since it seems to lose its hormonal dependency.

Carcinoma of the breast is another tumor that manifests hormone dependency in some patients. The picture is complicated, however, because the tumor seems to depend upon ovarian, adrenal, and pituitary hormones. The treatment is somewhat arbitrary; it is found that some patients are aided by the administration of estrogens, while others derive benefit from the removal of the ovaries, adrenal glands, or pituitary. In each instance the remission is unfortunately only temporary, for the treatment has an ameliorative effect but not a curative one.

Viral Infections

Fowl leukemia was shown to be transmissible by a virus in 1908 by Ellerman and Bang; a short time later fowl sarcoma was observed by Rous to be transmissible. Since then a number of animal tumors have been identified that can be transmitted by viruslike particles. One of the most interesting is the agent responsible for cancer of the breast in mice. This is known as the *Bittner factor* and is an agent that is secreted in the milk and infects the newborn suckling mice. The females that mature subsequently die of cancer of the breast. Infected males do not develop cancer unless given estrogens to encourage breast development.

The tumor-producing, or *oncogenic*, viruses that are now known fall into two groups:

DNA Oncogenic Viruses. The common wart in humans is caused by a papovavirus and may be regarded as a benign type of tumor. Rabbits suffer from a similar squamous-cell papilloma called the Shope papilloma; this ultimately becomes malignant and metastasizes as a squamous-cell carcinoma. This malignant propensity is not shown with human warts. The Epstein-Barr virus, which is associated with infectious mononucleosis, is thought to be a factor in the cause of Burkitt's lymphoma, but although the association is close, proof that it is the cause of the tumor is still lacking. Likewise, the herpes simplex virus appears to be more common in patients with cancer of the cervix; once again, the precise relationship is not clear.

Because viruses grow rapidly in cancer cells, it is difficult to be sure whether a virus found in association with a tumor is the cause of that tumor or merely a passenger that happened to be growing rather readily in the malignant cells. The *polyomavirus* is another oncogenic DNA virus that has been studied in great detail. It causes various types of tumors in many species of animals if injected into them. One of the curious features of this virus is that, having produced a tumor, it can no longer be found in the tumor cells. There is, however, evidence that parts of the viral genome are present. It seems that the DNA or part of the DNA of the virus becomes incorporated into the nuclear genetic material of the malignant or transformed cell (see below). The polyoma virus is closely related to a simian virus (SV-40), which is a common commensal found in monkey kidney cells. This emphasizes the danger of using animal tissue cultures when preparing vaccines for human use. Both the polyoma and the SV-40 viruses induce changes in cells growing in tissue culture. The cells show rapid, unruly proliferation and when implanted into an animal behave like malignant cells. This change is called *cell transformation* and is the *in vitro* manifestation of the development of malignancy.

RNA Oncogenic Viruses. These viruses differ from the DNA tumor viruses in that they commonly appear to produce tumors in their natural host; furthermore, the transformed cells regularly produce large quantities of infectious virus. The Rous virus belongs to this group, as does the virus that causes fowl leukemia. The mode of action of the RNA viruses is fascinating. It seems that the viral RNA leads to the production of DNA by means of a process of reverse transcription (Chapter 2). This DNA can then reproduce and finally become inserted into a host chromosome. The DNA, in fact, becomes part of the genetic make-up of the new cancer cell.

The Bittner virus is also an RNA virus, and contains an RNA-dependent DNA polymerase that catalyzes the synthesis of DNA. It has been found that the DNA synthesized by this virus is complementary to RNA extracted from human breast cancers. There is considerable evidence that human breast cancers contain an RNA oncogenic virus very similar to the Bittner factor. The precise relationship of the virus to the tumor is as yet undetermined. Particularly confusing is the observation that RNA virus particles can be found in normal cells. This has led to some interesting speculations. Perhaps infective virus could be generated by apparently uninfected cells. Possibly the *DNA provirus* exists in all normal cells as part of a normal gene pool — the so-called *oncogene*. Normally this is repressed, but under some circumstances — irradiation, the action of chemicals, etc. — the oncogene actively encodes for RNA virus particles. Another possibility is that informational transfer from DNA to RNA and back to DNA is a normal process. Disruption of this transfer mechanism, for example, by radiation or chemical damage, could result in an alteration of the genetic information encoded in a cell during its lifetime. Again, infective RNA virus could be formed.

Cancer Following Chronic Disease

It has often been taught that cancer follows prolonged stimulation of a tissue through "chronic irritation." Now that carcinogenic chemicals and agents have been discovered, it seems unlikely that pure physical irritation, acting alone, can produce cancer. Nevertheless, there are a number of conditions that may be regarded as precancerous, since the development of tumors is more common in the lesions than it is in normal tissue. Chronic skin ulcers from whatever cause are sometimes complicated by the later development of squamous-cell carcinoma. About 90 per cent of primary liver cell cancer in humans is superimposed on a previous cirrhosis (Chapter 33). Other examples in other organs could be quoted, but they are all rare, and it must be accepted that the great majority of human tumors apparently arise in previously normal tissue.

Early Stages in the Development of Cancer

In some organs cancer does not develop suddenly. Cancer of the epithelia of the skin and uterine cervix illustrates this well (Figs. 17–15 to 17–17). The first stage results in irregular maturation of the epithelial cells, and this *dysplasia* steadily progresses until the whole epithelium is replaced by

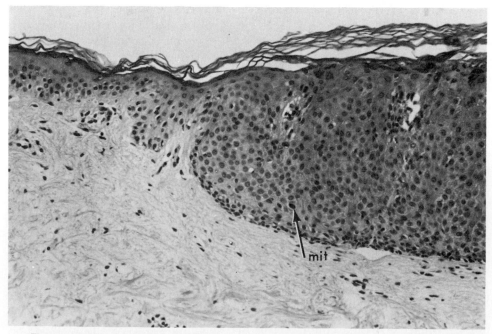

Figure 17–15. Epidermal dysplasia. The epidermis is seen to be markedly thickened; this acanthotic area ends abruptly where it becomes continuous with the normal epidermis. In addition to being abnormally thick, the affected epidermis contains occasional atypical mitoses (mit). The cells are also somewhat larger than normal and show delay in maturation. This is an example of mild dysplasia. The tissue was from a person having Bowen's disease (intraepidermal squamous-cell carcinoma) (× 250). Compare this photomicrograph with Figure 17–16.

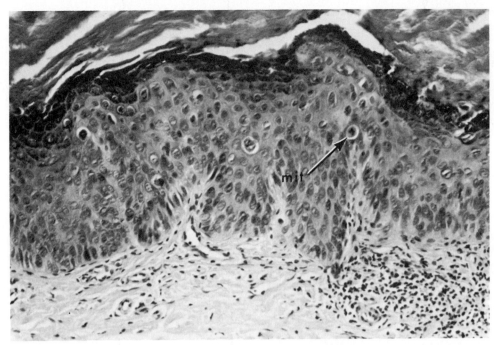

Figure 17–16. Epidermal dysplasia. The epidermis is acanthotic. Its cells are enlarged and show irregularity in size and shape. Mitoses can be identified (mit) and the keratin layer shows occasional remnants of nuclei, a condition termed parakeratosis (× 250). Compare the degree of dysplasia in this picture with that depicted in Figures 17–15 and 17–17.

atypical, pleomorphic cells that have the cytological features of carcinoma. At this stage the basement membrane is still intact, and the condition is called *carcinoma-in-situ.* The final stage results in invasion of the underlying connective tissues and subsequent metastasis. The whole process probably takes several years.

The cells of the cervix uteri are shed into the vaginal secretions; a smear from these can be examined for the presence of atypical cells. This examination forms the basis of exfoliative cytology, which was pioneered by Papanicolaou. By regular examination of "Pap smears" of adult women the early stages in the development of carcinoma can be detected, and the occurrence of invasive cancer can be prevented.

Carcinoma-in-situ is now recognized in other organs and has been studied more extensively in the skin, which is so easily examined. Bowen's disease and actinic keratoses provide good examples (Chapter 41).

Cancer is generally assumed to be due to a change in the character of the cells, which causes them to exhibit uncontrolled growth. The possibility that the connective-tissue stroma plays some part cannot be entirely ignored, because there are many examples in the embryological development in which the epidermis relies on the connective tissue for its stimulation and maintenance, and vice versa. The possibility that the essential change in cancer lies in the connective tissue has not been completely excluded. Nevertheless, it is generally assumed that the essential changes are in the cancer cell itself. The results of years of research have given us a vast amount of knowledge concerning the properties of such cells. These may be summarized as follows:

The Nature of Cancer

1. Morphological Abnormalities. The pleomorphic and bizarre appearances of malignant cells have already been described. It is by recognizing

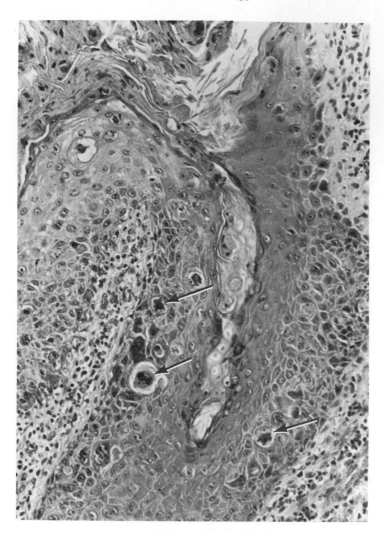

Figure 17–17. Carcinoma-in-situ. The epidermis contains many large atypical cells and abnormal mitoses (arrows). Parakeratosis is marked, and the entire epidermis has been thrown into folds (papillomatosis). Although the epidermal cells resemble those of a squamous-cell carcinoma, there is no invasion of the dermis (× 250). Compare this figure with Figures 17–9 and 17–16.

these changes that a pathologist is able to diagnose cancer from the Pap smear or a tissue section.

2. Biochemical Abnormalities. Malignant cells produce lactate at a higher rate than most normal cells. At the time of this discovery by Warburg this was thought to be a unique property of malignant cells, but it is now regarded as an expression of rapid growth rather than malignancy.

Many other biochemical changes can be cited. Some tumors produce substances normally found only in the fetus. The formation of alpha-fetoprotein by some liver cell cancers is an example of this reversion to a more primitive behavior. Likewise, carcino-embryonic antigen (CEA) is produced by many colorectal carcinomas. Some tumors produce enzymes or hormones that their parent cells were incapable of producing (page 236). These events all point to the conclusion that malignant cells can display a behavior that suggests *gene derepression*. Sometimes the detection of the abnormal product is useful in clinical diagnosis or in the detection of metastases following removal of the primary growth. However, there is no specific change such as the production of a chemical marker by which cancer can be detected. The changes described all appear to be differences from the normal quantitatively but not qualitatively. Hence, no specific "biochemical cancer test" is available.

3. Changes in Behavior in the Intact Animal. The usual relentless progressive growth, invasion of tissues, and metastases characteristic of malignant tumors have already been described.

4. Changes in Behavior in Vitro. Many changes have been observed in tissue culture. The cells appear to have attained potential immortality, since they can be grown indefinitely if subcultured at suitable times into an appropriate medium (see HeLa cells, Chapter 1). Normal cells tend to die after a limited number of mitoses. Malignant cells tend to pile up when grown on a glass surface because they show *decreased sensitivity to both contact inhibition* and *density-dependent inhibition of growth* (Chapter 7). Furthermore, malignant cells grow in a semisolid or fluid medium, whereas normal cells will grow only on a surface in a monolayer. This is described as *loss of anchorage dependence*.

Cells that exhibit these characteristics *in vitro* are termed *transformed cells*, and if implanted into a suitable intact animal behave in a malignant manner.

5. Antigenic Change. The immunological aspects of cancer have been extensively investigated. Some tumors appear to lose tissue-specific antigens because of their poor differentiation, and it has been proposed that they thereby escape the immunological surveillance activity of lymphocytes. There is indeed some increase in the incidence of malignant tumors in patients who are immunologically deficient, but in general there is little evidence of immunological incompetence in cancer patients, except as a terminal event.

Some tumors develop new antigens; the most important are *tumor-specific transplantation antigens*. These may be individual for the particular tumor (*e.g.*, tumors produced by chemical carcinogens), or they may be shared by all tumors produced by the same virus in a case of experimental animal tumors. The tumor antigen is immunologically quite distinct from viral antigens and will not cross-react with isolated virus.

An immunological reaction to these new antigens may be the means of holding some tumors in check — sometimes for many years. The heavy lymphocytic infiltrate around some tumors suggests that the cell-mediated immune response is involved in limiting the spread of these growths. Circulating immunoglobulins have been demonstrated against tumors, and it has been postulated that immune-complex formation can occur and account for some of the curious manifestations of cancer, such as those not directly explicable by the presence of tumor cells themselves (page 236).

6. Changes in Karyotype. It is tempting to regard neoplasia as due to a mutation, and it might be expected that some specific chromosomal abnormality would be found. In tumor cells there is often a great range in chromosomal abnormality in regard to number (aneuploidy), translocations, ring chromosomes, and many other complex deviations from the normal. Nevertheless, there is no constant change found in tumors that can be used as a tumor marker. The only well-known exception to this is the Philadelphia chromosome that is found in most cases of chronic myelogenous leukemia. Hence, the chromosomal abnormalities found in malignant cells must be regarded as secondary events, possibly due to the high mitotic rate, and not primary phenomena related to the cause of the neoplasia itself.

Whether a tumor commences in one cell or begins simultaneously in many cells has been argued for years. Recent studies of tumors in women have provided a partial answer. It has been found that with most tumors, all the tumor cells contain either the paternal X chromosome or the maternal X

Theories of Carcinogenesis

(see Lyon's hypothesis, Chapter 2). If the malignant change spreads from cell to cell like an infection, one would expect both types of cells to be involved. Thus, the tumor appears to be a clone of cells derived either from one cell or from a limited number of cells in one area. It seems likely that during the development of a tumor new clones evolve, each showing changes that enable it to replace its predecessors. Ultimately, the clone of malignant cells appears. Thus, cancer is a disease that evolves slowly, and it is not surprising that in those areas that have been intensively studied a sequence of premalignant changes can be found that ultimately progress through dysplasia to malignant tumor formation.

The nature of the change within the cancer cell is poorly understood, but two major theories have evolved:

1. *Genetic theory* — somatic mutation.
2. *Epigenetic theory* — aberrant differentiation.

In the somatic mutation theory it is supposed that there occurs some change in DNA that is inherited by all the progeny of the altered cells. There is much evidence to support this theory. Certain human tumors (*e.g.,* retinoblastoma) are inherited as mendelian dominant traits, and it may be supposed that some genetic abnormality predisposes the cells to a further mutation. A genetic mutation could be caused by a chemical carcinogen, or by incorporation of foreign genetic material in the form of a virus. Furthermore, there is close correlation between the mutagenicity and carcinogenicity of many chemicals. Nevertheless, the correlation is not absolute.

The *epigenetic theory* has many supporters. It presupposes that the basic genetic material of cancer cells is normal but the abnormality is in the expression of this genetic material. The cancer cell is assumed to result from the aberrant differentiation of the cell, with the defect lying anywhere from the transcription of DNA to RNA to the translation at the cytoplasmic level. The interposition of viral nucleic acid could upset this mechanism of differentiation. Chemicals likewise could modify the effect of genetic material by either turning off or modifying the effect of repressor genes. This theory would explain why some mutagens are not carcinogenic and vice versa. It also explains why some tumors produce fetal antigens and ectopic hormones, by suggesting that the normal genetic material is not basically altered but merely misused. This theory also explains why the evolution of a tumor is not an all-or-nothing affair but can proceed through a series of intermediate stages as genetic material is differently interpreted.

Further evidence in favor of the epigenetic theory of cancer comes from two different sources. It is possible to obtain early embryos of two separate strains of mice, fuse them together so that one embryo results, and finally allow this to develop within the uterus of another pregnant female. Such animals (termed allophenic) consist of clones derived from each of the separate strains. If mice of black and white hair strains are used, the resultant allophenic mouse has alternating black and white stripes, giving a tigroid appearance! This experiment has been extended to include fusion of a normal developing fetus of one strain of mouse with malignant tumor cells derived from a different strain of mouse. Completely normal baby mice are the result, and they contain differentiated cells derived not only from the normal embryo of one strain but from the malignant cells of the other. Hence, the malignant cells may be presumed to contain normal genetic material capable of supervising the normal development of all parts of the body.

A second piece of evidence in favor of the epigenetic theory of cancer is the observation that certain cases of neuroblastoma (a highly malignant tumor derived from primitive neuroblasts) can on occasions differentiate into a benign ganglioneuroma containing mature neurons. Indeed, sometimes the tumor shows spontaneous regression and self-cure. Again, this evidence suggests that the malignant tumors possess a normal genome but that differentiation is at fault. It is possible that these examples supporting the epigenetic theory are merely isolated rare events. On the other hand, they may indicate a more general principle that neoplastic, and particularly malignant, change is merely an example of aberrant differentiation much in the same way as metaplasia and hyperplasia are now regarded. This gives considerable hope for the future because it is conceivable that means may be found to persuade malignant cells to differentiate along normal lines and bring the neoplastic process to a halt. Such a line of treatment would be vastly superior to the modes of therapy currently used.

The present treatment for cancer consists of the radical removal of tumor by using either surgical resection or radiotherapy. These measures are effective only when the tumor is localized, but there is much evidence that cancer is not simply a local disease. Even if removal of the entire area is feasible, the presence of secondary deposits represents an unknown hazard. Since these deposits may remain dormant for many years, it is evident that an assessment of the effects of local treatment is very difficult. When the disease is clinically generalized, many cytotoxic drugs are available for use either separately or in various combinations. Often this holds tumor growth in check for many months, but complete cure is difficult to attain. Hormone therapy can produce some alleviation of symptoms in particular cases. *Interferon* has recently attained considerable notoriety as a possible treatment for cancer, and there is no doubt that in some instances it has produced remarkable regression or even cure of some cancers. Whether the effect is some direct influence on the malignant cells or, more likely, mediated by some immune response is not known.

The concept that the development of cancer can be held in check by an immunological response has led to attempts to cure cancer by stimulating the immune response. The current vogue for administration of BCG ("BCG" stands for bacillus Calmette-Guérin) to patients with terminal cancer is a reflection of this. Although some success has been obtained with particular tumors, the results on the whole are disappointing. The hypothesis that cancer is due to a breakdown in immunological surveillance is yet to be proved.

The most successful approach to the control of cancer at the present time lies in its prevention. Many known physical and chemical carcinogenic agents have already been described, and their avoidance can appreciably reduce the incidence of cancer. Each tumor must be considered separately; for instance, a reduction in the amount of cigarette smoking and atmospheric pollution would undoubtedly reduce the incidence of lung cancer, and the avoidance of undue exposure to radiation would reduce the incidence of leukemia.

A second method of cancer prophylaxis is the treatment of known precancerous lesions. A regular Pap smear can reduce the incidence of uterine cancer; once again, each individual type of tumor must be considered separately.

1. Compare the properties of a benign tumor with those of a malignant one.

2. Predict the microscopic appearance and the effects of a carcinoma of the rectum. How would these affect the patient? Where would you expect to find metastases?

3. Distinguish between the following:
   (a) a malignant tumor of ectoderm and a carcinoma
   (b) a malignant tumor of mesoderm and a sarcoma

Review Questions

4. Give three examples of a benign tumor that can cause death.

5. A patient who had had a mastectomy (removal of the breast) for carcinoma of the breast, develops metastatic carcinoma in the liver. Biopsy shows an adenocarcinoma. Postulate how this might have occurred.

6. Compare carcinoma with sarcoma.

7. Distinguish between a basal-cell carcinoma and
    (a) a squamous-cell carcinoma of the skin
    (b) a squamous-cell papilloma of the skin

8. Discuss the structure of the following tumors and indicate their probable cell of origin:
    (a) ovarian teratoma
    (b) neuroblastoma
    (c) squamous-cell carcinoma of the bronchus

9. How has the Lyon hypothesis been utilized in the investigation of the pathogenesis of tumors?

10. Compare the oncogenic DNA viruses with the oncogenic RNA viruses.

11. Distinguish between:
    (a) a procarcinogen and an ultimate carcinogen.
    (b) the process of initiation and that of promotion.
    (c) the genetic theory of cancer and the epigenetic theory

Selected Readings

Ackerman, L. V., and Rosai, J.: Surgical Pathology. 5th ed. St. Louis, The C. V. Mosby Company, 1974. A standard textbook covering the morphology of tumors and other aspects of surgical pathology.

Allen, D. W., and Cole, P.: Viruses and human cancer. New England Journal of Medicine, 286:70–82, 1972.

Devoret, R.: Bacterial tests for potential carcinogens. Scientific American, 241:40–49, 1979.

Editorial: Risk of cancer in ulcerative colitis. New England Journal of Medicine, 278:907, 1968.

Epstein, M. A.: The possible role of viruses in human cancer. Lancet, 1:1344–1347, 1971.

Farber, E.: Chemical carcinogenesis. New England Journal of Medicine, 305:1379–1389, 1981.

Fialkow, P. J.: The origin and development of human tumors studied with cell markers. New England Journal of Medicine, 291:26–35, 1974.

Gerald, P. S.: Origin of teratomas. New England Journal of Medicine, 292:103–104, 1975.

Guillino, P. M.: Angiogenesis and neoplasia. New England Journal of Medicine, 305:884–885, 1981.

Herbst, A. L., Kusman, R. J., Scully, R. E., and Poskanzec, D. C.: Clear-cell adenocarcinoma of the genital tract in young females. New England Journal of Medicine, 287:1259–1264, 1972.

Leading Article: Circulating cancer cells. Lancet, 2:84–85, 1967.

Leading Article: Geography of primary liver cancer. British Medical Journal, 1:381–382, 1970.

Leading Article: E. B. virus, Burkitt lymphoma, and nasopharyngeal carcinoma. Lancet, 1:218–219, 1971.

Leading Article: Viruses and human breast cancer. Lancet, 1:359–360, 1972.

Leading Article: Herpesvirus and cancer of the uterine cervix. British Medical Journal, 1:671–672, 1976.

Lukes, R. J., et al.: A morphologic and immunologic surface marker study of 299 cases of non-Hodgkin's lymphomas and related leukemias. American Journal of Pathology, 90:461, 1978.

Medline, A., and Farber, E.: The multi-step theory of neoplasia. In Anthony, P. P., and MacSween, R. N. M. (Eds.): Recent Advances in Histopathology. 11th ed. Edinburgh, Churchill Livingstone, 1981, pp. 19–34.

Nicholson, G. L.: Cancer metastasis. Scientific American, 240:66–76, 1979.

Ryser, H. J.-P.: Chemical carcinogenesis. New England Journal of Medicine, 285:721–734, 1971.

Temin, H. M.: On the origin of genes for neoplasia. Cancer Research, 34:2835–2841, 1974.

Todaro, G. J., and Huebner, R. J.: The viral oncogene hypothesis: new evidence. Proceedings of the National Academy of Science, 69:1009–1015, 1972.

U.S. Armed Forces Institute of Pathology: Atlas of Tumor Pathology. Series 1–2, Washington, D.C., 1949–1976. Many fascicles have been published and each covers the tumors of a particular organ or system.

Ionizing Radiations and Their Effects

CHAPTER 18

After studying this chapter the student should be able to:

- Define the terms atomic number, mass number, and isotope.
- Describe in simple terms the atomic structure of hydrogen and its two isotopes.
- Describe alpha particles, beta particles, gamma rays, and x-rays with respect to their
    - (a) physical nature
    - (b) powers of penetration
    - (c) ability to produce ionization and tissue damage
- Distinguish between the direct and indirect action of ionizing radiations.
- Describe the effects of irradiation on a cell and relate them to the stages of the mitotic cycle.
- Describe the relative sensitivities of cells when they are irradiated in the intact animal.
- Describe the effects of ionizing radiation on skin, gonads, lung, and bone.
- Describe the effects of total body irradiation with
    - (a) 500 rads
    - (b) 800 to 5000 rads
    - (c) more than 5000 rads
- Describe two important late effects of total body irradiation.
- List the factors that enable one to predict the radiosensitivity of a tumor.

Introduction

Although the damaging effects of ionizing radiation have been known since the discovery of x-rays and radium, it took the dramatic events of the atomic explosions at Hiroshima and Nagasaki to bring these to the fore. The effects of radiation vary from local tissue damage leading to ulceration that can terminate in cancer, to such disorders as leukemia and genetic damage. Since the physical properties of ionizing radiation have been well studied, it might be expected that the damage that the radiation produces and the mechanisms involved would be easy to explain. Such has not been the case, because the fundamental processes that occur in cells are poorly understood. Cancer produced by ionizing radiation is no easier to explain than that which evolves spontaneously or is produced by a chemical carcinogen.

Atoms are pictured as consisting of a nucleus containing closely packed protons and neutrons, around which are a number of orbiting electrons. Neutrons and protons are of equal mass, a proton having a unit positive charge, a neutron having no charge. An electron has a unit negative charge, and a mass of only 1/2000 of a proton. The *atomic number*, Z, of an element is defined as the number of protons in the nucleus; when the atom is in an electrically neutral state, the number of orbiting electrons is equal to the number of protons in the nucleus. The *mass number* of an element is the total number of protons and neutrons present in the nucleus (Fig. 18–1).

An element always has a particular atomic number, but various forms, or *isotopes*, can exist; these have differing mass numbers. Thus, the common

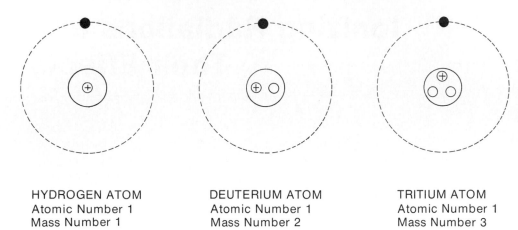

HYDROGEN ATOM
Atomic Number 1
Mass Number 1

DEUTERIUM ATOM
Atomic Number 1
Mass Number 2

TRITIUM ATOM
Atomic Number 1
Mass Number 3

Figure 18–1. Hydrogen and its isotopes.

form of hydrogen (mass number 1) has one proton in its nucleus and one orbiting electron. The isotope *deuterium* (mass number 2) has one proton and one neutron in its nucleus, whereas *tritium* (mass number 3) has one proton and two neutrons in its nucleus. Each has an atomic number of 1. Many other elements have isotopic forms and exist in nature as mixtures of these isotopes.

The various isotopes of a particular element behave similarly in chemical reactions but differ in certain physical properties that are related to mass. Some isotopes lose energy and mass spontaneously and emit radiations. Such *radioactive isotopes* are of great value in medicine. Some, such as radium, occur naturally, whereas others are man-made. Most of these radioactive isotopes give off three types of radiation:

1. *Alpha particles.* These consist of helium nuclei with two positive charges and a mass of 4.

2. *Beta particles.* These are electrons of negligible mass but each having one negative charge.

3. *Gamma rays.* These are electromagnetic waves of short wavelength. They are of a nature similar to x-rays.

X-rays are generated by allowing high-speed electrons to hit a target. Their energy is then changed into heat and electromagnetic waves of varying wavelengths, depending upon the voltage that is used to accelerate the electrons. When a low voltage, *e.g.,* 70 kilovolts (kV), is used, the x-rays have a long wavelength and a relatively poor penetrating power (they are said to be "soft"). X-rays of this nature are readily stopped by soft tissues and are used in diagnostic radiography. For cancer treatment, x-rays are generated at much higher voltage, are therefore of shorter wavelength, and penetrate the tissues of the body more readily.

Changes Induced in Matter by Passage of Ionizing Radiation

When ionizing radiation passes through matter, energy is absorbed. This leads to a variety of physicochemical events. Some molecules are excited, and ions and free radicals are formed. The changes vary with each particular variety of radiation.

Particulate Radiation.   The density of ionization for charged particles is *directly proportional to the square of their charge and inversely proportional to their velocity.* Thus, electrons and protons of equal velocity produce the same ion density; as they slow down, however, the density increases. Alpha particles (with their double charge and slow velocity) produce very dense ionization — hence, more damage.

Beta Particles. Because of their charge and negligible mass, beta particles are rapidly slowed down and give up energy to atoms through which they pass. They therefore have little power of penetration and can be used in the treatment of superficial tumors. Beta particles or artificially produced beams of electrons are used therapeutically in certain forms of skin tumors. Electrons generated at 2 MeV (million electron volts) have a maximum range of about 1 cm in soft tissues.

Alpha Particles. These have a double positive charge and a mass of 4. Their high charge and slow velocity means that they have little penetrating power. Alpha particles are readily stopped by the superficial layers of the epidermis; therefore, there is little danger of damage from an external radiating source. If taken internally, however, radioactive elements that emit alpha particles can cause serious damage.

Electromagnetic Radiation. Gamma rays and x-rays have much greater penetrating power than the particulate radiations. The shorter the wavelengths, the greater their penetration. It should be noted that the particulate radiations have a definite range of penetration, whereas the electromagnetic radiations are merely reduced in quantity. Thus, a particular thickness of a sheet of material (the half-value thickness) will reduce the intensity by half, a further thickness will reduce it by another half, and so forth. When gamma and x-rays traverse matter, they give up a quantity of energy and cause atoms to emit high-velocity electrons, which then behave like beta particles. Gamma and x-rays of high energy (short wavelength) produce fewer ionizations than do low-energy x-rays. They are therefore less destructive, since damage is caused by energy that is absorbed.

The net effect of these various changes is that molecules become more reactive, causing chemical changes to occur. Large molecules such as DNA and proteins can be affected by two separate processes:

Biological Effects of Ionizing Radiation

Direct Action. Chemical change may be caused by energy absorbed in the molecule itself.

Indirect Action. Alternatively, chemical change may be induced in a large molecule from the action of an adjacent ion or radical that had been produced by the effect of ionizing radiation on a nearby water molecule. Many of the biological effects of ionizing radiation are due primarily to the effects on water. Highly reactive ions are formed, in particular the free radicals $OH^{\cdot}$ and $H^{\cdot}$, which are electrically neutral but highly unstable. They react with water, particularly in the presence of oxygen, to form powerful damaging oxidizing substances such as $HO_2^{\cdot}$ and H_2O_2.

It is generally supposed that ionizing radiations initially produce an intracellular chemical change and that this leads to a *biochemical lesion*, which in turn produces morphological and functional changes in the affected cells. The nature of this biochemical lesion is poorly understood.

Although it would be desirable to explain cellular damage in terms of known physicochemical changes, this is not yet possible. With very high dosages, *e.g.*, on the order of 10,000 rads* or more, cells die regardless of their stage in the mitotic cycle. With a lower dosage of radiation, DNA synthesis is inhibited and mitosis is delayed. When DNA synthesis is resumed, it may not be followed by mitosis, resulting in the formation of giant nuclei. When

Effects on the Cell

---

*The original unit of measurement of radiation was the *Roentgen* (r), which was named after the discoverer of x-rays and was related to the number of ions produced in 1 ml of air. A more logical unit of measurement is the *rad*, which is related to the amount of energy absorbed per gram of substance radiated. "Rad" is an acronym for *r*adiation *a*bsorbed *d*ose.

mitosis does occur, various chromosomal abnormalities become apparent. Breaks in chromosomes are characteristic, and the fragments may reunite in an abnormal way or join other chromosomes. Sometimes these abnormalities are incompatible with life, and the cell dies.

Fractionated doses of radiation do not produce a strictly cumulative effect, and an intracellular mechanism seems to exist to correct radiation damage.

The sensitivity of cells to damage varies according to the stage in the mitotic cycle at which the radiation is given. Maximum sensitivity occurs in most cell types during mitosis itself. It follows that normal tissues with a high mitotic rate, *e.g.*, lymphoid and hematopoietic, are more sensitive than are those in which mitosis rarely or never occurs, *e.g.*, skeletal and cardiac muscle. Likewise, as a general principle malignant tumors are more sensitive than either benign tumors or the parent tissue of origin.

Two main theories have been proposed to explain the mechanism of cellular damage:

The Target Theory. This supposes that damage to cells is related to injury of a specific sensitive spot in the cell. Attractive as it may be to visualize a chromosome or a particular organelle as a target, there is little evidence to support this theory.

The Poison Theory. This supposes that ionization leads to the production of poisonous substances — usually powerful oxidizing agents — that then cause the cellular damage. There is considerable evidence that oxidizing substances are indeed formed in irradiated tissues. Thus, chemicals with a reducing action, *e.g.*, cysteine, give some degree of protection against ionizing radiation if they are present at the time of the initial irradiation. Furthermore, if tissues are irradiated in the absence of oxygen, they show considerably more resistance. This is probably because free oxygen is necessary for the production of oxidizing substances by ionizing radiation. This observation is of some importance in clinical radiotherapy, because many areas of a tumor are relatively hypoxic and conceivably could be protected during radiation therapy. Attempts have been made to overcome this by allowing patients to breathe pure oxygen under pressure during the actual administration of radiotherapy.

Effects on the Intact Animal

This important aspect of radiobiology is also the most difficult and least well understood. A remarkable feature is the delay in the appearance of radiation lesions. The actual damage caused by radiation must be almost instantaneous, and yet the effects may not be apparent for days, months, or even years. An experiment with amphibians has helped to explain this phenomenon. Frogs can be given a dose of radiation that will kill them within six weeks. If irradiated animals are kept at 5°C, they remain alive for several months, but on being warmed up, they die within six weeks. The experiments indicate that radiation damage manifests itself only when cells are active. This lends strong support to the concept that a biochemical lesion is produced. Such a lesion is not in itself harmful, but it produces effects when cellular activity commences. This goes some way toward explaining two of the phenomena of radiation damage:

1. Relative Sensitivity of Cells. In the human, the germinal cells of the ovary are the most sensitive. Then, in order from most to least sensitive, are the seminiferous epithelium of the testis, the lymphocytes, the erythropoietic and myeloid marrow cells, the intestinal epithelium, the muscle cells, and the nerve cells. This order of sensitivity to some extent parallels the rate of mitoses seen in the various tissues. Thus, the highly active intestinal epithelium is sensitive, and this explains the necrosis with its attendant gastrointestinal symptoms that follows total body exposure to ionizing radiation (page 264). Neurons, on the other hand, never divide and are relatively resistant.

2. The Chronic Nature of Radiation Lesions. When tissue is irradiated, several phases of damage occur. This is probably because different tissues have different rates of division and metabolic activity and therefore exhibit damage at different times. Hence, an irradiated area shows changes that persist for many weeks or months and have the characteristics of chronic inflammation. This inflammation can follow a single exposure of ionizing radiation.

When studying the action of radiation on any tissue, one must consider two main effects: (1) *the primary effect* of radiation on the tissue concerned; and (2) *the secondary effect*, which is due to damage to adjacent tissues. The most important example of this is damage to blood vessels, which generally results in thrombosis or gradual obliteration due to endarteritis obliterans. The ischemia that follows either event leads to necrosis. Some authorities attribute much of the beneficial effects of radiotherapy in cancer to this mechanism.

Skin. Following a single dose of ionizing radiation to the skin there is a phase of erythema beginning at about 10 days and showing all the features of acute inflammation. This phase is followed by pigmentation, due to melanin formation, causing the skin to acquire a dusky hue. With a heavy dosage, necrosis follows and an ulcer is produced. This heals slowly, and even when healed, the scar may subsequently break down, after only trivial injury. With a lower dose of irradiation of skin, a smoldering chronic inflammation ensues. This is made evident by fibrosis and endarteritis obliterans. Giant fibroblasts are often seen in the dermis. The hair follicles and sebaceous glands are more sensitive than the epidermis, and these structures tend to disappear. After several years, the area of irradiation appears atrophic. There is disturbance of pigmentation, and the area — although ischemic — shows the presence of dilated blood vessels (telangiectasia). The disturbed pigmentation (areas of hyperpigmentation and hypopigmentation) combined with atrophy and telangiectasia is called *poikiloderma* (Fig. 18–2). This is an unfortunate end-result, which is sometimes seen when a tumor such as a basal-cell carcinoma is treated by radiotherapy.

Effects of Irradiation on Individual Tissues

CASE HISTORY I. (See Figure 18–2). As a teenager and young woman, the patient had atopic dermatitis that was treated by local radiation and by many doctors. From repeated exposure to radiation, the patient developed severe radiodermatitis. During the previous 10 years several basal-cell carcinomas had appeared and had been treated by curettage or excision. The figure shows that a new tumor has developed and that necrotic facial bone is visible.

This patient's history illustrates many points:

1. It is dangerous to treat benign conditions with radiation, particularly in young people.

2. A patient can go from one physician to another, each being unaware of the treatment administered by the other. It was estimated that parts of this patient's face had received a total dose of over 11,000 rads. This is two to three times the dose commonly given to treat a malignant tumor.

3. Chronic ulceration is a feature of radiodermatitis.

4. Healing of radiation ulcers is slow, and skin grafting is often unsatisfactory because of the local ischemia.

5. Multiple tumors can develop in radiation-damaged tissues.

Gonads. The ovaries and testes are particularly susceptible to irradiation damage, and with a dose of over 500 rads, the germinal cells are destroyed and permanent sterility results.

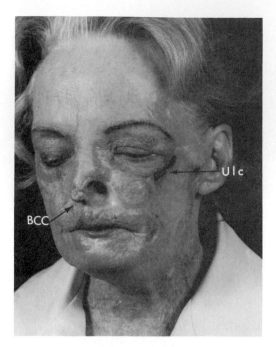

Figure 18–2. Radiodermatitis and its complications. This patient has severe dermatitis as a result of repeated radiation treatments for atopic dermatitis. A new basal-cell carcinoma (BCC) is present just above the right upper lip. A chronic indolent ulcer (Ulc) is present on the left cheek. The black tissue in the base of the ulcer is necrotic facial bone. Several attempts to close this defect by skin grafting have failed. Note that part of the nose has been lost. For further information, see Case History I.

Lungs. Irradiation of the lungs produces inflammatory changes that culminate in fibrosis. This is a complication of radiotherapy applied in the treatment of cancer of the lung or cancer of the breast (Fig. 18–3).

Bone. Irradiation of bone produces inflammatory changes that can persist for years and be punctuated by episodes of painful radionecrosis. Doses of over 1000 rads inhibit the growth of bone at the epiphyses, leading to stunted growth of the part affected.

CASE HISTORY II. (See Figure 18–3). The patient was a 39-year-old woman whose left breast had been removed for carcinoma. Since several axillary lymph nodes had been found to contain metastatic tumor, postoperative radiotherapy was given. She remained well for two years, but then began to experience fever, night sweats, and shortness of breath. A lung infection had been suspected, but in spite of extensive investigations, no definite diagnosis could be made. Thoracotomy and open-lung biopsy were performed in the hope that some treatable condition was present. The specimen showed extensive fibrosis consistent with radiation damage; in addition, however, carcinoma cells were present in lymphatic vessels. Death occurred three days later from respiratory failure. Necropsy revealed metastatic carcinoma in the lungs, mediastinal lymph nodes, liver, and vertebrae. No tumor was present in the mastectomy scar or the right breast. Radiation damage was marked in the left upper lobe of the lung (Fig. 18–3).

Effects of Irradiation on the Whole Body

When the whole body is exposed to irradiation, the effect is the sum total of the damage to all tissues. This is called the *radiation syndrome*. It has been studied extensively in animals, but in humans experience is limited only to those occasional accidents that have occurred in atomic experiments and to those individuals involved in the Japanese atomic explosions. It is convenient to describe the effects of total body irradiation under two headings: (1) those occurring during the first two months (immediate effects) and, (2) those occurring later (late effects).

Immediate Effects of Total Body Irradiation

Very Heavy Dosage (over 5000 rads per single exposure) — *the cerebral syndrome.* Death usually occurs within a day or two, with the patient developing shock, convulsions, and coma. The effects are due to a direct

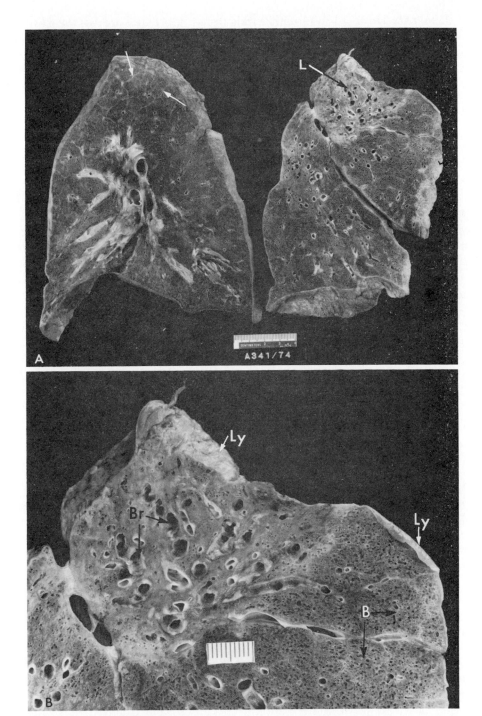

Figure 18–3.   Radiation fibrosis of lung.   Specimens of lung taken at necropsy from a patient who had died of respiratory failure. *A,* The cut surface of both lungs. The right lung exhibits prominent septa (arrows) that outline the lung lobules. Microscopically, these septa are shown to contain tumor. The apex of the left lung (L) is shrunken. *B,* The lung parenchyma is seen to have been destroyed and replaced by fibrous tissue. The bronchi (Br) are dilated, a condition called *bronchiectasis.* Below this, the lung is consolidated, but some dilated bronchioles (B) can be seen. Lymphatic vessels (Ly) on the pleural surface contain tumor. (For a more complete description, see Case History II.)

action on the central nervous system, since a similar syndrome results when the head alone is irradiated.

Moderate Dosage (800 to 5000 rads per single exposure) — *the gastrointestinal syndrome.* An initial phase occurs shortly after irradiation and is manifested as loss of appetite, nausea, and vomiting. The explanation for this is not known. The symptoms usually abate, only to recur some two to three days later, with intractable severity. Vomiting and diarrhea dominate the picture, and death occurs from dehydration and shock. These serious effects are due to necrosis of the intestinal epithelium.

Low Dosage (less than 800 rads per single exposure) — *the hematopoietic syndrome.* The initial phase of nausea and vomiting is less severe, and the subject may then appear to make a complete recovery. Two to three weeks later the results of bone-marrow aplasia become apparent. The serious effects of irradiation of this type are due to damage to the hematopoietic tissues. The granulocyte count falls after about one week and subsequently reaches very low levels. This predisposes the person to infection, particularly of the mouth and lungs. The lymphocytes show the earliest drop, and there is marked lymphopenia within a day or two. This is associated with an impaired immune response. The platelets also decrease in number, and there is marked thrombocytopenia within four weeks. This condition predisposes the victim to severe hemorrhage, often into the lungs. Although the red-cell precursors are highly radiosensitive, the mature red cells are resistant, and the effects of bone marrow aplasia on the peripheral count are delayed. Thus, the anemia is of gradual onset and is maximal at six to eight weeks in those individuals who survive the effects of agranulocytosis and thrombocytopenia. If the patient survives, the blood counts return to normal over a period of many months. In humans, 450 rads is generally taken as the dose that will kill 50 per cent of those exposed.

Late Effects of Total Body Irradiation. Those exposed to a sublethal dose may suffer from the following aftereffects:

The Carcinogenic Effect. Widespread irradiation of the bone marrow leads to an increased incidence of leukemia. This has been recorded in the survivors of the Nagasaki and Hiroshima atomic explosions and in patients with ankylosing spondylitis treated with radiotherapy. Likewise, local irradiation is followed by an increased incidence of malignant tumors at that site. Thus, carcinoma of the skin was reported as early as 1902 in workers who handled radioactive material or who were exposed to x-rays. Other examples are carcinoma of the thyroid following accidental irradiation of the gland for treatment of mediastinal lesions and osteosarcoma following local irradiation of bone lesions. Tumors have also been reported after the ingestion of radioactive substances such as radium and mesothorium, which are stored in the bones.

Genetic Effect. The ability of ionizing radiation to increase the rate of mutation is well established in microorganisms, plants, and animals. Mutations in the germ cells are of potential significance, since the new factor is handed down to subsequent generations. In clinical practice it is usual to protect the genitalia as much as possible during routine radiography for this reason.

Radiotherapy   The destructive effects of ionizing radiation on living cells, particularly those in an active state, have led to its widespread use in the treatment of malignant disease. Radiotherapy plays an important part in the curative treatment of some primary cancers, as well as in the palliation of those that have metastasized and are beyond the scope of surgical removal.

Tumors differ widely in their response to radiotherapy, and it is only after treatment has commenced that the effects can be assessed. Nevertheless, there are some guidelines that help one to predict the probable local results. The following factors are of importance.

Factors Influencing Response

The relative sensitivity of the normal tissue is often related to the radiosensitivities of the tumors derived from it. Thus, the lymphomas, like the parent lymphoreticular system, tend to be highly radiosensitive. Fibrosarcomas, on the other hand, are relatively radioresistant, like the normal fibroblast.

Tissue of Origin

Degree of Differentiation and Mitotic Activity. It is generally taught that within any tumor group the most undifferentiated tumors are also the most radiosensitive. As a generalization this is true; nevertheless, the histological features of a tumor are no sure guide to its sensitivity in practice. Thus, a well-differentiated squamous-cell carcinoma of the tongue or skin is usually highly responsive to treatment.

The Tumor Bed. The nature of the stroma supporting a tumor is also a factor of importance. If it is avascular as a result of previous radiation, the tumor tends to be more resistant. This has been attributed to the effects of hypoxia. It has been suggested that the stroma, particularly its lymphoid component, plays a part in restraining the growth of some tumors. Excessive irradiation, by destroying the stroma, might have a deleterious effect, since those tumor cells that survive are able to grow and subsequently metastasize.

Nature of the Individual Tumors. In practice, it has been found that certain tumors respond well, while others are resistant. Thus, most basal-cell and squamous-cell carcinomas of the skin are sensitive to treatment, whereas squamous-cell carcinoma of the lung is less responsive.

As with surgical treatment, the cure rate to be expected from radiotherapy must be considered in relation to the general properties of the tumor. Many malignant tumors (*e.g.*, the lymphomas) cannot be regarded as local diseases; although a tumor mass may respond remarkably well, the clinical course is characterized by the recurrence of the disease at other sites. Likewise, the oat-cell carcinoma of the lung is highly radiosensitive, and the local tumor masses in the chest melt with remarkable rapidity. Nevertheless, this tumor nearly always metastasizes widely, and death occurs from this generalized spread.

The Cure Rate

Radiotherapy is often effective as a palliative treatment, since it can reduce the size of a tumor mass and produce relief of symptoms. A mediastinal mass, such as that produced by oat-cell carcinoma or lymphoma, can obstruct the major blood vessels and trachea, producing grave respiratory difficulty: this condition can be alleviated by local irradiation. Bony metastases are often extremely painful, and the pain can be relieved by treatment. With relatively slow-growing tumors (*e.g.*, cancer of the breast and Hodgkin's disease), radiotherapy can hold the disease in check for long periods and give the patient several years of useful life. It may well be that radiotherapy and surgery are both forms of palliation that allow the body to retard the growth of a tumor; depending upon whether the malignant cells stay dormant for a short or long period, one may speak of a "5-year cure," a "10-year cure," and so forth. It is doubtful, however, that any of our present modes of treatment of cancer can be regarded as curative, if by "cure" one means the complete eradication of all malignant cells.

**Review
Questions**

1. A patient has a basal-cell carcinoma of the skin that forms a mass 1.0 cm in diameter and is about 0.25 cm thick. It is not attached to the underlying muscle. Would you expect this to be treated with
   (a) a beam of high-speed electrons
   (b) alpha particles
   (c) x-rays generated at 60 to 140 kV
   (d) x-rays generated at 2.0 MeV
   Give reasons for your choice.

2. Describe the changes that could be seen in the skin after the delivery of 1000 rads of x-rays (generated at 250 kV) to a rectangular area 4 × 5 cm after the following intervals of time:
   (a) 1 hour
   (b) 14 days
   (c) 1 year
   (d) many years

3. List the following tissues in their order of sensitivity to radiation: germinal cells of the ovary, epidermis, muscle cells, intestinal epithelium, and lymphocytes.

4. A scientist is accidentally exposed to 250 rads of total body irradiation. What are the probable effects of this accident on the patient? Is he or she likely to survive? From what might the person die?

**Selected
Readings**

Dalrymple, G. V., Gaulden, M. E., Kollmorgen, G. M., and Vogel, H. H., Jr.: Medical Radiation Biology. Philadelphia, W. B. Saunders Company, 1973. A reference book with an emphasis on the physicochemical changes produced in biological systems.

Finch, S. C.: The study of atomic bomb survivors. American Journal of Medicine, 66:899–901, 1979.

Leading Article: Hyperbaric oxygen and radiotherapy. British Medical Journal, 2:368, 1972.

Pollard, E. C.: The biological action of ionizing radiation. American Scientist, 57:206–236, 1969.

Prasad, K. N.: Human Radiation Biology. New York, Harper & Row, Publishers, 1974. A comprehensive but readable account of the subject in 508 pages.

Tievsky, G.: Ionizing Radiation. Springfield, Ill., Charles C Thomas, Publisher, 1962. An elementary account in 154 pages.

Warren, S.: The Pathology of Ionizing Radiation. Springfield, Ill., Charles C Thomas, Publisher, 1961.

Disorders of Fluid and Electrolyte Balance: Edema

After studying this chapter the student should be able to:

- Describe the three major fluid compartments of the body and indicate the volume of each in an average normal adult human being.
- List the important ions in each of the major compartments and describe the permeability of the membranes that separate the compartments.
- Discuss the value of expressing electrolyte concentrations in milliequivalents per liter.
- Give an account of the factors that maintain the body's content of water at a constant level.
- Describe the causes and effects of the following conditions:
    - (a) pure water deficiency
    - (b) pure water excess
    - (c) combined salt and water deficiency
    - (d) combined salt and water excess
- Describe the causes and effects of potassium depletion and of potassium excess.
- Define "acid" and "base."
- Describe four important buffer systems in the blood.
- Contrast respiratory acidosis with metabolic acidosis in terms of these factors:
    - (a) causes
    - (b) plasma bicarbonate levels
    - (c) arterial P_{CO_2}
    - (d) clinical effects
- Contrast respiratory alkalosis with metabolic alkalosis in terms of these factors:
    - (a) causes
    - (b) plasma bicarbonate levels
    - (c) arterial P_{CO_2}
    - (d) clinical effects
- Define "ascites," "hydrothorax," and "anasarca."
- List the types and causes of localized edema.
- List the types and causes of generalized edema.

Water is the principal component of the body and forms about 70 per cent of the lean body weight. Since adipose tissue contains little water, it follows that the water content of the average person is about 60 per cent of the body weight. The body can be discussed in terms of three "compartments" (intracellular space, interstitial space, and plasma), which are illustrated in Figure 19–1. Water is freely diffusible across the barriers that separate these various compartments; the volume of each is preserved by the osmotic, electrochemical, and hydrostatic forces acting upon it. With regard to osmosis, potassium, phosphate, and protein are important in the intracellular compart-

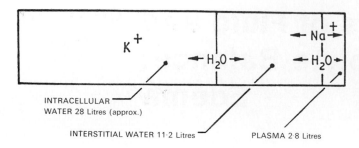

Figure 19–1. The fluid compartments of the body. This diagram shows the three compartments in which the body's water is accommodated. An excess or deficiency of water, which is freely diffusible, produces the greatest effects in the largest compartment—the intracellular space. Changes in sodium levels affect mainly the interstitial compartment.

INTRACELLULAR WATER 28 Litres (approx.)

INTERSTITIAL WATER 11·2 Litres   PLASMA 2·8 Litres

ment, whereas sodium, chloride, and bicarbonate are important in the interstitial and intravascular compartments.

Electrolytes

General Considerations

The biological effects of an electrolyte depend to a considerable extent on its equivalent concentration, *i.e.*, the number of particles present and the number of charges carried by each. It is therefore appropriate to describe the concentration of electrolytes in terms of milliequivalents per liter.

Expressing Electrolyte Concentration *in Milliequivalents per Liter*

To convert concentration of ions from mg per dl to mEq per liter, use this simple formula:

$$\frac{mg/dl}{\text{equivalent weight of ion}} \times 10 = mEq/L$$

The equivalent weight is 23 for sodium, 39 for potassium, 22.4 for bicarbonate (as ml CO_2 per dl), and 4.1 for protein. Expressing electrolyte concentrations in mEq per liter is more logical than expressing them in grams or milligrams per dl. It allows the importance of each electrolyte to be readily appreciated. Furthermore, since any solution must contain the same concentration of cations as anions, a balance can be struck between the two. This is shown in Table 19–1, which gives the composition of normal plasma.

It is evident that sodium is the all-important cation in the extracellular fluids and is balanced mainly by the combined concentration of bicarbonate and chloride. The "other anions," which are not measured directly, include HPO_4^{--} and SO_4^{--} as well as keto acids. It should be noted that the combined chloride and bicarbonate (131) subtracted from the combined sodium and potassium (147) is 16. This "anion gap" is normal. It is a useful figure to calculate, because an increase indicates the presence of an abnormal acid, *e.g.*, keto acids in diabetic acidosis and lactic acid in shock.

SI Units. The Système International (SI) units are in use in many countries, especially in Europe, and have certain advantages in that the degree of ionization of any molecule does not have to be known. Electrolytes are expressed in millimoles per liter. To convert concentration of substances (including ions) from mg/dl to mmol/L, use the following formula:

$$\frac{mg/dl}{\text{molecular weight}} \times 10 = mmol/L$$

It will be noted that the figures for sodium, potassium, chloride, and other univalent ions remain unchanged in mmol/L as compared with mEq/L. For large molecules, previously expressed in mg/dl, however, the figures are quite different. Thus, the normal blood glucose (molecular weight 180 daltons) level of 90 mg/dl becomes in SI units:

$$\frac{90}{180} \times 10 = 5 \ mmol/L$$

In this text the conventional units will be given followed by SI units in parentheses wherever appropriate.

TABLE 19–1. COMPOSITION OF NORMAL PLASMA

CATIONS (in mEq/L)		ANIONS (in mEq/L)	
Na^+	142	Cl^-	104
K^+	5	HCO_3^-	27
Ca^{++}	5	Other anions	7
Mg^{++}	2	Protein	16
TOTAL	154	TOTAL	154

Fluid Balance

General Considerations

The total water content of the body is maintained at a constant level by balancing intake with output.

Water is derived mainly by drinking fluid; the amount of this varies according to individual custom and habit. Some water is contained in food, and about 300 ml is derived from the oxidative processes of metabolism. Fluid is lost in the urine (about 1500 ml per day); some is lost in the expired air (about 700 ml per day); some is lost in the feces (about 200 ml per day); and a moderate quantity is lost by transpiration from the skin (300 to 500 ml per day). The mechanism by which fluid balance is attained can be considered under three headings.

1. Indirect Control. This includes the mechanisms that regulate sodium balance. Sodium cannot be retained without water (Fig. 19–2).

Aldosterone, a hormone secreted by the adrenal cortex, has the effect of increasing sodium reabsorption from the distal tubule of the kidney and thereby causes water retention as well. Sodium reabsorption from the prox-

Figure 19–2. Sodium retention. This diagram shows the means by which the body retains sodium after a sudden reduction in blood volume, *e.g.,* following a severe hemorrhage.

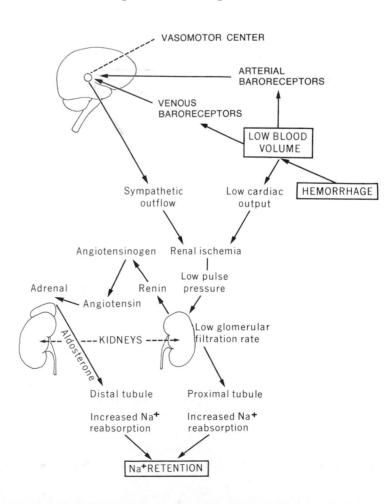

imal tubule is dependent to a large extent on the total glomerular filtrate. When the volume is reduced, as in shock and heart failure, sodium absorption is more complete, and water is also retained.

2. Renal Control. There are mechanisms that regulate the output of water by the kidney. The antidiuretic hormone (ADH) from the posterior lobe of the pituitary gland is important in this regulation. It acts by increasing water reabsorption from the collecting tubules of the kidney.

3. Thirst. Water intake is regulated by the sensation of thirst.

Water and sodium metabolism are so closely interrelated that it is convenient to consider them together.

Disturbances in Water and Sodium Balance

Pure Water Deficiency. This condition follows deprivation of water. It is seen in enforced starvation and in patients who are unable to swallow because of dysphagia, esophageal obstruction, or coma. It may complicate diabetes insipidus, a disease due to lack of antidiuretic hormone (ADH). Patients with this disease pass enormous quantities of urine — often 20 liters a day — instead of the normal 1 to 1.5 liters.

Effects. Since water can easily cross the membranes that separate the various fluid compartments, each is depleted in volume. The intracellular space, which is the largest compartment, is the most severely affected. Cellular dehydration causes intense thirst and eventually death.

Pure Water Excess. Excessive retention of water is called *water intoxication* and causes intracellular edema. It is encountered in patients who are given too much water too quickly. Rapid intravenous infusion of glucose solution is the common culprit, but even a large enema can lead to water intoxication in a susceptible patient, such as one in renal failure or in the immediate postoperative period, when water excretion is impaired. The effects of water excess are serious. Intracellular edema of brain and muscle causes vomiting, muscle cramps, headaches, convulsions, and — ultimately — death.

Combined Salt and Water Deficiency. Salt, or salt and water, deficiency is a common condition that is seen when there is a loss from any of the following:

1. The gastrointestinal tract, such as following severe vomiting or diarrhea.

2. The skin, such as following prolonged excessive sweating (heat exhaustion).

3. The kidney, such as following prolonged administration of diuretics for heart failure.

Effects. The effect of salt — or salt and water — deficiency is a reduction in the volume of the extracellular fluids. The interstitial fluid volume is reduced in amount, and the patient shows the clinical features of dehydration. The eyeballs are sunken, the skin is wrinkled, the tongue is dry, and the face is haggard. Surprisingly, thirst is often absent. The plasma volume is decreased, but vasoconstriction compensates for this. Since the veins are poorly filled, the blood pressure ultimately drops. Little urine is passed, and renal failure may be superadded. The reduction in plasma volume is detectable by a rise in the hemoglobin concentration (hemoconcentration). Unless relieved, this condition rapidly terminates in circulatory failure.

Combined Salt and Water Excess. This is invariably an artificially induced condition that is seen in patients with defective renal function who are given excessive amounts of saline solution, such as during the early postoperative period or during the course of acute renal failure.

Effect. The excess fluid is distributed mainly in the extracellular compartments, which therefore expand. The manifestations of this are an increased venous pressure and edema, both systemic and pulmonary (Chapter 30).

Potassium is an important intracellular ion; its level in the plama is low — 4.0 to 5.5 mEq/L (4.0 to 5.5 mmol/L).

Potassium Depletion.   Potassium can be lost from the body in the feces or in the urine. Chronic diarrhea, such as in ulcerative colitis, is a well-known cause of this depletion. Excess loss from the urine occurs in diabetes mellitus and following the use of certain diuretics (*e.g.*, chlorothiazide) in heart failure. Since cellular function is deranged, the effects of potassium deprivation are serious. In particular, the following structures are affected:

The Brain.   Apathy, confusion, and coma can occur.

The Kidney.   Damage to the tubules leads to polyuria and renal failure.

The Heart.   Irregularity of the heart rate, hypotension, and heart failure can result.

Muscles.   Intense weakness of the muscles is characteristic. If death results from this ion depletion, it is generally due to respiratory failure caused by weakness of the muscles of respiration. Smooth muscle is also affected, and paralytic ileus can follow.

Potassium Excess.   Retention of potassium is generally due to renal failure. Sometimes it is a complication of excessive potassium administration for potassium loss. The clinical manifestations of potassium retention are vague: mental confusion, apathy, and pains in the limbs. Although muscular weakness is also a feature, the most important complication is ventricular fibrillation; *sudden death* is not uncommon.

Disturbances of Potassium Balance

During metabolism, acidic substances are produced in large amounts. The most important of these is carbonic acid (H_2CO_3), which is the inevitable product of aerobic tissue activity. During anaerobic activity lactic acid is produced; phosphoric, sulfuric, and other acids are formed in smaller quantities. These acids are formed within cells and pass to the extracellular tissues, where they tend to increase the acidity. Nevertheless, cellular activity can take place only within a narrow range of acidity. The regulatory mechanisms by which this range is maintained are an aspect of homeostasis, which is of vital importance. In order to understand this process, it is essential to have a working knowledge of acids, bases, and buffers.

An acid is a molecule or ion that is capable of giving up a hydrogen ion (H^+, or proton). A base is a molecule or ion that is capable of receiving a hydrogen ion. Thus, in the equation

$$HB = H^+ + B^-$$

HB is an acid, whereas B^- is the base.

A strong acid is one that readily gives up its hydrogen ion. Thus, in the equation

$$HCl = H^+ + Cl^-$$

HCl is a strong acid and Cl^- is a weak base.

On the other hand, carbonic acid (H_2CO_3) is a weak acid:

$$H_2CO_3 = H^+ + HCO_3^-$$

The bicarbonate ion HCO_3^- is a strong base, because it accepts a hydrogen ion more readily than H_2CO_3 gives it up.

Acid-Base Balance

General Considerations

Maintenance of the pH of the Blood*

The normal blood pH ranges from 7.36 to 7.44. Survival is not possible outside the range of 6.8 to 8.0. To prevent changes of pH as much as possible, the body is provided with a series of *buffer systems*. These are chemical systems that are capable of "mopping up" excess hydrogen ions if the pH falls and of contributing hydrogen ions if the pH rises.

A physiological buffer consists of a mixture of a strong base and a weak acid; thus, in the dissociation equation

$$HB = H^+ + B^-$$

if B^- is a strong base, an excess of H^+ combines with it to form more of the weak acid HB.

The most important buffer in the extracellular fluids is the bicarbonate–carbonic acid combination.

$$H^+ + HCO_3^- \rightleftharpoons H_2CO_3$$

If hydrogen ions are added to plasma, more H_2CO_3 is formed. This passes to the lungs, where it dissociates, and carbon dioxide (CO_2) diffuses into the alveolar gas and is eliminated. The great importance of the bicarbonate ion lies not only in its buffering capacity but also in the extreme volatility of carbonic acid and the ease with which CO_2 is eliminated by the lungs.

Two other buffer systems in the extracellular fluids should be noted: monohydrogen phosphate and the plasma proteins:

$$H^+ + HPO_4^{2-} \rightleftharpoons H_2PO_4^-$$

$$H^+ + Protein^{n-} \rightleftharpoons HProtein^{(n-1)-}$$

An important means of buffering carbonic acid within the blood is found within the red cells, which contain not only hemoglobin, which acts as a buffer, but also the enzyme carbonic anhydrase, which accelerates the following reversible reaction:

$$CO_2 + H_2O \rightleftharpoons H_2CO_3$$

The carbonic acid then dissociates into bicarbonate and hydrogen ions:

$$H_2CO_3 \rightarrow HCO_3^- + H^+$$

The hydrogen ions are largely buffered in the red cells by the hemoglobin:

$$H^+ + Hb^- \rightleftharpoons HHb$$

The excess bicarbonate ions then diffuse into the plasma in exchange for chloride ions, which diffuse into the red cells. In this way the bicarbonate level in the plasma rises.

It is evident that the acids that are produced in the body or are ingested are eliminated by two routes: *the lungs*, as described above, and *the kidneys* (the cells of the distal tubules secrete H^+ ions).

Abnormalities of the pH of the Blood

An increase in the hydrogen ion concentration of the blood (pH less than 7.36) is called *acidemia*, whereas a decrease (pH over 7.44) is called *alkalemia*. Although the terms *acidosis* and *alkalosis* are sometimes used

---

*The pH of a fluid is the negative logarithm of the hydrogen ion concentration of a solution. The form $[H^+]$ is used to denote hydrogen ion concentration. In pure water at 25°C the following relationship exists:

$$[H^+] \times [OH^-] = 10^{-14}$$

That is, $[H^+] = [OH^-] = 10^{-7}$

Hence, pH = 7.0. At 37°C pH 6.8 corresponds to neutrality.

synonymously with acidemia and alkalemia, it is preferable to restrict them to descriptions of conditions in which there would be an appropriate change in pH if there were no compensatory mechanisms.

Respiratory Acidosis and Alkalosis. If there is hypoventilation of the lungs, CO_2 is retained and forms carbonic acid in the blood, which is a source of hydrogen ions. $[HCO_3^-]$ rises as well, but by a lesser amount. Hence, the pH of the blood decreases. This process is called *respiratory acidosis.* In a like manner, if there is hyperventilation, excess CO_2 is eliminated, and both carbonic acid and bicarbonate are reduced in the blood, causing an increase in the pH. This process is called *respiratory alkalosis.* It is evident that respiratory acidosis is directly related to hypoventilation of the lungs, with a resulting retention of CO_2 and a rise in the arterial P_{CO_2}. In respiratory alkalosis the reverse obtains, and there is a drop in arterial P_{CO_2}. A measurement of the arterial P_{CO_2} is therefore an accurate and useful method of assessing the respiratory component of acid-base balance.

Effects of Respiratory Acidosis. This condition results in vasodilatation, which is a direct effect of the raised P_{CO_2}. This vasodilatation may cause a rise in intracranial pressure. The level of plasma bicarbonate rises, and the plasma chloride drops proportionally.

Effects of Respiratory Alkalosis. Respiratory alkalosis is seen during hysterical hyperventilation, during work at high temperatures or at a high altitude, or during anesthesia when muscle relaxants are used and excessively vigorous artificial ventilation is applied. Peripheral vasoconstriction causes pallor of the skin. The lack of stimulation of the respiratory center by CO_2 causes a tendency toward respiratory arrest. *Tetany* is characteristic. This physiological response is identical with that seen in hypocalcemia. The symptoms are those of increased neuromuscular excitability. The most characteristic is spontaneous spasms of the hand muscles so that the fingers are extended and the palm hollowed. Generalized convulsions can occur.

Metabolic Acidosis and Alkalosis. If an excess of hydrogen ions is introduced into the blood, as a result of either ingestion or production of acidic substances, the bicarbonate of the plasma is replaced by chloride and other anions. There is a secondary fall in the P_{CO_2} to match this low concentration of bicarbonate, an effect produced by the low pH stimulating the respiratory center and causing overventilation. This is *metabolic acidosis.* Excessive ingestion of sodium bicarbonate leads to a rise in both the $[HCO_3^-]$ and the pH of the plasma. This is *metabolic alkalosis.*

Metabolic Acidosis. A fall in both pH and bicarbonate level of the plasma occurs under the following conditions: (1) *in shock* and *following a cardiac arrest,* when underprofusion of tissue leads to anaerobic metabolism and production of lactic acid *(lactic acidosis);* (2) *in severe diarrhea,* when there is a greater loss of hydroxyl (OH^-) ions than of hydrogen ions in the feces; (3) *in starvation* and *in uncontrolled diabetes mellitus,* when there is ketosis (the acetoacetic acids and β-hydroxybutyric acids provide the extra hydrogen ions); and (4) *in chronic renal disease,* and in conditions in which there is a failure of the distal tubules to excrete hydrogen ions (*e.g.,* renal tubular acidosis).

Effects of Metabolic Acidosis. The classic symptom of metabolic acidosis is "air hunger." Respirations are deep, rapid, and sighing. This is a compensatory mechanism, because it lowers the P_{CO_2} and thereby causes a respiratory alkalosis that tends to reverse the metabolic acidosis.

As the plasma bicarbonate falls, there is a corresponding rise in other plasma anions, particularly the chloride ions. In such cases there is a *hyperchloremic acidosis.*

Severe metabolic acidosis causes grave neurological symptoms that culminate in death. The heart's action is impaired, and a state of shock with low cardiac output and hypotension ensues. Metabolic acidosis is thought to potentiate traumatic and hemorrhagic shock, and it is one of the contributory factors in the development of irreversible shock (Chapter 21).

Metabolic Alkalosis. Both blood pH and blood bicarbonate level rise in this condition. Metabolic alkalosis occurs when there is excessive ingestion of bicarbonate or when there is excessive loss of acid from the body. The most common cause of this is persistent vomiting, such as with pyloric stenosis, when the ensuing loss of acidic gastric juice causes the alkalosis.

Effects of Metabolic Alkalosis. Tetany may occur. A fall in plasma chloride compensates for the rise in bicarbonate level.

Conclusion   It is evident from this brief account of electrolytes and acid-base balance that many abnormalities can occur in disease. With the aid of the modern clinical chemical laboratory the abnormalities can be measured and appropriate treatment can be instituted. In acute illness, serial estimations are often necessary to assess the effects of treatment. The "toxemias" that once afflicted patients having cholera, dysentery, and intestinal obstruction with vomiting are no longer mysterious, untreatable agents of death. Instead, these conditions are now known to be diagnosable, treatable upsets of the internal environment of the body.

Edema   As usually used, the term "edema" can be defined as an excessive accumulation of fluid in the interstitial tissues. Fluid is also particularly liable to collect in the various serous sacs, giving rise to *ascites, hydrothorax,* and *hydropericardium* (terms applied to effusions into the peritoneal, pleural, and pericardial sacs, respectively). When edema is generalized, it is called *dropsy* or *anasarca.* Of course, it is possible to have intracellular edema, as in hydropic degeneration of cells and in pure water intoxication. The remainder of this section, however, will be devoted to types of interstitial edema.

It is necessary first to understand the normal mechanisms regulating the distribution of fluid in the body.

Normal Mechanism of Control in the Systemic Circulation   Starling postulated that the movement of fluid between vessels and the extravascular spaces was determined by the balance of the hydrostatic and osmotic forces acting upon it (see Fig. 5–1).

Forces Tending to Move Fluid Out of the Blood Vessels Are the Following:

(a) *The hydrostatic pressure within the vessels*

(b) *The colloid osmotic pressure of the interstitial fluid*

Since the vascular wall is completely permeable to water and crystalloids, the only effective osmotic forces acting across the vessel wall are due to colloids — mainly protein — to which the vessel wall is not permeable. The interstitial fluids normally have a low protein content, and this is therefore not an important factor in the formation of the extravascular fluids under normal circumstances. Furthermore, those proteins that do escape from the blood vessels into the interstitial tissue spaces are removed by the lymphatic vessels.

Forces Tending to Move the Fluid into the Blood Vessels Are the Following:

(a) *The tissue tension.* This is normally low (3 to 4 mm Hg). Tissue tension is important in determining the distribution of edema. Thus, edema readily occurs in lax tissues such as the eyelids, over the sacrum, and in the

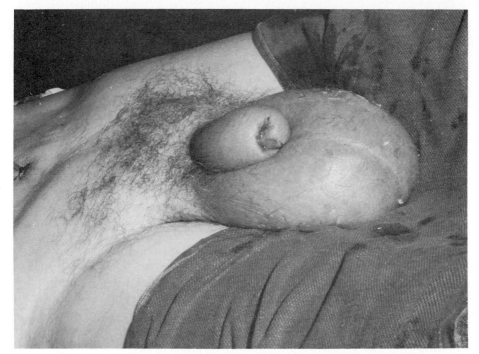

Figure 19–3.   Severe edema of the scrotum and penis.   The patient shows severe edema of the loose tissues of the scrotum and penis, whereas the more compact tissues of the thigh and abdominal wall are less affected.

genital area (Fig. 19–3). Tense tissues like the palms and soles do not readily become edematous. A rise in tissue tension is an important factor in limiting interstitial tissue fluid formation in the legs under normal conditions as well as in acutely inflamed parts.

(b) *The osmotic pressure of the plasma proteins.* This pressure is normally about 25 mm Hg and is due mainly to albumin. Since albumin does not normally pass through the vessel walls, the vascular permeability is important in regulating the distribution of fluids between the intravascular and extravascular compartments. In the event of an increase in the permeability, such as that occurring in acute inflammation, an exudate rich in protein is formed.

There are two types of edema:

An Exudate.   This is an accumulation of fluid in acute inflammation and is due to an increased vascular permeability. The fluid contains a high percentage of protein and has virtually the same composition as plasma.

A Transudate.   This is an accumulation of fluid due to hydrostatic imbalance between the intravascular and extravascular compartments. Since it occurs in the presence of a normal vascular permeability, the protein content of the fluid is low.

The importance of the lymphatic vessels should be remembered in any discussion of edema. They form an elaborate closed network in most tissues, and their function is to drain away fluid and protein.

When considering the cause of any type of edema, one should realize that the process is usually due to a combination of factors. Starling, who appreciated this, stated that dropsy was probably never due to the derangement of a single mechanism acting alone.

Types of Edema

Edema can be classified into local and generalized types. The localized varieties are the simplest to understand, because there are fewer factors involved in their pathogenesis.

Local Edema

Acute Inflammatory Edema.   This condition has been described in Chapter 5.

Hypersensitivity.   Edema is present in the lesions of type I and type III hypersensitivity reactions and in severe type IV reactions. It is due to an increase in vascular permeability.

Venous Obstruction.   A rise in venous pressure leads to an increase in capillary pressure, which in turn results in the formation of a transudate. Thus, in phlebothrombosis of the leg veins edema occurs but is rarely severe. Edema of the gut occurs in a strangulated hernia and in mesenteric venous thrombosis. It is this edema that causes further vascular impairment later resulting in infarction.

Lymphatic Edema.   Extensive lymphatic obstruction can produce an edema of high protein content. Because chronic lymphatic edema of the limbs stimulates connective tissue overgrowth, in due course there is such enlargement of the skin and subcutaneous tissues that the part becomes grossly distorted. This resulting grotesque deformity is called *elephantiasis*. It occurs in the legs as a complication of the lymphangitis from any cause, but is particularly severe in the lymphangitis associated with filariasis (Chapter 14). A similar condition can occur as a result of congenitally deformed lymphatics. Lymphedema of an arm is occasionally encountered as a complication of cancer of the breast when the lymphatic vessels are blocked either by tumor or by the fibrosis induced by radiotherapy.

Generalized Edema

Cardiac Edema.   In congestive heart failure there is retention of sodium and water that is first evident as an increase in body weight and later as a detectable edema. The distribution of this fluid is influenced by gravity. When the patient is ambulant, the legs are affected first, and swelling of the ankles is often the initial symptom. When the patient is in bed, the edema appears in the sacral and genital areas (Fig. 19–3). Firm pressure by a finger in an edematous area results in the formation of a pit that remains when the finger is removed. This "pitting edema" is characteristic of most forms of edema. Lymphedema is a major exception.

Renal Edema

Acute Glomerulonephritis.   Edema is often the first symptom of acute post-streptococcal glomerulonephritis (Chapter 35). The edema is often most apparent on the face and eyelids, but ankles and genitalia may also be affected. The reduced glomerular blood flow leads to a reduction in glomerular filtration rate, and this in turn causes sodium and water retention.

Nephrotic Syndrome.   The marked edema of the nephrotic syndrome is to a large extent due to the low plasma albumin level. In addition, there is a reduced blood volume, which stimulates the secretion of aldosterone from the adrenal cortex. This leads to sodium retention and therefore water retention. Hence, a salt-free diet, especially combined with a diuretic, causes considerable reduction in the amount of edema present.

Famine Edema (Nutritional Edema).   The edema that is seen after prolonged starvation is usually confined to the legs. At first sight, it would seem explicable in terms of the marked hypoalbuminemia that is usually present; on closer examination, however, one finds that there is no close correlation between the level of plasma proteins and the presence of edema. The precise explanation of famine edema is not known. An important factor appears to be loss of compact tissue — mostly fat — and its replacement by a loose connective tissue in which fluid can accumulate readily without any undue rise in tissue tension.

Marked edema is a feature of kwashiorkor (Chapter 23).

Unexplained Edema

Generalized edema sometimes occurs in the absence of any known cause. Although such cases are uncommon, they indicate that factors other than those already discussed may operate even in the common types of edema. A well-recognized condition, *cyclical periodic edema,* presents with recurrent attacks of edema involving skin, mucous membranes, and even internal organs. When the area involved is delimited to the subcutaneous tissues, it is called *angioedema.* The immediate cause of edema appears to be an increase in vascular permeability, but the precise cause is not known. In chronic urticaria there is edema of the dermis; again, the cause is rarely discovered.

Generalized edema is sometimes seen in terminal states, particularly in cirrhosis of the liver. The blood pressure is often low, and attempts to raise it and maintain an adequate urinary output by the administration of fluid only worsen the situation and increase the amount of edema. The mechanisms involved are complex and are not well understood.

Pulmonary Edema

This condition is considered in Chapter 30.

Conclusion

Although dropsy has been recognized as a symptom of disease since the beginning of medical history, it is evident that the mode of its formation is complex and often incompletely understood.

Review Questions

1. What is meant by the term "anion gap"? Describe how it is estimated as well as the significance of a raised value.

2. A woman sustains an abdominal injury in a car accident; one kidney is damaged and has to be removed. On the third postoperative day she is given a large water enema for constipation. Predict the possible consequences of this.

3. What type of acid-base imbalance would be expected in a patient who has just been resuscitated following a cardiac arrest?

4. Predict the effects of voluntary hyperventilation in a normal subject. (Warning! Do not attempt to hyperventilate anyone without supervision.)

5. A patient has nonpitting edema of one leg. Suggest some possible causes and discuss the pathogenesis.

6. How may fluid retention be detected in a patient with heart failure?

Selected Readings

Campbell, E. J. M., Dickinson, C. J., and Slater, J. D. H.: Clinical Physiology. 4th ed. Oxford, Blackwell Scientific Publications Ltd., 1974. See, in particular, Chapter 1, "Body Fluids"; and Chapter 5, "Hydrogen Ion (Acid:Base) Regulation."

Davenport, H. W.: A B C of Acid-Base Chemistry: The Elements of Physiological Blood-Gas Chemistry for Medical Students and Physicians. 5th ed. Chicago, University of Chicago Press, 1969.

Felver, L.: Understanding the electrolyte maze. American Journal of Nursing, *80*:1591–1595, 1980.

Robinson, J. R.: Fundamentals of Acid-Base Regulation. 5th ed. Oxford, Blackwell Scientific Publications Ltd., 1975.

Siggaard-Anderson, O.: The Acid-Base Status of the Blood. 4th ed. Baltimore, The Williams & Wilkins Company, 1975.

CHAPTER 20 Disorders of the Circulation

After studying this chapter the student should be able to:

- Distinguish between platelet aggregation and platelet adhesiveness.
- Define thrombosis and distinguish it from blood clotting.
- Describe the roles that the following chemicals play in the process of thrombosis: the prostaglandins, thrombin, and adenosine diphosphate.
- Outline the mechanism by which plasmin is formed.
- Describe Virchow's triad.
- Describe the common causes of thrombosis in an artery and list the possible effects on the tissue supplied.
- Compare phlebothrombosis with thrombophlebitis in terms of their causes and effects.
- List the circumstances under which thrombosis can occur in the heart.
- Describe the possible fate of a thrombus.
- Define hypoxia and list the four types.
- Define ischemia and classify its causes.
- Define embolus and classify emboli according to their composition.
- Describe the syndrome of massive pulmonary embolism.
- Describe the effects of a small pulmonary embolus.
- Define pyemia and describe its causes and effects.
- Outline the causes and effects of fat embolism.
- Define infarction and describe the process as it occurs in the following organs:
    - (a) heart
    - (b) spleen
    - (c) brain
    - (d) intestine
- Give examples of complications caused by arterial spasm.
- Distinguish between primary and secondary systemic hypertension.
- List the complications of systemic hypertension.
- Describe the main pathological and clinical features of malignant hypertension.

The publication of *De Motu Cordis* is generally conceded to be one of the great landmarks of medical research. In it, William Harvey propounded the theory of the circulation of the blood from the heart, through arteries, and to the veins. The missing link in this theory was the absence of any known connection between arteries and veins. Malpighi, who was born in the year of Harvey's publication, applied the compound microscope to the study of biological material and proved the existence of capillaries, thereby confirming Harvey's hypothesis. Today, although over 300 years of study have laid bare a wealth of information about the circulation, its disorders, particularly heart attacks and strokes, are still responsible for a vast amount of illness and death.

Normal Function   The function of the circulatory system is the maintenance of an adequate perfusion of blood to all tissues of the body. Each ventricular contraction ejects a quantity of blood into the aorta and causes a rise in systemic blood pressure. The aorta and its major branches are composed largely of elastic tissue; their expansion prevents an undue rise in pressure with each ventricular contraction (systole). The branches of these elastic vessels are the muscular arteries. It is by variation in the tone of their smooth-muscle walls that the amount of blood supplied to the various organs and tissues can be altered. The muscular arteries subdivide repeatedly, with blood next reaching the arterioles. These small muscular vessels provide the final mechanism by which blood is distributed to the tissues in response to their individual needs. The distribution of blood is in part regulated by the autonomic nervous system that acts on the smooth muscle of the arteries and arterioles, and in part by local mechanisms by which chemical agents, such as bradykinin, are released and act locally.

The blood flow in the major arteries is pulsatile. The elasticity of these vessels and the high resistance provided by the arterioles reduce the pulsation, so that in the capillaries and veins the blood flow is constant. It follows that blood escaping from damaged capillaries oozes out constantly, whereas blood from a cut artery spurts out.

Two obvious prerequisites of any circulation are the presence of a fluid and a means by which this fluid can be retained in the vessels should they be damaged. In the vascular system it is the platelets and the clotting mechanism that guard against the danger of hemorrhage. The deposition of platelets and fibrin effectively patches any minor defect, and even severed vessels are soon sealed off. The control of platelet deposition and fibrin formation is an excellent example of a homeostatic mechanism designed to prevent bleeding. Unfortunately, the intravascular deposition can sometimes becomes excessive, leading to the complete obstruction of the damaged vessel. This process is called *thrombosis*, a subject that must be studied in some detail. In order to understand thrombosis it is necessary first to describe the process of blood coagulation and the properties of platelets.

The Coagulation Mechanism.   Coagulation, or clotting, may be defined as the conversion of fibrinogen to a solid mass of fibrin. The mechanism is described in Chapter 26, and it is sufficient here to note that clotting can be initiated by clotting factors derived from either the blood (intrinsic) or tissues (extrinsic). The activation of the intrinsic system has two components:

1. Platelets that have become adherent to a surface liberate a lipid factor.
2. An abnormal surface activates Factor XII (Hageman factor).

Minor degrees of injury are constantly being sustained by blood vessels, and a layer of platelets is soon laid down to prevent hemorrhage. Endothelial cells cover this platelet deposit so that the smooth lining of the vessel is restored, further deposition ceases, and the process is brought to an end. The presence of naturally occurring anticoagulant substances, such as heparin and antithrombin III, and the constant bathing by the stream of blood tend to prevent clotting. Nevertheless, small quantities of fibrin are probably formed even under normal conditions, and there exists a *fibrinolytic mechanism* for its removal. The active agent *plasmin* is formed on the fibrin threads and leads to their dissolution (Fig. 20–1). Thus, three mechanisms normally prevent the intravascular accumulation of fibrin:

1. Endothelialization of both platelet deposits and areas of damage.
2. The fibrinolytic system.
3. Factors that limit the deposition of platelets (see below).

Under abnormal circumstances these mechanisms are inadequate, and intravascular coagulation becomes excessive.

Platelets.   Since platelets play an important role in thrombosis, their

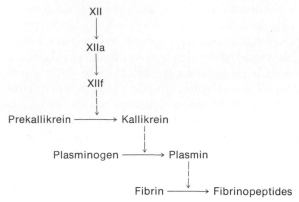

Figure 20–1. The blood fibrinolytic system. Plasmin is a fibrinolytic enzyme that digests fibrin to polypeptides (fibrinopeptides). It is formed from a precursor (plasminogen) by the action of the enzyme kallikrein, which itself is formed from a precursor by the activity of an activated component (Factor XIIf) of Factor XII (Hageman factor). Note that Factor XII activation also initiates the intrinsic clotting mechanism, and that kallikrein is one of the important components of the chemical mediators of acute inflammation. Transformations are depicted as solid lines, and enzymatic activities are shown as interrupted lines.

properties have been extensively studied. They are small nonnucleated structures present in the blood and have the property of sticking to each other (displaying *aggregation*) and of adhering to abnormal surfaces (showing *adhesiveness*).

Platelet Aggregation. Platelets aggregate immediately in the presence of adenosine diphosphate (ADP). This mechanism may be demonstrated *in vitro* by the addition of ADP to a platelet-rich preparation of plasma that is kept agitated. The aggregation can be detected by measuring the ensuing decrease in optical density of the plasma. An important property of thrombin is that it causes the release of ADP from platelets, and it therefore soon causes aggregation.

Platelet Adhesiveness. Experimentally, platelets are found to adhere to a variety of foreign surfaces. Thus, if a platelet-rich fluid is passed through a column containing glass beads, the platelets are found to adhere to the beads, and few are contained in the fluid that issues from the column. Since platelets also adhere to the walls of damaged blood vessels, it is believed that exposure of collagen in the vessel wall is an important factor in the ready adhesion of these structures; platelets readily adhere to collagen when tested *in vitro*. Adherent platelets swell and release a variety of chemicals *(platelet release reaction)*, including phospholipid (platelet factor 3, which plays a part in clotting), heparin neutralizing substance (platelet factor 4), 5-hydroxytryptamine (5-HT), and ADP. Ca^{++}, Catecholamines, PGF_2

Thrombosis

Pathogenesis of Thrombosis

Thrombosis may be defined as the formation of a solid mass in the circulation from the constituents of the streaming blood. The mass itself is called a thrombus. Thrombosis involves two distinct processes:

The Deposition of Platelets on a Vascular Surface. This occurs under three circumstances:

① When the endothelial lining is damaged or removed.

② With vascular stasis, when the platelets fall out of the axial stream and impinge on the wall.

③ In association with eddy currents, which deflect the platelets to an area on the wall.

Whenever any of these three factors operates to an excessive extent, an abnormal mass of platelets is formed. This is a *pale, or platelet, thrombus*. The small platelet thrombus that forms first is quite unstable, and platelets may break off and return to the circulation. The addition of a fibrin clot causes the thrombus to become stable (see below).

Platelets do not adhere to a normal intact endothelial surface; although this may be due to the active blood flow sweeping them along, there is also a possibility that a chemical mechanism is involved. This involves the formation of prostaglandins and is described in the next section.

The Formation of a Clot of Fibrin in Which the Blood Cells are Trapped. If the platelet thrombus is not speedily endothelialized, or if there is stasis, a blood clot is formed, and red and white cells are trapped in its meshes. Thrombin is potent in causing platelets to adhere to each other, and its liberation during the process of coagulation readily leads to a further deposition of platelets. In this way a large mass is built up. When blood clot is the major component, it is called a *red, or coagulation, thrombus*. Frequently the thrombosis is made up of both red clot and pale platelet components, and it is then called a *mixed thrombus* (Figs. 20–2 and 20–3).

The crucial feature of thrombosis is the deposition of platelets on a vascular surface. This can occur only in the presence of a flowing stream, and is therefore produced spontaneously only in the living animal. The clotting is a secondary phenomenon. It follows that the terms "clot" and "thrombus" are quite distinct; a thrombus contains a variable amount of clot, but the important feature is a platelet scaffold, which is lacking in a clot; it can be formed only *in vivo*. Clotting, on the other hand, may occur as part of thrombosis, and is also seen in a column of static blood *in vivo* or *in vitro*.

Since the cardinal process in thrombosis is the deposition of platelets on an intimal surface, it is evident that the integrity of the vascular system is all-important in preventing it. Two features of the vascular system that are important in preventing thrombosis are (a) the smooth endothelial lining, which diminishes frictional resistance between the wall and the circulating

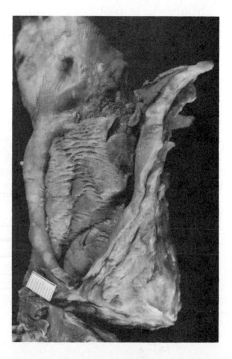

Figure 20–2. Thrombosis in aortic aneurysm. The aortic aneurysm has been opened to show adherent thrombus. The thrombus has a characteristic ribbed, or corrugated, appearance; this is quite different from the smooth, shiny surface of a postmortem clot.

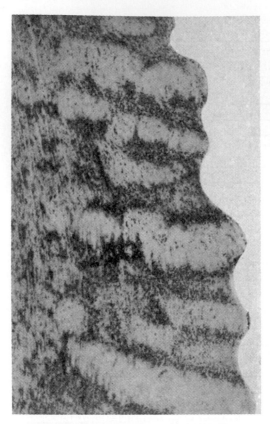

Figure 20–3. The structure of a thrombus. This is a photomicrograph of a thrombus and includes its free surface on the right. The thrombus consists of pale platelet laminae between which there is coagulated blood. Many white cells are adherent to the platelet laminae. Retraction of the clot leaves the laminae projecting from the free surface, and this is responsible for the ribbed appearance noted in Figure 20–2. The organized structure, with platelet laminae alternating with coagulated blood, distinguishes a thrombus from a blood clot, because it indicates that the structure has been formed from the elements of a flowing stream of blood. (From Hadfield, G.: Annals of the Royal College of Surgeons of England, 6:219, 1950.)

blood, and (b) the streamline of blood along the complex circulatory pathways, which moves the formed elements in a central axial stream (Chapter 5).

The speed of flow prevents local stasis, and the absence of irregularities in the walls does not allow the development of eddy currents. The streamline of blood can be threatened in a variety of ways, which are illustrated in Fig. 20–4. These lesions all lead to local stasis as well as to the formation of eddy currents, and the platelets that cover them are actually performing a remedial function. They serve to smooth out the contours of the wall and restore the streamline of blood in the vessel. The small amount of clotting factors that they generate is dissipated in the flowing blood, and they themselves are rapidly endothelialized. It is when this process is retarded that the platelet mass grows, clotting factors accumulate, much fibrin is produced, and thrombosis proceeds even to the extent of obliterating the vessel lumen.

Role of the Prostaglandins in Thrombosis

The prostaglandins are potent agents derived from 20-carbon polyunsaturated fatty acids that are present in the phospholipids of all cell membranes. They have been named by letter (approximately in order of discovery) and by figures 1 to 3 (according to the number of double bonds in the molecule). They are synthesized from *arachidonic acid*, which is released from cell-membrane phospholipid by the action of phospholipase A_2. The enzyme cyclo-oxidase converts arachidonic acid into the two unstable *prostaglandin endoperoxides*. In platelets these endoperoxides are converted into *thromboxane A_2* (TXA_2), which is a powerful agent that causes vasoconstriction and platelet aggregation.

PGE_2

When platelets adhere to a vessel wall, TXA$_2$ is formed, platelet aggregation is encouraged, and a platelet thrombus is formed. However, the endoperoxides formed by the platelets can also be used by cells of the vessel walls; these cells convert the endoperoxides into *prostacyclin* (PGI$_2$), which is a vasodilator and can inhibit platelet aggregation. A balance between the formation of thromboxane A$_2$ by the platelets and prostacyclin by the vessel wall may well be an important factor in determining the extent of thrombus formation. Damage to a vessel wall may impede prostacyclin formation and thereby encourage thrombus formation.

The vessel wall synthesizes prostacyclin from its own precursors, as well as from endoperoxides released by platelets. Thus, the continuous formation of prostacyclin may be an important homeostatic mechanism by which platelets that are forced onto the vascular endothelium (or onto areas of minimal damage) are prevented from building up an abnormal platelet thrombus. Prostacyclin in the circulation, partially derived from the lungs, appears to be an additional protective mechanism. When it is remembered that platelet deposition on arterial walls is thought to be a major factor in the pathogenesis of arteriosclerosis, it will be readily understood why research into the formation and properties of the prostaglandins is currently so active.

General Causes of Thrombosis

Three factors *(Virchow's triad)* must be considered in regard to the mechanism of thrombosis:

(1) **The Vessel Wall.** The various types of anatomical changes in the vessel wall that may lead to thrombosis are depicted in Figure 20–4. In general, these abnormalities play an important part in thrombosis involving the heart valves and ventricles. In the arteries, atheroma is by far the most common cause of thrombosis. In the veins, changes in the vessel wall are usually of much less importance.

(2) **The Flow of Blood.** The formation of *eddy currents* is important, for whenever the stream of the blood is disturbed the flow becomes turbulent, and platelets are thrown against the vessel wall and are deposited as a thrombus. This mechanism is important in fast-moving streams, *e.g.*, over the heart valves and in arteries. Slowing of the blood, or *stasis*, is the most

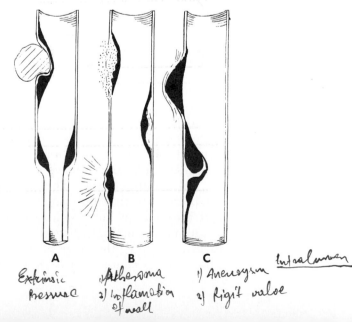

Figure 20–4. Vascular abnormalities that lead to thrombosis. This diagram shows seven different causes of a disruption of the normal streamlining of the blood flow, and the manner by which platelets (shown in black) are laid down to restore the architecture. *A*, Bulging due to external pressure and spasm. *B*, Endothelial damage in inflammation, an area of intimal thickening (*e.g.*, due to atheroma), and corrugation due to adjacent scarring. *C*, Aneurysm and a thickened, rigid valve. (From Hadfield, G.: Annals of the Royal College of Surgeons of England, 6:219, 1950.)

important cause of excessive thrombosis involving veins. It is also a factor in inducing thrombosis in the sac of an aneurysm as well as in the atria of the heart.

③ **The Constituents of Blood.** An increase in the platelet count, an increase in platelet adhesiveness, and a decrease in the clotting time — events that occur after trauma and bleeding — are sometimes important in inducing thrombosis. Likewise, increased viscosity of the blood due to hemoconcentration or polycythemia also leads to thrombosis. Other factors that may induce thrombosis are hyperlipidemia and administration of the birth control pill. The factors involved are complex and not completely understood.

It should be noted that usually more than one factor is implicated in the cause of thrombosis. For instance, there is regional stasis and a high platelet count after a surgical operation. Atheroma acts both by causing a loss of the endothelium and by inducing eddy-current formation.

Arterial Thrombosis

Thrombosis generally occurs in arteries as a complication of damage to the arterial wall; *atherosclerosis* is the most important cause, but *arteritis* also accounts for some cases. In an aneurysmal sac, thrombus deposition is a constant feature, and here stasis and eddy currents are important factors. These are considered in Chapter 29.

Effects of Arterial Thrombosis. Except for the aorta and its very large branches, arterial thrombosis results in the complete blockage of the vessel. The effects of this depend upon the local architecture. The following are possibilities:

① *No Effect.* When anastomoses are good, no ill effect is noted. Thus, if the radial artery is blocked, the hand is supplied by the ulnar artery because branches of the two vessels are normally joined together by *anastomotic channels*. These channels enlarge so that a *collateral circulation* develops. Blockage of either artery alone, therefore, leads to no serious aftereffects, provided the other vessel is not diseased.

② *Functional Disturbances.* Blockage of a major vessel may render tissue ischemic only with exercise. In coronary occlusion, which is an example of this blockage, the effect is pain on exercise (*angina pectoris*). Likewise, occlusion of the mesenteric artery can lead to pain after meals when the intestine exhibits marked peristalsis. Occlusion of the femoral artery can lead to pain on walking. This is called *intermittent claudication*.

③ *Cellular Degeneration.* Ischemia can induce enough hypoxia to cause the specialized cells of an organ to degenerate. This is a patchy affair and leads to atrophy. Often there is *replacement fibrosis* (*e.g.*, myocardial fibrosis); in the central nervous system there is *replacement gliosis*.

④ *Infarction.* The ischemia may be so severe that the whole area undergoes necrosis. This effect is called *infarction* and is considered later in this chapter.

Venous Thrombosis

Although disease of the vessel walls is uncommon, stasis is particularly evident in the veins, especially those of the legs. Thrombosis with a large element of clotting is therefore common. Two distinct entities can be recognized: phlebothrombosis and thrombophlebitis.

Phlebothrombosis. The commonest form of leg vein thrombosis is phlebothrombosis. This occurs in patients who are confined to bed, particularly if they are in heart failure or have been subjected to trauma, whether accidental or surgical. If the limb has been injured and immobilized (*e.g.*, a fractured femur), the stage is set for thrombosis, because the major cause of thrombosis is *venous stasis* (Fig. 20–5). A small thrombus forms at one site,

Figure 20–5. The pathogenesis of phlebothrombosis. *A,* An area of intimal damage is covered by a pale platelet thrombus. In the presence of a sluggish stream, this initiates further thrombosis. *B,* Upstanding laminae of platelets with intervening clot constitute the main thrombus. *C,* The lumen is occluded by further thrombosis. *D,* Blood *clot* forms to the next tributary. (From Hadfield, G.: Annals of the Royal College of Surgeons of England, *6*:219, 1950.)

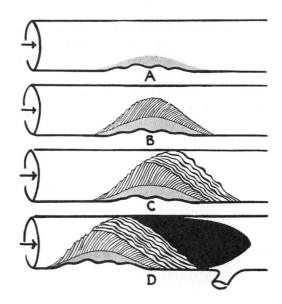

perhaps when the vein has been injured by pressure such as that produced by a pillow behind the knee. The flow of blood stops in the vein proximal to the thrombus, and the entire column *clots* (Fig. 20–6). This process can extend, or propagate, up to the iliac vein; as the clot retracts, it has minimal attachment to the vessel wall. The great danger then is embolism, for should the clot become detached, it would travel in the circulation to the right side of the heart and subsequently be ejected into the pulmonary artery. Here it would block either the main pulmonary trunk or one of its major divisions, leading to sudden death or infarction of the lung (see a discussion of this later in the chapter).

    Thrombophlebitis. Inflammation of a vein (phlebitis) can occur when there is an adjacent area of infection (*e.g.,* a boil). Thrombosis occurs

Figure 20–6. Propagation of clot in phlebothrombosis. *A,* Thrombus formation occurs at each entering tributary. This tends to anchor the clot. *B,* Clotting *en masse* in an extensive length of vein. This occurs when the circulation is very sluggish. The long propagated clot can easily become detached and lead to massive pulmonary embolism. (From Hadfield, G.: Annals of the Royal College of Surgeons of England, *6*:219, 1950.)

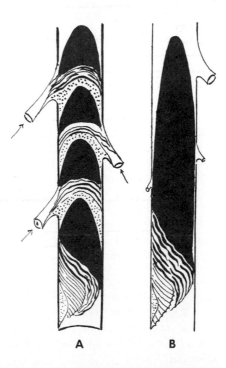

A   B

(*thrombophlebitis*) and is confined to the inflamed area of vein. A propagated clot does not form, and the risk of embolism is slight unless the thrombus itself becomes infected (see "Infected Emboli," page 291).

Thrombophlebitis affecting many veins at different times (called *migrating thrombophlebitis*) is an occasional manifestation of cancer, particularly cancer of the pancreas. The pathogenesis is not understood. The first description of this condition is attributed to Trousseau, a French physician, who observed it in himself and subsequently died of pancreatic cancer.

Local Effects of Venous Thrombosis.   In most tissues, because the veins show extensive anastomoses, venous thrombosis produces few obstructive effects. There are some exceptions to this. Obstruction of the superior mesenteric vein leads to intense engorgement of the intestine and edema of the gut wall. This blockage can be so marked that further blood flow through the part becomes impossible, and the intestine undergoes infarction. In the leg, venous obstruction can lead to some elevation of the venous pressure of the limb, an effect particularly marked if the subject stands for long periods. The result of this is edema of the ankles.

Cardiac Thrombosis

Thrombi may form in any of the chambers of the heart. The constant danger is their detachment and subsequent embolization. A common cause of atrial thrombosis is atrial dilatation secondary to mitral stenosis, atrial fibrillation, or heart failure. Ventricular thrombosis is most commonly encountered as a complication of myocardial infarction, either during the acute stage (see Fig. 28–6) or in an aneurysm that develops subsequently.

Thrombi on the heart valves (called *vegetations*) are a feature of acute rheumatic fever, infective endocarditis (see Fig. 28–3), and nonbacterial thrombotic endocarditis (Chapter 28).

Fate of Thrombi

Figure 20–7 summarizes the possible fate of a thrombus. These possibilities are further elaborated on below:

(1) Many thrombi undergo lysis and leave no trace of their previous existence. The fibrinolytic enzyme plasmin is probably important in removing thrombi (see Fig. 20–1).

(2) If an occluding thrombus in an artery or vein contains much clot, it retracts sufficiently for blood to pass by, in this way forming a new channel. It becomes endothelialized, and at that point *recanalization* is said to have occurred. In the pulmonary arteries a thin web of connective tissue may be all that remains of a previous life-threatening thromboembolism.

(3) A thrombus that is not removed may become organized into granulation tissue and subsequent scar tissue.

(4) Organized thrombi may become hyalinized and calcified. This response is common in the pelvic veins, and the *phleboliths* so produced may be seen on radiographic examination of the pelvis.

(5) Thrombi may be detached to form emboli — a process that is described later in this chapter.

Two important effects of thrombosis are occlusion of the lumen of the vessel involved and detachment from this to form an embolus. Vascular obstruction produces ischemia, which in turn leads to hypoxia.

Hypoxia

Hypoxia is a state of impaired oxygenation of the tissues.

Types.   Four types are commonly described:

1. *Hypoxic,* due to a low oxygen tension (PO_2) in the arterial blood. This form of hypoxia is a feature of some types of congenital heart disease and lung disease.

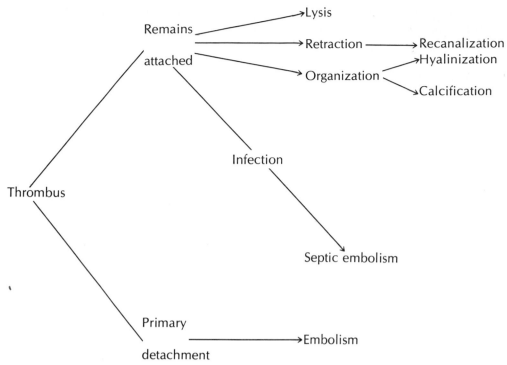

Figure 20–7.   Diagram illustrating the possible fate of a thrombus.

2. *Anemic,* due to an inadequate level of hemoglobin, which carries the oxygen in the blood stream.

3. *Stagnant,* or *ischemic,* due to an inadequate supply of blood to the tissues; this form of hypoxia may be due to a low cardiac output, as in heart failure, or to some local vascular obstruction.

4. *Histotoxic,* due to cellular poisoning, which prevents the uptake of oxygen (*e.g.,* cyanide poisoning).

Ischemia is a condition of inadequate blood supply to an area of tissue. It produces harmful effects in three ways:

Ischemia

Hypoxia.   A reduced oxygen supply is undoubtedly the most important factor in the production of damage in ischemic tissue. It is particularly important in active cells such as muscle and neurons. On the other hand, it plays no part in the lesions produced by pulmonary arterial obstruction because the alveolar walls derive their oxygen directly from the alveolar gas.

Malnutrition.   This is probably a factor of little importance, because the blood contains more nutrients than could be metabolized with the amount of oxygen it contains.

Failure to Remove Waste Products.   The accumulation of metabolites is the most probable explanation of pain in ischemic muscles. The presence of waste products or the failure to maintain important electrolyte balances is probably a factor in the pathogenesis of pulmonary infarction.

General.   Ischemia can be caused by an inadequate cardiac output. Not all tissues of the body are equally affected, because there is a redistribution of the available blood. The extremities — for instance, the fingertips and toes — tend to be most severely affected; in such cases the sluggish blood flow leads to peripheral cyanosis. (The term *cyanosis* refers to the blue color of tissues that is produced by the reduced hemoglobin in the vessels.)

Causes of Ischemia

Sudden cessation of the heart's action, such as may occur during the induction of anesthesia or as a result of coronary thrombosis, results in ischemia of all tissues in the body. The effects of this are confined to a single organ — the brain — which is particularly sensitive to hypoxia. If the arrest continues for 15 seconds, consciousness is lost; if the condition lasts for more than 3 minutes, irreparable damage is done. If the patient survives, the neurons degenerate and are replaced by glial tissue. If cardiac arrest lasts for more than 8 minutes, death is inevitable. It follows that *all persons who deal with patients should be capable of diagnosing cardiac arrest (absent heart sounds) and of dealing with it by the maneuvers of external cardiac massage and assisted respiration.*

Local.   By far, the most important cause of ischemia is obstruction of the arterial flow. Nevertheless, extensive venous and capillary obstruction can also produce ischemia.

Arterial Obstruction.   Most of the causes of obstruction have already been described. In review, they are:

Thrombosis.

Embolism.   The effects of an embolus are potentiated by the reflex spasm of the arterial wall and are completed by the rapid development of thrombus over the embolus.

Spasm.   See later in this chapter.

Atherosclerosis.   See Chapter 29.

Occlusive Pressure from Without.   Examples include tourniquets and ill-fitting casts.

Venous Disease.   Extensive venous obstruction leads to engorgement of the area drained by the affected veins. This may reach such an intensity that blood flow is impeded and ischemia results.

Capillary Damage.   See Chapter 29.

Embolism   An embolus is an abnormal mass of undissolved material that is transported from one part of the circulation to another. The most satisfactory classification is one based on the composition of the embolus.

Types of Emboli   Four distinct types may be recognized: *thrombi* and *clot; gas; fat;* and *tumor;* a fifth category — *miscellaneous emboli* — is also discussed.

Thrombus or Clot Emboli

Pulmonary Embolism.   The source of thromboemboli is generally one of the leg veins. If the embolus is large, it produces the syndrome of "massive pulmonary embolism." Either the main pulmonary trunk or many of its branches become plugged, so that the pulmonary circulation is greatly hindered (Fig. 20–8). The output of the right ventricle as well as that of the left ventricle drops precipitously. The effects of this drop are dramatic. The patient experiences sudden dyspnea and chest pain. Loss of consciousness and death may follow. The prevention of massive pulmonary embolism is the prevention of phlebothrombosis. A patient who is confined to bed must be given leg exercises to stimulate the venous circulation. Postoperative physical therapy and early ambulation have done much to reduce this complication of trauma and surgery. Anticoagulant drugs (*e.g.,* heparin) administered prior to surgery have been somewhat useful.

Small pulmonary emboli produce a different picture. If the subject is otherwise healthy, medium-sized pulmonary arteries can be obstructed without appreciable ill effect. Since the lung derives much of its oxygen from the alveolar gas, the area beyond a blocked artery does not become hypoxic. Nevertheless, the altered gas tensions in the tissue can lead to bronchospasm, with the result that the area ceases to be ventilated and may collapse. This

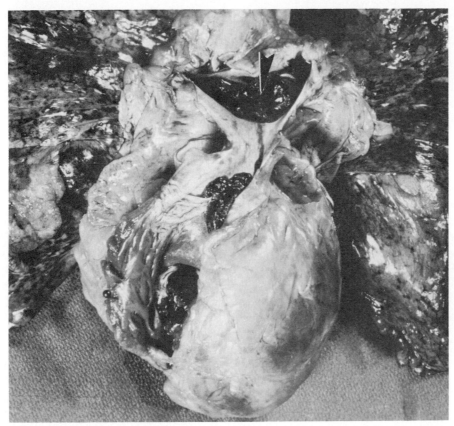

Figure 20–8. Massive pulmonary embolism. The right ventricle and pulmonary trunk have been opened to reveal a large embolus. Part of the embolus is sitting astride the division of the pulmonary trunk and is blocking both pulmonary arteries. This condition is known as a *saddle embolus* and causes sudden death.

area can become reinflated within a few hours. The transient radiographic shadows that can be seen following pulmonary embolism may be explained on this basis. At other times, the area becomes edematous; hypoxia is added to ischemia, and necrosis ensues. The end-result is infarction of the lung.

The circumstances determining whether infarction will follow pulmonary embolism are not clearly understood, but patients who are in heart failure or who are confined to bed seem to be most prone to this complication.

Systemic Embolism. The embolus usually arises from the heart, either in one of its chambers or from a valve. Thrombi attached to atheromatous ulcers in the aorta sometimes embolize distally.

Infected Emboli. If a thrombus contains pyogenic organisms, it tends to break up and produce multiple infected ("septic") emboli. Such a condition, which is called *pyemia*, is a complication of both acute endocarditis and thrombophlebitis in an area of suppurative inflammation (*e.g.,* acute appendicitis). If an infected embolus blocks a vessel supplying tissue that has a poor collateral circulation (*e.g.,* kidney), an infarct is produced, subsequently becomes infected, and a *septic infarct* results and soon suppurates. If the tissue has a good blood supply (*e.g.,* liver), no infarction occurs, but a local infection leads to abscess formation — a *pyemic abscess.* Thus, a complication of acute appendicitis is portal pyemia and multiple pyemic abscesses in the liver.

Gas Emboli

Air. Air may accidentally be introduced into a systemic vein during a surgical procedure. During operations on the head and neck, air may be sucked accidentally into the jugular vein and may then pass to the right side of the heart. Small quantities produce no adverse effect, but if a large quantity of air suddenly reaches the right ventricle, it becomes churned into a foamy mass that is compressed during systole but cannot be ejected. The cardiac output drops dramatically and sudden death ensues.

When a needle is introduced into the pleural cavity, as when fluid is aspirated, air may inadvertently be introduced into the pulmonary venous circulation and may reach the left side of the heart. From here it may travel to a coronary or cerebral vessel, occluding it. Even small quantities of air can produce serious, or even fatal, results in this manner.

Air embolism, either pulmonary or systemic, is a serious complication of open-heart surgery. All efforts must be made to exclude air from the circulation at the termination of the operation.

Nitrogen: The Decompression Syndrome. Bubbles of nitrogen appear in the circulation in those who, having been exposed to a high atmospheric pressure, are suddenly decompressed. This occurs in divers and tunnelers if they return to the surface too quickly. It is also seen in pilots if the cabin becomes decompressed at a high altitude. Nitrogen, being soluble in lipids, also appears as bubbles in the central nervous system. This particular effect may result in considerable damage to the spinal cord. The accompanying severe pain, which occurs most often in the joints, gives the condition its colloquial name "the bends." Permanent damage or death may ensue.

Fat Embolism. Globules of fatty marrow may enter small veins in the area of a fracture of a long bone. With multiple injuries, this embolization can be quite extensive. Usually the emboli are trapped in the lungs and, because of the enormous capacity of the pulmonary vascular bed, can produce little harmful effect. Small areas of collapse can be detected radiographically. Occasionally fat emboli traverse the pulmonary capillaries and enter the systemic circulation, where they produce the condition known as *systemic fat embolism*. Multiple emboli lodge in the kidneys, causing hematuria; in the brain, leading to severe neurological changes; and in the skin, causing petechial hemorrhages.

Tumor Emboli. It is probable that all malignant tumors invade the local blood vessels at an early stage of the disease and that isolated malignant cells are a frequent occurrence in the circulation. The majority of these emboli become impacted and are destroyed. A small percentage develop into metastatic deposits. Occasionally, a large mass of tumor invades a major vessel and becomes detached. Thus, in lung cancer a tongue of tumor can invade a pulmonary vein, become detached, pass into the systemic circulation, and block a large artery such as the femoral artery. The event is uncommon.

Miscellaneous Emboli. A variety of foreign bodies can act as emboli. For example, a portion of polyethylene tube may accidentally become detached and travel to the right side of the heart.

The condition described as *amniotic fluid embolism* is an occasional complication of pregnancy that follows escape of amniotic fluid into the veins of the uterus. It produces a syndrome characterized by shock and a generalized bleeding tendency. Although amniotic fluid does travel to the lungs, the syndrome is attributable not to embolism but rather to the initiation of intravascular clotting and fibrinolysis.

Infarction

Infarction is the circumscribed necrosis of tissue due to deprivation of its blood supply. The area of necrosis subsequently becomes organized into scar tissue. The process is as follows:

(a) Cells die in the area deprived of its blood supply. Blood, either from anastomotic vessels or from venous backflow, continues to seep into the

Figure 20–9. Pulmonary infarct.   This vertical section through the lung shows an area of hemorrhagic infarction involving the apex of the lower lobe (arrow). Note how the surrounding uninvolved lung has collapsed post mortem; this has left the infarct standing out in relief. The specimen is from a patient who had carcinoma of the lung.

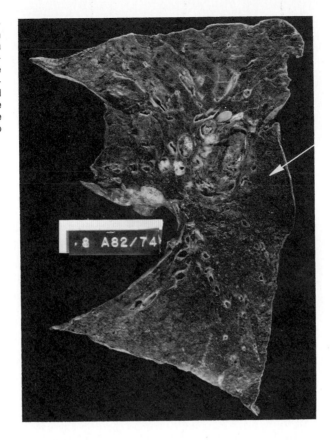

devitalized area for a short time. Thus, most infarcts contain a great deal of blood in the early stages and are swollen and red in color (Fig. 20–9). The red cells entering the affected area escape from the damaged capillaries and lie free in the dead tissue. Infarcts of lax tissue such as the lung and intestine are much more engorged than those of compact organs such as the kidney and heart. If an infarcted area adjoins a surface, the congested necrotic tissue oozes blood. Hence, with renal infarcts blood is present in the urine (*hematuria*), and with infarction of the lung the sputum is bloodstained (*hemoptysis*); a small bloodstained pleural effusion may also be detected.

(b) The dead tissue undergoes necrosis. In solid organs, the associated swelling of the cells tends to squeeze blood out of the infarct, which then becomes pale (Fig. 20–10). Infarcts of the spleen and kidneys characteristically show this color change and appear as pale, wedge-shaped areas of coagulative necrosis — the apex of such areas being a blocked supplying artery, the base being the capsule of the organ (Figs. 20–9 and 20–10). Infarcts of the heart are also pale, but their shape is more irregular owing to the arrangement of the vascular supply (see Fig. 28–4).

(c) Necrotic tissue undergoes progressive autolysis; red cells undergo hemolysis. Microscopically, the infarct shows a characteristic structured necrosis. The general outline of the cells is visible, but nuclei are either breaking up into fragments or have completely disappeared.

(d) At the same time the surrounding normal tissue shows an acute inflammatory reaction. Hyperemia gives the edge of the infarct a deep red color. Microscopic examination reveals an intense polymorph infiltration. Macrophages subsequently become the predominant cell and play an important part in removing the dead tissue. In pulmonary infarction the inflammation involves the parietal pleura, and this leads to *pain*, particularly on taking

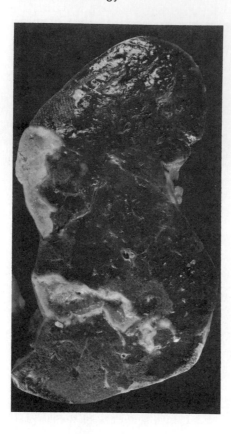

Figure 20–10. Splenic infarction. This section of spleen shows two pale areas of infarction. The specimen is from a patient who died of bacterial endocarditis.

a deep breath. Likewise, splenic infarction may cause pain in the left side of the abdomen.

(e) The infarct gradually shrinks and becomes replaced by granulation tissue that subsequently matures to scar tissue. The central portion of a large infarct may remain unorganized for many months and indeed may show dystrophic calcification and never become converted into scar tissue.

Infarcts in particular organs present certain characteristic features. For example, in the lung, the tissue is spongelike, and infarcts in it are always hemorrhagic. In the intestine, the necrotic bowel wall is soon invaded by putrefactive organisms and becomes gangrenous. In the limbs, sudden obstruction leads to infarction, which in turn is associated with infection and leads to *wet gangrene* (Fig. 20–11).

In the central nervous system, on the other hand, the process of infarction is somewhat different, because the necrotic tissue immediately undergoes liquefactive necrosis. The affected area may collapse and eventually be replaced by a glial scar, but if the infarct is large, the end-result is the formation of a cyst lined by glial tissue.

Vascular Spasm   Although vascular occlusion is generally caused by an organic lesion, there are a number of conditions in which spasm of the vessel wall plays a most important part. Either veins or arteries can be affected by spasm, but it is debatable whether capillaries are capable of independent contraction.

Venous Spasm   Trauma applied directly to the vessel wall can induce intense spasm. This may cause great difficulty during an inexpert venipuncture, *e.g.*, when a transfusion is set up or when blood is withdrawn from a vein. It is the reason why the novice has such difficulties in "taking blood."

Generalized venospasm occurs during hypovolemic shock, and it has also been postulated as occurring in heart failure.

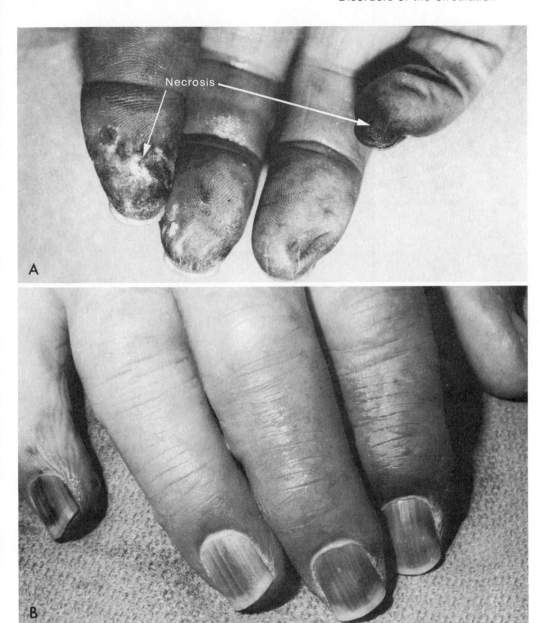

Figure 20–11.   Gangrene of the finger tips.   This patient died as a result of bleeding from esophageal varices secondary to alcoholic cirrhosis of the liver. He died in shock associated with severe and extensive edema of the subcutaneous tissues, ascites, and pleural effusions. Following the insertion of a needle to obtain a sample of arterial blood, the patient developed thrombosis of the right brachial artery and gangrene of the finger tips. There is blue-black discoloration of the tissues and necrosis of the finger pulps (*A*). Acute arterial obstruction associated with pre-existing edema has led to the condition of wet gangrene. The condition would have spread to involve the whole hand and even the arm, but death intervened. See also Figure 19–3.

Arterial Spasm

Trauma to an artery produces localized spasm; at times, this may be life-saving. There are many cases recorded in which whole limbs have been torn off (avulsed), and yet owing to the spasm of the main artery, the patient has not died of massive bleeding.

The ability of arteries and arterioles to contract can be used to advantage by a surgeon who is faced with severe bleeding during the course of an operation. It is a wise policy to pack the wound and await the onset of spasm rather than make heroic, though blind, efforts with a pair of hemostats.

Indeed, *anyone faced with bleeding from a wound should apply local pressure and await vasospasm, rather than panic or apply a tourniquet.*

Although arterial spasm as a response to trauma may be beneficial, it may sometimes be detrimental. Trauma to an artery, *e.g.,* by the close proximity to a bullet path, the jagged ends of a fractured bone, the pressure of a hematoma around a fracture, or the pressure of a plaster cast or tourniquet, may at times produce such persistent widespread spasm that the area involved becomes ischemic and infarcted. Because the process is often painless, the *pulse of a limb beyond an area of damage must always be carefully observed.* Absence of the pulse must be regarded seriously, and every effort should be made to relieve the spasm so that permanent damage will not occur.

Spasm of small arteries and arterioles is a feature of ergot poisoning and Raynaud's phenomenon (Chapter 1). It may lead to gangrene of the toes and fingertips. Widespread arteriolar spasm is a feature of shock (Chapters 21 and 28). It has also been incriminated as a cause of primary hypertension, which is discussed below.

Systemic Hypertension

High blood pressure, or systemic hypertension, is a common condition that is often discovered accidentally during a routine medical examination. It is normal for the systemic blood pressure to rise as a response to emotion and physical exercise. If a raised pressure is discovered, it is wise to check the measurement after the patient has been at rest for some time and has grown accustomed to the surroundings. Another factor to consider is the age of the patient. As people get older, the aorta becomes less elastic, and with each ventricular contraction the systolic blood pressure rises rapidly. However, the blood drains away normally through the arterioles to the venous system, and the diastolic blood pressure remains normal. In systemic hypertension the diastolic blood pressure rises. A rough guideline is that the systolic blood pressure should be less than 100 mm Hg plus age in years. There is, however, no sharp cut-off above which a patient may be regarded as having hypertension. A systolic pressure over 160 mm Hg with a sustained diastolic pressure over 95 mm Hg is usually taken as indicative of hypertension. The precise incidence of the disease is difficult to determine, but probably around 20 per cent of the population suffer from the disease to some extent or another.

Types of Hypertension

For practical purposes two types of hypertension can be recognized: primary hypertension and secondary hypertension.

Primary, or Essential, Hypertension.   This is the common form of high blood pressure, and it accounts for about 90 per cent of the cases. By definition its cause is unknown. Although an increase in cardiac output may play some part in the pathogenesis of hypertension, it is generally assumed that the cause of the increased blood pressure is an increase in peripheral resistance to blood flow. It is a condition that is more common in women than in men, and it is especially prevalent in North American Blacks. Primary renal or adrenal abnormalities have been postulated as causing this hypertension, but no conclusive evidence has been obtained.

Secondary Hypertension.   About 10 per cent of cases of hypertension fall into this secondary group. Renal disease is by far the most common cause, but it is also a feature of pheochromocytoma, a rare tumor of the adrenal gland, and is due to the effects of epinephrine and norepinephrine, which are secreted by the tumor. The hypertension is characteristically episodic. Hypertension is also a feature of some adrenal cortical tumors (Chapter 39).

Pathogenesis of Hypertension

As noted previously, it is generally assumed that the cause of the increased blood pressure is an increase in peripheral resistance to blood flow.

Many experimental models have been investigated in attempts to elucidate the nature of this resistance to blood flow in essential hypertension.

The classic experiments of Goldblatt proved that in the dog an obstruction to the renal artery blood flow could produce hypertension. This response is due to the release from the ischemic kidney of a proteolytic enzyme (called *renin*) that acts on a plasma globulin, angiotensinogen, to convert it into angiotensin I. Another plasma enzyme converts angiotensin I into angiotensin II, a peptide that induces vascular spasm and produces hypertension. Angiotensin II also stimulates the adrenal cortex to increase its secretion of aldosterone. This causes retention of sodium and water.

In humans, hypertension sometimes, but not always, occurs in acute and chronic glomerulonephritis, pyelonephritis, and other renal diseases. The mechanism producing the hypertension may or may not be similar to that operating in the Goldblatt experiment; present evidence is against such a pathogenesis, because in the majority of cases the plasma renin level is not elevated. In chronic renal failure retention of sodium and water leads to a rise in blood volume and cardiac output. Removal of sodium and water from the body by diuretics lowers the blood pressure. Hypertension with unilateral renal lesions, such as obstruction to the renal artery, is sometimes relieved either by unilateral nephrectomy or by correction of the arterial stenosis. Unfortunately, this treatment is not always successful, presumably because secondary vascular events have taken place in the other kidney by the time diagnosis is made.

The pathogenesis of primary systemic hypertension is not known. Retention of sodium, increased blood volume, and a rise in cardiac output have been postulated. Peripheral vasoconstriction is assumed to be secondary to this. Alternatively, a primary increase in the peripheral resistance may be the mechanism. Evidence for this being mediated by the renin-angiotensin mechanism is poor. A primary defect in the autonomic nervous system has been postulated, but its nature is not known. Perhaps stress triggers the mechanism, as suggested by the finding that hypertension is more common in individuals exposed to a high level of stress. Another possibility is that an abnormal sensitivity of the vascular smooth muscle leads to excess constriction in response to normal levels of vasoconstrictor substances such as epinephrine and angiotensin. A high level of sodium in the cells may be involved. It is known that hypertension is more common in individuals and races that have a high dietary sodium intake. Finally, there is the possibility that genetic influences are of importance. These are not well defined, and it is generally stated that the tendency to develop hypertension is multifactorial.

Effects and Complications of Hypertension

1. Hemorrhage. Weakened blood vessels tend to rupture more commonly in the hypertensive than in the normal subject; dissecting aneurysm of the aorta, ruptured berry aneurysm of the circle of Willis, and cerebral hemorrhage are all more common in the hypertensive subject.

2. Atherosclerosis. Atherosclerosis, with all its complications, is more common in patients with hypertension. Myocardial infarction and strokes bedevil the patient with hypertension.

3. Arteriolosclerosis. The small arteries of many organs show thickening of their walls, particularly the tunica intima, with hyaline material. This thickening is most marked in the arterioles of the renal glomeruli; gradually, as these vessels close down, the glomeruli and tubules that they supply become atrophic and are replaced by fibrous tissue. This scarring of the kidney is termed *nephrosclerosis*.

The arterioles of the retina share in this generalized process. The thickening of their walls and resulting ischemic changes in the retina constitute the features of *hypertensive retinopathy* (Chapter 42).

Arteriolosclerosis also affects the central nervous system. This sclerosis of the walls of the smaller arteries is presumed to be the cause of vague symptoms such as headache, lightheadedness, and giddiness. Personality changes and memory defects are also common. More severe lesions resulting from vascular occlusion or hemorrhage produce more definite effects, such as hemiplegia.

Heart Failure.   Systemic hypertension causes left ventricular hypertrophy and ultimately left ventricular failure (Chapter 28).

Malignant Hypertension

Hypertension, whether primary or secondary, may occasionally evolve into a malignant phase. The disease may also arise without pre-existing hypertension. The blood pressure becomes very high, causing necrosis of the arteriolar walls. Two organs are especially affected: the kidney and the brain. In the *kidney* the vascular changes cause hematuria and culminate in uremia. In the *brain* the changes cause hemorrhage and edema. Swelling of the optic discs (papilledema) is a useful sign of raised intracranial pressure; symptoms include mental confusion and epileptiform fits. The syndrome of malignant hypertension usually progresses rapidly over a period of several weeks and, unless treated expeditiously, results in death either from uremia, from an intracranial vascular catastrophe, or from heart failure.

The pathogensis of malignant hypertension is not understood. Blood renin levels are high, and presumably angiotensin causes vasoconstriction as well as retention of sodium and water via aldosterone secretion. The severe renal damage causes further renal ischemia, and a vicious circle ensues that ends in death.

Review Questions

1. Describe the way in which a thrombus differs from a clot.

2. List the steps that can be taken to avoid death from massive pulmonary embolism.

3. Compare the process of infarction in the kidney with that which occurs in the intestine.

4. Describe the role of thrombin in the formation of a thrombus.

5. Discuss the possible effects of thrombosis of the femoral artery.

6. Describe the possible effects of pulmonary embolism.

7. A 50-year-old man is found to have a systolic blood pressure of 170 mm Hg. Discuss possible causes of this.

8. Discuss the relationship between systemic hypertension and the kidney.

Selected Readings

Fleischner, F. G.: Recurrent pulmonary embolism and cor pulmonale. New England Journal of Medicine, *276*:1213–1220, 1967.
Leading Article: Fat embolism. British Medical Journal, *3*:476–477, 1970.
Leading Article: Prevention of deep-vein thrombosis: the way ahead. Lancet, *2*:693–694, 1971.
Leading Article: Fat embolism. Lancet, *1*:672–673, 1972.
Leading Article: Ischaemia of the intestinal tract. British Medical Journal, *4*:566–567, 1972.
Leading Article: Prevention of postoperative thromboembolism. Lancet, *2*:63–64, 1975.
Mitchell, J. R. A.: Prostaglandins in vascular disease: a seminal approach. British Medical Journal, *282*:590–594, 1981.
Moncada, S., and Vane, J. R.: Arachidonic acid metabolites and the interaction between platelets and blood-vessel walls. New England Journal of Medicine, *300*:1142–1147, 1979.
Salzman, E. W., Harris, W. H., and DeSanctis, R. W.: Reduction in venous thromboembolism by agents affecting platelet function. New England Journal of Medicine, *284*:1287–1292, 1971.
Sherry, S.: Thrombosis prevented. New England Journal of Medicine, *284*:1324–1326, 1971.
Walter, J. B., and Israel, M. S.: General Pathology. 5th ed. Edinburgh, Churchill Livingstone, 1979. See, in particular, Chapter 39, "General Features of Thrombosis and Its Occurrence in the Venous System"; Chapter 40, "Thrombosis in Arteries and in the Heart"; Chapter 41, "Embolism"; and Chapter 42, "Ischaemia and Infarction."

Shock and Hemorrhage

CHAPTER
21

After studying this chapter the student should be able to:

- Describe the metabolic changes that follow injury.
- Define the following terms: hemoptysis, hematuria, hematemesis, melena, petechia, ecchymosis, hematoma, hemothorax, hemopericardium, and hemarthrosis.
- List the causes of sudden severe bleeding.
- Describe the effects of an acute hemorrhage.
- Compare the clinical features of syncope with those of secondary shock.
- List seven important types of secondary shock and describe their pathogenesis.
- Discuss the concept of irreversible shock and describe its pathogenesis.
- List the organs that are frequently damaged in shock.
- Outline the treatment of shock.

Following major physical injury (*trauma*), there ensues a complicated series of changes from which scarcely any tissue of the body escapes. The nervous system responds promptly with an increased outflow of autonomic impulses. There is an immediate outpouring of catecholamines (epinephrine and norepinephrine) from the adrenal medulla. The other endocrine glands respond more slowly; stimulation of the hypothalamus leads to an increase in the secretion of ACTH from the pituitary gland, which in turn results in adrenal cortical overactivity. These changes assist the injured person to withstand trauma; this effect has been confirmed experimentally by the observation that the adrenalectomized animal is less able to withstand infection and trauma than is the normal animal.

One very obvious early effect of trauma involves the circulatory system. When the trauma is severe, a state develops from which some patients do not recover; this is called *shock*, and is characterized by inadequate perfusion of the tissues, hypotension, and depression of general metabolic activity. If the patient survives, metabolic changes follow that terminate in complete recovery. This is called the period of convalescence.

For descriptive purposes, it is convenient to consider the response to injury under three headings: The Metabolic Changes; The Circulatory Changes; and Shock.

The Metabolic Changes

The early response to injury is termed the low-flow, or ebb, phase. After severe injury it accompanies the state of shock. This phase is characterized by a reduction in the metabolic rate, a reduced body temperature, and an increased output of catecholamines from the adrenal medulla (Table 21–1). The increased blood level of catecholamines has several effects:

The Early or Ebb Phase

1. There is increased production of glucose in the liver from its glycogen stores (*glycogenolysis*).

2. Lactic acid is released from the muscles and is converted into glucose in the liver. The result of all this is *hyperglycemia* and possibly *glycosuria*. A

TABLE 21–1.   METABOLIC CHANGES FOLLOWING INJURY°

	LOW-FLOW PHASE	HIGH-FLOW PHASE
Metabolic rate	↓	↑
Body temperature	↓	↑
Catecholamine output	↑	Normal or slightly ↑
Blood insulin level	↓	↑
Blood glucose	↑	Normal or slightly ↑
Blood lactate	↑	Normal or slightly ↑
Blood fatty acid	↑	↓

°Modified from Ryan, N. T.: Metabolic adaptations for energy production during trauma and sepsis. Surgical Clinics of North America, 56:1073, 1976.

reduction in insulin secretion promotes the formation of glucose from noncarbohydrate sources in the liver (*gluconeogenesis*). This contributes to the hyperglycemia.

3. Catecholamines have a *lipolytic* effect, which means that fatty acids are released from the adipose tissue. The blood level of fatty acids is therefore raised. The metabolic acidosis that accompanies this ebb phase in patients in shock is considered in Chapter 19.

Convalescence   Assuming that the patient survives the initial phase and does not die of shock, there ensues a period of metabolic upset that has been termed the *high-flow phase*, or simply the *flow phase*. This has two components: (a) a *catabolic phase*, which is characterized by excessive protein breakdown and a negative nitrogen balance, followed by (b) an *anabolic phase*, during which the body's stores are replenished. These important metabolic changes are highly complex and are incompletely understood. They have been studied extensively both in animals and in human beings.

The Catabolic Phase.   During the catabolic phase there is increased glucose production in the liver (Table 21–1). This gluconeogenesis is fed by lactate, pyruvate, and alanine and other amino acids derived from muscle, which are used as substrates. The breakdown of muscle components, particularly the proteins, for use in energy generation leads to muscular atrophy and a consequent loss of weight. The nitrogen of the metabolized amino acids is excreted as urea, and the body enters a phase of *negative nitrogen balance*. The duration of this nitrogen loss varies with the extent of the trauma: after a minor surgical procedure it may last only a day or two, but with severe burns it can continue for 10 days or more. Fractures cause more disturbance than might be supposed from the clinical condition; suppuration may prolong the catabolic state for weeks. Two points should be noted:

1. The nitrogen loss cannot be abolished by increasing the protein intake; any extra protein in the diet is broken down and the extra nitrogen excreted. There is therefore no point in forcing patients to ingest protein during this phase.

2. The administration of carbohydrate reduces the nitrogen loss very considerably.

During the catabolic phase the production of insulin is increased two or three times above normal. Nevertheless, the tissues appear to be resistant to the action of insulin, and gluconeogenesis is stimulated by the unopposed action of cortisol. The relative lack of insulin activity is the probable mechanism by which amino acids are released from muscle. There is, however, sufficient insulin activity to inhibit lipolysis; hence, fatty acids are not released from the adipose tissues, and whereas the muscles waste as a result of protein loss, the adipose tissues remain intact. This contrasts to the situation encountered in simple starvation.

Mechanism of the Protein Loss.   The following should be noted:

1. The metabolic effects of injury are closely simulated by the effects of glucocorticoids.

2. The adrenal glands are known to enlarge following injury.

3. There is an increased secretion of adrenal cortical hormones after trauma.

4. Adrenalectomized animals do not show this nitrogen loss.

It would therefore not be unreasonable to assume that excessive adrenal function explains the loss of nitrogen, but that this is not the case is shown by the finding that adrenalectomized animals (and human subjects) on a constant maintenance dose of cortisol still show the same negative nitrogen balance when subjected to trauma. Thus, it appears that adrenal hormones are necessary for this metabolic change but do not directly produce it. It may be that they play a permissive role, but the increase in cortisol production is not the direct mechanism involved in the metabolic changes.

Other Metabolic Changes. *Sodium and Water Metabolism.* During the early period after trauma, the urine volume diminishes owing to an increased secretion of ADH, and sodium is retained by the kidneys as a result of increased aldosterone secretion (Fig. 21–1). This phase of sodium retention is a little shorter than the catabolic phase; it has been held that this is obligatory, and that the body is defenseless against overdosage, because it cannot excrete sodium and water.

There is a later return of sodium to the urine; unless there was excessive administration during the oliguric phase, its excretion is little increased.

Figure 21–1.   Mechanism of sodium retention.   Diagrammatic representation of the means by which the body retains sodium after a sudden reduction in blood volume, such as after severe hemorrhage.

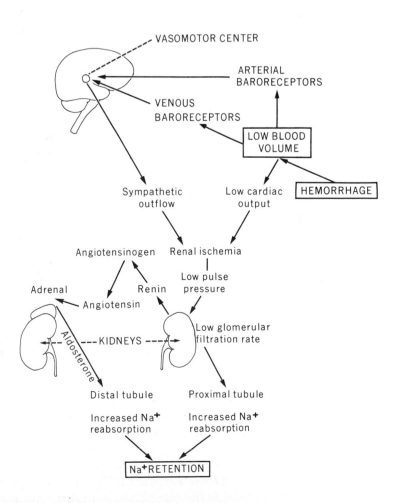

Potassium Metabolism. A negative balance occurs during the initial phase and is most marked on the first day. Because potassium is intracellular, it is presumed to be liberated at the same time that protein is metabolized.

Other Changes. There is an increased urinary excretion of *creatinine* (derived from the muscles), *phosphate,* and *sulfur.* This occurs *pari passu* with the excretion of nitrogen and potassium and is due to cellular breakdown.

Vitamin C is retained, its excretion in the urine being dramatically reduced. A scorbutic state may develop despite this careful guarding of the ascorbic-acid stores.

During this catabolic phase there is a marked loss of weight. A moderate *pyrexia* is invariable and is not due to concomitant infection.

The hematological changes are a moderate increase in the neutrophil polymorph count (neutrophilia) and a reduction in lymphocytes (lymphopenia) and eosinophils (eosinopenia). The platelet count is increased (Chapter 20). An interesting feature of severe trauma is the development of a progressive normocytic normochromic *anemia.* This is not due to iron deficiency; it may be that there is deficient hemoglobin synthesis during a period of general protein breakdown. *Sludging* may accentuate this anemia (page 308).

The Anabolic Phase. The final stage of convalescence is characterized by a positive nitrogen balance and a resynthesis of muscle protein. The changes noted during the catabolic phase are reversed, and the body returns to normal.

The Circulatory Changes

The changes in the circulation are seen most clearly following acute hemorrhage; this will therefore be described first.

Hemorrhage

Hemorrhage is defined as the escape of blood from the vascular system. The extravasated blood may escape to the exterior, or it may remain internal.

Types of Hemorrhage

External. Blood may be coughed up (*hemoptysis*), passed in the urine (*hematuria*), vomited (*hematemesis*), or passed in the feces either as fresh blood or, if from higher up in the intestinal tract, as a black, partially digested mass (*melena*).

Internal. Small flat hemorrhages, less than 2 mm in diameter, are called *petechiae* or *purpuric spots;* they are usually found in the skin and mucous membranes. A larger, more diffuse hemorrhagic area is called an *ecchymosis.* A *hematoma* is a discrete pool of blood, usually clotted, in a tissue. Collections of blood in natural spaces are named anatomically, *e.g., hemothorax* (in the pleural cavity), *hemopericardium, hemoperitoneum, hemarthrosis* (in a joint cavity), etc.

Causes of Acute Hemorrhage

Trauma. Penetrating wounds involving the heart or large vessels may result in the very rapid loss of large quantities of blood.

Inflammatory Lesions of the Blood-Vessel Wall. Inflammatory lesions may cause weakening of a vessel wall, usually arterial, with subsequent rupture. Aneurysmal dilatation may occur before the final rupture. The inflammation need not always be infective, *e.g.,* polyarteritis nodosa.

Neoplastic Invasion. Hemorrhage is a frequent result of malignant neoplasms. For example, it is often the terminal event in carcinoma of the tongue, in which it is due to rupture of the lingual artery; superimposed infection is a major factor in the weakening of the wall.

Other Vascular Diseases. Atheroma, with or without aneurysmal dilatation, is the most common cause. Aneurysms also fall into this category.

High Blood Pressure Within the Vessels.   Systemic hypertension may precipitate hemorrhage at sites of arterial weakness. Raised venous pressure with varicose-vein formation, *e.g.*, in the esophagus, is another important cause of severe hemorrhage.

Effects of Acute Hemorrhage.   The vascular system contains about 5 liters of blood, which are kept in motion by the action of the heart so that all tissues are adequately perfused. The amount of blood reaching any area is determined by two factors: the *diameter of the arterioles* supplying it and the *blood pressure.*

The effects of blood loss depend on the quantity of blood lost and the speed at which the loss occurs. If a small quantity of blood is lost suddenly, there is scarcely any effect on the circulation because the large venous system acts as a reservoir for blood. Consequently, when a small amount is lost, an increase in venous tone reduces the capacity of the venous system, so that there is no reduction in the volume of blood reaching the heart (the venous return). Thus, there is no reduction in the cardiac output. When a larger volume of blood is suddenly withdrawn, this reserve mechanism of the venous reservoir is inadequate. The venous return is diminished, the cardiac output falls, and the blood pressure would also fall were there no other compensatory mechanisms available. The next response to hemorrhage is a series of reactions designed to prevent any fall in blood pressure.

Following severe hemorrhage the fall in blood pressure is detected by the pressure-sensitive carotid sinus and other baroreceptors; these reflexly initiate a sympathetic outflow from the central nervous system (Fig. 21–2). The result is an increase in heart rate and constriction of the arterioles of the *skin, kidneys,* and *splanchnic area* both by direct action and by the indirect action of the adrenal medulla, which is stimulated to secrete epinephrine and norepinephrine. In addition, the reduced blood pressure acts on the kidney directly and causes a release of renin (Chapter 20). These mechanisms lead to an overall increase in the peripheral resistance, so that even with a reduced cardiac output, the systemic blood pressure is maintained at normal or near-normal levels. The maintenance of an adequate blood pressure allows the blood flow to the brain, the heart, and the respiratory muscles to remain virtually unaltered. However, the areas affected by arteriolar vasoconstriction tend to suffer; for example, the *skin* is cold and pale, the *kidneys* show a reduced urinary output (*oliguria*), and salivary gland secretion decreases, resulting in dryness of the mouth. Thus, the vasomotor response to acute hemorrhage causes a redistribution of blood, a mechanism that may be regarded as an emergency measure designed to keep the essential organs supplied with blood.

Mechanisms for Maintenance of the Blood Pressure

During the first few hours after bleeding the extravascular fluids pass into the blood stream, thereby restoring the blood volume. This can be demonstrated quite easily by checking the hemoglobin levels at intervals. Immediately after a sudden hemorrhage, the hemoglobin level is normal. During the next 8 hours it falls as dilution occurs. This process is largely complete by the end of 48 hours, by which time the hemoglobin level is a good guide to the extent of a previous blood loss. The transfer of extracellular fluid to the blood stream occurs as a result of the reduced capillary hydrostatic pressure, which is secondary to arteriolar vasoconstriction. Complete restoration of the plasma volume is dependent on replacement of the lost plasma proteins. These are manufactured for the most part in the liver and enter the circulation via the thoracic duct.

Restoration of Blood Volume

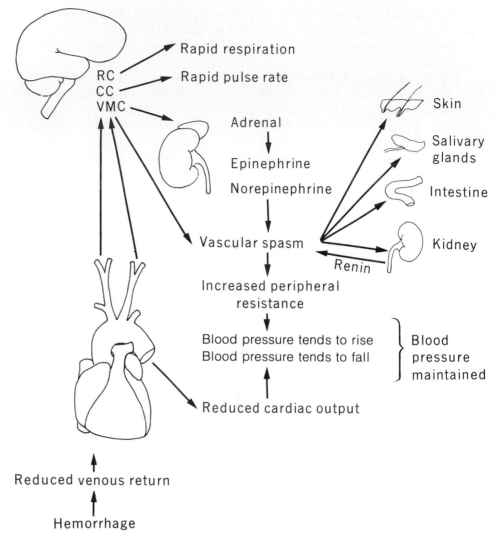

Figure 21–2. The cardiovascular effects of hemorrhage. Abbreviations: RC, respiratory center; CC, cardiac center; VMC, vasomotor center.

Changes in the Blood

Within a few minutes of bleeding, the clotting time is considerably decreased; during the next few hours, there is an increase in the level of platelets and neutrophils, which persists for several days. The restoration of the red cell count is a slow process, since the body has no reserve store of erythrocytes. New red cells have to be manufactured, and a normal count is not attained until four to six weeks later, regardless of the severity of the blood loss.

A normal adult can lose 500 ml of blood quite rapidly with little discomfort, a fact attested to by millions of blood donors. A sudden loss of 30 to 50 per cent of the blood volume (1.5 to 2.5 liters) can be fatal. However, such a loss spread over a day or so can be tolerated if the compensatory mechanism keeps pace with the blood loss. When the compensatory mechanisms are inadequate for this purpose, the patient sinks into a state described as shock, and this may be fatal.

Shock

Before the important subject of shock is discussed, the phenomenon of syncope will be described, since it has many features in common with shock and was at one time termed "primary shock."

Syncope, or a vasovagal attack, is better known as the common faint. The subject is invariably standing up; the initial symptoms are giddiness and lightheadedness. Shortly after this, consciousness is lost and the subject falls to the ground. Pallor of the skin is a striking feature; the body is bathed in a cold sweat. The blood pressure is low, and the pulse is weak, with its rate either slowed or normal. Syncope can occur following blood loss, but it can also be caused by pain or psychological factors. The very thought of having an injection or having blood withdrawn is enough to send some people into a faint. It is believed that syncope is caused by sudden autonomic overactivity that leads to vasodilatation in the muscles and pooling of blood there. The venous return is suddenly reduced and with it the cardiac output, blood pressure, and blood supply to the brain. The loss of consciousness in syncope is brief, and if the subject is laid horizontally, or attains that position spontaneously, he soon recovers. In rare cases death may occur — at least this is one suggestion for the rare cases of sudden death that occur unexpectedly, such as when a needle is introduced into the pleural cavity or during an attempted abortion. It has been reported that syncope occurring during induction of anesthesia may be fatal if the anesthetic is administered with the patient in the upright position, such as in a dental chair.

The remainder of this section deals with the much more serious condition of shock itself — or as it was once called, "secondary shock."

Shock is seen following many forms of injury; it may occur immediately, or it may happen after a period of comparative well-being. The patient lies still and listlessly; his temperature is subnormal, his skin cold and clammy, and his face ashen. Obvious cyanosis is often present, the blood pressure is low, and the pulse is rapid and thready. Little or no urine is passed.

In shock there is an inadequate blood supply to many tissues, leading to tissue hypoxia, metabolic acidosis, and defective function of the tissues concerned. Liver, lungs, heart, and kidneys are commonly affected, but under particular circumstances the effects of ischemia of other tissues (*e.g.,* retina, pituitary, and pancreas) may dominate the situation.

The clinical picture of shock may occur in a variety of conditions, and not surprisingly, these have all been assembled under the all-embracing title of "shock." Conditions that lead to a state of shock include:

Loss of blood
Trauma
Loss of plasma (*e.g.,* following burns)
Loss of fluid and electrolytes
Overwhelming infection
Acute heart failure
Generalized anaphylaxis

The inclusion of so many diverse conditions under the one heading of shock has tended to obscure our understanding of the condition. They all produce a similar clinical picture, but it is hardly to be expected that the mechanisms involved would be the same in each case. Furthermore, a state of shock can occur as a terminal event under many other circumstances, *e.g.,* after electrocution, overdose of drugs, drowning, or massive total body irradiation. To attempt to understand shock one must consider each condition separately.

Hemorrhagic Shock.   If the compensatory mechanisms following bleeding are inadequate to maintain an effective perfusion of the tissues of the body, a state of shock ensues (Fig. 21–3). Recovery may occur spontaneously or as a result of efficient treatment, such as transfusion; such shock is therefore

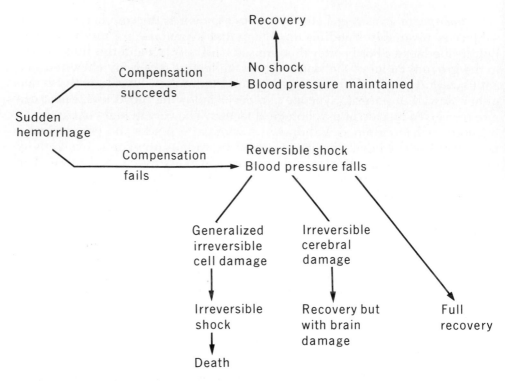

Figure 21–3. **The possible end-results of a sudden hemorrhage.**

said to be *reversible.* Occasionally, in spite of efficient, vigorous treatment, the blood pressure continues to fall, the patient's clinical condition deteriorates, and death ensues. This response, termed *irreversible* (or *decompensated) shock,* is considered later.

Traumatic Shock. The circulatory changes following trauma are very similar to those seen following hemorrhage. The possible mechanisms are:

Hemorrhage. It is often not appreciated that there is considerable bleeding into the tissues following any injury, even closed injuries such as a fractured femur. Much of the swelling that is seen around the fracture is due to blood that has poured into the adjacent tissues; some is due to inflammatory exudate, itself derived from the blood.

Infection. There is little doubt that the powerful exotoxins of the pathogenic clostridia exert a profound shocking effect. Gas gangrene, even in the absence of substantial tissue damage, causes shock and death.

Endotoxic Factor. The intravenous injection of endotoxins of the gram-negative bacilli leads to a shocklike state in animals. This is particularly marked following a second injection 24 hours after a previous one. The mechanism is not well understood, and the phenomenon is known as the Shwartzman phenomenon. Patients whose wounds are infected with gram-negative coliforms can suddenly develop shock as a result of endotoxemia or septicemia ("*septic shock*").

Inflammatory Exudate Formation. The outpouring of fluid into inflamed tissues is responsible for some of the swelling around injured parts and adds its quota to that of bleeding as a cause of reduction in blood volume.

In summary, *blood loss is the single most important factor in causing traumatic shock.*

Shock Following Thermal Burns. The severe shock that follows burns is largely related to the tremendous loss of plasma in the inflammatory exudate. At a later stage, bacterial infection, such as that with *Pseudomonas aeruginosa* and other coliforms, may play a part. An important point of difference from hemorrhagic shock is that there is concentration, rather than dilution, of blood. The hemoglobin level rises owing to this hemoconcentration.

Shock Due to Loss of Fluid and Electrolytes.   Loss of fluid or sodium can lead to such depletion of the extracellular tissue fluids that unless replacement therapy is instituted shock can develop as a result of an inadequate volume of circulating plasma. This condition is seen following persistent vomiting due to pyloric stenosis or intestinal obstruction, in cholera, and in any severe diarrhea (particularly in children).

Shock in Infection.   Shock is seen in a variety of infections. It is prominent in infections with the toxic organisms of diphtheria and gas gangrene, and it is also a feature of many other severe infections: pneumonia, peritonitis, typhoid fever, typhus, and others of a similar nature. In recent years, a new syndrome — endotoxic shock — has been recognized; it is caused by the sudden entry of gram-negative coliform organisms or their endotoxins into the circulation. It is a complication of any coliform infection and is usually a sequel to urinary tract infection. There is a sudden onset of profound shock; unless treated expeditiously, it causes high mortality.

The shock of infection has a complex pathogenesis: at least three factors must be considered:

1. *Pooling of blood.* Blood is sequestered in the splanchnic area because of vasodilatation. The effective blood volume is thereby reduced.

2. *Loss of fluid in inflammatory exudate.* In gas gangrene the profuse loss of protein-rich exudate is in part responsible for the hemoconcentration and the reduction of blood volume.

3. *Heart failure.* Some bacterial toxins (*e.g.*, diphtheria toxin) damage the myocardium, and an element of heart failure may further embarrass an already failing circulation.

Cardiogenic Shock.   Extensive myocardial infarction, sudden severe cardiac dysrhythmias, rupture of a valve cusp, and the sudden accumulation of fluid or blood in the pericardium can sometimes lead to a state of shock that resembles shock following trauma. This condition results from a low cardiac output, for it leads to underperfusion of tissues as an initial effect, and the resulting metabolic acidosis (see below) causes peripheral vasodilatation and pooling of blood. The shock that occurs following massive pulmonary embolism has a similar pathogenesis.

Anaphylactic Shock.   Generalized anaphylaxis occurs when an individual, already sensitized by IgE, encounters the specific sensitizing antigen. See Chapter 9 for a more complete discussion.

The Metabolic Upset During Shock

A patient in shock shows a profound reduction in metabolic rate (the nature of which is not well understood), but this reduction appears to be related to a block in carbohydrate utilization. In spite of cutaneous vasoconstriction — and therefore a reduction in heat loss — the patient's temperature tends to fall. An important effect of shock is that the underperfusion of tissues results in anaerobic glycolysis with the release of pyruvic and lactic acids into the circulation. A *metabolic acidosis* is characteristic of shock.

Summary of the Pathogenesis of Shock

It is evident that shock is essentially a state in which there is underperfusion of tissues. Shock may be mediated by the following:

1. Hypovolemia.   A low blood volume can occur after (a) hemorrhage (external or internal), (b) external loss of water and electrolytes (resulting from vomiting, diarrhea, diabetes insipidus, or the excessive use of diuretics), (c) rapid accumulation of inflammatory exudate (from burns and infection), and

(d) dehydration (heat exhaustion and inadequate fluid intake). If there is hemoconcentration, the increase in blood viscosity further impedes the peripheral circulation.

2. *Reduction of Effective Blood Volume Due to Internal Sequestration.* Peripheral vasodilation can result in pooling of blood so that the effective volume of circulating blood is decreased. The splanchnic area and skeletal muscle are the sites where vasodilation commonly occurs. This state has been called *peripheral circulatory failure* and is encountered particularly in endotoxic shock and metabolic acidosis.

3. *Cardiac Factors.* A state of low output can result from acute heart failure or from mechanical problems such as cardiac tamponade.

4. *Sludging.* If the flowing blood of a patient in shock is observed with a microscope, it will be seen that the red cells tend to flow in clumps rather than as individual cells. When this phenomenon was first described, the blood was said to be converted into a "mucklike sludge," from which comes the name *sludging*. The process differs from true agglutination in that the masses of red cells can be broken up mechanically *in vitro*. The cause of sludging appears to be an increase in the high–molecular-weight substance of the blood, and its effect is to impede the blood flow through tissues. Sludging therefore contributes to the poor perfusion of tissues in shock.

Irreversible Shock

Some patients with shock recover either spontaneously or as a result of treatment. Others steadily deteriorate in spite of all efforts to save them. It is commonly believed that there is a stage from which recovery becomes impossible. This is called *irreversible* or *decompensated shock*. The phenomenon can be demonstrated experimentally. If an animal is bled, it passes into a state of shock. It can be allowed to stay in a state of hypotensive hypovolemic shock for a few minutes and then be resuscitated by returning its own lost blood through a catheter. If the animal is allowed to stay in a state of shock for too long, the transfusion fails to reverse the shock, and its condition steadily deteriorates until death ensues.

The present concept of shock is that the major abnormality is the underperfusion of certain vital organs. If the state of shock is allowed to persist too long, there is permanent damage to tissues, and recovery is therefore impossible. The concept of irreversible shock as an entity is currently downplayed. One cannot deny that some patients reach a stage from which recovery is impossible, but the cause for this varies from case to case and is due to the summation of biochemical abnormalities, such as metabolic acidosis, and damage sustained by many tissues. Organs that show damage are the following:

Liver. It is common to find centrilobular necrosis in patients dying of shock.

Heart. Patchy myocardial infarction is common, and acute heart failure can be added to a state of shock produced by other mechanisms.

Lung. The important changes that take place in the lung are described in Chapter 30 under the heading of "Acute Adult Respiratory Insufficiency Syndrome."

Kidney. Oliguria and anuria are characteristic of shock. Acute tubular necrosis, which can become extensive, may lead to irreversible renal damage (Fig. 21–4).

CASE HISTORY I. (See Figure 21–4). The patient was a 40-year-old woman who had had a normal pregnancy until the thirty-first week of gestation. She was then found to be hypertensive (blood pressure raised to 240/120); she also developed abdominal pain and began to bleed from the vagina. Her condition was diagnosed as abruptio

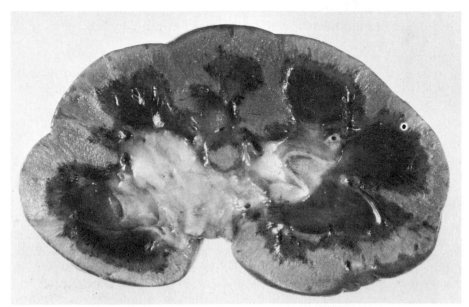

Figure 21–4. Cortical necrosis of the kidney. Specimen from a 40-year-old woman who died in renal failure. The specimen shows necrosis of the outer two thirds to three fourths of the cortex. The inner layer of the cortex and the medulla are congested. This is the most severe type of ischemic renal damage encountered in shock. The condition affects both kidneys equally and is similar to the changes seen in the rabbit in the generalized Shwartzman phenomenon. For a more complete description, see Case History I.

placentae (premature detachment of the placenta). An emergency cesarean section was performed, but it failed to save the child; there was also considerable loss of blood during the operation. The patient went into shock, developed anuria, and, in spite of peritoneal dialysis, experienced a rise in blood potassium to 7.0 mEq per liter (normal level is 3.5 to 5.5 mEq per liter). Her blood urea nitrogen also rose to 100 mg per dl (normal level is 10 to 20 mg per dl). She died in renal failure eight days after the onset of symptoms.

Gastrointestinal Tract.   Although the gastrointestinal tract is congested in shock, the blood flow through it is decreased. Patchy mucosal necrosis can occur in both the small and large intestine; the resultant bleeding may be severe and further complicate the clinical situation. Acute stress ulcers in the stomach and duodenum can cause further blood loss.

Pituitary.   Infarction of the pituitary is best known as a complication of shock following labor.

Eye.   Retinal ischemia can result in blindness.

Pancreas.   Patchy pancreatitis is not uncommon, but it is usually silent clinically.

It is evident that death from shock may occur for many reasons, either as a result of damage to some organ or from a metabolic upset secondary to this damage. From a practical point of view, the efficiency of treatment is of overriding importance, because many of the potentially lethal causes and effects of shock can be counteracted. Irreversible shock must be regarded as being almost always due to inefficient treatment.

The treatment of shock is a complex affair but includes the following: **Treatment of**

1. *Maintenance of adequate pulmonary ventilation.* Avoidance of any   **Shock** obstruction of airways can be life-saving; the inhalation of 30 per cent oxygen is helpful.

2. *Restoration of blood volume* by the administration of blood, water, or electrolytes, depending upon the circumstances. Fluid must be administered quickly, and the *central venous pressure* must be monitored with a catheter

placed in one of the large systemic veins. A rise in venous pressure indicates overburdening of the heart and the necessity for reducing the speed of fluid input.

Measurement of the central venous pressure has proved to be less useful than was at first hoped. An estimation of the *left atrial pressure* is now regarded as a more useful guide during the administration of intravenous fluids. The procedure is carried out by inserting a balloon-tipped catheter (*Swan-Ganz* catheter) into the right ventricle via an arm vein. On inflating the balloon, the catheter passes into the pulmonary artery and wedges in a branch of the vessel. A measurement of the wedged pulmonary arterial pressure is an accurate guide to the pressure in the left atrium.

3. *Correction of metabolic acidosis* by the intravenous administration of sodium bicarbonate solution.

4. *Maintenance of renal function.*

5. *Administration of drugs.* It is worth remembering that in any form of shock a drug administered by the subcutaneous or intramuscular route is liable to be absorbed slowly owing to the poor state of the circulation. Failure to get a satisfactory clinical response can lead to the need to readminister the drug. This, in turn, could lead to the formation of a large depot of the drug, which could subsequently be absorbed with fatal results.

Patients in shock are particularly sensitive to the effects of depressant drugs such as anesthetic agents. The place of morphine in shock should be limited to its use in alleviating severe pain and apprehension.

It was at one time recommended that norepinephrine and drugs with a similar action should be given with a view to causing vasoconstriction and a rise in blood pressure. Unfortunately, this treatment further imperils the blood supply to various vital organs — particularly to the kidney and intestine — and the use of these drugs is not now recommended. Indeed, *vasodilator* drugs are sometimes given. There are some authorities who recommend their administration with massive doses of glucocorticoids, although the mode of action of the steroids is by no means clear. Perhaps they reduce the sensitivity of vessel walls to epinephrine, and thereby prevent vasospasm in vital organs.

6. *Treatment of infection.* Although obvious enough in diseases like gas gangrene, infection following trauma may sometimes pass unnoticed and untreated.

7. *Treatment of mechanical complications.* The presence of shock may lead to a failure to appreciate the presence of remediable mechanical lesions such as a subdural hematoma, pneumothorax, and hemopericardium.

Conclusion   There are many features about shock that we do not understand. Nevertheless, vigorous, well-designed treatment can save many cases. "Shock" is not a diagnosis that should be accepted without qualification; it indicates that something is wrong — a low blood volume, metabolic acidosis, sludging, arterial desaturation, renal failure, pericardial hemorrhage, or some other drastic deviation from normal — all of which can be diagnosed and often treated. When a patient has very severe injuries, when shock has been present for some time, when patients are already ill with some other disease, and when a severe untreatable infection is present, death may be inevitable. The diagnosis of irreversible shock, however, should be made only after death has occurred.

Review Questions   1. A previously healthy 25-year-old man was involved in a brawl and was stabbed several times in the upper abdomen. He was admitted to the hospital and was given a laparotomy as part of his emergency treatment. The spleen was lacerated and had to be removed. Several puncture wounds of the intestine were located and were closed by sutures. The blood pressure, pulse rate, respiratory rate, and fluid balance were carefully monitored, and for 24 hours the patient did well. His condition then deteriorated, and he passed into a state of shock. Discuss the possible causes and indicate the investigations that might be helpful in managing this case.

2. Compare the general effects of a severe hemorrhage with those of a severe burn.

3. List the changes that occur in the constituents of the blood following the sudden loss of two pints of blood from a severed radial artery.

4. Explain why a patient may develop glycosuria following a severe injury.

Selected Readings

Baue, A. E.: Metabolic abnormalities of shock. Surgical Clinics of North America, 56:1059–1071, 1976.

Dowd, J., and Jenkins, L. C.: The lung in shock: a review. Canadian Anaesthetists' Society Journal, 19:309–318, 1972.

Federation Proceedings, 29:1832–1873, 1970. Report of a symposium entitled "Physiologic Basis of Circulatory Shock" in which various authors discuss different aspects of shock, including its treatment with glucocorticoids.

Herman, C. M.: Advances and newer concepts in shock. In Copper, P., and Nyhus, L. M. (Eds.): Surgery Annual. Vol. 4. New York, Appleton-Century-Crofts, 1974, pp. 1–49.

Jacobson, E. D.: A physiologic approach to shock. New England Journal of Medicine, 278:834–839, 1968.

Rutherford, R. B.: The pathophysiology of trauma and shock. In Zuidema, G. D., Rutherford, R. B., and Ballinger, W. F. (Eds.): The Management of Trauma. 3rd ed. Philadelphia, W. B. Saunders Company, 1979.

Ryan, N. T.: Metabolic adaptations for energy production during trauma and sepsis. Surgical Clinics of North America, 56:1073–1090, 1976.

Sevitt, S., and Stoner, H. B. (Eds.): The pathology of trauma. Journal of Clinical Pathology, 23 (Suppl. 4):1–214, 1971. This publication contains articles covering many topics, including the metabolic changes caused by trauma, fat embolism, and changes in coagulation.

Walt, A. J., and Wilson, R. F.: Treatment of shock. Advances in Surgery, 9:1–39, 1975.

CHAPTER 22 Fever and Hypothermia

After studying this chapter the student should be able to:

- Describe the physiological mechanisms by which the body's temperature is maintained within narrow limits.
- Define fever and hyperpyrexia.
- List ten causes of fever.
- Describe the central heat-regulating center and outline its mode of action
    - (a) under normal conditions
    - (b) in a patient with pneumonia
    - (c) in a patient with heat stroke.
- Compare bacterial pyrogens with endogenous pyrogens.
- Describe the circumstances under which malignant hyperpyrexia is usually encountered.
- Define hypothermia and describe the common causes and effects in infants and in adults.
- Give two examples of the value of induced hypothermia in medicine.

A rise in the body's temperature is so commonly found in illness that this response has been recognized since ancient times. Indeed, the term "fever" is sometimes used as being synonymous with disease. "Hayfever" and "cat-scratch fever" bear witness to this association, because in neither disease is fever an important feature. To avoid this confusion, the term "pyrexia" is commonly used in clinical medicine.

Before considering fever itself, one must understand the normal body temperature and the mechanism of its control.

The Normal Body Temperature

The most reliable method of taking the body's temperature is by placing a thermometer under the tongue with the lips closed. The temperature taken in this way varies from 36.1° to 37.4°C (97° to 99°F) and accurately reflects the temperature of the inside of the body (the *core temperature*). The maximum temperature is generally attained at about 6:00 P.M., whereas it is at its lowest at about 3:00 A.M. In women there is an elevation of the temperature during the middle of the menstrual cycle; its onset is thought to herald ovulation, and this rise in temperature has been utilized in the rhythm system of contraception. In unconscious patients it is convenient to take the temperature by placing a thermometer in the rectum; the readings obtained in this way are about 1°F higher than those taken by mouth. Measurement of temperature by placing the thermometer in the axilla or groin is quite unreliable, since it does not accurately reflect the core temperature. The surface skin temperature fluctuates widely and may approximate that of the external environment.

The maintenance of a constant body temperature is one aspect of homeostasis, and in humans it has obtained a high degree of efficiency. The importance of this is obvious when it is remembered that cellular activity involves many chemical reactions that are largely dependent upon enzymatic activity and therefore very susceptible to changes in temperature. The body's temperature is regulated by a heat-regulating center that initiates the various mechanisms to increase or decrease heat loss.

The constancy of the body's temperature is maintained by balancing the amount of heat produced in the body with that which is lost.

**Temperature
Regulation**

Sources of Heat.   The major source of heat is the body's metabolic activity. Heat production under fasting conditions with the individual at complete mental and physical rest is called the *basal metabolic rate* (BMR), which ranges from 1400 to 1800 Calories* per day. The heat released by the operation of the sodium pump (Chapter 2) in all cells is an important source of heat. In addition, heat is produced by other essential metabolic activity, *e.g.*, the beating of the heart and contraction of the diaphragm.

Under normal active conditions, additional heat is produced by exercise, which can be quite modest with sedentary workers (*e.g.*, 1000 Calories) or rather high in those engaged in heavy manual labor (*e.g.*, 6000 Calories). The heat produced by metabolism raises the temperature of the blood through the relevant organs. Thus, the blood leaving the brain and the liver is warmer than that entering them. Likewise, during manual work blood leaving the skeletal muscles is heated. The warm blood from these centers of heat production is distributed to the organs of heat loss. Of these, the skin is the most important.

Areas of Heat Loss.   Heat is lost from the blood as it perfuses the skin. Convection, radiation, and evaporation of sweat all play a part in the loss of heat. The latter is particularly important when the ambient temperature exceeds that of the body. Since the blood supply to the skin is regulated by the sympathetic division of the autonomic nervous system, the latter plays a dominant role in the maintenance of a constant body temperature. Some heat is also lost from the respiratory tract and mouth. In humans, this is a relatively constant amount, but in animals it can be increased considerably by panting.

Situated in the anterior part of the hypothalamus, in the *preoptic area*, is a group of nerve cells that is sensitive to the temperature of the arterial blood reaching it. When the temperature of the blood changes, impulses pass from this area to other parts of the hypothalamus. There are two main areas: (1) an anterior *heat-losing center,* which when stimulated leads to changes in the rest of the body, causing increased heat loss, and (2) a posterior *heat-promoting center,* which when stimulated leads to increased heat production and conservation (Fig. 22–1).

**The Central
Temperature-
sensitive Area**

Mechanism for Increasing Body Temperature.   The heat-promoting center acts mainly through the sympathetic division of the autonomic nervous system. Cutaneous vasoconstriction reduces the amount of heat lost from the skin, and blood diverted to the internal organs is insulated from the exterior by the subcutaneous fat. Furthermore, as the skin becomes cooler, the subject feels cold and may take appropriate voluntary action such as putting on extra clothing.

The increased sympathetic outflow causes an increased output of epinephrine and norepinephrine from the adrenal glands. These hormones increase the metabolic rate of all cells through a mechanism that is not well understood. Metabolism is further increased by a *generalized increase in muscle tone*. If these mechanisms are inadequate, muscle tone increases to the extent that stretch reflexes are elicited and *shivering* commences. As one group of muscles contracts, a stretch reflex of the antagonistic group is set in motion and initiates a fresh stretch reflex of the first group. This continuous shaking can increase the rate of heat production severalfold.

---

*The unit used in metabolic studies is the Calorie, which equals 1000 calories (spelled with a small "c"). One calorie is the quantity of heat required to raise the temperature of one gram of water 1°C.

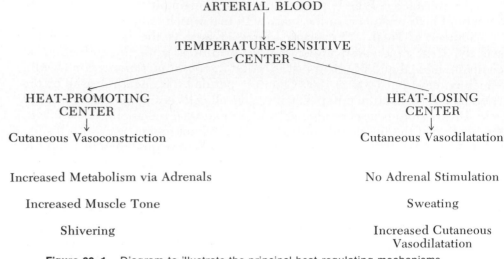

Figure 22–1. Diagram to illustrate the principal heat-regulating mechanisms.

Mechanism of Decreasing Body Temperature. When the body's temperature tends to rise, there is a withdrawal of sympathetic vasoconstriction activity, the skin becomes warm, and heat is lost. The subject feels hot and may remove clothing, retire to the shade, or take other appropriate action. If this regulating mechanism does not suffice, the heat-loss center initiates sweating from the eccrine glands. Evaporation of this fluid requires heat, but an additional effect of sweating is the local release of bradykinin from the glands. This induces further vasodilatation and heat loss.

Peripheral Temperature Receptors

The heat-regulating mechanism is also influenced by impulses received from the peripheral receptors in the skin. This influence can be demonstrated by an experiment in which the blood to one arm is occluded by a cuff and the arm is then immersed in cold water. Within seconds the skin of the opposite arm undergoes vasoconstriction, indicating that a nervous reflex is involved rather than a change in blood temperature. After a while, this vasoconstriction wanes, but on restoration of the circulation, a more prolonged period of vasoconstriction ensues as the cooled blood of the limb reaches the hypothalamus and activates the central mechanism directly.

Fever

Fever, or *pyrexia,* may be defined as an elevation of the body's temperature following a disturbance of the regulating mechanism. When the temperature reaches or exceeds 40°C (104°F), the condition is called "hyperpyrexia."

Heat Stroke. Some rise in body temperature normally occurs during extreme exercise, because the heat-eliminating mechanisms cannot immediately keep pace with the excessive heat production in the muscles. When the environment is hot and humid, even mild exercise can cause a marked rise in body temperature. Sometimes the heat-regulating mechanism breaks down under these circumstances and the temperature rises. This condition of *heat stroke* or *sun stroke* occurs most commonly in elderly individuals with pre-existing chronic disease; unless it is promptly treated, the temperature continues to rise, reaching 43°C (109.4°F) or even more. Patients become comatose, often have convulsions, and may have permanent brain damage if they survive. Heat stroke must therefore be treated most energetically with tepid sponging or immersion in cold water until the temperature approaches normal.

Two other effects of exposure to a high environmental temperature should be noted.

Heat Cramps.   Heat cramps are characterized by painful cramps of the voluntary muscles and usually follow strenuous exercise. They are apparently due to local loss of sodium and chloride.

Heat Exhaustion.   Heat exhaustion or heat collapse is the most common heat syndrome. It usually affects elderly individuals who are unable to adapt to a high external temperature. The pathogenesis is not clear. Weakness, headache, nausea, and vomiting are followed by collapse and hypotension. The body's temperature is either normal or low, as it is in other forms of shock. Patients with heat exhaustion are generally depleted of salt and water owing to prolonged sweating combined with inadequate fluid and salt intake. Whether this is the major cause of the condition is not clear, but certainly fluid and electrolyte imbalance should be corrected as part of the treatment of the condition.

Infection.   Infection is the most common cause of fever; the pattern of the temperature chart is sometimes characteristic of a particular disease. The relapsing course of malaria and brucellosis are examples of this. So also are the two phases of fever that characterize dengue. With some acute infections, particularly if there is an initial septicemia as in urinary tract infections and lobar pneumonia, the onset of fever is sudden. The following stages are recognized:

The Cold Stage.   At the onset of the illness, the patient experiences an intense feeling of cold. There is peripheral constriction, which is manifested by pallor, and the patient starts to shiver. The teeth chatter, and the patient shakes all over with the familiar condition called a "rigor." The increased muscular activity combined with reduced heat loss causes the temperature to rise. The blood pressure and pulse rate also rise. In general, there is an increase in pulse rate of about 10 beats per minute for each 1°F rise in temperature (18 beats per minute per 1°C). In children, the rigor may be replaced by a convulsion.

The Hot Stage.   As the temperature approaches its peak, the peripheral vasoconstriction relaxes, and the patient feels dry and warm. The amount of heat lost now balances that formed, and the temperature remains constant. It must be noticed that the thermostat of the heat-regulating mechanism is still under control but is geared to maintain the temperature at a higher level than normal. The normal daily variation in temperature is seen, so that the highest levels occur during the evening. This phase can last for several hours or days.

The Sweating Phase.   The temperature begins to fall, and the patient soon experiences a sensation of intense heat. The patient feels the urge to throw off clothing and sweats profusely, and then the temperature returns to normal. When this phase occurs over a short period, the termination is described as "crisis." This is particularly characteristic of lobar pneumonia and attacks of malaria. In some illnesses, the pyrexia subsides slowly (such as in typhoid fever), and its termination is described as "lysis."

In old age and in debilitated subjects, no fever may occur even with severe infections. This absence of response is said to be of poor prognostic import. It is the opposite of childhood response to infection — with children, even a trivial infection can cause a high fever.

Chronic infections frequently cause fever, and the prolonged rise in metabolic rate combines with loss of appetite to produce wasting. Chronic pulmonary tuberculosis provides an example of this; the emaciated appearance of the patients earned the terms "consumption" and "phthisis" for the disease.

Infarction.   A mild fever is commonly seen in patients with infarction, such as of the lung or the myocardium.

Tumors.   Some tumors are particularly liable to produce pyrexia, even in the absence of a complicating infection. It is a well-known feature of Hodgkin's disease as well as of carcinoma of the kidney.

Hemorrhage.   Fever may follow bleeding, particularly bleeding into the gastrointestinal tract or the peritoneal space. Sudden bleeding from a ruptured ectopic pregnancy, for example, can produce acute abdominal pain, distention, and fever, which might mimic an infection.

Brain Damage.   Any cause of brain damage (*e.g.*, bleeding, infection, or infarction) can lead to an upset of the central heat-regulating mechanism, either by damaging the hypothalamus directly or by interfering with the outflow of autonomic nervous impulses.

Injury.   Fever lasting for several days often follows mechanical trauma, such as a crushing injury.

Severe Anemia.   During phases of acute hemolysis, fever is sometimes prominent.

Miscellaneous Conditions.   Fever is a prominent feature of acute gout and some of the collagen diseases (*e.g.*, lupus erythematosus and rheumatic fever). An adverse reaction to a drug is an important cause. In most instances, the disease is accompanied by an inflammatory reaction, and the fever is probably related to this (see below).

Diagnosis of Fever

Disease is so often accompanied by fever that the pyrexia itself is sometimes the presenting symptom.

Fever or pyrexia of unknown origin (*FUO* or *PUO*) is a common clinical problem, and accurate diagnosis demands considerable clinical skill combined with laboratory aids. A good history combined with a knowledge of epidemiology will sometimes suggest the correct diagnosis (see Case History I and Fig. 22–2).

CASE HISTORY I.   The patient was a 69-year-old man who had gone on an African safari for one month. While there, he had occasional attacks of diarrhea and had developed a chronic cough, which was productive of a large amount of sputum. He gave a history of having had such severe night sweats on several occasions that the whole bed had been soaked. Before leaving Africa, he developed a superficial skin infection between the fourth and fifth fingers of his right hand. Two days after arriving in Canada he was brought into the emergency ward, having collapsed at home while unpacking a suitcase. He had struck his head and had lost consciousness for about 20 minutes. He complained of a mild headache, had a temperature of 102°F, and had a laceration of the left frontal area of the scalp. Infection was noted on the hand, and the fever was attributed to this infection. He was given penicillin and sent home. The next day he felt quite well, but the following day he was found by a friend to be drowsy, although still responsive and able to watch a hockey game. The next morning he was found unconscious and was again admitted to a hospital — this time, in a coma. Blood and urine were obtained for culture, and numerous biochemical tests were ordered. In view of the history of cough and drenching night sweats, the possibility of pulmonary tuberculosis was considered; a radiograph of lung, however, revealed no evidence of disease. Cerebrospinal fluid was obtained by lumbar puncture and revealed an elevated protein content (56 mg per 100 ml). The patient was noted to be slightly jaundiced. Before the results of the various tests were obtainable, a blood film was examined and was found to contain a large number of malaria parasites (see Fig. 22–2). A diagnosis of malignant malaria with cerebral involvement was made, and emergency treatment with the antimalarial drug chloroquine was undertaken. Nevertheless, the patient rapidly deteriorated, developed hypotension, and died within four hours. This case illustrates how a good history and a knowledge of diseases endemic to particular geographic locations can help in arriving at a diagnosis. Attributing fever and loss of consciousness to a minor skin infection was a mistake that cost this patient his life.

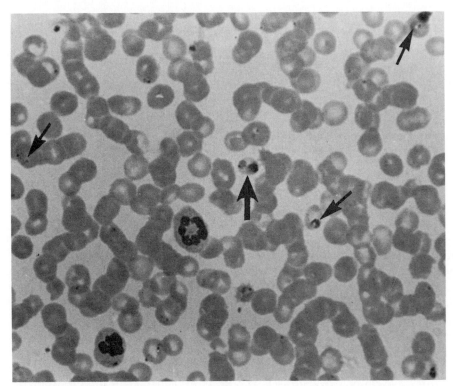

Figure 22–2. Blood film from patient with malignant tertian malaria. Numerous ring forms (small arrows) of *Plasmodium falciparum* are present in blood film. Particularly characteristic is the presence of two or more organisms in one red cell (large arrow). Blood film stained by Giemsa stain (× 1000).

A fever combined with a heart murmur suggests bacterial endocarditis; repeated blood cultures must be performed for an accurate diagnosis. Pulmonary tuberculosis can be remarkably silent but will be revealed by an x-ray. Fever in a patient past the age of 40 should lead to a search for occult cancer, fever in a child might suggest leukemia, and fever in a young adult might cause suspicion of infectious mononucleosis. In the diagnosis of PUO the physician's skills and knowledge can thus be taxed to the extreme (see Case History II).

CASE HISTORY II. A 30-year-old male was admitted to the hospital for the investigation of fever. Five weeks before admission, he had developed severe pain in the back, which had been relieved by aspirin. Two weeks later, the pain recurred and radiated toward the sternum. Although a heart attack was suspected, an electrocardiogram showed no abnormality; his serum enzymes were also normal. He had several bouts of fever during the next three weeks. On examination in the hospital he was found to be a pale, sallow, somewhat overweight man, who was sweating profusely and in moderate distress. His temperature on admission was 105°F, and his pulse was 120 beats per minute; blood pressure was 115/65 mm Hg. A murmur was heard over the precordium, and bacterial endocarditis was considered a possible cause. Numerous blood cultures were performed, all of which were sterile. Analysis of the urine was normal; culture was sterile. No obvious site of infection could be found clinically. The fever dropped to 100°F with aspirin but recurred each evening while the patient was in the hospital. Numerous other investigations were performed, including radiographs of the chest and vertebrae and an intravenous pyelogram. Blood was taken for the Widal, Weil-Felix, and brucella agglutination tests. Radiographs of the abdomen revealed no evidence of a subphrenic abscess such as might occur following a perforation of appendix, peptic ulcer, or diverticulum of the colon. All agglutination tests were negative, as was the VDRL test. A blood count was, however, unusual. In spite of the patient's having a fever, he had a total white count of 4400 with 95 per cent neutrophils and 4 per cent band forms. The platelet count was 95,000. Systemic lupus erythematosus was first considered, but since no anti-DNA antibodies were present in the blood, this condition was eliminated from consideration. In view of the unusual blood findings, a bone marrow puncture was performed, and the smear revealed almost complete replacement of normal marrow cells by primitive blast cells. There were a few normal erythroid precursors and virtually no megakaryocytes. In cases such as this, at times it is not possible to decide whether the cells are lymphoblasts or myeloblasts. The terms *stem cell leukemia* or *blast cell leukemia* are therefore convenient. About a week after admission, the patient still had a fever at night, and he developed ulceration of the mouth. He was treated with a variety of chemotherapeutic agents in courses over the next few months, but he died eight months after the first admission with bronchopneumonia. This case illustrates how malignant disease — in this case leukemia — can closely mimic infection by virtue of fever that is a presenting and constant feature.

Pathogenesis of Fever

The intravenous injection of gram-negative organisms produces a rigor and a sharp rise in temperature. This response appears to be due to lipopolysaccharide substances that are part of the bacterial body and are called *bacterial pyrogens*. They are thought to act indirectly by causing polymorphs to release an *endogenous pyrogen* that circulates in the blood and acts on the heat-regulating center. There is evidence that in humans a similar endogenous pyrogen can be released from monocytes as well as from polymorphs. The actual mode of action of endogenous pyrogens is complex. It appears that the substance acts on the heat-regulating center and sets its thermostat to a higher level. It is clear that the common pathogenesis of fever is the release of endogenous pyrogens from inflammatory cells. The precise action of endogenous pyrogens is probably an indirect one mediated by the release of local transmitters such as 5-hydroxytryptamine, a thermogenic amine, and a number of prostaglandins. As noted in Chapter 5, prostaglandin formation is inhibited by aspirin, and this action may well explain how this time-honored remedy acts to lower the body's temperature in fever.

The bacterial pyrogens are heat stable and are of importance because they can produce febrile reactions if present in the fluids used in intravenous therapy, which, though sterile, may still cause a sharp rigor (Chapter 26). The fluids used for injection purposes must be carefully prepared by distillation to insure the exclusion of all bacterial products. Such pyrogen-free fluids must always be used.

The fact that fever often accompanies necrosis, such as in tumors and infarcts and following hemolysis of red cells, suggests that dead tissue contains pyrogenic substances. Pyrogens similar to those of bacteria have been isolated.

Certain steroid hormones can produce a rise in body temperature, and it is believed that the release of progesterone is responsible for the temperature rise that occurs during the menstrual cycle.

In the fully anesthetized patient, the heat-regulating mechanism is not functioning. The body therefore becomes poikilothermic (like the body of an amphibian) and takes up the temperature of the surrounding atmosphere. The patient must therefore be protected against hyperpyrexia as well as hypothermia.

Fulminating or *malignant hyperpyrexia* is a rare but important condition in which there is a rapid rise in temperature during the administration of general anesthesia. The progress of the pyrexia is extremely rapid, and unless vigorous cooling is employed, the patient dies from hyperpyrexia and cardiac arrest. In most cases, the skeletal muscles show increased tension; it is believed that excess heat is produced in them. The precise cause of this condition is not known; in many instances, however, it is related to a type of muscle disease or myopathy that can be detected before surgery by finding an elevation of the serum levels of creatine phosphokinase, an enzyme that is released from damaged muscle. Sometimes there is a family history of myopathy.

Although recent work has shed some light on the mystery of fever, much has yet to be illuminated. It would be satisfying to believe that a rise in temperature in infection is a beneficial reaction designed to aid the body's defenses. There is, however, little evidence to support this. As yet, we must regard the maintenance of a normal temperature as an important homeostatic mechanism for the proper functioning of the body. Any marked departure from the normal appears to be, at best, of no value and, at worst, deleterious to well-being. There is some indication that fever is of benefit in virus infections. It seems that fever stimulates interferon production of infected cells and so may limit the course of the disease.

Hypothermia

Hypothermia may be defined as a body temperature below 35° C (95° F). It is an important cause of death in cold climates, especially of infants and the aged, and it has been utilized as an adjunct to anesthesia.

Hypothermia in Infants

Newborn infants are particularly susceptible to cold, because of the relatively high ratio of surface area to body mass, the paucity of subcutaneous fat, and the low production of heat by physical means because of the inability to exercise or shiver. Furthermore, the thermoregulatory mechanism is relatively inefficient at birth and remains so for several hours.

During the first few weeks of life, infants need constant warmth, especially when ill. In cold countries open windows, lukewarm baths, and power cuts can cause inconvenience to adults but can be fatal to infants.

The early signs of cold injury are lethargy and difficulty in feeding. Indeed, the child has a still, serene appearance, and the cheeks, nose, and extremities have a flush that deludes the onlooker into believing all is well. The cry is like a whimper, and the body feels cold. Later, bradycardia and edema of the eyelids and extremities occur. In the worst cases, the subcutaneous fat becomes hard.

Hypothermia in Adults

Hypothermia can occur in adults in a number of circumstances. Immersion hypothermia is one of the lethal factors in shipwreck. Hypothermia is an important complication of myxedema and hypopituitarism, and it also occurs in patients with widespread eczema and generalized erythroderma. In widespread skin disease, the passive diffusion of water through the epidermis is greatly increased, and heat is lost by both evaporation and convection.

The most important example is the spontaneous hypothermia that occurs in old people — usually women — who live alone in poorly heated rooms and are poorly clothed. Undernutrition is often an additional factor; in persons who are in both calorie- and protein-deficient states, the basal metabolic rate is decreased. Hypothermia in the aged is sometimes a complication of senile dementia or the effects of depressant drugs like alcohol and chlorpromazine that have dulled the mind. There is sometimes a severe precipitating infection such as pneumonia.

The patient with hypothermia looks ill. There is a corpselike chill of the body, and the rectal temperature can be as low as 21°C (70°F). The skin is pale, and the subcutaneous tissue is pliant and doughy. The patient remains still; muscles are rigid, and shivering is absent. The tendon reflexes are sluggish, and there is bradycardia, sometimes with atrial fibrillation. Since peripheral edema and puffiness of the eyelids are common, myxedema may be simulated. Oliguria (diminished urine output) is common, respiration is depressed, and death often occurs from cardiac arrest.

It is easy to overlook hypothermia, in both infants and adults. Clinical thermometers that register as low as 24°C (75°F) should be available and used if the circumstances raise the possibility of hypothermia.

Induced Hypothermia

Some animals have acquired the ability to hibernate for long periods in a state of hypothermia as a useful adjunct to survival in winter. From experimental work carried out on small animals, it has been found that they can be cooled below 0°C (32°F) if they are made first to ingest propylene glycol. Mice can be kept in suspended animation for about one hour and then reanimated by artificial respiration and microwave diathermy. Larger animals do not tolerate this treatment so well and usually die within a few days. A lesser degree of hypothermia has been used as an adjunct to cardiac surgery. If the body's temperature is lowered, cardiac arrest can be tolerated for about one hour. The development of extracorporeal circulatory systems has allowed profound hypothermia to be used in open-heart surgery. In one method, the blood is cooled rapidly by passage through a heat exchanger and the circulation is maintained extracorporeally. At the temperature of 12.7° to 15°C (55° to 59°F), the circulation is stopped, and the heart is opened in a bloodless field. When the operation is finished, the blood is rewarmed, the heart is defibrillated, and a normal circulation is restored. Extracorporeal circulations are now so efficient that hypothermia is less commonly used or is merely used as an adjunct to this procedure.

Local Hypothermia

Extreme cold causes tissue damage; when the part is rewarmed, an acute inflammation follows and blisters occur. Direct damage to the capillaries is prominent, and vascular occlusion contributes to tissue necrosis. This type of cold injury is called "frostbite" and in cold climates is not uncommon following accidental exposure to cold. Usually, the toes, fingers, ears, and nose are affected. Deliberate application of extreme cold (cryosurgery) is used therapeutically in surgical practice. Solid carbon dioxide and liquid nitrogen are commonly applied to warts and other skin tumors. Various types of probes that are refrigerated by liquid nitrogen have been devised for applying cold to deeper tissues. They have been used to treat eye tumors as well as intracranial surgery. At present, the use of cold is confined to special centers; the late effects are still being assessed.

Review Questions

1. Write an outline of the investigations that should be performed on a patient with pyrexia of unknown origin (PUO).

2. It is often assumed that fever indicates infection. Discuss this proposition, and give some examples of conditions in which fever is a manifestation of a noninfective process.

3. Compare the temperature-regulating mechanisms of an infant with those of an adult.

4. A patient develops a rigor following an intravenous injection of 500 ml of glucose solution. List the possible causes.

Selected Readings

Guyton, A. C.: Textbook of Medical Physiology. 6th ed. Philadelphia, W. B. Saunders Company, 1981. See in particular Chapter 72, "Body Temperature, Temperature Regulation, and Fever."

Noble, E.: Malignant hyperthermia need not be lethal. The Canadian Nurse, 76:33–37, 1980.

Petersdorf, R. B.: Alterations in body temperature. In Isselbacher, K. J., et al. (Eds.): Harrison's Principles of Internal Medicine. 9th ed. New York, McGraw-Hill Book Company, 1980, pp. 53–60.

Petersdorf, R. B.: Chills and fever. In Isselbacher, K. J., et al. (Eds.): Harrison's Principles of Internal Medicine. 9th ed. New York, McGraw-Hill Book Company, 1980, pp. 60–67.

Rae, D.: Accidental hypothermia. The Canadian Nurse, 76:28–33, 1980.

Disorders of Nutrition CHAPTER 23

After studying this chapter the student should be able to:

- Describe the metabolic effects of starvation.
- Distinguish between nutritional marasmus and kwashiorkor.
- Define obesity.
- Describe the differences between lifelong obesity and adult-onset obesity.
- List the endocrine disorders that are associated with obesity.
- List the complications of obesity.
- Classify and list the vitamins that are required by humans.
- Describe the sources of vitamin A and discuss the effects of vitamin A deficiency and excess.
- Describe the sources of vitamin C and give an account of scurvy.
- Classify beriberi according to its several forms and describe the features of each type.
- Describe the effects of riboflavin deficiency.
- Outline the main features of pellagra.
- Describe the effects of pyridoxine deficiency.
- Describe what is meant by a trace element.
- Describe the syndromes that are known to be caused by a deficiency of a trace element.

The most important disorders of nutrition relate to a deficiency or an excess of those components of the diet that provide both energy and the materials for the synthesis of proteins, carbohydrates, and fats. *Starvation* and *obesity* will be described first. The role of *vitamins* will then be considered. Finally, a note has been added concerning the *trace elements* — the note is short, for, although these elements are probably of great importance in the human body, remarkably little is known about their role in health and disease.

STARVATION

With the world population expanding at an estimated rate of 70 million each year, it is likely that malnutrition will become increasingly common. The effects of total starvation will first be described.

Metabolic Changes During Starvation

The body's store of glucose and glycogen is sufficient for only 1 day's metabolic needs. The protein supply and the triacylglycerols of adipose tissue provide enough energy for an additional 2 to 3 months in the average individual. For a fat person there are enough energy reserves for about 1 year's survival.

Immediate Changes in Starvation. The brain normally uses only glucose as fuel; after the first day of starvation the blood glucose level is maintained by new glucose formation in the liver, in which amino acids are used as fuel. The amino acids are provided by the breakdown of protein. Because the nitrogen component is excreted as urea, the body is in negative nitrogen balance.

The triacylglycerols of adipose tissue are broken down to glycerol and fatty acids. Fatty acids are converted into ketone bodies in the liver, and these are used directly by most organs of the body instead of glucose.

Later Changes in Starvation. After the first week of starvation the breakdown of protein declines rapidly. A change occurs in the brain's metabolism such that it is able to utilize ketone bodies, particularly beta-hydroxybutyrate, instead of glucose. Starvation can now continue until all the stores of body fat are utilized. When the supply of fat has been exhausted, only protein remains. The muscle masses decline and death soon follows.

During starvation the body conserves energy by reducing energy output. The starved individual is apathetic and lacks interest in life. Hypothermia is a danger in cold climates. This picture of starvation differs from that of the patient with anorexia nervosa, who is usually restless (Chapter 39).

Loss of water is a characteristic feature of early starvation. Its cause is unknown. For individuals who try weight-reducing diets this loss provides false encouragement during the first few days of the regimen. In starvation the kidney is unable to concentrate urine, and polyuria results.

The edema of starvation affects the dependent parts and appears to be due to the laxity of the subcutaneous tissues.

The wasted appearance of the starving person is all too familiar. The lax, dry skin and wasted muscles are matched by wasting of the internal organs. In particular, with advanced starvation the intestine becomes increasingly thin; hence, when treating a starving patient one must give frequent small feedings if the person's life is to be saved.

Protein-Calorie Malnutrition in Childhood

Protein-calorie malnutrition is regarded as a spectrum of disease with marasmus at one end and kwashiorkor at the other end.

Nutritional Marasmus

Marasmus is the name given to starvation in infants. It is due to deficiency of both protein and calories and is encountered in infants under 1 year of age. It is a common condition in the developing countries and is usually due to cessation of breast feeding when the mother again becomes pregnant. The child exhibits the wasted appearance of starvation and in addition shows lack of growth. In those who survive, dwarfism is a frequent complication. As with starvation in adults, the marasmic child is more susceptible to infection; tuberculosis and dysentery often complete the lethal process initiated by starvation.

Kwashiorkor

This is a syndrome observed in children between the ages of 1 and 3 years. Its name is derived from a local African word denoting illness in a child displaced from the breast by a subsequent pregnancy.

Kwashiorkor is due to a low protein intake and the presence of an adequate carbohydrate supply. It is characterized by a fatty liver and marked edema of the subcutaneous tissues. The inadequate protein supply leads to defective pigment formation; consequently, the hair becomes pale and even red in African children, and the skin is often depigmented and shows hyperkeratosis and flaking.

OBESITY

Obesity has been a problem of mankind since time immemorial, for evidence of it has been found in the relics of the Stone Age, in ancient Egyptian mummies, and in Greek sculptures. It is now rampant in the affluent world, as a walk down any main street in North America will bear witness. It has been estimated that approximately 20 per cent of middle-aged males and 40 per cent of middle-aged females are obese.

There is no precise definition of obesity, since there is no sharp cut-off from those individuals who are well covered and considered normal to those who are obese. For practical purposes an obese individual can be defined as one having a body weight over 20 per cent above mean ideal body weight based on height, build, and age. Life insurance companies have compiled tables giving such mean ideal body weights. The measurement of skin fold thickness over various parts of the body using simple calipers provides another guide. Skin fold thickness at the triceps greater than 23 mm for men and greater than 30 mm for women indicates obesity.

The number and variety of published weight-reducing diets and the existence of weight-losing clinics and spas bear witness to our lack of comprehension of this topic and the ineffectiveness of treatment.

Pathology and Pathogenesis

Two clinical types of obesity can be recognized:

1. Lifelong Obesity. Although of normal weight at birth, these individuals tend to be heavy as children and to have large spurts of weight gain during puberty, and in women during pregnancy. Fat tends to be widely distributed, affecting limbs as well as trunk. Eventually, these individuals tend to be grossly overweight, and weight reduction is a lifelong losing battle. A possible explanation for this type of obesity is that there is an increased number of fat cells *(adipocyte hyperplasia)*. The number of adipocytes appears to be fixed early in life. In the normal individual, adipose cell proliferation occurs during the first two years of life and again at puberty. In obese children, the number of adipose cells continues to increase throughout childhood.

2. Adult-Onset Obesity. These individuals are of normal weight until the age of 20 to 40 years and then steadily become obese. This "middle-aged spread" is associated with deposition of fat, predominantly in a central location. Hence, the increase in thickness of a scapular skin fold is greater than that of measurements taken over the triceps or ulna. The *number of fat cells is normal,* but they are overdistended with neutral fat. This is in contrast to persons with lifelong obesity, in whom there is fat cell hyperplasia.

The reasons for developing "middle-aged spread" are poorly understood: too little exercise, social customs, overeating, and overdrinking may all play a part. The key to the answer must be a knowledge of the mechanism by which food intake is adjusted to energy output. The presence in the hypothalamus of a feeding center and a satiety center has been postulated, but these centers are ill-defined and their regulation is not understood. Eating habits, emotional state, social custom, olfactory impulses, and visual temptations all influence an individual's desire to start eating, and indicate when he should stop. There can be no doubt that excess of calorie intake over energy expenditure results in excess fat deposition. When a steady state is attained, energy input again equals output, but the adipose cells remain overloaded and the feedback mechanism by which overfilled adipocytes inhibit appetite is defective. Unfortunately, we are quite ignorant of the mechanism involved.

Certain known causes of obesity will be listed, but they are rare.

1. Inheritance. There are strains of rats that are genetically destined to develop obesity due to adipose-cell hyperplasia. A human counterpart is possible, but the situation is obscured because environmental influences may override genetic traits. Obesity in a family may be the effect of adipose-cell hyperplasia induced by overfeeding in childhood.

2. Hypothalamic Lesions. See Chapter 39.

3. Hyperinsulinemia. This is usually due to a tumor of the islets of Langerhans.

4. Hypothyroidism. Obesity can result from hypothyroidism, but it is rarely marked. The popular treatment of obesity by administering thyroid hormone is not only dangerous but also quite ineffective.

5. Cushing's Syndrome. The distribution of fat in this condition is quite characteristic (Chapter 39).

6. Hypogonadism. Although eunuchs tend to be somewhat overweight, there is little evidence of hypogonadism in the common type of obesity.

Effects of Obesity

The effects of obesity are severe, for not only is life expectancy reduced but so also is the quality of life. Complications of obesity may include:

1. Diabetes Mellitus. In obese individuals there is insulin resistance due to tissue insensitivity to this hormone. It appears that there is a decreased number of insulin receptors on the adipocytes. Hyperinsulinemia results, and eventually diabetes mellitus of the insulin-independent (maturity-onset) type develops.

2. Atherosclerosis. Obese individuals develop hyperlipoproteinemia of a pattern that predisposes them to develop atherosclerosis.

3. Systemic Hypertension. This coupled with atherosclerosis renders the obese person particularly vulnerable to ischemic heart disease and cerebrovascular accidents.

4. Osteoarthritis. This degenerative disease affects particularly the large weight-bearing joints.

5. Hypoventilation (Pickwickian Syndrome). This syndrome is discussed in Chapter 30.

6. Operative Risks. The obese person is at risk following surgery not only because of ventilatory problems, but also because of the purely mechanical factors that the surgeon encounters when trying to enter an obese abdomen.

7. Miscellaneous. Intertrigo, varicose veins, gallstones, hernias, and toxemia of pregnancy are all more common in the obese than in the normal subject.

THE VITAMINS

Definition and Classification

Vitamins are organic substances that the body cannot manufacture and that are necessary for normal metabolism; only ten such substances are known. If these substances are present in insufficient quantity, disease results. The ten vitamins essential for good health are listed in Table 23–1.

Causes and Effects of Individual Vitamin Deficiencies and Excesses

Vitamin A (Retinol)

Vitamin A is one of the fat-soluble vitamins. In herbivorous animals the colored pigments (carotenoids, such as carotene) of plants and vegetables are converted into vitamin A in the intestine, are absorbed, and subsequently are stored in the liver. Humans acquire their supply either directly from the carotenoids in vegetable matter (*e.g.,* carrots, beet root, and green vegetables in general) or indirectly from animal or dairy products. The concurrent absorption of fat and the presence of bile salts in the intestine favor vitamin A absorption.

Causes of Vitamin A Deficiency. This is usually due to a deficient diet. This nutritional problem usually occurs in Indonesia, parts of Asia, India, the

TABLE 23–1. THE ESSENTIAL VITAMINS

FAT-SOLUBLE	WATER-SOLUBLE
Vitamin A	Vitamin C
Vitamin D	Vitamin B Complex
Vitamin K	Thiamine
	Riboflavin
	Niacin
	Pyridoxine
	Cobalamin (B_{12})
	Folate

Middle East, and Latin America: it is almost unknown in North America and Europe. Vitamin A deficiency does, however, occur as a complication of the malabsorption syndrome; indeed, the blood level of carotene or vitamin A is used as a measure of the degree of malabsorption occurring.

Effects of Vitamin A Deficiency

The Eye. Vitamin A forms an essential component of rhodopsin, a pigment in the rods of the retina. By absorbing light, rhodopsin initiates an electrical impulse that is transmitted to the brain and is interpreted as light. The first sign of vitamin A deficiency, therefore, is *night blindness.* Apart from this known biochemical action of vitamin A, its other functions remain a mystery in spite of much research. It is known that vitamin A regulates the structure of certain epithelial cells. In vitamin A deficiency, the epithelia of the genitourinary tract, the trachea, the nose, and the conjunctiva tend to undergo *squamous metaplasia.* The most important effect is in the eye. The conjunctival epithelium loses its mucus-secreting goblet cells and becomes keratinized, thereby taking on the characteristics of epidermis. The lacrimal ducts are affected in the same way, so that the eye becomes dry and subject to cracking and infection. The condition is called *xerophthalmia.* In due course the cornea becomes cloudy; with infection it can soften *(keratomalacia),* causing the globe to be perforated. The lens can be extruded, and blindness results. Indeed, vitamin A deficiency is a leading cause of blindness in the world.*

Other Effects. The replacement of respiratory epithelium (with its goblet cells and cilia) by keratinized squamous epithelium is a factor in the production of respiratory infections (see Fig. 30–8). Nevertheless, in the presence of a normal amount of vitamin A there is no evidence that an excessive intake can prevent respiratory infections. The time-honored tradition of administering children large quantities of vitamin A (in cod-liver oil) to prevent colds and respiratory infections appears to be quite ill-founded. Indeed, such a practice can cause toxic effects (see below).

In spite of the dramatic changes seen in epithelium in vitamin A deficiency, the biochemical nature of the defect is quite unknown. If a small piece of skin is grown in organ culture and is subjected to vitamin A deficiency, it soon shows hyperkeratosis. If an excess quantity of vitamin A is now added to the medium, the epithelium changes to a goblet-cell, mucus-secreting type. There is no evidence, however, that excess vitamin A in humans can convert normal keratinized epidermis into mucus-secreting epithelium.

Toxicity of Vitamin A

Acute Toxicity. Very large doses of vitamin A are toxic and can cause an increase in intracranial pressure with headache, blurring of vision and vomiting. This effect has been noticed by Arctic explorers after eating the livers of polar bears or bearded seals, which are very rich sources of vitamin A.

Chronic Toxicity. Chronic poisoning is sometimes encountered in children given the vitamin to treat acne or to prevent colds. The condition is easily overlooked, because the symptoms are vague and include loss of hair, dry skin, hyperpigmentation of the skin, liver damage, bone pains, and psychiatric symptoms.

---

*Other common causes are trachoma, diabetes mellitus, onchocerciasis, gonococcal ophthalmia, injury through accidents, cataract, and glaucoma. Although smallpox has now been eradicated, blindness caused by past cases of the disease is still common.

Vitamin D   Vitamin D is present in all fat-containing animal products, but its richest source is cod-liver and halibut-liver oil. Vitamin D is also formed in the skin by the action of ultraviolet light on 7-dehydrocholesterol. Vitamin D exists in several forms. The most active compounds are formed by the liver and kidney.

The main action of vitamin D is to maintain calcium balance by aiding in the absorption of calcium from the intestine. The effects of hypovitaminosis D — that is, rickets and osteomalacia — are considered in Chapter 40.

Hypervitaminosis D. Toxic doses of vitamin D can cause hypercalcemia and metastatic calcification (Chapter 40). Vomiting, diarrhea, drowsiness, and renal failure are the main clinical features.

Vitamin K   Vitamin K is widely distributed in vegetable and animal foods. It is also synthesized by bacteria in the gut. Vitamin K deficiency is considered in Chapter 26.

Vitamin E   Vitamin E includes a group of fat-soluble substances (tocopherols) that act as antioxidants. Various vitamin E deficiency states are recognized in animals. In humans, vitamin E deficiency has been described in premature infants and in patients having cystic fibrosis with severe steatorrhea (Chapter 33). There is unfortunately no good evidence that excess vitamin E can ward off old age, coronary disease, or the other ills that are associated with the aging process.

Vitamin C (Ascorbic Acid)   Humans share with other primates and the guinea pig the feature of being among the few mammals that cannot synthesize vitamin C. The main dietary sources are citrus fruits, currants, berries, green vegetables, and potatoes.

Vitamin C is needed for the synthesis of collagen; a deficiency of this vitamin causes *scurvy*. The effects in adults are different from those encountered in children.

Adult Scurvy.   The outstanding feature is swelling and bleeding of the gums. This is seen only in those who have teeth, and it is associated with infection. Wound healing is impaired (Chapter 7). Bleeding into the skin is characteristic and is first detected around the hair follicles. Bleeding may also occur into the joints, the gastrointestinal tract, and elsewhere.

In the past, scurvy has plagued sailors on long sea voyages, because the disease first becomes manifest after a person has been on a deficient diet for about 2 months. For example, Vasco da Gama is reported to have lost 100 men of his 160-man crew on his trip around the Cape of Good Hope (1497). Lind, a British naval surgeon, introduced oranges, limes, and lemons into his sailors' diet in 1747, and he thereby earned the nickname of "limey" for his countrymen.

Infantile Scurvy.   Milk and milk products are often a poor source of vitamin C; consequently, scurvy can develop in infants at about the age of 8 months. There is impaired osteoid formation, and the epiphyses can become dislocated. An outstanding feature is subperiosteal hemorrhages, which are extremely painful. Bleeding can occur elsewhere, but gum lesions are not seen unless the teeth have erupted.

Vitamin B Complex   **Thiamine.**   Thiamine is a coenzyme necessary for several steps in carbohydrate metabolism. In the absence of this vitamin, lactic and pyruvic acids accumulate rather than enter the Krebs cycle. The vitamin is widely distributed in foodstuffs. Thiamine deficiency was once prevalent in the Orient, where polished (highly milled) rice formed the staple diet (the process of milling removes most of the thiamine from the rice). Thiamine deficiency is now much less common in the world, but it is still encountered in the Orient, particularly in persons of all ages living in isolated communities, in infants, and in pregnant women. In North America it is sometimes encountered in chronic alcoholics.

Effects of Thiamine Deficiency.   The early symptoms of thiamine deficiency (called beriberi) are vague: weakness, swelling of the ankles, "pins and needles" (paresthesia), and numbness of the legs. At any time, one of the two major severe forms may develop:

Wet Beriberi.   In this form it is theorized that the accumulation of lactic acid and other vasodilator chemicals causes so much vasodilatation that a form of high-output heart failure develops. The outstanding features are extensive edema and accumulation of fluid in the serous sacs. Sudden death from heart failure is not uncommon.

Dry Beriberi.   The outstanding feature of this form is degeneration of nerve fibers, particularly of the peripheral nerves (polyneuropathy). Numbness and anesthesia are the results of sensory nerve damage, whereas weakness and muscle wasting are the effects of motor nerve involvement. The patient eventually becomes bedridden.

Two other effects of thiamine deficiency are noteworthy:

Infantile Beriberi.   Infants with a low thiamine intake can develop acute beriberi between the ages of 2 and 6 months. The sudden development of heart failure, which is often fatal, is characteristic.

Wernicke's Encephalopathy and Korsakoff's Psychosis.   These conditions, described in Chapter 44, may occur with other forms of beriberi, but in Europe and North America they are invariably encountered in alcoholics.

Treatment of Beriberi.   Beriberi responds promptly to thiamine administration; with the wet form, early treatment is essential, since sudden death is common. Likewise, in Wernicke's encephalopathy, delay may lead to irreparable brain damage.

Riboflavin.   Riboflavin is a constituent of many foods and is a component of several enzymes that play a vital role in metabolism. Yet the lesions associated with its deficiency are ill-defined. A sore mouth is an early symptom. The angles of the mouth become macerated and later develop cracks (*angular stomatitis or perlèche),* the lips become sore, dry, and cracked (*cheilosis),* and the tongue becomes smooth and sore (*glossitis).* A scaly dermatitis, resembling seborrheic dermatitis, develops later and affects the face and the scrotum or vulva.

Niacin.   Niacin is a generic term that includes nicotinic acid and nicotinamide. As with thiamine and riboflavin, this vitamin is widely distributed in plant and animal food and is also a component of important enzymes. Deficiency of niacin causes *pellagra,* a disease so named because of the rough skin (from the Italian *pelle agra,* or "rough skin") that is present. Pellagra is a disease of poor peasants who subsist chiefly on maize (American corn). Although this cereal contains niacin, the vitamin is in a bound form. Furthermore, maize is deficient in tryptophan, an amino acid from which the body can manufacture niacin.* Indeed, pellagra is probably caused by a lack of niacin, tryptophan, and riboflavin, perhaps combined with an excess of toxic or antivitamin substances.

Pellagra was once common in Spain and Italy. It became widespread in the United States in the early 1900s but it has been largely swept away by

---

*Strictly speaking, niacin should not be labelled a vitamin, since it can be manufactured from tryptophan in the body. However, 60 mg of tryptophan is needed to produce 1 mg of niacin, and by convention niacin is always included in the list of vitamins necessary for humans.

improved economic circumstances. Nevertheless, it is still sometimes encountered in chronic alcoholics.

Symptoms. The symptoms of pellagra are most easily remembered as the *four D's:*

Dermatitis. Erythema, superficially resembling a sunburn, is present on the sun-exposed areas. This may progress to blistering and a chronic type of dermatitis.

Diarrhea. Diarrhea is common, as is a smooth, sore tongue of "raw beef" appearance.

Dementia. Mental symptoms are common; they may be in the form of acute delirium or a chronic manic-depressive state followed by progressive dementia.

Death. Death was a common end-result of pellagra before the advent of vitamin therapy.

Pyridoxine (Vitamin B$_6$). Pyridoxine is also a component of important coenzymes. Dietary deficiencies are unusual, but pyridoxine deficiency has been reported as a complication of drug therapy — particularly with the administration of isoniazid, which is used in the treatment of tuberculosis. It has also been reported as a complication of taking the birth control pill. A seborrheic type of facial dermatitis, angular stomatitis, sore tongue, and anemia are the main effects.

It is evident from this short account that thiamine, riboflavin, niacin, and pyridoxine are widely distributed in food and that deficiencies are due to an unbalanced or inadequate diet. Such dietary deficiencies are generally the effect of poverty, ignorance, or alcoholism. It follows that multiple deficiencies are often present in the same patient. Hence, it is common and acceptable practice to treat a patient with a prescription containing a mixture of all members of the vitamin B complex.

Cobalamin (Vitamin B$_{12}$) and Folate. These vitamins are necessary for red-cell maturation. The absence of these substances leads to a megaloblastic anemia (Chapter 26).

MINERALS

Electrolytes

Sodium, potassium, magnesium, and chlorine are generally available in abundance and are considered in Chapter 19. Calcium metabolism is considered in Chapter 40.

Trace Elements

Inorganic elements that are present in the tissues in trace amounts (micrograms to picograms per gram of wet tissue) are termed trace elements. The following are thought to be essential to life: chromium, cobalt, copper, fluorine, iodine, iron, manganese, molybdenum, nickel, selenium, silicon, tin, vanadium, and zinc.

The precise role of these elements is incompletely understood. The metals are often involved in the activation of enzymes or are part of the enzyme molecule itself. Disease can occur as a result of a direct excess or deficiency of a trace element, or more often there is an imbalance among several metal ions wherein an excess of one affects the function of another. Hence, simple measurement of the concentration of one ion does not necessarily reflect its activity in vivo. Furthermore, the actual measurement of trace elements is technically difficult and not within the expertise of most pathology laboratories. It is therefore not surprising that, with the exceptions of iodine and iron, the syndromes of trace element excesses or deficiencies are not well documented.

Zinc deficiency has been reported in childhood as a cause of retarded growth and hypogonadism. A better documented syndrome is *acrodermatitis enteropathica,* which is characterized by severe diarrhea, loss of hair (alopecia), and ulceration around the body orifices and on the extremities. The disease is apparently caused by zinc deficiency in patients with an autosomal recessive defect. The possible role of zinc in wound healing is mentioned in Chapter 7.

Copper deficiency is rare in humans but has been reported as a cause of anemia and leukopenia.

1. Describe the changes that occur in the metabolism of the brain during starvation.

2. You encounter a patient with gross obesity. Describe the features in the patient's history and general appearance that would give you a lead as to the cause and pathogenesis of the condition.

3. Describe the effects of vitamin deficiency on the skin and the mucous membranes.

4. Describe the effects of thiamine deficiency and indicate the circumstances under which it might be encountered in North America.

5. Give a brief account of the importance of zinc in the human diet.

Cahill, G. F.: Starvation in man. New England Journal of Medicine, *282:*668–675, 1970.

Hirsch, J.: The adipose-cell hypothesis. New England Journal of Medicine, *295:*389–390, 1976.

Leading Article: Laboratory tests in protein-calorie malnutrition. Lancet, *1:*1041–1042, 1973.

Lehninger, A. L.: Biochemistry. 2nd ed. New York, Worth Publishers, Inc. See Chapter 13, pp. 335–360, for a description of the vitamins and pp. 840–845 for a description of starvation.

Mason, J. B., Hay, R. W., Leresche, J., et al.: Treatment of severe malnutrition in relief. Lancet, *1:*332–335, 1974.

Truswell, A. S.: Nutritional factors in disease. *In* Macleod, J. (Ed.): Davidson's Principles and Practice of Medicine. 13th ed. Edinburgh, Churchill Livingstone, 1981, pp. 83–127.

CHAPTER 24

Metabolic Disorders

After studying this chapter the student should be able to:

- Describe how the level of blood glucose is regulated.
- List the hormones and their actions that are involved in glucose homeostasis.
- Classify the types of diabetes mellitus.
- Distinguish between insulin-dependent and insulin-independent diabetes mellitus with respect to:
  - (a) age of onset
  - (b) etiology
  - (c) pathogenesis
- Outline the laboratory tests used in the diagnosis of diabetes mellitus.
- List the complications of diabetes mellitus.
- Describe the causes and effects of hypoglycemia.
- Describe the clinical and pathological features of gout.
- Distinguish between primary gout and secondary gout.

GLUCOSE METABOLISM

The most important upset of glucose metabolism is diabetes mellitus. The frequency of this disease, which affects about 3 per cent of the population, has stimulated a vast amount of research into glucose metabolism. Yet even today there are many aspects of the disease that are incompletely understood.

Glucose is used as a fuel by many cells of the body and is the only substance used by the brain under normal circumstances. Hence, the maintenance of a blood glucose level within narrow limits (55 to 90 mg/dl or 3.0 to 5.0 mmol/L in the fasting subject) is an important homeostatic mechanism. The blood level is mainly regulated by the balance between the production of insulin, which lowers the blood glucose level, and the activity of the liver, which can either store glucose as glycogen or produce glucose from glycogen (*glycogenolysis*) or noncarbohydrate sources (*gluconeogenesis*). Following the absorption of glucose from the intestine, the rise in the blood glucose level stimulates the secretion of insulin from the pancreatic islets by a direct action. Furthermore, various intestinal hormones are released, and these also act on the pancreatic islets to promote secretion. Insulin enhances the entry of glucose into cells by aiding its transport across cell membranes. This is particularly important in resting muscle and fat cells, which are the *insulin-dependent tissues*. Following the ingestion of 100 g of glucose only about 15 per cent enters these tissues along insulin-dependent pathways. An additional 25 per cent escapes from the splanchnic bed and is utilized to meet the ongoing glucose needs of insulin-independent tissues, especially the brain. From 55 to 60 per cent of the glucose absorbed is retained in the liver, for there is no barrier to its entry into liver cells and this organ is well situated anatomically to intercept glucose from the portal vein and prevent it from entering the systemic circulation. In the liver, glucose is utilized in the synthesis of glycogen and triglycerides. It follows that in the normal person, even after a carbohydrate meal, the blood glucose does not rise above 160 mg/dl (9 mmol/L), this forms the basis of the glucose tolerance test.

In this test a fasting subject previously on an adequate carbohydrate diet is given 100 g of glucose by mouth. The blood glucose should not exceed 90 mg/dl (5 mmol/L) at the start of the test nor 160 mg/dl (9 mmol/L) an hour later. It should have returned to normal after 2 hours. When the blood level of glucose exceeds 180 mg/dl (10 mmol/L), glucose escapes into the urine because the renal tubules are no longer able to reabsorb the excessive amount that is present in the glomerular filtrate. *Glycosuria* therefore results.

In the fasting state the liver and insulin-dependent tissues (resting muscle and fat) show little glucose uptake. The insulin-independent tissues, particularly the brain, show a continued glucose uptake, and the normal blood glucose level is maintained by release of glucose from the liver.

Secretion and Actions of Insulin

Insulin is synthesized in the beta cells of the islets of Langerhans as pro-insulin, a polypeptide chain, the head and tail of which are united by two disulfide bonds. By the action of peptidases the middle segment (termed the C peptide) is excised, leaving the two ends of the molecule to form the A and B chains of the insulin molecule. They remain united by the original disulfide bonds. The formation and excretion of C peptide have been used as a measure of the rate of insulin synthesis. The major stimulus for both synthesis and release of insulin is hypoglycemia. Gastrin, secretin, and other intestinal hormones also stimulate the islets of Langerhans, and the release of these hormones following oral administration of glucose plays a minor role in promoting insulin secretion.

The target cells of insulin are the adipose tissues and muscle, both of which have specific insulin receptors. Glucose transport into the cells is enhanced, and glycogen synthesis is increased. Insulin promotes the synthesis of protein from amino acids and inhibits the breakdown of neutral fat (*lipolysis*).

Furthermore, insulin has two important effects on the liver. Glycogenolysis is inhibited by small doses of insulin, whereas larger doses inhibit gluconeogenesis. The net effect of insulin is to lower the blood glucose level; since the half-life of the hormone is about 3 minutes, the continuous and varying secretion of insulin is the main regulatory mechanism by which the blood glucose level is normally maintained within narrow limits.

Other Hormones Affecting Glucose Metabolism

Five other hormones have important effects on glucose metabolism:

Glucagon. This hormone is secreted by the alpha cells of the islets of Langerhans and is released whenever the blood glucose level drops below 80 mg/dl (4.5 mmol/L). Its main action is to stimulate the liver to break down glycogen into glucose, which is then released into the blood. Lipolysis is stimulated in the adipose tissues. It is evident that glucagon counterbalances the actions of insulin.

Epinephrine. Epinephrine raises the blood glucose level by promoting glycogenolysis in the liver and muscles.

Pituitary Growth Hormone. This hormone opposes the actions of insulin, thereby raising the blood glucose level.

Adrenoglucocorticoids. These decrease glucose utilization in muscle and fat. Gluconeogenesis in the liver is stimulated and the blood glucose level rises.

Somatostatin. This hormone of the hypothalamus inhibits the release of insulin from the islets of Langerhans.

Diabetes Mellitus

The discovery of insulin by Banting and Best appeared to provide both an explanation of the pathogenesis of diabetes mellitus and an effective treatment. Ironically, this outstanding discovery tended to retard further research into the true nature of the disease, so that even today its precise pathogenesis is not understood. It has become evident that insulin deficiency is only one factor in the disease. Many diabetics need insulin in quantities far in excess of those required by totally pancreatectomized individuals. Some diabetics have a normal blood insulin level or even one that is above normal. Moreover, although insulin therapy can prolong the life of some diabetic subjects, it fails to prevent premature death from some of its cardiovascular complications. The life expectancy of a diabetic is still below that of the normal individual.

Definition and Types of Diabetes Mellitus

Diabetes mellitus may be regarded as a syndrome characterized by relative or absolute deficiency of insulin. Three main types of disease may be recognized.

1. Spontaneous Diabetes Mellitus.   Over 90 per cent of diabetics fall into this group. It is probably a heterogeneous collection of diseases, but for simplicity it can be divided into two main types:

(a) *Type I or Insulin-Dependent Diabetes Mellitus (IDDM).*
(b) *Type II or Insulin-Independent Diabetes Mellitus (IIDM).*

2. Diabetes Mellitus Associated with Other Endocrine Disorders.   In these conditions there is an overabundant production of hormones that counteract the actions of insulin.

3. Diabetes Mellitus Associated with Pancreatic Disease.   Diabetes is occasionally encountered as a complication of chronic pancreatitis, hemochromatosis, cystic fibrosis, or total pancreatectomy performed for carcinoma.

Spontaneous Diabetes Mellitus

Since the earliest descriptions of diabetes mellitus, it has been recognized that the disease is familial and that it could occur either in a severe lethal form or as a mild affliction associated with gluttony, obesity, and somnolence. It is now evident that spontaneous diabetes mellitus is not an entity in itself but a collection of separate diseases with many overlapping features. Two types will be described, but this must not be regarded as an absolute classification, because future research will no doubt unfold the truth.

Type I or Insulin-Dependent Diabetes Mellitus (IDDM).   This type of diabetes generally begins abruptly and is often called juvenile-onset diabetes, since it generally commences before the age of 30 years. The symptoms are thirst (*polydipsia*), increased volume of urine produced (*polyuria*), weight loss in spite of a good appetite, blurring of vision, general lassitude, and sometimes a craving for sweet beverages. Nausea, vomiting, coma, and death follow within weeks or possibly months. Only insulin therapy can save these patients.

Etiology.   Type I or IDDM is strongly associated with certain HLA haplotypes (*e.g.*, B8, Bw15, Dw3, and Dw4). There are several explanations for this association:

1. The haplotypes are closely linked with other, as yet unidentified, genes that are held responsible for the disease.

2. The haplotypes associated with the Ir gene render the subject susceptible to certain viral infections that cause the destruction of the islets.

3. The immune state is so primed that autoantibodies against islet tissue can be formed. This could follow damage to the islets by viral infection or possibly by some chemical poisons.

Histologically the islets show cell degeneration and infiltration with lymphocytes. These changes are consistent with an infection or an autoimmune process. In support of the latter concept is the observation that 60 to 85 per cent of patients have demonstrable autoantibodies in their serum that react to islet cell components.

Pathophysiology. In fully developed Type I diabetes mellitus the blood level of insulin is very low. The uptake of glucose by muscle and fat cells is low, and the liver manufactures glucose from glycogen and noncarbohydrate sources — mostly amino acids derived from muscle, which therefore wastes.

In this type of severe diabetes mellitus there is hyperglycemia even in the fasting state. Following a carbohydrate meal the blood glucose level rises even higher, since in the absence of insulin the storage of glycogen in the liver is inhibited. The presence of glucose in the urine necessitates an increased volume in order to contain it, an effect called *osmotic diuresis*. This leads to a loss of water and electrolytes, and the patient becomes dehydrated and thirsty, hence the polyuria and polydipsia. The fluctuating levels of blood glucose lead to osmotic effects in the lens and humors of the eye. This causes blurring of vision.

In the absence of insulin, lipolysis in the adipose tissue is accelerated. The released fatty acids are utilized by the liver to form acetylcoenzyme A. Although normally this could enter the Krebs cycle, in the absence of insulin it is converted into ketone bodies (β-hydroxybutyrate, acetoacetate, and acetone) (see Fig. 2–10). Finally, with low insulin levels the use of ketone as a fuel by peripheral tissues is inhibited. The net effect of these changes in fat metabolism is hyperketonemia (and ketonuria) and a metabolic acidosis that is responsible for diabetic ketoacidotic coma and death.

It is evident that in diabetes mellitus of this type the body's metabolism is geared to maintaining a high blood glucose level, even though this exceeds the renal threshold. The body literally starves in the midst of plenty, as fats and proteins are converted into glucose, only to be passed in the urine and lost from the body. Loss of weight and hunger are therefore characteristic symptoms.

Type II Diabetes Mellitus or Insulin-Independent Diabetes Mellitus (IIDM). This type of diabetes mellitus can occur at almost any age but is most common after the age of 40 years and is therefore commonly called maturity-onset diabetes. The disease has an insidious onset, and its symptoms are mild. Ketoacidosis is uncommon. Often the disease is detected by biochemical examinations prompted by the onset of one of the complications of the disease.

Etiology. Type II diabetes mellitus is a familial disease, but the precise mode of inheritance is not known. Hence, the disease is usually described as being multifactorial, with genetic and environmental factors playing a part. There is no association with HLA types as in Two I diabetes mellitus.

Pathophysiology. In Type II diabetes mellitus the blood insulin levels may be low, normal, or high. In the early stages of the disease the pancreas is slow to respond to the rise in blood glucose that follows a carbohydrate meal. Hence, hyperglycemia results but is transient because it stimulates the islets of Langerhans to produce excess insulin, and this results in *hypoglycemic attacks*. This phase of the disease is temporary.

Histological examination of the pancreas gives no clues to the nature of the defect. The islets may appear normal, or in the later stages of the disease they may be atrophic with fibrosis or infiltration by amyloid tissue.

Since absolute lack of insulin does not seem to be the cause of Type II diabetes mellitus, some other factor must be in operation. The presence of insulin antagonists or excess of secretion of glucagon have been proposed but appear not to be major factors.

Insulin resistance of tissues is the major abnormality. It has been suggested that peripheral tissues show a decrease in the number of insulin receptors per cell. A complicating factor is *obesity*, for it is known that obesity itself causes insulin resistance.

Patients with Type II diabetes mellitus do not generally require insulin therapy. Often their disease can be managed by drugs or diet alone. In particular, those patients who are obese are greatly helped if they can lose weight.

In summary, it may be supposed that some individuals have a genetic fault that prevents the islets from producing adequate insulin when the demand for this hormone increases. Resistance of the tissues to insulin occurs with obesity. Whether the tendency to develop obesity in diabetes mellitus is itself inherited is undecided. Obesity could be an effect of the disease, because there is sufficient insulin in Type II diabetes to inhibit lipolysis in fat cells. Hence, wasting is not a feature of this type of the disease. The situation is clearly complex, because 20 per cent of Type II diabetics are not obese, and some other cause for insulin resistance must operate. Pregnancy is one factor that can cause such insulin resistance. The differences between the two types of diabetes are summarized in Table 24–1.

Diagnosis of Diabetes Mellitus

Three stages of the disease are recognized:

Prediabetes.   The subject has the inherited tendency to develop the disease but has neither symptoms nor detectable biochemical abnormality. Diagnosis is impossible until after the subject has developed diabetes.

Chemical Diabetes.   Symptoms are absent, and the fasting blood-sugar level is normal. The glucose tolerance test is, however, abnormal. A random blood-glucose determination is of little value in diagnosis at this stage. To avoid the tedious three-hour glucose tolerance test, one may take a single blood sample two hours after a carbohydrate meal as a screening test.

Overt or Clinical Diabetes.   Symptoms are present, the fasting blood glucose is raised, and glycosuria is present.

Complications of Diabetes Mellitus

Diabetic Ketosis and Coma.   This is most common in the growth-onset type of the disease and may be precipitated by a diabetic patient's failure to administer his insulin. Vomiting and abdominal pain may be severe enough to mimic an abdominal emergency. *This mimicking of one condition by another underlines the need to perform a routine urinalysis in all ill patients.*

Hyperosmolal Coma.   Very high blood-glucose levels (*e.g.*, over 1000 mg per dl) can produce such a diuresis and an elevation of blood osmolality that hypovolemic shock and cerebral dehydration lead to coma, even in the

TABLE 24–1.   COMPARISON BETWEEN INSULIN-DEPENDENT DIABETICS AND INSULIN-INDEPENDENT DIABETICS*

	INSULIN-DEPENDENT DIABETICS TYPE I	INSULIN-INDEPENDENT DIABETICS TYPE II
Age of onset	Usually under 30	Usually over 40
Ketoacidosis	Common	Rare
Body weight	Thin	80% are obese
Prevalence	0.5%	2–4%
Genetics	HLA-associated in 40–50%	Familial but not HLA-associated
Circulating islet cell antibodies	50–85%	Less than 10%
Treatment with insulin	Necessary	Usually not required

*Modified from Felig, P., Baxter, J. D., Broadus, A. E., and Frohman, L. A.: Endocrinology and Metabolism. New York, McGraw-Hill Book Company, 1981, page 799.

absence of ketosis. The condition is not common. It usually occurs in the maturity-onset type of diabetes.

Susceptibility to Infection. Diabetic subjects are particularly liable to recurrent infections of various types. These may be pyogenic, and skin infections such as recurrent boils should alert one to the possibility of an underlying diabetes mellitus. Recurrent cystitis, particularly in women, is common, as is candidal vaginitis. This is one of the causes of vulval itching (pruritus vulvae), which is a common complaint of patients with this disease. It is an old observation that diabetics are particularly susceptible to tuberculous infection of the lungs.

Vascular Disease. Diabetics are liable to develop more severe atherosclerosis than are nondiabetic subjects of a like age. Indeed, among diabetics myocardial infarction is the most common cause of death and is almost as frequent in females as in males. Involvement of the major vessels to the legs contributes to peripheral vascular disease. This may culminate in gangrene.

In addition to changes in the large vessels, the small vessels show a characteristic thickening of the intima. This constitutes *diabetic microangiopathy*. The changes can be seen in almost all tissues and combined with atherosclerosis are a major cause of the peripheral vascular disease described above. Nevertheless, the major effects of diabetic microangiopathy are borne by the kidneys, the eyes, and the nerves.

Renal Disease. The microangiopathy affects both the arterioles supplying the glomeruli and the vessels in the glomeruli themselves. The nephrotic syndrome may develop in some patients. Ultimately the vessels become thickened, basement-membranelike material accumulates between the capillaries, and the whole glomerulus becomes converted into an eosinophilic hyaline mass. This is associated with the development of chronic renal failure, and indeed this is a common mode of death in diabetes mellitus. There has been much argument in the past as to whether these vascular changes are caused by the hyperglycemia and other effects of the disease or whether they are associated with the primary defect. The matter is undecided, but there is little firm evidence that the methods of controlling diabetes now available can prevent the development of microangiopathy, particularly as it affects the kidneys and leads to renal failure.

Neuropathy. Diabetic microangiopathy can affect the nerves in a variety of ways. Most common is *diabetic polyneuropathy*, in which the axons of the sensory nerves "die back" from the periphery; that is, degeneration appears to begin in the distal portions of the axons and gradually spread more proximally. This results in a symmetrical loss of sensation of the hands and feet, giving the so-called stocking-and-glove effect. There is loss of sensation, which paradoxically is sometimes associated with spontaneous pain. The lack of pain sensation in the feet can lead to unnoticed injuries. Infection and gangrene can then follow. The polyneuropathy seen in diabetes mellitus is very similar to that which can occur in alcoholism, nutritional deficiencies, and uremia. Sometimes the neuropathy affects one nerve, and this is presumably the result of ischemic damage of a more localized nature. Neuropathy affecting the autonomic nervous system can lead to many diverse effects. Neuropathy affecting the gut may cause constipation or alternatively diarrhea and malabsorption syndrome. Difficulty with emptying the bladder can be another effect and can be complicated by urinary tract infection.

The balance between insulin and glucose requirements is easily upset by trauma and infection. Any diabetic patient who is subjected to surgery should therefore have skilled medical treatment.

Surgery and Diabetes Mellitus

Hypoglycemia

If the blood glucose is below 50 mg per dl, particularly if its fall is rapid, symptoms of hypoglycemia develop. These consist of sweating, hunger, mental confusion, and — in severe cases — coma, convulsions, and death. Common causes of hypoglycemia include:

1. Insulin Overdosage. All diabetic subjects on insulin therapy should be warned of the effects of hypoglycemia.

2. Diabetes Mellitus. In the early stages in the development of diabetes mellitus, the hyperglycemia that follows a meal may lead to such a delayed and excessive secretion of insulin by the pancreas that hypoglycemia follows.

3. Tumors of the Islets of Langerhans. An islet-cell tumor (adenoma or carcinoma) can cause periodic attacks of hypoglycemia.

PURINE METABOLISM

Gout

Clinical Features

Gout is a disease of great antiquity and is characterized by a high blood uric acid level (*hyperuricemia*) accompanied by recurrent attacks of acute arthritis. Deposits of urates are found in the joint cartilages, and these lead to chronic arthritis. Nodular deposits of monosodium urate are also found in connective tissues around the joints as well as in some nonarticular cartilages, particularly those of the external ear, where they are called *tophi*. The clinical features of gout were well recognized by Hippocrates; the classic features were described by Sydenham, who himself was a sufferer. The initial attack invariably affects the great toe and is characterized by the sudden onset of severe pain and inflammation. Rigors and fever accompany the attack, which usually subsides within a few days. It responds well to the administration of colchicine, a drug introduced into North America by Benjamin Franklin, who was yet another famous sufferer of gout, and still used today. Repeated attacks of arthritis occur and affect other joints; ultimately, a chronic arthritis develops in all four limbs, particularly in the distal joints. Urates are also deposited in the kidney, leading to renal damage and ultimately to renal failure. About one third of the patients develop kidney stones composed of urates.

Pathogenesis

Uric acid is the end-product of the metabolism of the purines derived from nucleic acid. Most of this uric acid is of endogenous origin, but some is exogenous, being derived from the diet. Two types of gout are recognized:

Primary Gout. This is a heterogeneous group of inborn errors of metabolism. In some types there is an overproduction of uric acid that is sometimes accompanied by a failure to recycle purines in the formation of new nucleic acid. In other types there is impaired renal excretion. Primary gout is familial and tends to affect males more often than females. The precise biochemical error causing most familial forms of gout is not understood. There are, however, some rare types of gout in which the enzyme defect is known.

Secondary Gout. As in primary gout, the secondary variety can be due either to increased production of uric acid or to decreased excretion of uric acid. Widespread malignant disease, such as leukemia and polycythemia — particularly if treated with cytotoxic drugs — is a common cause of secondary gout; this is due to overproduction of uric acid. Chronic renal failure, particularly if it is due to hypertension, and chronic lead poisoning can lead to typical attacks of gout through retention of uric acid.

The precise reason for the deposition of urates in joints, tendons, and cartilages is not understood. The acute attacks are believed to be due to the deposition of urate crystals in the joint spaces. These crystals are phagocytosed by polymorphs. Lysosomal enzymes are then released and mediate the local inflammatory reaction as well as the rigors and fever.

1. Explain why thirst is a common symptom of diabetes mellitus.

2. A patient who is known to have diabetes mellitus is found unconscious. Discuss the possible causes and indicate the test that would help in the differential diagnosis.

3. A patient is suspected of having diabetes mellitus. After a long wait in the outpatient clinic, he is finally examined at 11:30 A.M., and blood and urine samples are taken. No glucose was found in the urine, and the blood-glucose level was subsequently reported as being 100 mg/dl. Discuss the significance of these laboratory findings.

4. Discuss the relationship between the amount of body fat and diabetes mellitus.

5. Describe the symptoms of gout and indicate why the disease sometimes occurs as a complication of leukemia.

Review Questions

Baird, J. D.: Diabetes mellitus. *In* Macleod, J. (Ed.): Davidson's Principles and Practice of Medicine. 13th ed. Edinburgh, Churchill Livingstone, 1981, pp. 500–530.

Cahill, G. F., and Soeldner, J. S.: Diabetes, glucagon, and growth hormone. New England Journal of Medicine, *291*:577–578, 1974.

Foster, D. W.: Diabetes mellitus. *In* Isselbacher, K. J., et al. (Eds.): Harrison's Principles of Internal Medicine. 9th ed. New York, McGraw-Hill Book Company, 1980, pp. 1741–1755.

Leading Article: Pathogenesis of diabetes mellitus. British Medical Journal, 3:594, 1971.

Lehninger, A. L.: Biochemistry. 2nd ed. New York, Worth Publishers, Inc., 1975, pp. 810–822, 845–849.

McCormick, J. H., and Nuki, G.: Gout. *In* Macleod, J.: Davidson's Principles and Practice of Medicine, 13th ed. Edinburgh, Churchill Livingstone, 1981, pp. 635–639.

Robbins, S. L., Angell, M., and Kumar, V.: Basic Pathology, 3rd edition, Philadelphia, W. B. Saunders Company, 1981, pp. 135–151.

Selected Readings

The Plasma Proteins: Amyloidosis

After studying this chapter the student should be able to:

- Describe five methods used to separate the plasma proteins.
- List the causes of hypoalbuminemia.
- Classify the types of hypergammaglobulinemia.
- Outline how the erythrocyte sedimentation rate (ESR) test is performed, give the normal values, and indicate its usefulness.
- Classify amyloidosis and outline the main features of each group.
- Describe the effects of amyloid infiltration on the
    - (a) Heart
    - (b) Kidney
    - (c) Liver
- Outline what is known about the composition of amyloid.

The Plasma Proteins

The blood stream forms the major route by which the secretions of one organ can travel to distant parts of the body and influence other organs and tissues. It is not surprising, therefore, that an analysis of the blood itself has proved to be a rewarding pursuit and has shed light on many bodily functions. The fluid and electrolyte components have already been discussed in Chapter 19; in this chapter, the plasma proteins will be described. One great advantage of investigating the plasma proteins rather than tissue proteins is that blood is readily available and can be obtained easily with little inconvenience to the patient.

Methods of Separation

The plasma proteins have been classified in various ways; unfortunately, the terminology is quite complex. In order to understand the classification, it is essential to have an elementary knowledge of the physicochemical properties of the proteins, because the name attached to a particular member is often a reflection of the method used in its identification.

Knowledge of the evolution of the present rather complex system is instructive. *Fibrinogen* presents no great problem; it is a protein that forms an insoluble fibrin clot during coagulation. Until the middle of the last century the remaining serum was thought to contain a single protein called "albumin." It was then shown that by half-saturation of the serum with ammonium sulfate part of the protein could be precipitated (now called *globulin*), leaving the remainder in solution (the *albumin*). Estimation of these three fractions is a useful first step in clinical investigation. The normal levels are the following:

Albumin	4.0–5.7 g/dl	(40–57 g/L)
Globulin	1.3–3.0 g/dl	(13–30 g/L)
Fibrinogen	0.1–0.5 g/dl	(1–5 g/L)
TOTAL	6.2–8.2 g/dl	(62–82 g/L)

Figure 25–1. Cellulose acetate electrophoresis of serum. On the left, electrophoretic strips from eight separate sera are shown. The anode is on the left, and the dense band that has moved furthest to the left is due to albumin. No. 8 is normal serum, whereas Nos. 4 and 7 show a diffuse increase in the γ globulins. Each shows the picture of a polyclonal gammopathy. No. 1 shows a dense band in the γ-globulin area. The density of the bands of strip No. 1 is depicted in graphic form on the right. The various serum proteins are in the same relative positions on both the strip and the graph. The sharp spike in the γ region is characteristic of a monoclonal gammopathy. (From Hall, C. A.: Neoplasms of the blood. *In* Halsted, J. A., and Halsted, C. H. [Eds.]: The Laboratory in Clinical Medicine. 2nd ed. Philadelphia, W. B. Saunders Company, 1981, p. 476.)

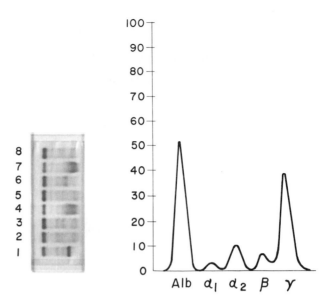

In aqueous solutions at a suitable pH, the proteins have a negative charge, so that when they are placed in an electric field, they migrate toward the anode. Individual proteins move at a particular rate dependent, to a great extent, upon their size and electrical charge. The test, called *electrophoresis*, is conveniently performed on strips of filter paper, starch gel, or cellulose acetate; an electric current is passed for a suitable time, the strip is dried, and the separated proteins are stained (Fig. 25–1). When serum undergoes electrophoresis, the albumin travels fastest as one large band. The globulins on the other hand separate into three major groups, which have been designated α globulin, β globulin, and γ globulin. In fact, each of these bands can be resolved into numerous smaller bands, each composed of a distinct protein. It is the separation and identification of the globulins that have presented the greatest challenge to the ingenuity of the biochemist. Immuno-electrophoresis, illustrated in Figure 25–2, is an invaluable technique. The protein fractions are separated by electrophoresis and then identified immunologically.

Another method of plasma protein separation uses a high-speed ultracentrifuge. Large molecules tend to settle quickly, whereas small ones can be spun down with greater difficulty. The various fractions that can be obtained are measured in *Svedberg units*. The large globulin molecules, termed *macroglobulins*, are spun down in the 19S fraction. This fraction contains an important group of antibodies, which are therefore designated IgM. The more abundant IgG forms the 7S fraction.

Some proteins precipitate out in the cold. These are called *cryoglobulins;* an abnormal increase in concentration *(cryoglobulinemia)* can cause trouble because of vascular obstruction when the hands are exposed in cold weather. Finally, some proteins contain either lipid or carbohydrate. The former are called *lipoproteins*, and the latter are termed *glycoproteins*.

It is evident that an individual chemical protein can be described in a number of ways. Thus, a single protein may be a macroglobulin in the 19S range, a γ globulin, and also a glycoprotein. This protein may also be an antibody and therefore an immunoglobulin. The function of a particular protein is yet another way in which it may be described.

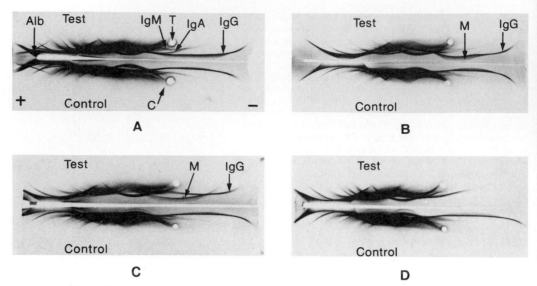

Figure 25–2. Immunoelectrophoretic patterns in disease. The technique is illustrated in *A.* The test is performed in an agarose gel. Test serum is placed in well "T," and a control normal serum is placed in well "C." A current is passed for a suitable period, and then the proteins tend to migrate toward the anode (+). Albumin (Alb) migrates most quickly, whereas IgG moves most slowly; under the conditions of the test, some IgG actually moves towards the cathode. The separated plasma components are demonstrated by placing antiserum to whole plasma down the central strip. From there the antibodies diffuse to form precipitin lines with each separated protein. The sheet is stained and photographed. *A,* The IgG band is heavier than that of the control and is closer to the central strip. Serum tested here was from a patient who has systemic lupus erythematosus and a polyclonal hypergammaglobulinemia. The IgA and IgM bands are clearly shown. *B,* An M protein is present and distorts the normal IgG band. The serum is from a patient with multiple myelomatosis and an IgG M protein. *C,* An M protein is present and is in the position of the normal IgA band. Note how the normal IgG band crosses the M protein. The serum is from a patient with multiple myelomatosis producing an IgA M protein. *D,* Note the deficiency of the IgG band. From a patient with congenital hypogammaglobulinemia. (Courtesy of Dr. K. C. Carstairs.)

Albumin Albumin, like most of the plasma proteins (with the notable exception of the immunoglobulins), is produced in the liver.

Hypoalbuminemia. Chronic liver disease, especially in the terminal phases, is often accompanied by hypoalbuminemia resulting from underproduction of this protein. Similarly, during starvation the plasma albumin level tends to fall rather more quickly than the other plasma protein levels. For reasons that are not well understood, the albumin level also falls during infections, especially if severe and in an acute phase; following trauma, including surgery; and following tissue necrosis, particularly if extensive, *e.g.,* a myocardial infarct. This appears to be due to increased catabolism and is accompanied by a rise in the α_2-globulins and fibrinogen. This has been termed the *acute reaction to stress.* Although the response is quite nonspecific — being mediated by the release of adrenal hormones — it forms the basis for a common pathological test—the *e*rythrocyte *s*edimentation *r*ate (ESR), which is discussed later in this chapter.

Hypoalbuminemia also occurs whenever there is excessive loss of albumin from the body. This is seen under several circumstances:

1. With the *nephrotic syndrome,* when large quantities are lost in the urine.

2. With *chronic loss of inflammatory exudate* from the body. Common examples are draining abscesses, extensive burns, and severe, infected wounds.

3. With *protein-losing enteropathy*, which is an uncommon cause of hypoalbuminemia and is due to loss of protein into the intestine. This syndrome is associated with a variety of gastrointestinal lesions, including gastric cancer, Crohn's disease, and ulcerative colitis.

Effects of Hypoalbuminemia. Albumin is a small molecule (molecular weight: 70,000) and is in high concentration in the plasma. It therefore constitutes the major noncrystalloid component of plasma. As would be expected, hypoalbuminemia leads to edema (Chapter 19).

Hyperalbuminemia. This occurs whenever there is hemoconcentration, due either to lack of water intake or to excessive water loss.

The globulins include a wide array of plasma proteins. The immunoglobulins form a major component: mostly they are present in the gamma fraction, but they are also found to a lesser extent in the beta fraction. The normal level appears to be maintained by the body's contact with microorganisms, particularly those in the intestine. Thus, in germ-free animals the γ globulin level is maintained at about one fifth of normal. When the intestinal flora of such animals is restored, the plasma proteins return to normal.

Hypergammaglobulinemia. Hypergammaglobulinemia is invariably due to an increase in the level of immunoglobulins. Two major patterns are described below:

Polyclonal Gammopathy. An increase in the gammaglobulins is seen in many chronic infections when there is a prolonged and marked immune response. Chronic tuberculosis, lepromatous leprosy, and kala-azar can be singled out as typical examples. It is also characteristic of those diseases in which the production of autoantibodies is a major component. Systemic lupus erythematosus is the prototype of this type of disease. Hypergammaglobulinemia is also characteristic of sarcoidosis; the pathogenesis, however, is obscure. The electrophoretic pattern in these conditions is that of a broad-based elevation of the γ globulins. There is an elevation in the levels of all classes of immunoglobulins, and it is assumed that many clones of antibody-forming cells are stimulated. Hence, the term *polyclonal gammopathy*.

Monoclonal Gammopathy. In some cases of hypergammaglobulinemia, it is found that the increase in gammaglobulin is due entirely to an increase in one particular protein belonging to *one* of the major classes — IgA, IgG, IgE, IgM, or IgD — and furthermore consists of either the lambda or the kappa variety. The supposition is that the globulin is produced by one particular clone of antibody-forming cells. Monoclonal gammopathy is usually associated with malignancy of the lymphoreticular system. The most common example is that of multiple myelomatosis, which is described elsewhere, but it is also seen in a variety of other malignant lymphomas and occasionally other malignant tumors. The term *M protein* (derived from *M*ultiple *M*yelomatosis; *M*alignant lymphoma; *M*alignant tumor) is therefore sometimes applied to an abnormal homogeneous protein, which appears as a spike on electrophoresis, in contrast to the broad-based increase seen in the polyclonal gammopathies (Fig. 25–1). The finding of such a spike in a case of hypergammaglobulinemia leads the physician to search for malignancy — particularly malignant lymphoma — in the patient.

The lipoproteins form a complex group of proteins and have now been divided into five major types. Elevated levels of some of these types are associated with the development of atherosclerosis, particularly coronary atherosclerosis, which causes heart attacks. Some cases of hyperlipoproteinemia are familial and are therefore genetically determined. Nevertheless, in most instances the hyperlipoproteinemia appears to be secondary to some

The Globulins

The Lipoproteins

other disease, particularly diabetes mellitus, alcoholism, and the nephrotic syndrome. In addition, the precise pattern of an individual's lipoproteins is influenced by his diet. This complex subject is of tremendous interest, since it is possible that by detecting a dangerous pattern of hyperlipoproteinemia at an early stage, treatment by diet or drugs can correct the abnormality and avert or delay subsequent heart attacks.

The Erythrocyte Sedimentation Rate (ESR)

When a column of blood rendered incoagulable with an anticoagulant such as citrate or oxalate is allowed to stand vertically, the red cells steadily gravitate downward, because their density is greater than that of the plasma. The speed at which this sedimentation occurs is dependent on several factors, the most important of which are the degree of rouleaux formation and the extent of sludging. In *rouleaux formation*, the red cells pile one on the other like an orderly pile of plates; in *sludging*, the massing of red cells with mutual adhesion is much more irregular and more closely resembles that of agglutination, except that the clumps of cells can be readily separated. Any increase in the plasma content of high–molecular-weight substances (*e.g.*, the macroglobulins and fibrinogen) is found to increase the ESR. The low–molecular-weight albumin *delays* red cell sedimentation. For this reason, a raised ESR is particularly characteristic of the acute reaction to stress (noted on page 340), macroglobulinemia, and hypoalbuminemia.

The ESR is normally higher in women than men, and it shows a significant rise with age. The upper limits of normal based on the commonly performed Westergren method* may be taken as 15 mm for men and 20 mm for women under the age of 50 years, and 20 mm and 30 mm, respectively, for those over that age. It is usually raised during infection and after tissue necrosis, *e.g.*, myocardial or pulmonary infarction. Presumably, an alteration in the balance between the plasma components is responsible, but the precise alterations concerned are ill-defined and rarely investigated. The nonspecific nature of the ESR limits its value in diagnosis; nevertheless, it is a useful investigation. It is of interest to note that the erythrocyte sedimentation rate was once introduced as a test for pregnancy, since ESR is elevated in this condition.

The presence of a raised ESR must always be taken to indicate disease, provided anemia and pregnancy are first excluded. Also, administration of birth-control pills is reported to raise it slightly. However, a normal ESR does not rule out organic lesions. A patient with a small carcinoma of the breast or lung often has a normal ESR. The ESR is of value in following the course of a known disease, such as tuberculosis and rheumatoid arthritis. Sequential measurements provide a useful indication as to the activity of the disease and its response to treatment. In the Wintrobe method of measuring ESR, the tube contains 1 ml of undiluted oxalated blood and is graduated from 1 to 100. The method has the advantage that after the ESR is read, the tube can be centrifuged and the packed cell volume can be measured. The normal level is 0.40 to 0.54 (Chapter 26).

It should be noted that the precise values of the ESR depend very much on the technique employed. The Westergren and Wintrobe methods give

---

*In the Westergren method the column of citrated blood is 200 mm in height. As the red cells sediment, a clear zone of plasma appears on top of the red-cell mass. The ESR is reported as the distance from the top of the plasma to the top of the red-cell mass at the end of one hour. The Wintrobe method uses a smaller tube (100 mm in height) and oxalated blood. It is less accurate but has the advantage of permitting the hematocrit to be measured by centrifuging the tube after a reading of the ESR at one hour. Partial clotting of a blood sample and other errors in technique can influence the ESR. An unexpected result should always be checked by repeating the test.

different figures. When using a laboratory, one must learn to appreciate the normal range of its findings.

Amyloid is an eosinophilic, hyaline material that is deposited in the extracellular spaces. It reacts with iodine in acid solutions to give a blue color; this superficial resemblance to starch led Virchow to call it starchlike or "amyloid." At a neutral pH it stains a mahogany-brown color with iodine. Amyloid is commonly identified in histological sections by the fact that it takes up the stain Congo red. When viewed under ordinary light the amyloid is pink in color, but with polarized light this changes to apple green.

Amyloid is not normally present in the body in detectable amounts; its deposition in the tissues constitutes the condition of amyloidosis.

Amyloidosis

Four types are recognized, although the distinction between them is not rigid. In all of them there are deposits of amyloid in many tissues.

Generalized Amyloidosis

Primary Amyloidosis. Generalized amyloidosis may occur as an idiopathic condition. The distribution is usually different from that of secondary amyloidosis (described below). Deposits tend to occur in mesenchymal tissues such as the tongue, respiratory tract, and heart. Liver, spleen, and kidney may be involved, although less extensively than with secondary amyloidosis. Amyloid is a rigid material, and its presence interferes with the mechanical activity of muscle. Hence, amyloidosis of the tongue interferes with swallowing, whereas the condition with cardiac involvement leads to intractable heart failure.

Secondary Amyloidosis. Deposits of amyloid are found beneath the endothelium of blood vessels and sinuses of liver, spleen, kidney, intestine, and many other organs but in smaller quantities (Figs. 25–3 and 25–4). The

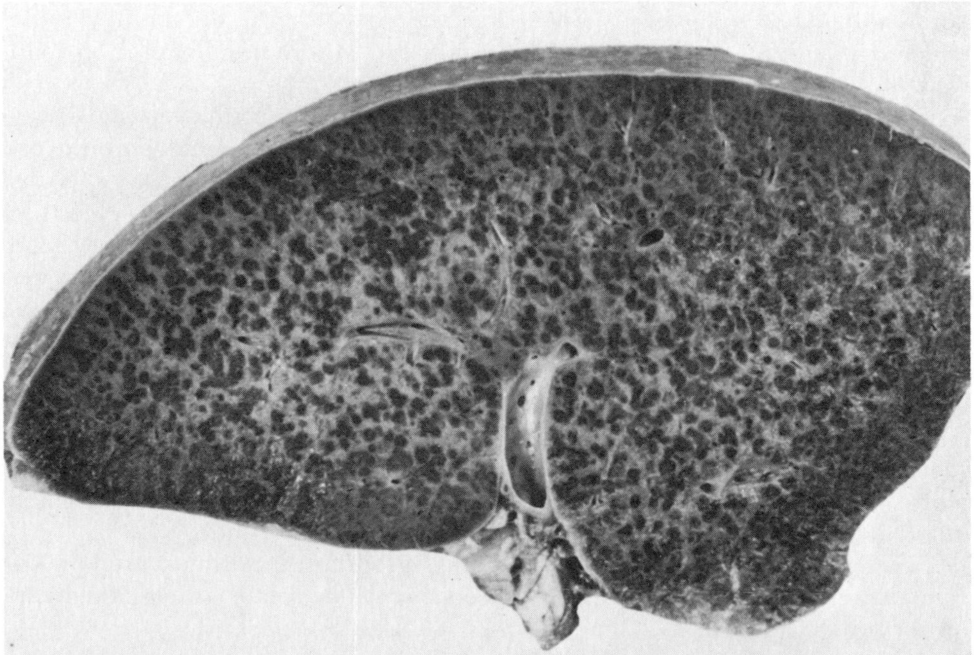

Figure 25–3. The spleen in amyloidosis. The patient had suffered from rheumatoid arthritis; during the last few months of her life, she developed the nephrotic syndrome (albuminuria, hypoalbuminemia, and edema). At necropsy, heavy deposits of amyloid were found in the liver, spleen, and kidneys. Smaller amounts were present in the intestine, lung, thyroid, and adrenal glands. The specimen pictured here is a cut surface of the spleen and has been treated with an iodine solution. Many dark, firm, semitranslucent nodules of amyloid material can be seen. These deposits have been likened to grains of sago. This type of splenic involvement, therefore, is commonly referred to as a "sago spleen."

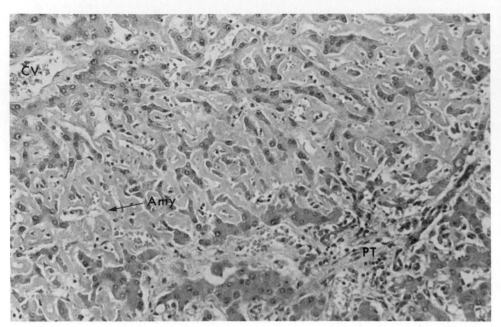

Figure 25–4. The liver in amyloidosis. There is extensive deposition of amyloid (Amy) around the liver sinusoids. This deposition has compressed the liver cells, many of which are small; others have disappeared completely. The liver cells around the central vein (CV) and the portal tract (PT) present a more normal appearance. A liver with this degree of involvement is enlarged, hard, and easily palpable. Nevertheless, clinical evidence of liver failure is generally lacking because of the reserve capacity of this organ (×250).

liver and spleen become enlarged and hard as the parenchyma is replaced by amyloid; such is the reserve of these organs that there is little functional derangement. The same response does not occur with the kidneys: the affected glomeruli leak protein. The nephrotic syndrome (Chapter 35) and renal failure result and prove fatal.

Causes. Generalized amyloidosis used to be encountered most frequently in patients with chronic suppurative infections (*e.g.*, chronic osteomyelitis and thoracic empyema), chronic tuberculosis, and tertiary syphilis with gummas. Presumably, the long-continued antigenic stimulation leads to the formation of amyloid. The presence of a soluble precursor in the blood would explain why amyloid is deposited in organs with a high reticuloendothelial cell content and in the kidney. Today generalized amyloidosis is associated with one of the following conditions: rheumatoid arthritis, lepromatous leprosy, and malignant disease (particularly Hodgkin's disease). It is also found in patients with large chronic bed sores associated with paraplegia and urinary tract infection.

Amyloidosis Associated with Multiple Myeloma. Amyloidosis is much more common in patients with multiple myelomas than with other malignant disease. Its distribution is similar to that of primary amyloidosis.

Heredofamilial Amyloidosis. Several hereditary syndromes are known. Each has characteristic features and affects particular organs, such as the heart or peripheral nerves.

Localized Amyloidosis   Amyloid can be deposited diffusely in one particular organ (*e.g.*, the heart, where it can lead to heart failure), or it can form tumorlike masses at any site (*e.g.*, lung, larynx, tongue, or bladder). Indeed, amyloidosis can mimic many diseases, thereby underlining the need for obtaining histological confirmation of the diagnosis of any mass. One cannot assume that all masses are neoplasms.

Amyloid is a protein that has two components. The minor one, called the *P component*, consists of rod-shaped structures made up of doughnut-shaped subunits piled up one upon another. These subunits are made up of part of the first component of complement (C1, Chapter 9). The major component of amyloid is a *non-branching fibril* that has a particular physicochemical configuration known as a β-pleated sheet. It has been found that many proteins, *e.g.*, insulin and calcitonin, can be partially digested to yield a β-pleated sheet that will aggregate *in vitro* to form a type of "amyloid." Analysis of the amyloid in human disease has revealed that two main chemical types occur:

Amyloid of Immunoglobulin Origin.   This type of amyloid consists of the light chains of the immunoglobulin molecule or part of the light chains. It is found in the amyloid deposited in patients with multiple myeloma, and the amino-acid sequence of the amyloid is identical to that of part of the M protein present in the blood and the Bence-Jones protein found in the urine. These are products of the tumor cells.

Amyloid of immunoglobulin origin is also found in primary generalized amyloidosis, and it is likely that some, perhaps all, patients with primary amyloidosis will eventually develop multiple myeloma or some similar malignancy of immunoglobulin-producing cells.

Amyloid of Unknown Origin (AA).   The amyloid of secondary amyloidosis has no amino-acid sequences in common with immunoglobulin and is of unknown origin — possibly it is derived from the breakdown of tissue in the areas of disease that are associated with the amyloidosis. It has been found that the blood of patients with secondary amyloidosis contains a soluble component (termed SAA) that is related in composition to the amyloid itself.

It has been proposed that in generalized amyloidosis there is a circulating component, either of immunoglobulin origin or SAA, that can leave the circulation and form the insoluble β-pleated protein termed amyloid. Possibly, local reticuloendothelial cells play a part in this process by partially degrading the soluble protein. Nevertheless, it remains a mystery why amyloid should be laid down in some organs but not in others, and in some patients but not in others with apparently similar conditions.

Other Types of Amyloid.   The amyloid found in the islets of Langerhans appears to be derived from insulin, while that present in the stroma of medullary carcinoma of the thyroid is formed from calcitonin. Analysis of the amyloid in cardiac amyloidosis and in some cases of heredofamilial amyloidosis has revealed yet other types of amyloid. It is evident that we have a lot to learn about the pathogenesis of amyloidosis, particularly of the localized forms.

1. An antibody to the red-cell antigen A may be described as a macroglobulin, an IgM protein, a glycoprotein, and a component in the 19S fraction. Explain what is meant by each of these descriptive terms.

2. An apparently healthy 54-year-old man was found to have an ESR of 75 mm. The result of immunoelectrophoresis of his serum is shown in Figure 25–5 together

Figure 25–5.   Immunoelectrophoresis of serum.   The serum labeled "test" is from the patient described in question 2. A normal control serum is included for comparison.

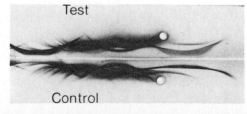

with that of a normal serum. Comment on these laboratory results and speculate on the diagnosis.

3. A patient is found to have albuminuria and a plasma albumin level of 1.5 g/dl (15 g/L). A renal biopsy was attempted, but no suitable tissue was obtained. A biopsy of the rectal mucosa revealed infiltration by amyloid. Electrophoresis showed a spike in the γ region, and immunoelectrophorèsis confirmed that this was an IgG protein. Discuss the diagnosis.

4. A 22-year-old married woman is found to have an ESR of 27 mm (Westergren method). What significance should be attached to the results of the test?

Selected Readings

Glenner, G. G., and Page, D. L.: Amyloid, amyloidosis, and amyloidogenesis. International Review of Experimental Pathology, 15:2–92, 1976.

Halsted, J. A., and Halsted, C. H. (Eds.): The Laboratory in Clinical Medicine. 2nd ed. Philadelphia, W. B. Saunders Company, 1981. See pp. 124–127 for a description of the hyperlipoproteinemias and pp. 575–577 for a discussion of the erythrocyte sedimentation rate.

Katz, A., and Pruzanski, W.: Newer concepts in amyloidosis. Canadian Medical Association Journal, 114:872–873, 1976.

Murphy, K. E.: Amyloidosis, a deadly disease. American Journal of Nursing, 80:1336–1338, 1980.

Stirling, G. A.: Amyloidosis. In Harrison, C. V., and Weinbren, K. (Eds.): Recent Advances in Pathology, No. 9. Edinburgh, Churchill Livingstone, 1975, pp. 249–272.

Disorders of the Blood CHAPTER 26

After studying this chapter the student should be able to:

- Outline the stages in the formation of the red cells and the white cells and indicate the sites of hematopoiesis.
- Describe the mature red cell and the abnormal forms that are encountered in disease.
- List the normal values of the red-cell count, the hemoglobin content of blood, the packed cell volume (PCV), the mean corpuscular hemoglobin concentration (MCHC), and the white-cell count.
- List the requirements for red-cell formation and describe the fate of old, worn-out red cells.
- Indicate the clinical features of anemia and describe the five main types of this condition (as outlined in this chapter) in terms of the following factors:
    - (a) causes
    - (b) blood picture
    - (c) pathological findings in organs other than blood
- Describe the main features of the red-cell fragmentation syndrome.
- Define polycythemia and distinguish between the primary and secondary forms.
- Define the following terms and give at least one cause of each: leukocytosis, leukopenia, neutropenia, lymphocytosis, monocytosis, eosinophilia, and pancytopenia.
- Classify the leukemias and describe the salient features of each type.
- Describe the outstanding features and important causes of the following conditions:
    - (a) bone marrow aplasia
    - (b) hypersplenism
    - (c) leukoerythroblastic anemia
- Describe the clotting mechanism and differentiate between the intrinsic system and the extrinsic system.
- Classify the bleeding diseases and give examples of each type.
- Briefly describe the following tests and indicate the value of each in assessing the cause of a bleeding disease:
    - (a) platelet count
    - (b) clotting time
    - (c) bleeding time
    - (d) capillary fragility test
    - (e) partial thromboplastin time
    - (f) prothrombin time
- Describe the ABO and Rhesus blood groups and outline the way in which a sample of blood is typed.
- List the hazards of blood transfusion and indicate how they may be avoided.

The formed elements of the blood consist of the red cells *(erythrocytes),* the white cells *(leukocytes),* and the *platelets.* In the fetus, blood formation *(hematopoiesis)* takes place in the bone marrow (in the medullary cavity of the bones), liver, spleen, and other organs. After birth, the extramedullary sites disappear, so that within a few weeks blood formation occurs only in the bone marrow. As the child develops, the blood-forming tissue in the long bones is replaced by fatty marrow, so that by the time adulthood is reached the main source of blood cells is the red marrow of the ribs and the vertebral column. The marrow of the long bones is available for extension of hematopoietic tissues should a need arise for increased production.

THE RED CELLS

Development

The earliest recognizable precursor of the blood cells is a large cell with abundant basophilic cytoplasm and a nucleus containing one or more nucleoli. This cell is termed a *stem cell.* The first recognizable red-cell precursor is termed a *pronormoblast;* its cytoplasm contains many ribosomes but no hemoglobin. As hemoglobin is formed, the cytoplasm becomes more eosinophilic and the nucleus becomes condensed (a process called pyknosis). Such a cell is termed a *normoblast;* early, intermediate, and late stages are recognized. Ultimately, the nucleus is extruded, and the cell assumes the flattened shape of the mature erythrocyte.

The Mature Erythrocyte. The red cell is a biconcave disc and is conveniently examined by making a smear of blood on a glass slide and staining with one of the Romanowsky stains* (Fig. 26–1). The average diameter of a red cell when examined in this manner is 6.7 to 7.7 μm. Young red cells have a faint basophilia in the cytoplasm that is due to remnants of rough endoplasmic reticulum. Such cells are termed *reticulocytes.* Normally less than 2 per cent of the total red cells are reticulocytes, and an increase in their number generally indicates a more rapid production of cells such as occurs in hemolytic anemia or after a hemorrhage. Reticulocytosis is also seen whenever an anemia is treated successfully, such as when an iron-deficiency anemia is treated with iron. Under normal conditions the nucleated red cells are prevented from leaving the bone marrow; however, with extremely rapid erythropoiesis, particularly if it is occurring in abnormal sites such as the liver and spleen, nucleated red cells can appear in the circulation. A good example of this phenomenon is *hemolytic disease of the newborn* (page 356).

Examination of the Red Cell. The normal red-cell count is 4.6 to 6.2 $\times$ 10^{12}/L in males;† the normal hemoglobin content is 14 to 18 g/dl. In women the red-cell count is 0.5 $\times$ 10^{12}/L less and the hemoglobin level is 2 g/dl lower. A useful and accurate measurement is the hematocrit reading, or packed cell

---

*These stains, which include Leishman, Jenner, and Giemsa, consist of blended mixtures of methylene blue and eosin.

†The red-cell count has commonly been expressed as the number of cells in millions per cu mm of blood. In the SI (*Système International,* or International System) units now in common use it is expressed in number of cells $\times$ 10^{12} per liter (L). In SI units the normal red-cell count is 4.6 to 6.2 $\times$ 10^{12}/L; in the previous system it was 4.6 to 6.2 million/cu mm. Note that 100 ml is now 1 deciliter (dl). Note also that 1 cu mm is also written as 1 mm^3 or 1 μL.

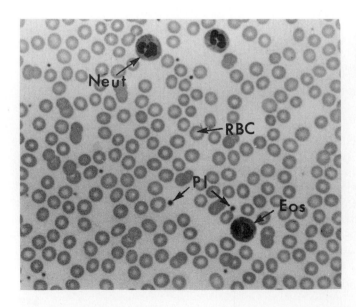

Figure 26–1. Normal blood film. The red blood cells (RBC) are of uniform diameter and evenly stained. The central, pale-staining area is due to their biconcave shape. Also shown are two neutrophil polymorphs (Neut), one eosinophil (Eos), and several platelets (Pl) ($\times$600).

volume (PCV). In this test a thin, cylindrical, graduated Wintrobe tube is filled with blood and centrifuged for half an hour at 3000 revolutions per minute. In the adult male the PCV is 0.40 to 0.54, meaning that 40 to 54 per cent of the blood volume consists of red cells.

There are three *absolute values* in common use:
Mean corpuscular volume (MCV), which is obtained thus:

$$\frac{\text{Volume of packed red cells (L/L)} \times 1000}{\text{Red cell count } (\times 10^{12}/\text{L})}$$

The result is expressed in 10^{-15}L, or femtoliters (fl).
Mean corpuscular hemoglobin (MCH), which is obtained thus:

$$\frac{\text{Hemoglobin (g/L)}}{\text{Red cell count } (\times 10^{12}/\text{L})}$$

The result is expressed in $10^{-12}/\text{g}$ or picograms (pg).
Mean corpuscular hemoglobin concentration (MCHC), which is obtained thus:

$$\frac{\text{Hemoglobin (g/dl)}}{\text{Volume of packed red cells (L/L)}}$$

This is expressed in grams of hemoglobin per deciliter of packed red cells (g/dl).

The MCHC is an index of the concentration of hemoglobin in the red cells. The normal range is 32 to 36 g/dl, and a value less than 32 g/dl indicates underhemoglobinization of the cells and suggests impaired hemoglobin synthesis, a condition often caused by iron deficiency. The normal absolute values are summarized in Table 26–1.

With experience, it is possible to get a great deal of information merely by examining a well-stained blood film with a microscope. The normal red cell is described as *normocytic* and *normochromic*. If it is smaller than normal, it is called *microcytic;* if larger than normal, *macrocytic*. If the cell is poorly hemoglobinized, it looks pale and is termed *hypochromic*. The normal cell is fully saturated with hemoglobin, and therefore hyperchromia cannot occur. If the cells vary greatly in size, the term *anisocytosis* is used. The presence of irregularly shaped cells is called *poikilocytosis. Burr cells* have projections or spikes arising from their surface; *sickle cells* have an elongated shape; *spherocytes* are spherical, rather than being flat discs. Spherocytes look abnormally small and stain darkly in a blood film. Another interesting pathological variant is the *target cell,* in which a small central dot of hemoglobin is seen; this is separated from the outer rim by a wide clear area (Fig. 26–2).

TABLE 26–1.   CHARACTERISTICS OF THE NORMAL RED BLOOD CELL

Packed Cell Volume	0.40 to 0.54 (no unit is necessary, but liter per liter is implied)
Mean Corpuscular Volume (MCV)	80 to 96 fl
Mean Corpuscular Hemoglobin (MCH)	27 to 31 pg
Mean Corpuscular Hemoglobin Concentration (MCHC)	32 to 36 g per dl
Mean Corpuscular Diameter (MCD)	6.7 to 7.7 μm

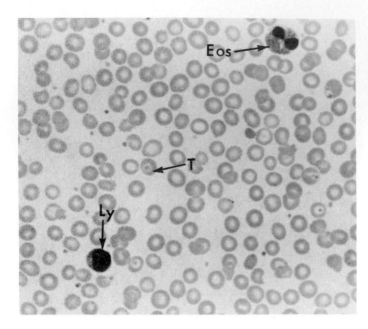

Figure 26–2. Blood film from patient with iron-deficiency anemia. The red cells are hypochromic, and the central pale-staining area is more pronounced than normal. The cells that exhibit a central dot are called target cells (T). Also shown is an eosinophil (Eos) with a typical bilobed nucleus and a small lymphocyte (Ly) (×600).

Requirements for Red-Cell Formation

Hemoglobin consists of protein (globin) combined with heme, an iron-containing porphyrin.

In starvation, inadequate globin production can result in anemia. Under most circumstances, however, it is the formation of heme and maturation of the cells that are most important for the formation of healthy red cells; for this the following components are required (Table 26–2).

Iron. Each heme molecule contains one atom of iron; without this, hemoglobin cannot be formed. Iron is absorbed from food in an ionic form by the mucosal cells of the duodenum and upper small bowel. Heme, derived from hemoglobin and myoglobin in the diet, can be absorbed directly.

The manner in which iron is absorbed is not well understood, but it is known that there is a mechanism by which the amount absorbed can be regulated. Thus, in iron deficiency states, if there is accelerated erythropoiesis, the amount of iron absorbed in the gut is increased. On the other hand, if the body is overloaded with iron, the amount absorbed is decreased.

Once absorbed, iron combines with an iron-free protein (termed *apoferri-*

TABLE 26–2.   REQUIREMENTS FOR RED-CELL FORMATION

REQUIREMENT	Marrow Changes	RESULT OF DEFICIENCY Blood Changes	Other Changes
Iron	Normoblastic hyperplasia	Hypochromic microcytic anemia	Oral mucosal atrophy
Folic acid	Megaloblastic hyperplasia	Normochromic macrocytic anemia	Oral mucosal atrophy
Vitamin B$_{12}$	Megaloblastic hyperplasia	Normochromic macrocytic anemia	Oral mucosal atrophy; subacute combined degeneration of cord

tin) to form *ferritin,* the storage form of iron in the body. Much of this is stored in the reticuloendothelial system, where it is available for hemoglobin and myoglobin synthesis.

Vitamins. The most important vitamins essential for blood formation belong to the B complex vitamins: *folic acid* and *vitamin B₁₂.* Both are necessary for the proper development of the normoblast. If either substance is deficient, the normoblast develops abnormally; that is, it remains large and the nucleus has an abnormal stippled appearance of its chromatin. Such a cell is termed a *megaloblast,* and the red cell that it produces is large (a *macrocyte*). Both vitamins are present in the diet and are absorbed in the small bowel. The two vitamins differ in that folic acid is taken up directly, whereas vitamin B₁₂ cannot be absorbed unless bound to a complex mucoprotein secreted by the gastric mucosa. This substance is called *intrinsic factor.* It follows that gastric secretion is essential for the absorption of vitamin B₁₂.

Vitamin C. Although this vitamin is also required for red-cell production, deficiency is rarely a factor in human disease.

Other Substances. These include *copper* and *cobalt,* but although deficiency in the experimental animal causes anemia, their role in human disease is debatable. *Thyroxin* is necessary for red-cell formation, and it is not surprising that anemia is encountered in myxedema. Likewise, *androgens* stimulate erythropoiesis and are used in the treatment of some types of aplastic anemia. *Glucocorticoids* can also stimulate red-cell formation. Anemia is seen in hypopituitarism, and polycythemia is a feature of Cushing's syndrome (Chapter 39). Erythropoietin is a hormone formed in the kidney as well as in other organs, and increased production leads to increased erythropoiesis. The stimulus for its formation is hypoxia.

Disposal of the Red Cell

The normal life span of the red cell is about 120 days. As cells age, they become fragmented and are taken up by the reticuloendothelial cells (Fig. 26–3). Hemoglobin is split into globin and heme. The globin is degraded and returned to the body's pool of amino acids. The iron portion of the hemoglobin is split off and combined with apoferritin to form ferritin, which is stored for further use. The porphyrin nucleus is metabolized to bilirubin, which passes into the blood stream, becomes attached to albumin, and is excreted by the liver. Normally there is very little free hemoglobin in the plasma, and any that does appear is immediately removed by combination with a globulin component of the plasma called *haptoglobin.* Any large excess of hemoglobin in the circulation is oxidized to heme and combined with albumin to form *methemalbumin.* Both the haptoglobin and the albumin complexes are removed by the reticuloendothelial cell so that none escapes into the urine. It is only when both these binding proteins are exhausted that free hemoglobin appears in the blood (*hemoglobinemia*) and in the urine (*hemoglobinuria*). Massive sudden destruction of red cells must occur before this is evident (see "Blackwater Fever," Chapter 15).

The Anemias

Anemia is defined as a condition in which there is *a fall in the quantity of either red cells or hemoglobin in a unit volume of blood in the presence of a low or normal total blood volume.* The question of blood volume is important in relation to pregnancy. A moderate fall in the level of the red cell count and hemoglobin is common during the last part of pregnancy and is followed by a slow recovery in the puerperium. There is a raised blood volume in pregnancy, and it is probable that much of the "physiological anemia" is due to simple hemodilution. Nevertheless, iron deficiency can also occur.

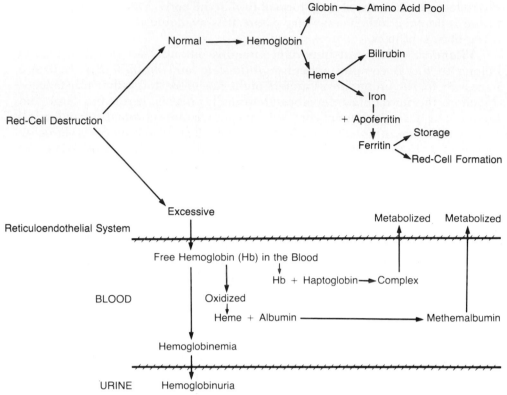

Figure 26–3. Diagram showing the fate of destroyed red blood cells and their contained hemoglobin.

The main clinical features of anemia are the following:

1. *Pallor*, best detected in the conjunctiva, nail bed, or mucous membrane of the mouth. Pallor of the skin, particularly of the face, is a deceptive sign. It can be absent in some patients with anemia and yet present in many pale-skinned normal people.

2. *Tiredness, easy fatigability*, and *generalized muscular weakness* are common symptoms; the pathogenesis, however, is not clear. Such symptoms are also common in psychoneurotic patients who are not anemic.

3. *Shortness of breath* and *palpitations* are common. They are related to tissue hypoxia and an increased cardiac output. *Heart failure* can occur.

4. *Angina pectoris, intermittent claudication*, and *giddiness* are due to tissue hypoxia in organs in which the blood supply is already impaired by arterial disease.

The pathological effects of anemia are attributable to cellular hypoxia. At necropsy there is severe fatty change of the liver, heart, and kidneys, and death is usually attributed to heart failure.

TABLE 26–3. THE ANEMIAS

TYPE	BLOOD PICTURE	
Posthemorrhagic	Normochromic	Normocytic
Iron deficiency	Hypochromic	Microcytic
Megaloblastic	Normochromic	Macrocytic
Hemolytic	Normochromic	Normocytic
Bone-marrow deficiency	Normochromic	Normocytic

The classification of the anemias is somewhat unsatisfactory, but for practical purposes the following groups can be recognized (Table 26–3).
1. Acute posthemorrhagic anemia
2. Iron deficiency anemia
3. Megaloblastic anemia
4. Hemolytic anemia
5. Bone-marrow inadequacy anemia

The pathogenesis of the anemia that results from a sudden hemorrhage is described in Chapter 21. The anemia is normocytic and normochromic, provided the patient is not iron deficient as a result of previous blood loss or other disease. Within a few days a reticulocytosis occurs, and recovery proceeds to completion within about six weeks.

Acute Posthemorrhagic Anemia

Causes
Chronic Blood Loss. This is the most important cause of iron deficiency anemia. Common examples are bleeding from a chronic peptic ulcer, gastrointestinal cancer, or hemorrhoids. In women, menorrhagia is an important cause of blood loss, whereas in underdeveloped countries ankylostomiasis takes its toll.

Iron Deficiency Anemia

Defective Iron Absorption. This may be secondary to dietary deficiency and is quite common in infants. It should be remembered that milk contains very little iron. Nutritional deficiency combined with the increased demand for iron by the growing fetus is a common cause of anemia in pregnancy. In the elderly an inadequate diet can also lead to iron deficiency anemia.

Defective iron absorption is a feature of the malabsorption syndrome (Chapter 32). Thus, it accompanies many intestinal diseases and is also a common feature following gastrectomy because of the "intestinal hurry" that follows this operation.

Pathological Findings. The bone marrow undergoes hyperplasia that is of the normal normoblastic type. Red marrow extends into the shafts of the long bones. In the peripheral blood there is a moderate anemia in which the red-cell count is relatively less reduced than the hemoglobin level. *The red cells are markedly microcytic and hypochromic*, and target cells may be present (see Fig. 26–2). The reticulocyte count is low, unless there has been a recent hemorrhage.

Other features of iron deficiency sometimes accompany the anemia. Sometimes there is diffuse hair loss. The *nails* tend to become brittle and spoon-shaped. The most common *oral manifestation* is loss of the filiform papillae of the tongue, which consequently appears smooth and red. Mucosal atrophy can extend into the pharynx. Both in the mouth and pharynx this atrophy is sometimes complicated by the development of squamous-cell carcinoma (see Plummer-Vinson syndrome, Chapter 31).

Megaloblastic anemia is due to a deficiency of folic acid, vitamin B_{12}, or both. It is characterized by an abnormal type of erythropoiesis in the marrow.

Megaloblastic Anemia

Causes
Dietary Deficiency. This is quite common in underdeveloped countries, where the anemia is often due to an inadequate intake of folic acid.

Pregnancy. Folic-acid deficiency resulting from poor diet is sometimes precipitated by the extra demands of the fetus in pregnant women.

Gastric Disease. The intrinsic factor of the stomach is necessary for vitamin B_{12} absorption from the bowel. Therefore, total resection of the stomach must in time lead to vitamin-B$_{12}$ deficiency. However, the body's stores of vitamin B$_{12}$ are so great that it takes up to 5 years for anemia to develop. The most important gastric disease to produce megaloblastic anemia is *pernicious anemia*, an idiopathic condition in which there is progressive atrophy of the gastric mucosa. The stomach fails to secrete pepsin, hydrochloric acid, and finally intrinsic factor itself. The disease is familial and appears to have an autoimmune component; autoantibodies against parietal cells of the gastric mucosa and against intrinsic factor itself are usually detectable in the patient's serum.

Intestinal Malabsorption.   Failure to absorb folic acid and vitamin B$_{12}$ is a feature of the malabsorption syndromes. The defect may be related either to the bowel disease itself or indirectly to an alteration in the intestinal flora (Chapter 32).

Drugs.   Certain drugs, particularly anticonvulsants used in epilepsy treatment and the antimetabolites of the antifolic acid type used in cancer treatment (*e.g.*, methotrexate), can cause megaloblastic anemia if given over a prolonged period.

Pathological Changes.   The peripheral blood shows a severe anemia in which the *red-cell count is relatively more reduced than the hemoglobin level*. The red cells are conspicuously large (a condition called *macrocytosis*) and appear normally colored; they show marked *poikilocytosis* and *anisocytosis*. It is common to find both the white cells and platelets reduced in number. The bone marrow is markedly hyperplastic and contains many megaloblasts (Fig. 26–4).

The other effects depend on the cause of the anemia. Vitamin B$_{12}$ is essential for the proper functioning of the central nervous system; without it, *subacute combined degeneration* of the spinal cord can occur. With this form of degeneration there is demyelination of the posterior and lateral columns of the cord. It does not occur in pure folic-acid deficiency.

There is sometimes a superficial stomatitis; the tongue is smooth and denuded of papillae, having a characteristic raw, beefy appearance.

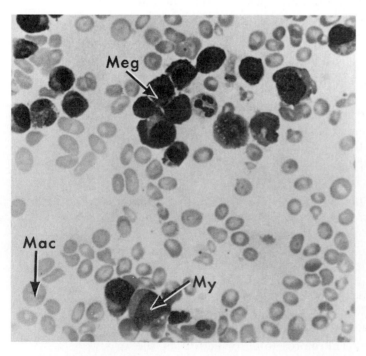

Figure 26–4. Bone marrow smear from patient with megaloblastic anemia. The red cells show great variation in size. Some are large (Mac), whereas others are small and are irregularly shaped. The number of nucleated red-cell precursors is increased, and a group of megaloblasts is present (Meg). Also shown are a number of myelocytes (My) (×600).

The term *hemolytic anemia* is applied to those conditions in which there **Hemolytic** is an increased rate of red-cell destruction. This destruction is due either to an **Anemia** intrinsic defect in the red cells themselves or to some extracorpuscular factor acting on normal red cells. If the defect is primarily corpuscular, the red cells of a patient will not survive long when they are transfused into a healthy recipient; on the contrary, normal cells transfused into a patient will not be destroyed. If the cause of the hemolysis is extracorpuscular, normal red cells will be eliminated in the same way as those of the patient, whereas the patient's red cells will survive well in a normal recipient.

The increased red-cell destruction stimulates new red-cell formation, which is manifested by a reticulocytosis.

Causes

Corpuscular Defects.   In northern European races the most important cause is a spherical malformation of the red cells that causes the condition of *hereditary spherocytosis* or *acholuric familial jaundice.* The abnormal cells are liable to become trapped and destroyed in the spleen so that splenectomy is usually effective in allaying the anemia while having no effect on the spherocytosis.

The Hemoglobinopathies.   The hemoglobinopathies are a group of conditions in which the red cells contain an abnormal form of hemoglobin.

In *sickle cell anemia* the cells containing the abnormal hemoglobin HbS become sickle-shaped and are destroyed in the spleen when deprived of oxygen. This condition occurs almost exclusively in Blacks. Many other abnormal types of hemoglobin have been found — their presence sometimes leading to a hemolytic anemia. The best known is hemoglobin C, which leads to an anemia that is less severe than that of sickle cell disease.

In the *thalassemia syndromes* the red cells of a patient contain various types of hemoglobin that are normally present only in the fetus. The most common variant of the syndromes is *thalassemia major,* in which the red cells usually contain much fetal hemoglobin (Hb-F). The disease is the common hemoglobinopathy of the Mediterranean races and causes severe anemia.

It should be noted that the hemoglobinopathies can occur in combination to produce complex syndromes. Thus, it is not uncommon to find sickle cell defect and hemoglobin C disease in the same person.

Enzyme-Deficient Red Cells.   It was the finding that some Black Americans were very liable to have a severe hemolytic anemia following the administration of certain drugs (*e.g.,* the antimalarial pamaquine) that led to the discovery that certain individuals have hereditary enzyme defects. The most important defect is a deficiency of glucose-6-phosphate dehydrogenase (G6PD) in their red cells. Many variants of G6PD deficiency have been described; these are inherited as dominant X-linked characteristics. Occasionally they lead to a chronic anemia, but more usually the defects become apparent as acute hemolytic anemia following ingestion of drugs or contact with a particular substance, such as the fava bean. The latter phenomenon is seen in some Mediterranean races; the anemia following contact with the bean is reputed to be the reason why Pythagoras counseled his followers never to walk in bean fields.

Extracorpuscular Defects

Autoantibodies.   The most important antibodies that act on red cells are autoantibodies that usually occur idiopathically but may on occasion develop during the course of some other disease such as mycoplasmal pneumonia, lupus erythematosus, or a reticuloendothelial neoplasm. Two types of autoantibodies are described below:

Complete Autoantibodies.   These antibodies agglutinate red cells directly in a saline suspension; they are termed *complete antibodies*. Most of these are not active at body temperature but cause agglutination at room temperature. Such antibodies are therefore called *cold antibodies*. Although readily detectable in the laboratory, they have a feeble *in vivo* activity and consequently tend to cause comparatively mild hemolytic anemia.

Incomplete Autoantibodies. The most important autoantibodies do not agglutinate red cells in a saline suspension. They are, however, readily adsorbed onto the red cell surface, which thereby becomes coated with autoantibody. If an antihuman γ-globulin serum (obtained by immunizing a rabbit against human globulin) is added to a suspension of these coated cells, the cells undergo immediate agglutination. This antiglobulin technique is known as the *direct Coombs' test.**

Most incomplete antibodies act maximally at 37°C, and are therefore also called *warm antibodies*. Although they do not hemolyze red cells *in vitro*, the coated red cells *in vivo* are damaged and are readily destroyed. Warm antibodies therefore lead to severe hemolytic anemia.

Alloantibodies.† The blood group antibodies can also cause a hemolytic anemia under special circumstances. For example, in Rh-hemolytic disease of the newborn, an Rh-negative woman married to an Rh-positive man produces an Rh-positive fetus. During the last part of pregnancy — and particularly during labor — a leak of fetal red cells into the maternal circulation is quite common. The mother is thereby stimulated to produce Rh antibodies. Although the first child escapes damage, future Rh-positive fetuses may be attacked by maternal Rh antibodies that cross the placenta. The fetus develops a severe hemolytic anemia, characterized by numerous nucleated red cells in its circulation (*hemolytic disease of the newborn*). In severe cases the fetus is stillborn; generalized edema due to heart failure is a prominent feature. Less severely affected infants survive but are jaundiced and may suffer brain damage. (kernicterus; see "Hemolytic Jaundice," Chapter 33).

An advance of great importance was the discovery that the administration of human γ-globulin containing anti-Rh antibody of high activity can prevent sensitization of Rh-negative mothers by Rh-positive fetal cells, provided it is given within 72 hours of delivery or abortion. The passively administered anti-Rh antibodies probably coat the Rh-positive fetal cells and prevent them from providing an adequate antigenic stimulus. In this way sensitization does not occur.

Other important extracorpuscular factors that may lead to hemolytic anemia are the toxins of organisms such as *Clostridium welchii,* drugs such as sulfonamides, severe burns that damage the red cells locally, and finally the malarial parasite, which directly attacks the red cells (Chapter 15).

Red-cell Fragmentation Syndrome. Red cells that are subjected to excessive physical trauma in the circulation may undergo premature fragmentation and lysis. This has been described following prolonged jogging and is

---

*In the *direct Coombs' test*, a sample of a *patient's red cells* that have been washed in saline is mixed with Coombs' reagent (antihuman γ-globulin). A positive test is indicated by agglutination due to the presence of a coating of antibody on the red cells. In the *indirect Coombs' test*, a sample of a *patient's serum* is mixed with a suspension of suitable red cells. These are washed in saline and then mixed with Coombs' reagent. Agglutination indicates the patient's serum contains antibodies capable of adhering to the red cells. In Rh sensitization of pregnancy, the mother's serum is tested for antibodies (the indirect Coombs' test), whereas the baby's cells are submitted to a direct Coombs' test.

†An alloantibody is an antibody present in one member of the species, which is capable of reacting specifically with an antigen present in some other members of the same species. The term isoantibody was previously used in this connection, but it has been discarded so that the terms will parallel those used in transplantation immunology.

also encountered in association with abnormalities of the heart and great vessels in which extreme turbulence appears to be the damaging factor. It is most commonly seen following the insertion of a synthetic valvular prosthesis. Red-cell fragmentation is also seen in association with small vessel disease *(microangiopathic hemolytic anemia)*. This occurs in disseminated intravascular coagulation (page 366), and a particular example of this is the *hemolytic uremic syndrome,* which is an acute condition occurring in the great majority of cases in infants and young children. There is an acute hemolytic anemia, a low platelet count, and acute renal failure. The cause of this disease is not known, but it commonly follows a bacterial or viral infection.

Pathological Findings.   *In hemolytic anemia the red cells are typically normochromic and normocytic. The outstanding feature of the disease is a high reticulocyte count*, which indicates active erythropoiesis. The reticulocyte count may even reach 30 per cent of the total cell count. The bone marrow shows marked normoblastic hyperplasia.

In hemolytic anemia there is overproduction of bilirubin; jaundice is present in most patients. When the hemolytic process is sudden and severe, hemoglobinemia may occur, leading to hemoglobinuria. This response is unusual, except in the most severe cases such as in patients having blackwater fever. The presence of much free hemoglobin in the blood, particularly when the hemolysis has been caused by an immunological reaction, may cause renal vasoconstriction, anuria, and renal failure.

Anemia is frequent in many chronic diseases such as rheumatoid arthritis, leukemia, renal disease, and chronic suppurative infections. *The anemia found with these diseases is normocytic* and *normochromic* and is not attended by any significant reticulocytosis. Some deficiency or toxemia probably impairs red-cell production, but the mechanism is not known. **Bone Marrow Inadequacy Anemia**

Two other types of anemia come into this category and are described later: bone marrow aplasia (aplastic anemia) and bone marrow replacement (leukoerythroblastic anemia).

Polycythemia is a condition in which the red-cell count is raised in a unit volume of blood in the presence of an increased total blood volume. It must be distinguished from hemoconcentration, such as that occurring in burns, in which the red-cell count is increased because of a decrease in the plasma volume. **Polycythemia**

Polycythemia may be secondary to chronic hypoxia. It is therefore a feature of chronic lung disease and cyanotic congenital heart disease. Some degree of polycythemia is normal in those who live at a high altitude.

As a primary condition *(polycythemia vera)*, the normoblastic proliferation of the erythropoietic element of the bone marrow appears to be of a neoplastic type. The red-cell count can reach $10 \times 10^{12}/L$ (10 million/μl) and there is often a considerable increase in both white cells and platelets, a change not encountered in secondary polycythemia. Indeed, some cases terminate as myelocytic leukemia, and it is reasonable to classify the disease as one example of a myeloproliferative disorder (page 363). Polycythemia vera is generally a disease of middle-aged or elderly people, and thrombotic complications are common because of the high viscosity of the blood. Mesenteric venous thrombosis, coronary artery thrombosis, and cerebral thrombosis are common terminal events.

Important white cells are the granulocytes, the lymphocytes, and the monocytes (Figs. 26–5 and 26–6). **THE WHITE CELLS**

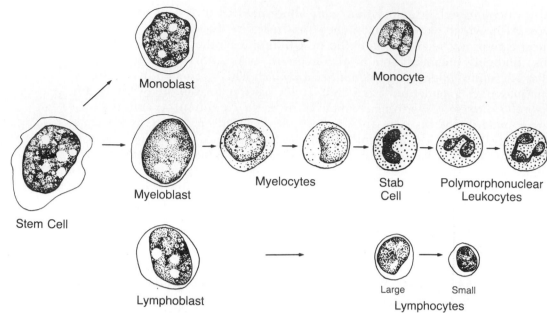

Figure 26–5. Development of the white cells. The monoblast and myeloblast are depicted as being derived from a common pluripotential cell called a stem cell. The lymphoblast is derived from its own stem cell. The three blast cell types cannot be distinguished easily from each other on morphological grounds. The myelocyte matures to a stab- or band-form; the nucleus of the mature polymorph is formed by subsequent lobulation. (Drawn by Margot Mackay, Department of Art as Applied to Medicine, University of Toronto.)

Development

The precursor cell of the granulocyte is the *myeloblast*, a cell that closely resembles the pronormoblast. As it matures, it loses its nucleoli and is then termed a *promyelocyte*. When specific cytoplasmic granules — neutrophilic, eosinophilic, or basophilic — appear, the cell is called a *myelocyte*. The indented nucleus of the late or metamyelocyte is ultimately drawn out into two or more discrete lobes joined by fine chromatin threads. This is the mature *polymorphonuclear granulocyte* ("polymorph"), so called because of the shape of its nucleus. Most granulocytes have fine lilac-colored granules and are called *neutrophils*. A few are *eosinophils*, which have large red granules, and the least common is the *basophil*, which has very large purple granules. The development of the granulocytes occurs in the bone marrow, and under normal conditions only mature cells appear in the peripheral blood.

The precursor cells of lymphocytes and monocytes are called *lymphoblasts* and *monoblasts*. As these cells mature, they lose their nucleoli; in the case of the lymphocyte, the cytoplasm becomes sparse as the nucleus condenses and becomes hyperchromatic.

Normal White-Cell Count and Its Variations in Disease

The total white-cell count in the blood is 4 to 11 × 10^9/L (4000 to 11,000/μl).* The range of the differential count for the adult is as follows:

Neutrophils	40 to 75% (2.0 to 7.5 × 10^9/L or 2000 to 7500/μl)
Eosinophils	1 to 5% (0.05 to 0.4 × 10^9/L or 50 to 400/μl)
Basophils	0 to 1% (up to 0.1 × 10^9/L or 100/μl)
Lymphocytes	20 to 45% (1.5 to 4 × 10^9/L or 1500 to 4000/μl)
Monocytes	3 to 7% (0.2 to 0.8 × 10^9/L or 200 to 800/μl)

---

*The white-cell count has commonly been expressed in number of cells per cubic millimeter (abbreviated cu mm or μl) of blood. In the SI units now in common use it is expressed in number of cells × 10^9 per liter (L.). Thus, the normal white-cell count is 4 to 11 × 10^9/L or in the previous system 4000 to 11,000/cu mm. or 4000 to 11,000/μl.

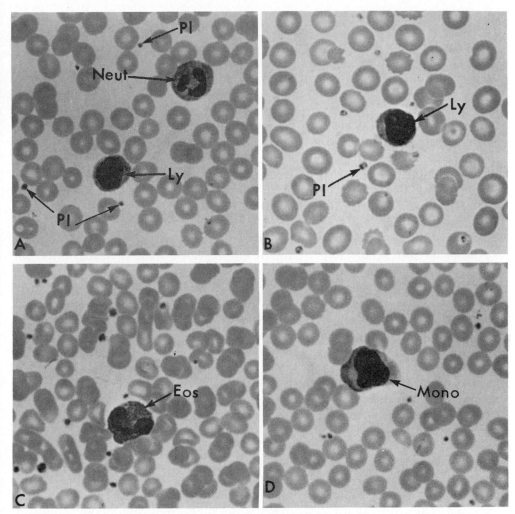

Figure 26–6. Normal white cells in the peripheral blood. *A,* The neutrophil polymorph (Neut) has a typical lobed nucleus and fine cytoplasmic granules. The small lymphocyte (Ly) has a deeply staining nucleus and scanty cytoplasm. A number of platelets (Pl) are present. *B,* Typical small lymphocyte (see also Review Questions). *C,* Eosinophil with coarse granules (Eos). *D,* Monocyte (Mono). The cell is larger than a lymphocyte and has more abundant cytoplasm (×960).

The suffix *-cytosis* implies an excess of cells, *e.g., leukocytosis* indicates an increased total white-cell count, and *lymphocytosis* indicates an increase in the number of lymphocytes. The suffix *-penia* means a decrease in the relevant cells, *e.g., leukopenia* means a decrease in the number of white cells, and *lymphopenia* is a decrease in the number of lymphocytes. *Neutrophilia* is sometimes used as an alternative to neutrophil leukocytosis. Likewise, *neutropenia* denotes a reduction in the total number of neutrophil polymorphs, and the term *agranulocytosis* is commonly used as a synonym. The figures in parentheses in the range listed above indicate the absolute number of cells present. This is a more useful figure than the percentage. Thus, if there is a drop in the number of neutrophils, the percentage of lymphocytes increases — a condition called a *relative lymphocytosis.* The term, however, is misleading, since the actual number of lymphocytes can remain unchanged. The main variations in the white-cell count are as follows:

Neutrophil Leukocytosis (Neutrophilia). This common condition is usually due to infection. The highest counts are seen when the organism concerned is one of the pyogenic bacteria, *e.g.,* staphylococci, pneumonococci, and coliforms.

Other important causes are *massive tissue necrosis,* such as after a myocardial infarct; *uremia; acute gout, severe hemorrhage and hemolysis; rapidly growing malignant tumors* and *neoplastic disease of the marrow,* such as chronic myelocytic leukemia and polycythemia vera.

At one time a classification of the maturity of neutrophils based on their nuclear segmentation was very much in vogue. The results were expressed in tabular form, with the left-hand side of the page listing the most primitive cells and the more differentiated cells being on the right-hand side. Although this detailed accounting is now obsolete, the term "a shift to the left" is still useful in denoting an increase of young forms of polymorphs in the blood, such as occurs in the leukocytosis of infection. In extreme cases metamyelocytes and even myelocytes may enter the blood. This *leukemoid blood picture* can sometimes closely mimic leukemia itself.

Neutropenia.   A reduction in the number of neutrophils is seen in infections such as typhoid fever and malaria. It is also a common feature of the prodromal period of many viral diseases. Any overwhelming infection, whatever the cause, also reduces the neutrophil count.

Other causes of neutropenia are hypersplenism, bone marrow aplasia, and acute leukemia.

Regulation of the Neutrophil Count.   The neutrophil count can be altered by two regulatory mechanisms:

1. *Release of neutrophils from the reserves.* Of the neutrophils in the blood, over half are in a "marginated pool" adherent to the walls of the blood vessels, particularly in the lungs. These can be released rapidly; this release accounts for the leukocytosis that occurs during exercise and following the administration of epinephrine. The second reserve is in the bone marrow, where the number of neutrophils sequestered is about 10 times the total number of cells present in the blood. The mechanism of their release is poorly understood, but various neutrophil releasing factors have been described.

2. *Increased production of neutrophils in the bone marrow.* Various stimulating factors (*e.g.,* chalones) and inhibitory factors have been described. Their role, if any, in the regulation of the neutrophil count in health or disease is not clear.

Lymphocytosis.   An absolute lymphocytosis is not common. It is seen in *whooping cough* and in *infectious mononucleosis.* In the latter disease the lymphocytes are atypical and somewhat resemble monocytes. This disease, which is common in young adults, is thought to be caused by the Epstein-Barr virus. The illness usually commences with a sore throat, which is followed by enlargement of cervical lymph nodes, and later by the appearance of the characteristic cells in the blood. An interesting feature is the presence in the serum of antibodies that agglutinate sheep's red cells to high titer. These antibodies may be detected by the *Paul-Bunnell test.* A variant of this test utilizing horse red cells is in common use and is termed the monospot test. During convalescence specific antibodies to the Epstein-Barr virus appear in the blood as well as the heterophilic antibodies described above. An illness clinically resembling infectious mononucleosis can occur in cytomegalovirus infection and in toxoplasmosis. In such cases the Paul-Bunnell test is negative.

Another important cause of lymphocytosis is chronic lymphocytic leukemia.

Monocytosis.   An increased number of monocytes is typically seen in some protozoal diseases, *e.g.,* malaria and leishmaniasis. It is a feature of monocytic leukemia and also of some chronic bacterial infections, *e.g.,* tuberculosis.

Eosinophilia. This condition, which is characterized by the formation and accumulation of a large number of eosinophils in the blood, is encountered in atopic conditions, particularly bronchial asthma, hay fever, and urticaria. It is also a feature of helminthic infections, particularly when the parasites are migrating through the blood stream and tissues.

The Leukemias

Leukemia is a condition in which there is a widespread proliferation of white cells and their precursors throughout the tissues in the body. There is usually an increase in the number of circulating white cells also. The cause of leukemia is unknown, but it has been found that there is an increased incidence following exposure to ionizing radiation. In birds and mice the cause appears to be viral.

The leukemias are classified according to the rapidity of progression of the disease and the type of cell involved:

Chronic Leukemia

(a) Chronic myelocytic leukemia (also called chronic myelogenous or myeloid leukemia)

(b) Chronic lymphocytic leukemia

Acute Leukemia

(a) Acute myeloblastic leukemia (also called acute myelogenous or myeloid leukemia)

(b) Acute lymphoblastic leukemia (also called acute lymphocytic leukemia)

Chronic Myelocytic Leukemia

This is a disease of middle life and is characterized by an enormous leukocytosis, the white-cell count reaching 1000×10^9/L (1 million/μl) on occasions. The predominant cell is the neutrophil polymorph, but metamyelocytes and myelocytes are also present. Coincidental with the leukocytosis is a progressive anemia and a gradual fall in the platelet count.

Clinically, the patient has immense enlargement of the spleen, and to a lesser extent, the liver. Death usually occurs within three to five years and may be heralded by an acute exacerbation in which the blood stream is flooded with myeloblasts.

Chronic Lymphocytic Leukemia

This is usually a disease of later life, and there is a marked lymphocytosis with a total white-cell count ranging up to 250×10^9/L (250,000/μl). Most of the cells in the blood stream are mature lymphocytes, but there are a varying number of lymphoblasts. There is a progressive anemia and thrombocytopenia.

Since the condition affects lymph nodes primarily, the patient usually presents with generalized lymphadenopathy. The spleen and liver are enlarged, but to a lesser extent than with myeloid leukemia. As with the latter disease, death usually occurs within five years and is due to anemia and secondary infection.

Acute Leukemia

The two types of acute leukemia are best considered together because they resemble each other very closely. In the acute leukemias the white-cell count may vary from less than 1×10^9/L (1000/μl) to over 100×10^9/L (100,000/μl). When there is a raised count, the blood is invariably flooded with primitive blast cells, and it is often difficult or even impossible to be sure whether these are myeloblasts or lymphoblasts. Sometimes the cells have the features of monocytes and the disease is labelled *acute myelomonocytic* or *monoblastic leukemia*. The monocyte and myeloblast have a common stem cell of origin and "acute monocytic leukemia" is now regarded as a variant of acute myeloblastic leukemia. Occasionally the blast cells cannot be identified, and the term *stem cell leukemia* is used. However, in most cases there is also an increased number of more mature cells, thereby helping in the differential diagnosis.

In acute leukemia the primitive white cells replace the mature ones, and the polymorph count is invariably reduced (agranulocytosis). This leads to an impaired defense against infection, so that gingivitis and bronchopneumonia are common.

In acute leukemia there is rapidly progressive normocytic, normochromic anemia and severe thrombocytopenia.

Acute leukemia occurs at all ages. In childhood it is usually lymphoblastic, but in adult life the myeloblastic variety is more common. Clinically, it is not possible to distinguish between the two types. The onset is usually sudden, the main features being high fever, a generalized bleeding tendency, progressive anemia, and necrotic infective lesions of the mouth and throat. Acute leukemia can therefore closely mimic an acute infectious disease.

Most patients with acute leukemia die within six months, usually as a result of infection or bleeding into vital areas such as the central nervous system. Intensive modern therapy has increased the average survival considerably. As many as 50 per cent of patients may survive five years, and perhaps one third of children with acute lymphoblastic leukemia can now be cured.

Changes in the Organs in Leukemia.   The pathological course of leukemia is a monotonous infiltration of leukemic cells into numerous organs, which become enlarged, soft, and pale. Lymph nodes, spleen, and bone marrow are particularly involved and are crowded out by the responsible cells. No organ is exempt from this infiltration; massive local involvement is particularly characteristic of acute leukemia. Other changes found are those associated with infection and hemorrhage.

Bone Marrow Aplasia

When the bone marrow ceases to release mature elements into the circulation, there is a serious drop in the blood count, and the condition is described as *aplasia*. Sometimes the failure of division occurs at the "blast" stage; in such cases no mature elements are present either in the peripheral blood or in the bone marrow. At other times there is a failure in division at a later stage of hematopoiesis, so that the marrow, although crowded with maturing cells, is unable to release them into the circulation. This is called *maturation arrest*.

Aplasia of the marrow may involve all three elements, thereby leading to a diminution of all cells of the blood *(pancytopenia)*, or it may affect only one of these elements. *Pure red-cell aplasia* is very uncommon, but aplasia of the granulocytes *(agranulocytosis)* is an important condition. Whether a *pure platelet aplasia* occurs is doubtful; in idiopathic thrombocytopenic purpura (page 366) the platelets are destroyed after they have been released from the bone marrow.

Pancytopenia

Aplasia affecting all the formed elements of the marrow can be due to ionizing radiations or drugs, of which the most important are chloramphenicol, the sulfonamides, phenylbutazone (used in the treatment of arthritis), gold salts (used in the treatment of rheumatoid arthritis), and the cytotoxic drugs (used in the treatment of cancer). It is also a rare complication of miliary tuberculosis. In some patients, no cause can be found, and the condition must be termed "idiopathic." Some instances of the last group eventually turn out to be leukemia. An occasional cause is hypersplenism, which is described later in this chapter.

Hematologically, there is an anemia with no reticulocytosis, a leukopenia, and a thrombocytopenia. If the bone marrow is found to be hypocellular, the prognosis is poor. On the other hand, cases of maturation arrest have a better prognosis.

Aplasia of the white-cell elements is a serious complication of therapy with certain drugs, particularly thiouracil (used in the treatment of thyrotoxicosis), phenylbutazone, and chlorpromazine (used as a tranquilizer). Agranulocytosis also occurs as a result of the use of anticancer drugs. Some cases occur with hypersplenism, whereas others are idiopathic.

Agranulocytosis

The chief effect of agranulocytosis is a tendency for infection to develop; consequently, ulcerating infective lesions occur in the mouth and throat, gastrointestinal tract, and vagina. Overwhelming infection with bronchopneumonia is the usual end-result.

The function of the spleen in relation to blood formation is ill-understood. It is active in removing defective and aging red cells from the circulation, and it is possible that it exerts an inhibitory effect on the formation of white cells and platelets in the marrow.

Hypersplenism

Occasionally conditions leading to gross splenomegaly give rise either to marrow aplasia affecting any or all of the formed elements of the blood or to a hemolytic anemia. If the blood disorder abates after removal of the spleen, the condition is diagnosed as hypersplenism. The precise mechanism is not understood, and the condition is described in the splenomegaly of many conditions, *e.g.*, cirrhosis of the liver, schistosomiasis, and leishmaniasis.

The normal bone marrow is sometimes crowded out by foreign elements such as metastatic carcinoma or myeloma. This results in a typical blood picture of *leukoerythroblastic anemia*. This consists of a normocytic, normochromic anemia in which there are many nucleated red cells (normoblasts) in the blood. There is a moderate to considerable polymorph leukocytosis, and many myelocytes and metamyelocytes are also present in the blood.

The Syndrome of Bone Marrow Replacement

In a number of instances a leukoerythroblastic anemia is present in the face of fibrosis of the bone marrow *(myelosclerosis)*. This condition has been grouped with polycythemia vera and leukemia under the all-embracing heading of *myeloproliferative disorder*.

Platelets are small discs devoid of a nucleus that are formed in the bone marrow by fragmentation of the cytoplasm of large multinucleate cells termed *megakaryocytes*. Platelet adhesion and aggregation have already been described in Chapter 20 in relation to thrombosis. In this section we shall consider the platelets and the clotting mechanism, particularly in relation to the defects that lead to a bleeding tendency.

THE PLATELETS AND CLOTTING FACTORS

Blood clotting itself is a very complex mechanism (Fig. 26–7). In essence it consists of a conversion of *fibrinogen (factor I)* to fibrin by the action of thrombin. This enzyme exists normally as an inert precursor, *prothrombin (factor II)*, which is activated to thrombin by *prothrombinase*, which itself is generated by the interaction of activated *factor X* (designated *Factor Xa*) with *factor V*, platelet factor 3, and calcium ions *(factor IV)*. This sequence is called the common pathway and can be initiated by two completely separate mechanisms, the intrinsic (blood) system and the extrinsic (tissue) system (Figs. 26–7 and 26–8).

The Clotting Mechanism

The Intrinsic System. In the intrinsic (blood) system, contact with an abnormal surface leads to the activation of *factor XII* to factor XIIa. This

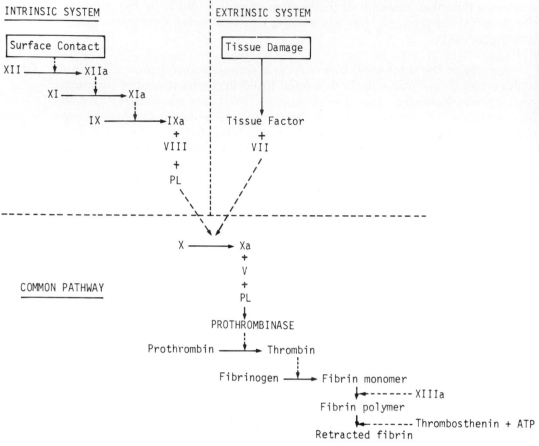

Figure 26–7.   A simplified diagrammatic representation of the blood clotting mechanism.
The three pathways are separated by interrupted lines. Solid arrows indicate transformation,
interrupted arrows denote actions. PL denotes platelet factor 3. Not shown in the diagram is the
calcium which is required for most of the steps shown. (After Marcus, A. J., *in* New England Journal of Medicine, *280*:1213, 1969.)

activates *factor XI*, and factor XIa activates *factor IX*. Factor IXa in conjunction with factor VIII and platelet phospholipid activates factor X.

The Extrinsic System.   In the extrinsic (tissue) system, tissue damage
results in the release of a tissue factor rich in phospholipid. It is called *factor
III*. This in conjunction with *factor VII* activates factor X, which, as already
described, is involved in the production of prothrombinase via the common
pathway.

The tissue factor is found in large amounts in the brain, extracts of which
are used as a source of it in various laboratory tests, such as the prothrombin
time. The venom of the Russell viper is also rich in it.

The two pathways of blood clotting are both important, for a derangement
of either leads to a serious defect in hemostasis. The intrinsic system develops
much more slowly than the extrinsic one, but both are initiated by tissue
damage, either by releasing tissue factor or providing an abnormal surface. In
both systems there is activation of factor X, and from then on there is a final
common pathway involving factor V, platelet factor 3, calcium ions, prothrombin, and fibrinogen.

It should be noted that factors II, VII, IX, X, XI, XII, and XIII are all
enzymes; they are of a class called *serine esterases*. Digestive enzymes and
complement enzymes are also members of this class. Characteristically they
are all stored as an inactive precursor, activated by a given stimulus, and then

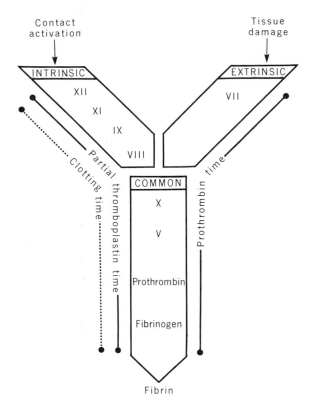

Figure 26–8. The interpretation of screening tests of blood clotting. (Modified from Bithell, T. C., and Wintrobe, M. M. *In* Wintrobe, M. M., et al. (Eds.): Harrison's Principles of Internal Medicine, 7th ed. New York, McGraw-Hill Book Company, 1974. Copyright © 1974 by McGraw-Hill, Inc. Used by permission of McGraw-Hill Book Company.)

undergo a cascadelike activation. Thus, the activation of the various factors involved in clotting is believed to follow a *cascade sequence,* many of the factors being substrates that are activated by a preceding enzyme.

The earliest phase of the intrinsic system is slow, but once thrombin is formed the process is greatly accelerated — indeed, there is a real cascade, for thrombin potentiates the activity of factors V and VIII. It also causes platelets to aggregate and so increases the amount of lipid factor 3. This is called the *autocatalytic action of thrombin.* Interestingly, thrombin also destroys factors V and VIII after potentiating their reactivity; in this way fibrin formation is stopped when a high concentration of thrombin has been achieved.

It should be noted that the plasma clotting factors (all globulins) are given Roman numerals. They are also given alternative names: factor VIII is antihemophilic factor; factor IX is Christmas factor; and factor XII is Hageman factor. The personal names refer to the surnames of the patients in whom a deficiency of the particular factor was first described. The latest factor described is *factor XIII* (fibrin-stabilizing factor), which converts soluble fibrin into insoluble, or stabilized, fibrin.

When small blood vessels are damaged, the injured vessels are sealed by a mass known as a *hemostatic plug.* At first this consists of platelets, but soon this is consolidated by fibrin formation. Finally the entire aggregate contracts, probably owing to the contractile protein in the platelets called *thrombosthenin.* Thrombin released during clotting causes further platelet deposition as well as fibrin formation. Defects in the intrinsic system of blood clotting, such as in hemophilia (page 366), do not prevent the formation of a hemostatic plug, and therefore the bleeding time is normal (page 367). However, the plug is not stable, and rebleeding occurs later. Serious bleeding can therefore follow the infliction of a wound such as that caused by dental extraction. A third cause of bleeding is some abnormality in the vessels themselves.

The Bleeding Diseases

Bleeding Due to Platelet Deficiency

The normal platelet count is 150 to 440 × 10⁹ per liter (150,000 to 440,000 per μl), with an average of 250 × 10⁹/L. It is raised after injuries and operations (especially splenectomy). A count below 100 × 10⁹/L is designated *thrombocytopenia.*

A low platelet count (thrombocytopenia) leads to spontaneous bleeding into the tissues with the production of small petechiae. In the skin the condition is called *purpura.* Spontaneous hemorrhage also occurs into the gastrointestinal and urinary tracts.

Thrombocytopenia may occur as an idiopathic condition *(primary thrombocytopenic purpura),* usually in young people. This is due to the formation of an IgG autoantibody that is directed against platelets and causes them to be destroyed in the spleen. Sometimes the condition remits spontaneously or following splenectomy, but relapses are common, and death not infrequent.

As a secondary condition, thrombocytopenia occurs in leukemia (especially the acute variety), marrow aplasia, and hypersplenism, and following the administration of certain drugs.

Bleeding Due to Defects in the Clotting Mechanism

Clotting mechanism defects are manifested by massive bleeding into the tissues and from the body orifices. Purpura is unusual, but intractable postoperative hemorrhage is characteristic and serious: fatal bleeding can occur even after a trivial operation or injury.

The following disorders are important:

Hemophilia A.   A hereditary disease characterized by spontaneous or traumatic hemorrhages, this is due to a deficiency of factor VIII. It affects only males, since it is inherited as an X-linked recessive trait (Chapter 3). Bleeding is often severe; a special feature is bleeding into joints (hemarthrosis), which is usually recurrent and leads to extensive damage to the affected joints. The disease can now be treated by giving the patient preparations of plasma containing concentrated factor VIII.

Hemophilia B or Christmas Disease.   This condition is due to a deficiency of factor IX. Its mode of inheritance and clinical manifestations are indistinguishable from those of hemophilia A.

Deficiencies of the Vitamin K–Dependent Coagulation Factors.   The two common causes are liver failure and a deficiency of vitamin K. This vitamin is used by the liver for the synthesis of prothrombin as well as for the synthesis of other clotting factors. The vitamin is fat soluble, and its absorption is aided by the presence of bile salts. Consequently, it is poorly absorbed in obstructive jaundice, and this is one of the factors in the bleeding tendency that complicate obstructive jaundice and chronic liver disease.

Vitamin K deficiency also occurs in the newborn because of an inability of the infant to synthesize the vitamin in its bowel. If the mother's intake is also deficient, a serious bleeding state may occur — *hemorrhagic disease of the newborn.* Another cause of hypoprothrombinemia is the administration of dicumarol anticoagulants, which inhibit the synthesis of clotting factors in the liver. These drugs are used as a treatment of phlebothrombosis and myocardial infarction.

Hypofibrinogenemia.   A deficiency of fibrinogen is usually acquired as a result of tissue factor entering the circulation. Such an event sets up intravascular clotting, causing the residual blood to become incoagulable. In addition, there is usually an activation of plasminogen so that fibrinolysis and fibrinogen destruction occur together with the clotting. The condition is called *disseminated intravascular coagulation, consumptive coagulopathy,* or the *defibrination syndrome* and is characterized by severe bleeding. It is encountered most commonly as a complication of pregnancy, when amniotic fluid enters the circulation and sets up both clotting and fibrinolysis. It also follows severe trauma, lung operations, and incompatible blood transfusions. The condition is a rather uncommon feature of widespread disseminated cancer.

This type of bleeding usually takes the form of purpura, but more extensive bleeding can occur into the tissues as well as into organs to produce hematuria and hematemesis.

Bleeding Due to Vascular Disease

A common form of vascular damage is the vasculitis that is due to the deposition of immune complexes. This occurs in immune-complex disease and is also a feature of certain infections (*e.g.*, gonococcal) and other types of septicemia. Ingestion of drugs such as aspirin is another cause of vascular damage mediated by an immunological mechanism.

Important Tests in Bleeding Diseases

1. Platelet Count.   The normal platelet count is 150 to 440×10^9/L.

2. Clotting Time.   This is the time taken for a specimen of whole blood to clot *in vitro* at 37°C. The normal time is 5 to 10 minutes. The clotting time is prolonged if there is a deficiency in any of the factors involved in the intrinsic clotting system or in the common pathway. The test is insensitive, and a normal result can be obtained even in the presence of a very low level of some clotting factors. The clotting time is prolonged when a circulating anticoagulant such as heparin is present in excess. The test is therefore widely used to control heparin therapy. The clotting time is greatly prolonged in hemophilia A and Christmas disease.

3. Bleeding Time.   The time taken for a small skin puncture to stop bleeding is termed the *bleeding time*. It varies from 1 to 9 minutes and is prolonged when there is a lack of platelets. In hemophilia it is normal, but it is prolonged in thrombocytopenia.

4. Capillary Fragility Test.   A sphygmomanometer (blood pressure) cuff is placed around the arm and inflated to a pressure of 100 mm Hg for five minutes. If the test is positive, the skin of the arm below the cuff shows a petechial eruption. A positive test indicates platelet deficiency, because normally the platelets seal off any defects caused by a sudden rise in blood pressure. The test is also positive if the vessels themselves are abnormal, *e.g.*, in scurvy.

5. Partial Thromboplastin Time (PTT).   This is the time required for plasma to clot in a glass tube when an extract of brain, called *cephalin,* is added in the presence of calcium chloride. The cephalin provides excess phospholipid and makes the test independent of the platelet count. The PTT is a sensitive measure of the factors concerned in the intrinsic and common pathways.

6. Prothrombin Time (PT).   In this test equal amounts of brain extract containing tissue factor, calcium chloride, and plasma are incubated, and the time required for clotting to occur is recorded. The test is measured against the time needed for a normal sample of plasma to clot. The prothrombin time is a measure of the factors concerned in the extrinsic system (factor VII) and in the common pathway (factors X, VII, and prothrombin). The intrinsic system is bypassed.

The PT and PTT together can give a fair indication of the nature of a clotting defect (Fig. 26–8 and Table 26–4). If both PTT and PT are normal, the defect is probably in the vessels or in the platelets. If either PTT or PT is prolonged, there is probably a defect in the clotting system. If both PTT and PT are abnormal, the defect is most likely in the common pathway, whereas if the PTT is prolonged and the PT is normal, the defect is probably in the

TABLE 26–4. THE BLEEDING DISEASES

DISEASE	PLATELET COUNT	CLOTTING TIME	BLEEDING TIME	CAPILLARY FRAGILITY TEST	PARTIAL THROMBOPLASTIN TIME	PROTHROMBIN TIME
Primary thrombocytopenic purpura	↓	N	↑	↑	N	N
Hemophilia	N	↑	N	N	↑	N
Christmas disease	N	↑	N	N	↑	N
Deficiency of the vitamin K–dependent coagulation factors	N	N	N	N	↑	↑
Disseminated intravascular coagulation	↓	↑	↑	↑	↑	↑

intrinsic system. The combination of a prolonged PT and a normal PTT is rare and indicates a deficiency of factor VII.

The red cells contain many antigens, but for practical purposes those concerned with the ABO and Rhesus blood groups are the most important.

THE BLOOD GROUPS AND BLOOD TRANSFUSION

The ABO System

Antigens of the ABO system are glycoproteins and are derived from a basic antigen called the H substance. Under the influence of the *A* or *B* gene, the H substance is converted into either A or B antigen. At birth there are no corresponding antibodies in the plasma, but within six months the antibodies corresponding to the antigens not present in the red cells make their appearance. These antibodies, called *alloantibodies*, are capable of agglutinating the red cells of normal people who are of a different blood group and of not agglutinating the red cells of persons having the same blood group as that of the individual tested. The following table describes the distribution of ABO antigens and antibodies.

BLOOD GROUP	ANTIBODIES NORMALLY PRESENT IN PLASMA
A	Anti-B
B	Anti-A
AB	None
O	Anti-A and Anti-B

The antibodies probably develop as a result of blood group–specific substances that are produced by bacteria in the intestine. The infant presumably forms antibodies against those antigens to which it is not immunologically tolerant.

To perform a blood grouping, one must treat a suspension of red cells with anti-A and anti/B sera, each derived from a donor with a high titer of these antibodies. If anti-A serum alone agglutinates the cells, the sample is of blood group A; if anti-B serum alone does it, the sample is of blood group B. If the cells are agglutinated by both anti-A and anti-B, the sample is of group AB, and if by neither anti-A nor anti-B, the sample is of group O. Similarly, with stock suspensions of cells of known blood group, it is possible to detect the appropriate antibodies in the patient's serum and to do the "reverse grouping."

The Rhesus System

About 85 per cent of the white population of the world has a red-cell antigen that was first noted in Rhesus monkey red cells. This is called the Rh antigen; cells containing it are called Rhesus positive (or Rh positive). Rh-negative individuals do not normally have Rh antibodies in their plasma, but if they are immunized by Rh-positive cells, they may form antibodies very easily. Such immunization can follow a mismatched blood transfusion or can occur after the pregnancy of an Rh-negative woman bearing an Rh-positive fetus. Many Rhesus antigens have been discovered: C, D, E, c, among others. The most important of these is D; cells containing it correspond to the original Rh-positive cells.

Other Blood Groups

Human red cells contain many antigens other than those belonging to either the ABO or the Rh systems. At least 10 other blood group systems are known. Occasionally antibodies to these antigens are a cause of transfusion reaction.

Blood Transfusion

Indications

Blood transfusion is an essential and common procedure in clinical practice. Not only is it mandatory for restoring the blood volume after severe hemorrhage, but it is also used extensively in major operative procedures. In anemia packed cells should be given rather than whole blood, which contains unwanted plasma. Surplus plasma can always be used by blood banks for other purposes, such as the preparation of factor VIII concentrates. Whenever possible, it is desirable to treat anemia with the specific agent in short supply, *i.e.*, iron or vitamin B_{12}, unless the patient's life is in danger.

Various blood components are available from transfusion centers; these are useful in restoring deficient clotting factors, such as factor VIII in hemophilia A.

Cross Matching

The important elements to consider are the donor's red cells and the recipient's plasma. As a general rule, the donor's plasma is not important because, with rare exceptions, the antibodies it contains are so diluted by the recipient's plasma that they are not likely to react with the recipient's cells. It is always preferable to use the blood of exactly the same ABO and Rh groups as those of the recipient, but group O Rh-negative blood can be given in an emergency in which delay might lead to death from exsanguination (extensive blood loss). Under all other circumstances a cross matching is essential. To do this matching, cells of the donor are mixed with the serum of the recipient; no agglutination should occur.

Hazards of Blood Transfusion

Incompatible Reactions. These are usually due to the rapid destruction of the donor's red cells by the recipient's plasma such as when group A cells are transfused into a group O patient. The antigen-antibody reaction leads to agglutination of the red cells, causing blockage of capillaries and the release of vasoconstrictor substances and leading to widespread vascular phenomena. There is initial pain along the vein, followed by facial flushing, headache, a sense of constriction around the chest, and backache. In severe cases, renal vascular spasm combined with free hemoglobin in the blood lead to acute renal failure and death from uremia.

Bacterial Contamination of the Blood. This is usually due to the accidential introduction of coliform organisms in the transfusion fluid.

Diseases Introduced from the Donor. The most important of these are viral hepatitis, syphilis, and malaria.

Febrile Reactions. These are usually due to the presence in the recipient of anti–white cell antibodies that have been formed as a result of previous transfusions or pregnancy. This type of febrile reaction may be quite severe, but it generally responds to simple treatment such as the administration of aspirin. Although febrile reactions themselves are of little importance, each must be investigated; fever, although not dangerous in itself, may be a component of an incompatible transfusion. Future transfusions can be given with blood from which the white cells have been removed in order to avoid additional febrile reactions.

Febrile reactions may be also due to the presence of gram-negative endotoxin present either in the transfusion fluid or in the apparatus. Modern disposable apparatus and properly prepared fluids have largely eliminated this complication.

Allergic Reactions. These are usually urticarial and are due to some antigen present in the donor's plasma to which the recipient is hypersensitive.

Overloading the Circulation. Transfusing an excess volume of blood can lead to heart failure and can be avoided by slow transfusion. Pulmonary edema is the usual manifestation of this complication.

Air Embolism.   With modern equipment this is a rare event.

Thrombophlebitis.   This response (inflammation of a vein with associated thrombus formation) follows the local irritation of the vein by the needle or cannula.

Transfusional Hemosiderosis.   Repeated transfusions are liable to lead to iron overload with hemosiderin deposited in many tissues, including the liver, where it may set up fibrosis.

Sensitization.   The transfusion of blood carrying antigens not present in the recipient may stimulate the production of alloantibodies against the foreign antigens. These alloantibodies to red cells, white cells, platelets, or plasma protein antigens may complicate future transfusions or pregnancies (see also hemolytic disease of the newborn, mentioned earlier).

In modern centers, blood transfusion is a life-saving procedure, but it must never be forgotten that the possible complications are numerous and occasionally fatal. Except under emergency conditions transfusion should never be attempted without expert supervision. Any patient receiving a blood transfusion must be carefully and repeatedly watched so that the early signs of any complication can be detected. The nursing attendants play a vital role in the teamwork that transfusion requires. A particular function that deserves special stress involves the correct identification of specimens. More serious complications of blood transfusion result from giving a unit of blood to the wrong patient than are due to errors of grouping or cross matching. The wrong Smith can soon become a dead Smith!

Review Questions

1. Distinguish between normoblastic and megaloblastic hyperplasia of the bone marrow.

2. A 45-year-old woman who had had indigestion for several months suddenly vomited about 250 ml of blood. This was repeated 12 hours later, and she was admitted to a hospital shortly afterwards. Investigations revealed the following: hemoglobin, 8.5 g/dl; mean corpuscular hemoglobin concentration (MCHC), 25 g/dl; and a reticulocyte count of 8 per cent. What conclusions can be drawn from these findings?

3. Describe the association of anemia with red cells containing:
   (a) An abnormal type of hemoglobin
   (b) An abnormal enzyme

4. A woman gives birth to a child with generalized edema, severe anemia, and nucleated red cells in the peripheral blood. The direct Coombs' test on the baby's blood is positive, and the mother's blood group is AB, Rh negative. Describe the pathogenesis of the baby's anemia assuming that:
   (a) It is the mother's second child.
   (b) It is the mother's first child.

5. A 25-year-old man develops a sore throat, general malaise, and enlarged lymph nodes of the neck. Discuss the differential diagnosis if:
   (a) The total white-cell count is 2.5×10^9/L and the neutrophil polymorphs constitute 25 per cent of the total.
   (b) The total white-cell count is 1.0×10^9/L, and 20 per cent of the cells are large mononuclear forms with obvious nucleoli.
   (c) The total white-cell count is 15×10^9/L, and many of the cells are lymphocytes that are atypical but do not contain nucleoli.
   (d) The total white-cell count is 20×10^9/L and 90 per cent of the cells are polymorphs. No atypical cells are present.

6. Examine the red cells in Figure 26–6B. What type of anemia does the morphology of the cells suggest? What might be the cause of the anemia and how could the diagnosis be substantiated?

7. List the important steps that should be taken before a patient is given a blood transfusion.

Selected Readings

Cullino, L. C.: Preventing and treating transfusion reactions. American Journal of Nursing, 79:1935–1936, 1979.

de Gruchy, G. C.: Clinical Haematology in Medical Practice. 4th ed. Oxford, Blackwell Scientific Publications, 1978.

Kazak, A.: Processing blood for transfusion. American Journal of Nursing, 79:931–934, 1979.

Leading Article: Prevention of haemolytic diseases of the newborn due to anti-D. British Medical Journal, 282:676–677, 1981.

Leeson, T. S., and Leeson, C. R.: Histology. 4th ed. Philadelphia, W. B. Saunders Company, 1981. Note, in particular, Chapter 8, "The Circulatory System."

Silver, R. T.: Morphology of the Blood and Marrow. New York, Grune & Stratton, Inc., 1970, 125 pp. A well-illustrated, short account of common blood disorders.

Wintrobe, M. M., Lee, G. R., Boggs, D. R., Bithell, T. C., Athens, J. W., and Foerster, J.: Clinical Hematology, 7th ed. Philadelphia, Lea & Febiger, 1974, 1896 pp. Useful for reference.

The Collagen Vascular Diseases

After studying this chapter the student should be able to:

- List the major collagen vascular diseases and discuss the validity of grouping them under one heading.
- Describe the main features of chronic discoid lupus erythematosus and systemic lupus erythematosus.
- List the autoantibodies that may be found in the various collagen vascular diseases.
- Describe the lesions of dermatomyositis.
- Distinguish between morphea and progressive systemic sclerosis. Describe the main lesions of each disease.
- Describe the main features of
    - (a) The classical type of polyarteritis nodosa
    - (b) Three variants of polyarteritis

The term *collagen disease* was coined to describe a group of disorders in which the primary lesion appeared to be damage to collagen. *Lupus erythematosus, dermatomyositis, progressive systemic sclerosis,* and *polyarteritis* are now included in this group, and each will be described in this chapter. *Acute rheumatic fever* and *rheumatoid arthritis* can also be included, but they are described in Chapters 28 and 40.

The evidence for these diseases being primary disorders of collagen is by no means convincing, but because they all possess certain features in common it is convenient to group them together. Since blood vessel involvement is as constant a feature as collegen damage the term *collagen vascular disease* is currently used.

Lupus Erythematosus

Chronic Discoid Lupus Erythematosus (DLE)

This type of lupus erythematosus has been recognized for many years by clinical dermatologists as a skin condition that occurs particularly on the exposed areas of the body and is worsened by exposure to sunlight. The lesions consist of well-defined, erythematous, scaly papules and plaques. The epidermis shows atrophy, and as the lesions heal there is scarring. When the scalp is involved, there is loss of hair (alopecia). Indeed, lupus erythematosus is an important cause of alopecia with scarring; the lesions are very similar to those produced by scleroderma of the scalp. Chronic discoid lupus erythematosus may progress to the systemic disease, but this occurs only rarely.

Systemic Lupus Erythematosus (SLE)

In systemic lupus erythematosus there are widespread lesions affecting many organs. The skin may show lesions identical to those of chronic discoid lupus erythematosus, or it may merely show redness (erythema) and edema of the sun-exposed areas. Typically, it affects the nose and both cheeks, thereby giving the classic "butterfly rash." Other important features of systemic lupus are arthritis, pericarditis (Fig. 5–6A), pleurisy, endocarditis, and glomerulonephritis. It is the kidney lesions that commonly cause the patient's death from renal failure (Fig. 35–3). Systemic lupus erythematosus varies considerably in severity. The onset may be acute with fever, malaise, a low white cell count (leukopenia), elevated ESR, joint pains, lymphadenopathy, and skin rashes. On the other hand, the disease may be insidious, often with the development of a skin rash, which is later to be followed by evidence of other organ involvement. Raynaud's phenomenon is common. When there is involvement of the brain there can be a severe psychotic illness, and the disease may commence in this way.

A prominent feature of SLE is the presence of many autoantibodies in the serum. Acute hemolytic anemia can occur, confirmed by a positive Coombs' test. The standard serological tests for syphilis are sometimes falsely positive. The rheumatoid factor is present in about 30 per cent of cases.

The important antibodies, from a diagnostic point of view, are those that react specifically with nuclear antigenic components. Antinuclear protein and anti-DNA antibodies can be demonstrated in most cases of the active disease. The antibodies may be detected by immunofluorescence: the patient's serum is applied to a section or smear of tissue, and the anti-DNA antibody that adheres to the nuclei is detected by subsequently applying fluorescein-labeled anti-IgG and examining the tissue by ultraviolet microscopy. A less sensitive method of detecting these antibodies is to search for the LE cell phenomenon. This was the first specific laboratory test described in the diagnosis of SLE. When normal human leukocytes are incubated for about two hours with the serum of a patient with SLE, some neutrophils are found to contain a homogenous basophilic mass of nuclear material. Such neutrophils are called *LE cells*. The mass is derived from a necrotic leukocyte nucleus that has been acted upon by antinuclear antibody. Its subsequent phagocytosis by a polymorph produces the LE cell.

Systemic lupus erythematosus affects females far more often than males, and Blacks more often than Whites. It can occur at any age, but most cases are in the 20–40 age bracket. The cause and pathogenesis of the disease are not understood. A disease very similar to it, and encountered in Aleutian minks, is caused by a viral infection. Viruslike particles can be found in the lesions of human SLE, but they have not been cultured and their nature remains undetermined. There seems little doubt that SLE is a disease in which many autoantibodies are formed, particularly against nucleic acid, but whether the antigen is the patient's own nucleic acid or whether it is foreign — possibly viral — nucleic acid is not known. It is probable that the disease occurs in persons who are genetically susceptible, since there is an increased incidence of autoantibodies and autoimmune diseases in relatives of patients with SLE. It may well be that in these susceptible individuals various factors can trigger the formation of autoantibodies, and that immune-complexes damage the blood vessels of the skin, kidney, and other organs to produce the syndrome of SLE.

The precipitating factor may be a viral infection, administration of a drug (Chapter 9), or exposure to sunlight.

The cutaneous lesions of chronic discoid lupus erythematosus cannot be distinguished from those found in some cases of SLE. Nevertheless, the two diseases appear to be distinct entities, but their interrelationship remains to be clarified.

Dermatomyositis   The combination of muscle inflammation (myositis) causing progressive weakness of the proximal limb muscles and a variety of skin rashes constitutes this extraordinary disease. The occurrence of edema and erythema, giving a heliotrope discoloration, particularly around the eyes, is characteristic. Skin and muscle biopsies help establish the diagnosis. The disease may run a fulminating, fatal course, or it may be chronic. In patients over the age of 40 years, dermatomyositis is often associated with a malignant tumor of some internal organ. Hence, a thorough search for carcinoma should be undertaken. Specific signs or symptoms may indicate where this might be; the common sites, however (*e.g.*, lung, gastrointestinal tract, and kidney), should always be investigated.

Scleroderma

Like lupus erythematosus, scleroderma can occur in two forms. The purely cutaneous disease is called *morphea*. The skin becomes thickened and ultimately densely fibrous. Small plaques may occur at any site, or the disease can be widespread and affect areas of skin. In the latter type, Raynaud's phenomenon is common (Chapter 29).

In the systemic variety of scleroderma, called *progressive systemic sclerosis*, not only is the skin involved but so also are the internal organs. Particularly involved are the esophagus and other parts of the gastrointestinal tract, which show fibrosis and impaired peristalsis, thereby leading to obstruction. Fibrosis can occur in the lungs, and the effects of aspiration are added to this. Systemic sclerosis is often associated with Raynaud's syndrome; indeed, some authorities maintain that in most instances idiopathic "Raynaud's disease" is but an early manifestation of systemic sclerosis, and that given time other manifestations of the disease will appear. Vascular involvement is usually not a feature except in the kidney, and in this organ progressive vascular obstruction leads to renal failure in a considerable number of patients.

Polyarteritis Nodosa

Classical Polyarteritis Nodosa

This type of polyarteritis, first described in the last century, usually affects middle-aged males and is characterized by an arteritis involving many organs. The inflamed arterial walls become necrotic and infiltrated with both inflammatory cells and fibrin, which gives the appearance of *fibrinoid necrosis*. The weakened vessel wall bulges, and the aneurysms so formed are responsible for the designation "nodosa." The lumen of the affected vessels becomes obstructed by thrombus, and the disease is characterized by ischemia and infarction affecting many organs, particularly nerves, spleen, and kidney. Renal failure, often with hypertension, is a common end-result of this fatal disease.

Variants of Polyarteritis Nodosa

The classic polyarteritis nodosa described above is relatively uncommon, but many variants have been described recently. Often, when the vessels affected are small, the term *microscopic polyarteritis* has been applied to these lesions. In some of them, the precipitating cause appears to be an infection, whereas in others hypersensitivity to a drug has been implicated. In none of them is the pathogenesis at all clear; an immune complex type of vasculitis has been postulated, however. Some of the recognized syndromes are as follows:

Lethal Midline Granuloma.   This disease usually affects young males. It commences with bleeding from the nose and is characterized by a vasculitis with much necrosis affecting the nose and nasopharynx. This terrible disease produces extensive necrosis and gangrene affecting the nose and nasopharynx. Without treatment, death is invariable and results from local infection, massive bleeding, or bronchopneumonia.

Progressive Allergic Granulomatosis.   This variant usually commences with asthmatic attacks and pneumonia. Infarcted areas, which are found in the lung, excite a granulomatous reaction that closely resembles tuberculosis histologically.

Wegener's Granulomatosis. This disease is defined as a microscopic polyarteritis affecting kidneys, lungs, and upper respiratory tract. In the last site, the lesions resemble those described in lethal midline granuloma. Death is usually due to renal failure.

It is not clear whether these variants of polyarteritis represent a single disease or are completely separate entities sharing one morphological component — namely, a necrotizing vasculitis. Certainly necrotizing vasculitis can occur in other conditions. Thus, it is a prominent component of septicemia due to *Pseudomonas aeruginosa* and gonococcal septicemia (see Fig. 29–6). It is also a feature of the Arthus reaction, and it is encountered in rheumatoid arthritis, lupus erythematosus, and systemic sclerosis.

Summary   The validity of grouping these diseases under the heading of collagen vascular disease is dubious. Mixed cases occur, and patients appear who exhibit features of several diseases. Thus, some have lesions of scleroderma with vasculitis, or lupus erythematosus with rheumatoid arthritis. The occurrence of these mixed connective tissue diseases suggests that there is a common mechanism, but it does not prove a common cause. The presence of non–organ-specific autoantibodies is another feature that these diseases have in common, being the most striking in lupus erythematosus and the least evident in polyarteritis. Until the origin and pathogenesis of these diseases are discovered, it is convenient to refer to the group collectively as the "collagen vascular diseases" since they share many features. Thus, they are all *multisystem diseases,* since they produce widespread lesions affecting many organs, and often they exhibit marked constitutional effects such as fever, raised erythrocyte sedimentation rate (ESR), and hypergammaglobulinemia. This tendency is least marked in systemic sclerosis. All the diseases respond to glucocorticosteroid therapy as well as to other immunosuppressants such as azathioprine. Presumably, these act by suppressing autoantibody formation, thereby inhibiting the formation of new lesions. Once again progressive systemic sclerosis is the odd man out and is least responsive to therapy.

Review Questions

1. A young woman has developed an erythematous scaly rash on her face, the V of her neck, and her forearms. She feels tired and generally unwell. What tests could usefully be carried out to substantiate a diagnosis of systemic lupus erythematosus (SLE)?

2. A 56-year-old man has developed marked weakness of his shoulder and back muscles. He cannot easily sit up in bed or stand without assistance. The illness began several weeks ago and has been accompanied by redness and swelling around the eyes and on the hands and forearms. What tests could be performed to help establish a diagnosis of dermatomyositis? What other examinations should be carried out?

3. What symptoms and pathologic lesions can systemic lupus erythematosus and progressive systemic sclerosis have in common?

Selected Readings

Leading Article: Wegener's granulomatosis. Lancet, 2:519, 1972.

Peltier, A. P., and Estes, D.: Antinuclear antibodies. *In* Ioachim, H. L. (Ed.): Pathobiology Annual. Vol. 2. 1972, pp. 77–109.

Talbott, J. H.: Collagen-Vascular Diseases. New York, Grune & Stratton, 1974, 285 pp. All the topics mentioned in this chapter are described in detail in this book.

Diseases of Individual Organs

PART II

Diseases of the Heart   CHAPTER 28

After studying this chapter the student should be able to:

- Relate the development of the heart to the common types of developmental heart disease.
- List the main features of Fallot's tetralogy and of coarctation of the aorta.
- Describe the main features of acute rheumatic fever and discuss the immediate and long-term effects of this disease on the heart.
- Indicate the importance of nonbacterial thrombotic endocarditis.
- Contrast acute infective endocarditis with subacute infective endocarditis.
- Describe calcific aortic stenosis.
- Discuss the effects of myocardial ischemia and describe in detail the clinical and pathological features of myocardial infarction.
- Describe the changes in blood enzyme levels that are of value in the clinical diagnosis of acute myocardial infarction.
- Define chronic cor pulmonale and indicate the mechanisms involved in its evolution.
- List the causes and effects of stenosis and regurgitation of each of the four heart valves.
- Describe the pathophysiology and effects of the major cardiac dysrhythmias.
- Draw a typical electrocardiogram of each type.
- List the cardiac reserves.
- Describe the causes and effects of left ventricular failure, right ventricular failure, and congestive heart failure.
- Describe what is meant by a "cardiomyopathy."
- List the causes of acute cardiac tamponade.
- List the causes of acute pericarditis.

Diseases of the heart are a common cause of human ill health and death. In the neonatal period, congenital disease accounts for many deaths, whereas a heart attack *(myocardial infarction)* is one of the chief causes of death in men between the ages of 30 and 50 years in the Western civilized world.

Diseases of the heart may affect primarily the pericardium, the myocardium, or the endocardium — in particular, the endocardium that covers the valves. These structures may be attacked separately or in combination. The types and causes of heart disease are therefore many and varied; the effects, however, are few and stereotyped. Since the heart is a pump, it follows that the diseased and failing heart often pumps inefficiently. The consequences of this are circulatory disturbances that together constitute the syndrome of *heart failure*. This complex of disturbances will be described later, after individual diseases of the heart have been considered.

DEVELOPMENTAL ANOMALIES

The heart develops early in fetal life, and most of the developmental anomalies are therefore present at birth. This group of diseases is commonly called "congenital heart disease," and it is present in about 1 per cent of infants at birth. Without effective treatment at least 40 per cent of the infants so afflicted die during the first five years of life — most, in fact, during the first few months. Many developmental anomalies are known; until recently, however, their recognition was largely a matter of academic interest, particularly to the embryologist. Now, fortunately, since cardiac surgeons are able to offer a chance of cure, their interest is more than academic. Many techniques have been developed to assist in accurate diagnosis during life. Only a few of the common anomalies will be described.

Septal Defects

Since the heart develops from a single tube, a failure in the formation of the septa dividing the left and right chambers is not uncommon. In *atrial septal defects* some blood passes from the left atrium to the right atrium and from there into the right ventricle and the pulmonary circulation (Fig. 28–1A). The output of the right ventricle is several times greater than normal, but so long as it copes with this additional work, the patient is not seriously handicapped. This is indeed the most common congenital cardiac anomaly in adults and is not accompanied by cyanosis, as long as the shunt remains from left to right.

Ventricular septal defects are also common (Fig. 28–1B); if small, they cause little functional disturbance. With large defects the results are serious. There is a large left-to-right shunt that puts a strain on the left ventricle, because in addition to the shunted blood, it must eject an adequate amount of blood into the aorta if life is to be sustained. In time, the left ventricle fails. Furthermore, the right ventricle is subjected to the high pressure of blood coming from the left side so that the pulmonary circulation works at a high pressure. As long as the shunt is from left to right, the patient has no cyanosis. However, in response to the high pressure the pulmonary vessels become narrowed. The pulmonary resistance increases, and the right ventricular pressure rises even higher. The shunt then changes from left-to-right to right-to-left, and cyanosis ensues. Ventricular septal defects illustrate one of the complexities of treatment in congenital heart disease. If the defect is closed when the patient is young, he may develop normally and live to old age. If treatment is delayed until the blood flow is from right-to-left because of increased pulmonary resistance, then closure of the defect causes rapid heart failure and death.

Pulmonary Stenosis

An unequal division of the truncus arteriosus may result in the development of a large aorta and a correspondingly small pulmonary artery and valve (pulmonary stenosis) (Fig. 28–1C).

Transposition of the Great Vessels

Owing to a failure of rotation, the aorta can arise from the right ventricle and the pulmonary artery can arise from the left ventricle. If this were the only anomaly, life would not be possible — a complementary defect must also be present. The patient's survival after birth depends upon there being some communication, *e.g.*, a septal defect, between the two sides of the heart (Fig. 28–1D). Transposition of the great vessels is one of the common fatal anomalies in children under one year of age.

Dextrocardia

Occasionally the heart develops as a mirror-image of the normal. If this mirror-imaging involves all organs *(complete situs inversus)*, the patient lives a normal life, since there are no other abnormalities. If only the heart is affected, the results are serious, because other defects are also present.

Multiple Defects

Developmental anomalies are often multiple. Malformations may be found not only in other organs but also in the heart itself. A common combination is the *tetralogy of Fallot* (Fig. 28–1E), which consists of the following:

(a) Pulmonary stenosis.
(b) Ventricular septal defect.
(c) Overriding of the interventricular septum by the aorta, so that blood from both the right and left ventricles enters the aorta.
(d) Hypertrophy of the right ventricle — this is compensatory.

ATRIAL SEPTAL DEFECT

VENTRICULAR
SEPTAL DEFECT

PULMONARY STENOSIS

Aorta PA RV LV **A**

Aorta PA RV LV **B**

Aorta PA RV LV **C**

TRANSPOSITION OF
THE GREAT VESSELS

FALLOT'S TETRALOGY

PATENT DUCTUS
ARTERIOSUS

Aorta PA RV LV **D**

Aorta PA RV LV **E**

Aorta PA RV LV **F**

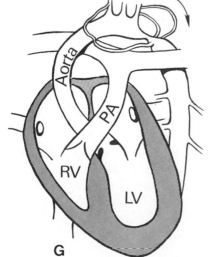

COARCTATION
OF THE AORTA

Aorta PA RV LV **G**

Figure 28–1.

The effects of Fallot's tetralogy illustrate many of the features of developmental heart disease and will be considered in some detail in the following paragraphs.

Murmurs.   These are often loud and may be heard over the precordium with the aid of a stethoscope. They may even be felt as *thrills*.

Central Cyanosis.   Since blood from the right ventricle enters the aorta directly, there is a considerable right-to-left shunt. The arterial blood is not fully oxygenated, and this causes central cyanosis. Patients with Fallot's tetralogy are born as "blue babies." Central cyanosis affects all tissues — skin, mucous membranes, tongue, and the others. Central cyanosis is also found in severe lung disease as well as in direct vascular shunts. It should be contrasted with peripheral cyanosis, which is due to stagnation of the blood in vessels of the skin. Peripheral cyanosis is never seen in the mucous membranes, which have an active blood supply, and this forms a useful clinical point of differentiation.

Polycythemia.   This condition (an increase in the total red cell mass of the body) is due to hypoxia of the bone marrow.

Clubbing of the Fingers and Toes.   This abnormality is generally seen when cyanosis is present and of long duration. The pathogenesis is obscure; it also occurs in other diseases, *e.g.*, chronic suppurative lung diseases, lung cancer, and bacterial endocarditis.

Underdevelopment.   Unless the heart defects are corrected, the child shows poor physical development. Early death from infection or heart failure is usual.

Squatting.   Patients tend to assume a squatting position after exertion, because this gives them relief from breathlessness.

Hypoxic Spells.   A sudden increase in the amount of cyanosis can lead to cerebral hypoxia.

Patent Ductus Arteriosus

In the fetus, blood that reaches the right ventricle by-passes the unexpanded lungs because of the high resistance of the pulmonary circulation. The blood passes from the pulmonary artery into the aorta through the patent ductus arteriosus. After birth, as the pulmonary circulation opens up, the ductus normally becomes obliterated, but occasionally this fails to happen and it remains patent (Fig. 28–1*F*). The left-to-right shunt that develops puts a strain on the left ventricle, which in due course may fail. In addition, pulmonary hypertension ensues, and this places a burden on the right ventricle. In addition to these hemodynamic effects, a patent ductus arteriosus presents yet another hazard to life. An *infective endarteritis* analogous to bacterial endocarditis may develop at the site of the ductus.

Coarctation of the Aorta *

The process of obliteration that affects the ductus may involve the aorta and may then lead to the formation of a stricture. This generally occurs beyond the subclavian arteries, so that blood reaches the upper half of the body normally by the arch of the aorta and its major branches, but it arrives at the lower half of the body only via collateral vessels (Fig. 28–1*G*). This condition is important for two reasons: (1) the area of stenosis may become infected, and (2) systemic hypertension may occur in the upper part of the body, leading to left ventricular hypertrophy and failure. Unless it is treated, life is seldom prolonged over the age of 40 years.

The diagnosis of coarctation of the aorta should be suspected if systemic hypertension can be measured in the patient's arms, and yet no pulse can be felt in the femoral or other leg vessels.

---

*Although not strictly a disease of the heart, this topic is described here for convenience.

Acute rheumatic fever is a disease of childhood and generally affects those between 5 and 15 years of age. It typically occurs two to three weeks after a streptococcal sore throat and is currently believed to be due to an immune-complex reaction between large amounts of streptococcal antigen and antibody present in the patient's serum. The soluble antigen-antibody complexes appear to localize in the small blood vessels of the heart and joints and by activating complement lead to tissue damage. The reason for the localization of the lesions in rheumatic fever is not known. Patients with rheumatic fever generally have a neutrophil leukocytosis, a raised ESR, and a high or rising antistreptolysin O titer *(ASO titer)*. The latter is an antibody to streptolysin O, a hemolysin produced by *Streptococcus pyogenes.*

The disease is characterized by *fever,* flitting *pains and swelling of the joints, subcutaneous nodules* (particularly over the bony prominences), and most important, *involvement of the heart.* Since *pericarditis* sometimes occurs, the two roughened surfaces of pericardium cause a characteristic rubbing noise that can be heard with a stethoscope. Some degree of heart failure is common and occasionally is fatal. At necropsy the heart is dilated, but the myocardium appears surprisingly normal. The characteristic lesion is a chronic inflammatory focus called an "Aschoff's nodule," which occurs between muscle bundles. Dilatation of the valve ring can lead to mitral regurgitation, which contributes to heart failure.

The most important lesions of acute rheumatic fever are those of the valves, which are swollen. Where the valve cusps meet there are depositions of thrombi on the endocardial surface — depositions called *vegetations,* which appear as small nodules along the line of valve closure. The mitral and aortic valves are most commonly affected by this *endocarditis.* Even though most other lesions of acute rheumatic fever undergo resolution, those of the valves do not. They tend to progress to a state of chronic inflammation, and the cusps become thickened, fibrosed, and contracted *(chronic rheumatic endocarditis).* Adjacent cusps adhere to each other, rendering the orifices stenotic, while the rigid leaflets and thickened chordae tendineae of the mitral valve lead to regurgitation (Figs. 28–2 and 28–3). If the aortic valve is affected, it is also rendered both stenotic and regurgitant.

Not all patients who suffer from an attack of acute rheumatic fever have persistent heart valve damage. Nevertheless, the disease has a tendency to recur, and with each attack valvular damage increases. Since the disease is precipitated by streptococcal infection, long-term antibiotic therapy is often instituted as a prophylactic measure.

In those patients unfortunate enough to progress to chronic rheumatic heart disease, mitral stenosis is the commonest valvular lesion found. Blood is dammed back in the left atrium, which becomes dilated; its wall becomes hypertrophied. Stasis may lead to the formation of thrombus on the wall of the atrium, particularly if there is atrial fibrillation (page 393). Pulmonary venous congestion follows. The effect of this is to make the lungs more rigid, so that breathing is more difficult and requires more effort. This alteration causes shortness of breath and distress *(dyspnea).* Intra-alveolar bleeding leads to *hemoptysis,* and gradually to brown induration of the lungs (page 398). In mitral stenosis the left ventricle is under no strain and is therefore small. However, should there be an additional factor of regurgitation or an aortic valvular lesion, the left ventricle would become enlarged and might subsequently fail. The back-pressure effect on the lungs eventually leads to pulmonary hypertension and right ventricular failure.

In chronic rheumatic heart disease the valves of the left side are much more frequently affected than are those of the right. Aortic lesions can occur alone or, more commonly, combined with mitral damage.

ACQUIRED HEART DISEASE

Rheumatic Heart Disease

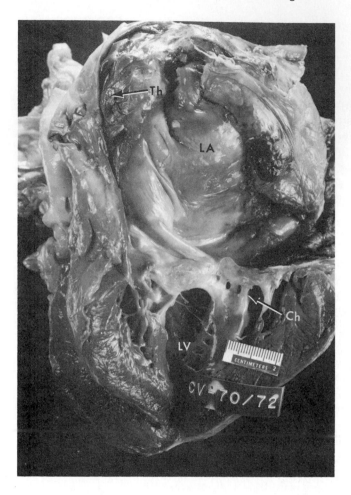

Figure 28–2. Mitral stenosis due to chronic rheumatic disease. The heart has been opened by an incision passing from the left atrium (LA) to the apex of the left ventricle (LV). The left atrium is enormously dilated, and thrombus (Th) is adherent to its walls. The mitral valve is markedly fibrosed, and its chordae (Ch) are greatly thickened and shortened. The left ventricle shows no abnormality, thereby indicating that the major function effect of the valvular lesion was that of stenosis. (Courtesy of Dr. M. D. Silver.)

Nonbacterial Thrombotic Endocarditis

Small warty vegetations along the line of closure of the mitral or aortic valves are a fairly common finding at necropsy. These vegetations are sterile and are of importance in two respects. First, they occasionally become detached and embolize to the brain. About 10 per cent of cerebral embolism has been attributed to this mechanism. Second, the vegetations may form a focus (commonly called a *nidus*) for the development of infective endocarditis. Nonbacterial endocarditis has been called "terminal" or "cachectic" endocarditis, but of necessity, the lesions can be found only at necropsy. Probably they occur quite frequently.

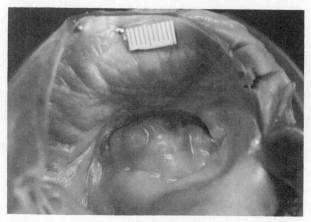

Figure 28–3. Mitral stenosis due to rheumatic heart disease. The mitral valve is viewed from the left atrium. Fusion of its cusps and fibrosis have combined to produce the characteristic rigid "fish mouth" or "buttonhole" stenotic deformity. (Courtesy of Dr. M. D. Silver.)

In this condition the valve cusps are inflamed and covered by thrombus, and the whole area is invaded by organisms.

Infective
Endocarditis

Acute Infective Endocarditis.   During the course of septicemia, organisms may invade the heart valve and produce an endocarditis that is characterized by the deposition of large, friable thrombi on the valve surfaces (Fig. 28–4). The valves themselves may undergo destruction and then rupture. The clinical condition is generally overshadowed by a septicemia, but the presence of heart murmurs is characteristic: frequently, they change in character as vegetations form or the valves rupture. Pyemia occurs as fragments of infected thrombus become detached and enter the arterial circulation, usually the systemic. The infecting organism in acute infective endocarditis is generally *Staphylococcus aureus* or the pneumococcus. Unless vigorous and efficient antibiotic treatment is instituted early, acute bacterial endocarditis is invariably fatal.

CASE HISTORY I. (See Figure 28–4)   The patient was a 63-year-old man with a 15-year history of essential hypertension and a five-year history of intermittent claudication. Investigation revealed blockage of the bifurcation of the abdominal aorta. A by-pass operation was performed by insertion of an aortoiliac synthetic (Dacron) prosthesis. For the next four years the patient was able to walk without pain; then the claudication returned. Surgery was again performed, and the prosthesis was found to be obstructed by thrombus. The prosthesis was replaced. As a result of the previous surgery, many peritoneal adhesions were present. Unfortunately, the small bowel was accidentally opened during the operation. The tear was sutured, but the fecal contamination led to a postoperative wound infection. In spite of vigorous antibiotic therapy and surgical drainage of abscesses, the patient's condition steadily deteriorated and he died four months after the operation. On several occasions during the course of his illness *Escherichia coli* and *Candida* species had been isolated from the blood.

At necropsy septic infarcts and pyemic abscesses were found in the brain, myocardium, kidneys and spleen. These were related to endocarditis involving the mitral valve (Fig. 28–4).

Subacute Infective Endocarditis.   The adjective "subacute," hallowed by tradition, is meaningless. The course of this disease is chronic.

Figure 28–4. Candida endocarditis. The heart has been opened to show the mitral valve, the left atrium (LA), and the left ventricle (LV). Friable vegetations (Veg) are present on the anterior cusp of the mitral valve; *Candida* was identified in the vegetations both by culture and in histological sections. The necropsy findings (see Case History I) indicate that this was an example of acute infective endocarditis. Nevertheless, the long clinical course was more suggestive of the subacute variety. Chemotherapy modifies the clinical and pathological findings; it is now more useful to describe endocarditis in terms of the infecting organism rather than as "acute" or "subacute." (Courtesy of Dr. M. D. Silver.)

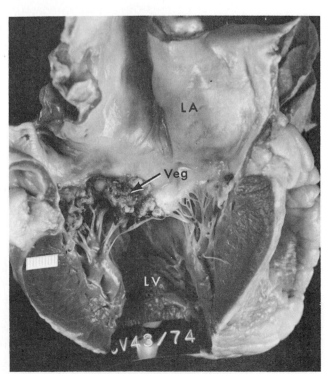

The disease commonly affects a valve that has been previously abnormal as a result of either rheumatic disease or congenital malformation. Any heart valve can be affected, but the mitral and aortic are most frequently involved. The valve is covered by large, red, friable vegetations that are liable to break off and embolize. Histologically, the thrombi contain numerous bacterial colonies that are well protected from the blood stream. Vegetations are attached to the valve by means of granulation tissue, which is neither profuse nor deeply penetrating into the vegetation. The organisms are once more beyond the reach of the blood. The poor vascularity of the valve cusp is probably the explanation for this inadequate organization. It is a good example of frustrated repair, and as such it is typical of chronic inflammation.

One of the curious features of this disease is that the organism is of relatively low virulence and is able to survive in the presence of a high degree of immunity. Its inaccessibility in the thrombus appears to be the explanation of this feature.

Clinical Features.   The disease runs a chronic course; unless early, prolonged, and effective treatment is instituted, the patient dies within one year — usually of heart failure due to valvular destruction or cicatrization, or of a progressive glomerulonephritis, probably of an immune-complex type. Pyrexia of unknown origin is a common presentation of the disease; weight loss and anemia are constant features. The chronic bacteremia is responsible for reticuloendothelial hyperplasia, which accounts for the splenomegaly. Clubbing of the fingers is common, and multiple embolic phenomena are characteristic. Large emboli may cause infarction of the brain, intestine, kidney, or spleen, whereas smaller emboli produce kidney lesions that lead to hematuria. Petechial hemorrhages in the skin and under the nails are sometimes seen. Although the emboli contain bacteria, they behave as if they were sterile. When the infected thrombi leave the heart, the bactericidal action of the blood appears to be adequate to destroy the organisms.

A positive blood culture is necessary for a diagnosis of subacute bacterial endocarditis. *Streptococcus viridans* is the common causative organism. Nevertheless, because the disease is so serious, treatment should be commenced without waiting for bacteriological confirmation if the clinical picture suggests the condition.

Prior to the days of antibiotics, the disease was invariably fatal. With modern treatment, a cure is possible, but the healed valves are often grossly distorted, show calcification, and may require surgical excision and replacement to prevent the occurrence of heart failure.

Endocarditis Following Implantation of Artificial Valves.   The cardiovascular surgeon can now replace damaged valves by prosthetic valves of ball or flap design. The thrombus that forms around the rim of these devices, particularly where sutures are inserted, forms a nidus for infection. The endocarditis can cause local destruction, causing the artificial valve to become partially detached and to leak.

Calcific Aortic Stenosis

This condition usually affects elderly men and appears to be a degenerative condition arising in a congenitally abnormal valve. Usually the valve has two cusps rather than the customary three. The aortic valve cusps become calcified and fused together, producing a tight stenosis. The left ventricle is hypertrophied, but in spite of the overaction of this chamber, an inadequate amount of blood is pumped into the aorta. In particular, the blood supply to the coronary vessels is impaired, and these patients are in constant danger of sudden death. Surgical replacement of the diseased valve by a homograft or a plastic prosthesis is therefore indicated.

Two coronary arteries supply the myocardium with blood. These vessels are particularly liable to be affected by atheroma, which causes narrowing of their lumina and subsequent myocardial ischemia.

The incidence of ischemic heart disease steadily increased after 1920, until by 1960 the disease had reached almost epidemic proportion. Tobacco smoking, a sedentary life, gasoline fumes in the air, a diet containing too much saturated animal fat, the stress of modern life, and other factors were all blamed for the increased death rate from myocardial ischemia. Nevertheless, the evidence for any of these factors playing a significant role was not convincing. Quite unexpectedly, since 1965 the incidence of ischemic heart disease in North America has decreased. The reason for this change is not known, for there appears to have been no great change in life style to explain it.

Effects of Myocardial Ischemia

Gradual Coronary Occlusion. Slow occlusion of the coronary arteries leads to increasing ischemia; at first, this has no obvious effect on the heart. Some patients notice pain on exercise (called *angina pectoris*); characteristically, this is felt in the center of the chest and sometimes radiates into the neck and down the inner aspect of the left arm. The pain comes on with exercise, particularly in cold weather, and after a heavy meal. It can also be precipitated by emotional stress. The pain is thought to be due to accumulation of metabolic substances produced by muscle contracting under ischemic conditions. What is not understood is why only some patients with coronary disease experience angina.

Invariably, the pain of angina pectoris is relieved by resting and by placing a tablet of nitroglycerin under the tongue. This drug is readily absorbed from the buccal mucosa and appears to act by causing peripheral vasodilatation, which lowers the systolic blood pressure and lessens the load on the left ventricle.

The morphological effects of gradual coronary occlusion are patchy necrosis of heart muscle and replacement fibrosis. At necropsy, the fibrosis is the most evident feature. Nevertheless, myocardial infarction can occur in the absence of complete coronary occlusion (see below).

Sudden Coronary Occlusion. Myocardial infarction or an acute fatal *dysrhythmia* is the common effect. These conditions are described below.

Extensive myocardial necrosis occurring suddenly is seen under the following circumstances:

1. *Following coronary artery thrombosis,* which is itself secondary to atherosclerosis. In the past it has often been assumed that nearly all myocardial infarcts were due to coronary thrombosis; the two terms (myocardial infarction and coronary thrombosis) are thus commonly used almost interchangeably. It is now realized that thrombosis is not always present, and it may even occur in the coronary artery after the infarction has already taken place.

2. *With coronary artery stenosis only.* When no thrombus can be found, it is assumed that some additional factor is concerned. Additional strain on the left ventricle may occur if blood pressure rises suddenly or if there is an increased heart rate (tachycardia). Sudden lowering of the blood pressure, as is seen in shock, is also a factor, since although it diminishes the load of the left ventricle, the blood flow through the coronary arteries is diminished even more so.

3. *With neither coronary artery stenosis nor coronary artery thrombosis.* Severe hypotension (as occurs in shock) and anemia may be present in some cases, but in others no explanation can be found. Multiple small platelet

emboli or thrombi have been postulated, and their early dissipation can explain why they are not found at necropsy.

4. *Coronary Artery Spasm.* It is now well established that vascular spasm (demonstrated by coronary angiography) is sometimes the cause of angina pectoris, and this may explain not only cases of sudden death due to acute dysrhythmia but also those cases of myocardial infarction in which no coronary artery blockage can be demonstrated.

It may come as a surprise to realize that in spite of the enormous amount of money and time spent in investigating myocardial infarction, the pathogenesis is still not understood. Perhaps this is why we have not yet found a means for decreasing its incidence.

Clinical Features of Myocardial Infarction. The sudden onset of severe pain in the center of the chest (retrosternal) is characteristic of myocardial infarction. The pain is not relieved by rest or nitroglycerin, and its severity may cause the patient to sweat. Although the typical heart attack is accompanied by severe pain, it is not uncommon for the pain to be relatively mild and atypical. Pain may be situated in the upper abdomen and therefore be mistaken for gastritis. Occasionally, the attack is not accompanied by any pain, and the presence of massive infarction comes as a surprise at necropsy of a patient who died of heart failure for unknown reasons.

Electrocardiographic Changes. Myocardial ischemia and infarction produce changes in the electrocardiogram (ECG*) that are of great diagnostic value (Fig. 28–10D) and from which an idea of the site and extent of the damage can be assessed. Repeated ECGs are of particular value in following the progress of the patient. As with most investigations, the method is not infallible. A patient can die of myocardial infarction and yet have equivocal findings on electrocardiography. Likewise, a patient dying of some disease can have chest pain and ECG changes "typical" of a myocardial infarct, and yet at necropsy no infarction can be found.

Effects of Acute Myocardial Ischemia

Acute Functional Derangements. Acute ischemia may cause sudden death. The left ventricle fibrillates in some cases, whereas in others ischemia of the conducting system causes heart block. Sudden death is most common during the first 24 hours after the onset of ischemia, and the value of acute coronary care units is that immediate external cardiac massage or defibrillation can save the life of a number of these patients. These patients need not necessarily develop subsequent infarction: the acute ischemia may have been transient enough to allow the muscle fibers to survive. It is obvious that the sooner an effective cardiac output is re-established, the less likely there is to be permanent myocardial or cerebral damage. Hence, it is essential that all medical personnel at all levels should be trained in the techniques of cardiopulmonary resuscitation.

Heart Failure. Acute heart failure, due directly to myocardial damage or to dysrhythmia, can produce a low cardiac output and a state of *shock* (Chapter 21). Persistent low blood pressure *(hypotension)* is serious and may lead to renal ischemia, oliguria, renal failure, and fluid retention.

Infarction. If the patient survives, the heart muscle subjected to prolonged ischemia undergoes necrosis. The infarct appears as a firm, yellow area of coagulative necrosis with some surrounding hemorrhage and later inflammation (Figs. 28–5 and 28–6). An increase in the white-cell count and a slight fever are manifestations of this inflammation.

Enzyme Changes in the Diagnosis of Myocardial Infarction. Necrotic heart muscle releases enzymes into the blood stream, and their detection is a

---

*Some doctors use the letters EKG instead of ECG in order to avoid possible confusion with EEG (electroencephalogram), which sounds rather similar.

Figure 28–5. Recent myocardial infarction. The specimen shows part of the wall of the left ventricle. The recent infarct (Inf) is pale and has a hemorrhagic border. The lesion is about ten days old. Fibrosis in other areas (Fib) is the result of a previous heart attack.

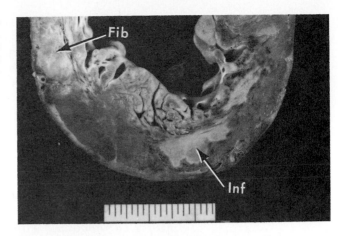

useful diagnostic procedure (Chapter 4). The *creatine phosphokinase (CPK)* is the most specific, and its blood level rises within 6 hours, peaks at 24 hours, and returns to normal by 72 hours. CPK is also present in skeletal muscle, and an intramuscular injection (*e.g.*, of a pain-relieving drug) can cause a considerable rise. The CPK isoenzyme MB is virtually specific for myocardium, but its estimation is expensive and not a routine procedure in most centers. The *serum glutamic-oxaloacetic transaminase (SGOT)* level rises in about 12 hours, peaks at 36 hours, and gradually falls by about the fifth day following infarction. The enzyme is also present in liver cells, and very high blood levels suggest liver damage. This could be due to acute congestion and hypoxia secondary to the heart failure precipitated by a myocardial infarction. The *lactic dehydrogenase (LDH)*, particularly the isoenzyme LDH 1, predom-

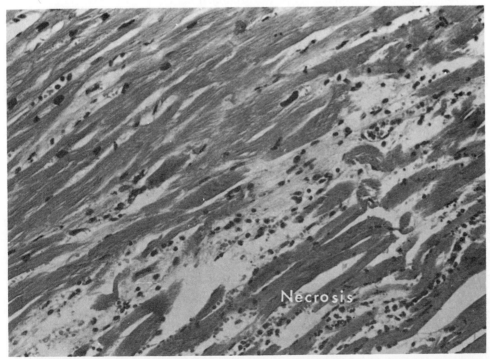

Figure 28–6. Myocardial infarction. The muscle fibers on the right-hand side are shrunken and show intense staining with eosin. Between the fibers there is an infiltration by polymorphonuclear leukocytes. A number of red cells are also seen extravasated in the interstitial tissue. Compare these fibers with the normal ones in the upper left part of the picture. This section was taken at autopsy from a man who eight days previously had sustained an intense crushing pain in the chest and shortly afterward had developed cardiac shock that was not alleviated by treatment (× 250).

inates in the heart and red cells. Its level rises slowly after a myocardial infarct, peaks at 48 hours, and may not return to normal for 1 to 3 weeks. It is evident that the significance of enzyme levels in an isolated sample of blood can be difficult to assess. In the diagnosis of a patient with suspected myocardial infarction it is advisable to examine samples of blood over a period of several days.

Nuclear Imaging. Technetium-labelled pyrophosphate and diphosphonate accumulate in ischemic or infarcted myocardial fibers, and "hot spots" indicative of damage can be detected by scanning for radioactivity.

Three early complications of myocardial infarction, described below, should be noted:

Pericarditis. This condition occurs if the infarct involves the pericardial surface.

Mural Thrombosis. This is seen if the infarct involves the endocardium (Fig. 28–7). Portions of this thrombus may break off and embolize to systemic organs (*e.g.,* the brain and the kidneys), thereby producing serious and sometimes fatal results.

Rupture. Occasionally, the necrotic muscle ruptures, causing acute hemopericardium and sudden death. Both this complication and systemic embolism are likely to occur at the end of the first week. Rupture of an infarcted papillary muscle leads to sudden mitral insufficiency, heart failure, and death.

About 70 per cent of patients with coronary thrombosis survive their first attack. The infarct organizes to produce a fibrous scar (Fig. 28–8), which may later bulge and lead to an *aneurysm of the left ventricle.* The aneurysm itself may subsequently rupture, but this is an uncommon event. Usually the patient who has had a myocardial infarct is left with some heart damage, and further episodes of infarction are not uncommon.

In the past it has been customary to keep patients at rest for several weeks following myocardial infarction. At that time it was assumed that the heart needed rest for healing to occur. Medical personnel now realize that this rest is unnecessary. It is common practice to keep the patient in bed for two weeks only and then to allow increasing exercise. This program of moderate exercise has not increased the death rate and has diminished the incidence of complications of bed rest, *e.g.,* pulmonary embolism.

Figure 28–7. Myocardial infarction with extensive mural thrombosis. The dilated left ventricle has been opened, and part of its lateral wall has been swung over to the left. The anterior cusp of the mitral valve (Mit) is clearly shown. Part of the aorta is included in the specimen, and the orifices of the two coronary arteries (Cor O) can be seen immediately above the three cusps of the aortic valve. There is extensive infarction (Inf) of the left ventricular wall immediately adjacent to the endocardium. Attached to the infarcted muscle there is dark mural thrombus. Both coronary arteries were markedly stenosed by atheroma, but no occluding thrombus was present. It is not uncommon to find this pattern of myocardial infarct in the absence of a thrombosed coronary artery.

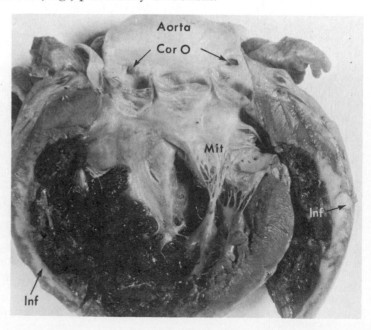

Figure 28–8. Myocardial fibrosis. The specimen is an oblique section through part of the wall of the left ventricle. White fibrous scar tissue has replaced much of the muscle in the lower part of the specimen. This was the end-result of an infarct several years prior to death.

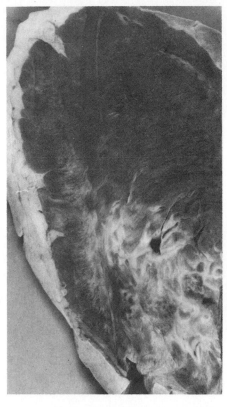

The presence of systemic hypertension puts a strain on the left ventricle. The muscle fibers enlarge, and this leads to *concentric hypertrophy* of the left ventricle. In due course, often after many years, the left ventricle fails. Attacks of paroxysmal nocturnal dyspnea may occur (Chapter 30). The reason why hypertrophic muscle fibers eventually work inefficiently is not known. One explanation is that no new capillaries are formed to provide them with an adequate blood supply. Another factor may be the development of coronary artery atheroma, which frequently complicates hypertension.

The detection of systemic hypertension is important because effective drug therapy is available and heart failure can be averted.

Hypertensive Heart Disease

Cor pulmonale may be defined as enlargement of the right ventricle secondary to disease or dysfunction of the lungs. The effect on the heart is mediated by *pulmonary hypertension.* The increased pressure in the pulmonary artery is caused by one of three mechanisms. The pulmonary vasculature may be *blocked by material within the lumen* (e.g., thrombus or, rarely, tumor emboli); the vessels may go into *spasm,* an effect generally caused by local tissue hypoxia; finally, the pulmonary vessels may fall victim to *local destructive disease, e.g.,* a type of chronic inflammation such as tuberculosis.

In *acute cor pulmonale* the right ventricle is acutely dilated and fails owing to an acute obstruction to the pulmonary arterial system. The most common cause is massive pulmonary embolism. A sudden severe attack of bronchial asthma is a less common cause.

In *chronic cor pulmonale* the right ventricular muscle undergoes hypertrophy secondary to chronic pulmonary hypertension. Causes may be listed:

1. Multiple repeated small pulmonary embolisms.

2. Primary pulmonary vascular disease. Occasional examples of polyarteritis affecting the lung are encountered but are not common. In *idiopathic*

Cor Pulmonale

pulmonary hypertension no cause for the small vessel disease can be found.

3. Chronic obstructive lung disease and any other chronic disease that is accompanied by lung destruction, *e.g.*, chronic pulmonary tuberculosis and pneumoconiosis (Chapter 30). Hypoxia adds the effect of vascular spasm to the vascular destruction caused directly by the disease.

4. Impaired pulmonary ventilation from whatever cause, *e.g.*, severe kyphoscoliosis (Chapter 40), muscular paralysis, or obesity (see "Pickwickian Syndrome," Chapter 30).

Chronic cor pulmonale is often associated with secondary polycythemia caused by chronic hypoxemia. This increases the viscosity of the blood and adds an additional strain on the already overtaxed right ventricle. Right-sided heart failure eventually ensues.

Valvular Disease of the Heart

It is convenient at this point to summarize the valvular defects. Details of these will be found in other parts of the book.

Mitral Valve Disease

Mitral Stenosis. This defect is the most common valvular disease of the heart and is nearly always due to chronic rheumatic endocarditis (Figs. 28–2 and 28–3).

*Mitral Regurgitation.** Some degree of mitral regurgitation is common in chronic rheumatic mitral stenosis. It is also seen in heart failure when dilatation of the mitral ring leads to valve dysfunction. Occasionally, mitral regurgitation results from infarction of the papillary muscles holding the valve cusps. The regurgitation can be due to dysfunction or to actual rupture of the papillary muscles. A recently recognized cause of mitral regurgitation is *myxomatous degeneration* of the valve cusps themselves (Chapter 4). The valves become thin and floppy; they bulge or prolapse into the left atrium during ventricular systole, and regurgitation results. This is called the *mitral valve prolapse syndrome.* Ulcerating endocarditis is a rare cause of mitral regurgitation.

Aortic Valve Disease. Aortic stenosis is usually combined with aortic regurgitation in chronic rheumatic heart disease. Congenital stenosis can affect either the valve itself or, when the stenosis is produced by muscular hypertrophy *(congenital subaortic muscular stenosis)*, the region below the valve. Calcified aortic stenosis is seen in old age, and most cases are probably the end-result of fibrosis in a congenitally bicuspid aortic valve. Some calcific aortic stenoses are probably examples of healed endocarditis.

Aortic Regurgitation. There are a number of conditions in which the elastic tissue of the aorta and the aortic ring are so weakened that the ring becomes dilated. The valve cusps fail to meet, causing severe regurgitation to result. Syphilitic aortitis and medionecrosis of the aorta fall into this group. Syphilitic aortitis is now a rare disease, but a similar type of aortitis with aortic regurgitation is encountered in *rheumatoid arthritis* and *ankylosing spondylitis.* Sufficient dilatation to cause regurgitation is also seen in hypertension.

Tricuspid Valve Disease. Tricuspid stenosis is generally of rheumatic origin, but it is rare. Tricuspid regurgitation, which is more common than stenosis, is generally due to dilatation of the valve ring in right-sided heart failure.

---

*The terms insufficiency or incompetence are sometimes used to denote regurgitation. Strictly interpreted, however, they could also include stenosis. Regurgitation is more explicit and will be used in this book.

Pulmonary Valve Disease.   Pulmonary stenosis is nearly always congenital in origin. Sufficient rheumatic endocariditis to cause deformity is rare.

The term "dysrhythmia" is used to describe any condition in which the heart is beating either too quickly, too slowly, or irregularly. The impulse that initiates cardiac contraction commences in the sinoatrial (S-A) node in the right atrium, spreads throughout the atria to the atrioventricular (A-V) node, and then travels down the conducting bundle of His to reach the two ventricles via the two major branches of the bundle of His. This regular spread of electrical impulse can be interrupted in many ways by various pathological conditions. Only some of the most common disorders will be described here (Figs. 28–9 and 28–10).

Ectopic Beats.   An ectopic beat arises prematurely from a site other than the S-A node. It may be in the atria, in the A-V node, or in the ventricle (Fig. 28–10*C*). Distinction between these types can be made only by study of the electrocardiogram. Following the ectopic beat there is a compensatory pause before the next normal heart beat. This sometimes produces the feeling of the heart "turning over," but apart from this, ectopic beats produce no symptoms. They are common in normal people, but they can also be an indication of myocardial disease. This association with myocardial disease applies particularly to the ventricular ectopic beats, which are seen in patients with myocardial ischemia and in those who have taken too much digitalis.

Paroxysmal Tachycardia.   In this condition there are attacks of rapid heart action resulting from a regular succession of ectopic beats that last for a few seconds or as long as several days. *Paroxysmal atrial tachycardia* is the most common type and is generally not associated with heart disease. The *ventricular type* is more usually seen in patients with ischemic disease; like ventricular ectopic beats, this condition may precede ventricular fibrillation in patients with myocardial infarction.

Atrial Fibrillation.   This is a common and important disorder. It appears to be due to multiple ectopic foci discharging at variable rates in the atria.

Cardiac Dysrhythmias

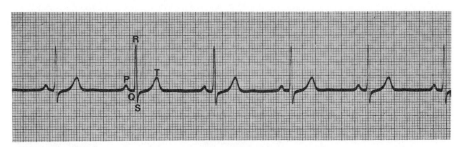

Figure 28–9.   The normal electrocardiogram (ECG). The electrocardiograph is a meter that amplifies and records the differences in electrical potential between two points (bipolar leads) on the surface of the body. Originally three standard leads were used (lead I, left arm—right arm, lead II, left leg—right arm, and lead III, left leg—left arm), but the "unipolar" or V leads are now commonly used. An exploratory electrode is placed on various parts of the chest wall; for example, VI lead is placed on the fourth right intercostal space near the sternum, and the second electrode is kept at zero potential.

The electrocardiogram is representative of the electrical activity in the heart, and this triggers muscular activity. P, the first wave, represents passage of activity through the atria (depolarization), and triggers atrial contraction. The QRS complex represents ventricular excitation corresponding to ventricular systole. The T waves represent ventricular recovery, or repolarization. The Q wave is a small negative deflection and is often absent. With the graph paper used for the standard electrocardiogram, each small square of the abscissa is 1 millimeter and represents 40 msec. The heart rate can be estimated by counting the number of millimeters between two consecutive R waves (or other portions of the complex) and dividing 1500 by this number. In the record shown above, the distance between each R wave is 29 or 30 millimeters, and this corresponds to a heart rate of just over 50 beats per minute. (Courtesy of Dr. R. S. Baigrie.)

Rapid fibrillary waves take place rather than normal atrial contraction, and the multiple impulses that reach the A-V node (up to 600 per minute) cannot all be conducted to the ventricles. Approximately 100 to 160 reach the ventricles at a completely irregular rhythm. Because not all ventricular contractions are powerful enough to open the aortic and pulmonary valves, the pulse rate as felt at the wrist is less than that heard at the apex of the heart. Rheumatic heart disease, particularly mitral stenosis, is the most common cause of atrial

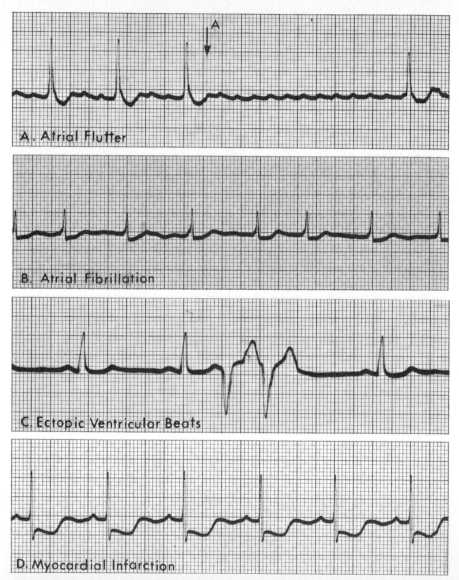

Figure 28–10.   Abnormal electrocardiograms.   *A, Atrial flutter.* Normal P waves are absent and are replaced by a flutter wave occurring at approximately 300 per minute. Some impulses reach the ventricles and lead to ventricular complexes. At point A, pressure was applied to the carotid sinus, and this produced reflex vagal activity. The effect of this was to produce a temporary heart block, and for a period there was ventricular standstill. *B, Atrial fibrillation.* In this electrocardiogram no P waves can be seen, and the irregular atrial fibrillation indicates chaotic atrial activity. The ventricles respond in an erratic manner, so that the heart rate in addition to being fast (95 beats per minute) is irregularly irregular. *C, Ectopic ventricular beats.* Two ectopic beats are shown in which the QRS complex is abnormal. This abnormality is a reflection of the beats arising within the ventricles themselves, and not being a response to normal stimulation from the atria. *D, Myocardial infarction.* The outstanding feature of this electrocardiograph is depression of the ST segment. This change was seen shortly after an acute myocardial infarction. In other leads there was ST segment elevation, and analysis of the changes in the standard leads can give a good indication of the site of the infarct. (Courtesy of Dr. R. S. Baigrie.)

fibrillation, but in older patients ischemic heart disease, systemic hypertension, and thyrotoxicosis are other important causes.

Atrial fibrillation is generally treated by the administration of digitalis, which acts by impairing conduction in the bundle of His. Fewer impulses reach the ventricles, causing them to be slowed, so that each contraction is more effective. The atrial fibrillation itself is not terminated. Indeed, to try to stop the fibrillation itself may precipitate detachment of a mural thrombus from the atrium.

Atrial Flutter. This form of dysrhythmia is less common than atrial fibrillation. The atria contract at a rate of about 300 beats per minute, being stimulated by a rapidly firing ectopic pacemaker. Atrioventricular block results in a slower ventricular rate (Fig. 28–10A).

Ventricular Fibrillation. This is a most serious condition, and it is generally the immediate precursor of death in myocardial infarction. Immediate external electrical defibrillation is the most effective treatment if equipment is available.

Heart Block. The term "heart block" is used to describe depression of conduction between the atria and the ventricles. In the early stages, the time required for the impulse to reach the ventricles is merely prolonged, but as the condition progresses, occasional impulses fail to reach the ventricles and a beat is dropped. When conduction is completely blocked, there is *complete heart block;* no impulses from the atria reach the ventricles, which then beat at their own intrinsic rate of about 40 beats per minute. The chief causes of heart block are ischemic heart disease and an overdose of digitalis. When complete heart block occurs suddenly, the ventricles may not start to beat for several minutes, and the patient rapidly loses consciousness and develops convulsions. These episodes are known as *Stokes-Adams attacks.*

Effects of Cardiac Dysrhythmias. Irregular or rapid cardiac contraction may lead to a sensation in the chest that is described as *palpitation.* If the heart rate is either very rapid (*e.g.,* over 160 beats per minute, as in paroxysmal tachycardia and atrial fibrillation) or very low (*e.g.,* below 40 beats per minute, as in complete heart block), the cardiac output is diminished particularly on exercise. If the heart is otherwise normal, this change in rate may be of no immediate consequence, but if it is superadded to some other heart disease, the results can be serious. Tachycardia increases the heart's requirements for oxygen, and the energy expended is wastefully used by ineffective contractions. Furthermore, during tachycardia the coronary blood flow is decreased. Most of the coronary blood flow takes place during diastole, so that with tachycardia diastole is shortened and the blood flow is diminished. The heart muscle therefore has an increased need for oxygen at the same time that its supply is reduced. The ischemia that results further impairs myocardial activity and can lead to necrosis, either patchy or massive.

Heart Failure

The major contractile element of the heart is the muscular walls of the two ventricles. When the muscle is relaxed (*diastole*), blood flows into the ventricles; the flow is aided to some extent by atrial contraction. When the ventricular muscle contracts (*systole*), the atrioventricular valves close, and a volume of blood (the cardiac output) is forced past the pulmonary and aortic valves into the main arteries. At the end of systole some blood remains in the ventricles; this is called the *residual volume.* Under resting conditions the venous return to each ventricle is about 5 liters per minute, but with exercise this increases to 25 liters or more. Cardiac output is correspondingly increased by utilizing the three *cardiac reserves* described below:

1. The increased filling of the ventricles stretches the heart muscle fibers, causing an increase in the force of the next contraction. This response

is known as *Starling's law of the heart,* which states that *the energy of contraction is proportional to the initial length of the cardiac muscle fibers.* In spite of the increased venous return of exercise, the pressure of blood in the atria does not rise under normal circumstances.

2. Increased sympathetic tone causes an increase in the strength of cardiac contraction. This reduces the residual volume, and therefore increases the amount of blood ejected with each systole. A change in the force of contraction of the heart without a corresponding change in the initial length of the muscle is termed an *inotropic effect.* The alkaloids of digitalis are used in heart failure because they have an inotropic effect.

3. Increased sympathetic tone also causes an increase in heart rate, *e.g.,* from the normal 70 beats per minute to over double that figure.

The venous return to the right ventricle is the amount of blood draining from all the tissues of the body except the lungs, and this is directly related to the arterial supply to these tissues. The blood supply of a tissue is determined mainly by local self-regulatory mechanisms that are designed to ensure sufficient blood flow to satisfy the activity of the tissue at all times. The venous return, and hence the cardiac output, is governed mainly by extracardiac factors — namely, the metabolic requirements of the body as a whole. By using the reserves described above, the normal heart can cope with any normal load placed upon it. When it fails to do this, the result is heart failure, because in the presence of an adequate venous return it fails to supply the needs to the body. At first the effects of this are seen only during exercise, but as the failure increases, the effects are apparent even at rest. Either the left or the right ventricle may fail separately; more usually the heart fails as a whole. The condition is then called *congestive heart failure.*

Effects of Right Ventricular Failure

Rise in Central Venous Pressure.   A failure of the right ventricle to eject all the blood it receives leads to distention of the right atrium by a back-pressure effect. The pressure in the great veins rises, and the jugular veins are seen to be distended with blood when the patient sits up in bed. To some extent this aids heart function, because by stretching the heart muscle the raised pressure increases the force of contraction. Eventually, however, a point is reached beyond which increased stretching causes a *decrease* in cardiac contraction (Fig. 28–11). Exercise, by increasing the venous return, further reduces the cardiac output and forces the patient to be bedridden. Once past this critical point, therapeutic bleeding increases the cardiac output by reducing the venous pressure. (This is the basis of the time-honored practice of bleeding as a treatment of heart failure.) A similar effect can be obtained by applying tourniquets to the limbs to obstruct the venous return and to allow pooling of blood in the peripheral vessels. In right-sided heart failure all the organs of the body are congested because of the increased venous pressure. This effect is particularly evident in the liver, where the center of the lobules is congested and red. Congestion is also apparent in the skin, especially of the face.

Cyanosis.   The sluggish circulation allows the blood to become deoxygenated as it passes through the tissues; this response is apparent in the skin as a bluish discoloration known as cyanosis. Cyanosis is evident when the capillary blood contains more than 5 grams of reduced hemoglobin per dl. Cyanosis due to stasis is known as *peripheral cyanosis,* and it should be contrasted with the type (central cyanosis) that occurs when venous blood is directly shunted into the systemic arterial system, as in some types of congenital heart disease. Peripheral cyanosis is not necessarily due to heart disease and occurs in other conditions when the circulation is sluggish. It is also seen in shock, whenever there is some local cause of venous obstruction,

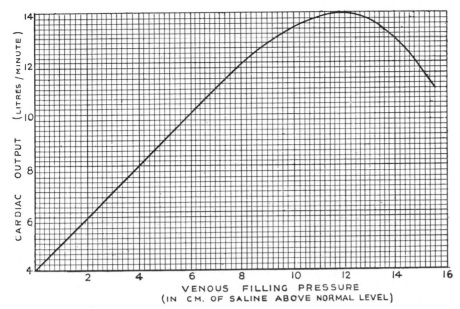

Figure 28-11.   Relationship of cardiac output to venous filling pressure (Starling's curve). (From Wood, P.: Diseases of the Heart and Circulation. 2nd ed. London, Eyre and Spottis Woode, 1956.)

as well as when the blood becomes viscous. Stasis in the skin vessels sometimes occurs as a response to cold in people who are otherwise normal. Indeed, it is a common experience to see some degree of cyanosis of the ears, nose, and finger tips on a cold winter's morning.

Polycythemia. An increased red-cell count occurs as a result of bone marrow hypoxia.

Edema. Edema of the dependent parts is a prominent sign of heart failure. If the patient is up and about, swelling of the ankles is first apparent, whereas if he is in bed, swelling of the tissues over the sacrum and external genitalia occurs most often. The pathogenesis of the edema is complex. In part it is due to the chronic passive venous congestion; this, in itself, is not the complete answer, however. It certainly helps to account for the *location* of the fluid accumulation — be it in the sacral region or legs — but it does not explain *why* the fluid accumulates. In right ventricular failure the output of the heart is inadequate for the needs of the body, and this results in peripheral vasoconstriction, which allows the blood to be most economically distributed. The mechanism is analogous to that which is seen in shock (Chapter 21). The redistribution of blood appears particularly to affect the kidneys and results in a more complete reabsorption of sodium. This causes concurrent water retention and an increase in volume of the extracellular fluids. This increased volume appears as edema. The importance of sodium retention in the pathogenesis of cardiac edema is reflected in treatment. Diuretics that cause excretion of sodium are of great use in treatment of cardiac edema. Likewise, a diet low in salt is frequently prescribed with advantage.

Rise in Pulmonary Venous Pressure. With the onset of left ventricular failure the left atrial pressure increases, and the atrium together with the pulmonary vessels becomes distended with blood. As in mitral stenosis, dyspnea ensues. The rise in pulmonary venous pressure is extremely serious, because of the imminent danger of pulmonary edema. The edema of the lungs may accumulate slowly, but sometimes acute attacks occur, particularly at night. This reaction, which is called *paroxysmal nocturnal dyspnea*, is a

Effects of Left Ventricular Failure

life-threatening event. The patient wakes up in the early hours of the morning with a sense of breathlessness and acute oppression of the chest. He becomes acutely distressed and coughs up the blood-stained watery sputum that is characteristic of severe acute pulmonary edema. Spasm of the bronchi is often a feature, and the condition resembles bronchial asthma to the extent that it sometimes is called *cardiac asthma.* The pathogenesis of acute paroxysmal dyspnea is only partially understood. It seems to be precipitated by a sudden sympathetic overactivity. Intense constriction of the peripheral systemic blood vessels drives the blood from the systemic circulation to the pulmonary circuit. The excess blood distends the pulmonary vessels, and there is a transudation of fluid into the alveoli to produce edema. Morphine quiets the patient and has a dramatic ameliorative effect, whereas epinephrine can be fatal. This effect is extremely important to remember, because in bronchial asthma epinephrine is helpful, whereas morphine is dangerous.

Chronic venous congestion of the lungs results in rupture of some capillaries, and blood-stained sputum (hemoptysis) is produced. Some of the extravasated blood is converted into hemosiderin, and the lungs become brown and slightly fibrotic (see Fig. 30–5). This is called "brown induration of the lungs," and it is characteristic of long-standing left ventricular failure (and mitral stenosis).

When considering the pathogenesis of heart failure (whether it is left or right), one must remember that the output of both ventricles is the same over any reasonable period of time. In left ventricular failure, the left ventricle is functioning with the aid of increased venous filling pressure, but the right ventricle, on the other hand, is working normally. This leads to a redistribution of blood, more being retained in the pulmonary circuit than is normal. As noted above, this produces congestion of the lungs, and ultimately there is a rise in pulmonary arterial pressure. Eventually this causes the right ventricle to fail as well, and congestive heart failure ensues.

Congestive Heart Failure

In congestive heart failure, both ventricles of the heart fail together, and the effects are a combination of those described under the separate headings of left and right ventricular failure. The inadequate output of the left ventricle leads to sympathetic overactivity with resultant peripheral vasoconstriction. In particular, the vessels of the skin tend to be constricted, causing stasis in the skin; this response leads to peripheral cyanosis. The lessened blood supply to the liver leads to atrophy and necrosis of the cells in the center of the classic liver lobules. This change contributes to the appearance of the characteristic "nutmeg" liver of heart failure (Figs. 28–12 and 28–13). The kidneys respond to the redistribution of blood by salt and water retention, but they show no morphological evidence of this malfunction. The brain receives an adequate supply of blood until the terminal stages of heart failure. Loss of consciousness tends to be a terminal event.

The Causes of Heart Failure.   Although the heart has adequate reserves that enable it to cope with any demand for additional work, it is not capable of maintaining a high output for any length of time. In the face of a continuous demand for additional work, it eventually fails. Thus, failure may be the result of *overburdening due to a sustained increase in ventricular pressure.* This increase in pressure occurs in systemic and pulmonary hypertension and also in aortic and pulmonary stenosis.

Overburdening due to a sustained increase in cardiac output is another important cause of heart failure. In mitral regurgitation the left ventricle is forced to eject a large volume of blood, partly back into the left atrium and partly into the aorta. Aortic regurgitation also causes an increase in left ventricular output, because during diastole blood from the aorta flows back

Figure 28–12. The liver in heart failure. This specimen shows the characteristic "nutmeg appearance" of chronic venous congestion in the liver. The dark areas consist of regions where liver cells have undergone necrosis and in which there is intense congestion. They are classically described as the center of the liver lobules, but in fact they correspond more accurately to the peripheral parts of the liver acinus (see Fig. 33–1). (From Robbins, S. L., and Cotran, R. S.: Pathologic Basis of Disease. 2nd ed. Philadelphia, W. B. Saunders Company, 1979.)

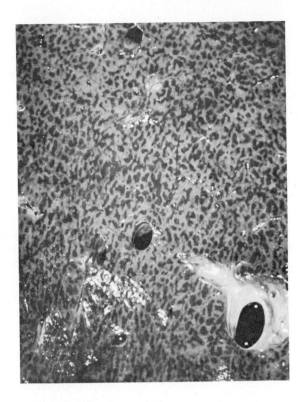

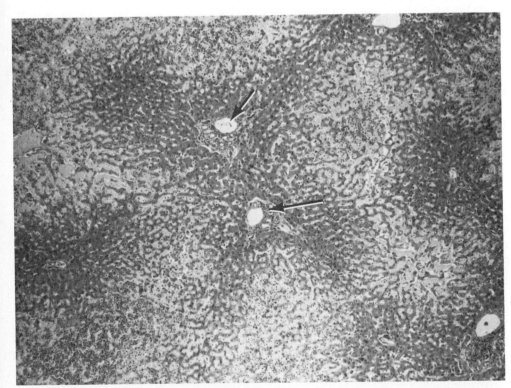

Figure 28–13.   The liver in congestive heart failure.   Two portal triads are indicated by the arrows; radiating from them are columns of relatively normal liver cells. These are in zone 1 of the Rappaport acinus. The liver cells in zones 2 and 3 have undergone necrosis, and these zones are intensely congested. Correlate this appearance with Figure 28–12 (× 60).

into the left ventricle. With each ventricular systole a large volume of blood must be ejected so that the effective output remains normal. In time, both mitral and aortic regurgitation lead to left ventricular failure. Likewise, pulmonary and tricuspid valve regurgitation leads to right ventricular failure.

Another example of overburdening due to an increased cardiac output is seen in a group of diseases in which the resting cardiac output is above normal. This occurs under a variety of conditions. In *anemia,* for example, the tissues require an increased volume of blood to compensate for its low oxygen-carrying power. In *thyrotoxicosis* the metabolic needs of the tissues are increased. In cases in which a large *fistula* exists between an artery and a vein the shunt diverts so much blood that the cardiac output must be increased to meet the demands of the rest of the body. There are some common diseases (*e.g., chronic lung disease* and *advanced liver disease*) in which the cardiac output even at rest is high for no very obvious reason. Whenever the resting cardiac output is increased, the heart copes with the load for a while, but it ultimately fails. Even in failure the output may be above that of the normal resting cardiac output, and for this type of condition the term *high-output failure* is used. Although the cardiac output is raised relative to the normal, it is still insufficient to meet the demands of the body. In the more common type of heart failure, termed *low-output failure,* the cardiac output is less than that of a normal person of similar stature.

Myocardial Disease

Myocardial ischemia is a common cause of heart failure. Acute infarction, described previously, may precipitate acute heart failure. Repeated infarcts, or gradual coronary occlusion causing fibrosis, may put such a strain on the remaining muscle fibers that failure ultimately occurs.

If one examines the heart muscle from a patient in failure due to hemodynamic conditions, it is disappointing to find that no abnormality can be detected. The muscle fibers may be hypertrophied, but this does not explain why they failed, nor does a biochemical examination elucidate the problem. We have to admit that the heart that fails in hypertension or valvular disease appears normal microscopically, but it does not behave normally. Obviously, our methods of examination are crude and not suited to detecting the lesion involved.

There are, however, many diseases in which the myocardium appears to be directly affected and which explain the cause of heart failure. The most important of these is when the muscle becomes hypoxic as a result of coronary artery disease; this has already been considered in detail. Some poisons seem to affect the heart directly: alcohol is one such poison. Likewise, various types of myocarditis are known. Viruses (particularly Coxsackie) are the most common cause, but bacteria, protozoa, fungi, and helminths (*e.g.,* Trichinella) can all cause myocarditis. In South America trypanosomiasis (Chagas' disease) is important. Amyloidosis is a rare cause of heart failure. When all known causes have been eliminated from consideration, there remains a group of conditions in which the heart fails for no detectable reason. The heart is large, dilated, shows no valvular or coronary disease, and yet it fails. This is a fascinating residual group which, for want of a better name, is called *cardiomyopathy.* The diagnosis is one of exclusion. In some instances the disease seems to be the result of an inherited factor; for the most part, however, we must confess our complete ignorance as to its nature. When all the above morphological cardiac factors causing heart failure have been excluded, there remain four other very common contributory factors that do not themselves cause heart failure but rather enhance it when it is due to some other factor. These factors are *anxiety, pyrexia, pregnancy,* and *dysrhythmias. Anxiety* raises the heart rate and blood pressure, thereby adding an additional burden to the left ventricle. By raising the metabolic rate *pyrexia* causes an increase in cardiac output. *Pregnancy* increases the strain as a result of an increased blood volume and the necessity for supplying blood to the fetus. The effects of *dysrhythmias* have been considered earlier in this chapter.

The pericardial sac normally contains 30 to 50 ml of fluid, and its smooth lining aids the functions of the heart. An excessive amount of fluid within the pericardial sac occurs under three circumstances:

1. Hydropericardium.   A transudate of low specific gravity may accompany any type of generalized edema, *e.g.*, in heart failure or in the nephrotic syndrome.

2. Pericardial Effusions Due to Pericarditis (see below).

3. Hemopericardium.   Pure blood or blood clot in the pericardium generally results from the rupture of a myocardial infarct or of the outer wall of a dissecting aneurysm of the aorta. Trauma is a third cause and may be inflicted by a stab wound, or by the physician's needle when he inadvertently tears a coronary vessel when attempting to obtain fluid from the pericardial sac.

The effect of excess fluid in the pericardium depends on the quantity of fluid present and the speed with which it accumulates. A slow accumulation of 3000 ml can be tolerated, since the pericardial sac gradually stretches. Rapid accumulation of even 200 ml can lead to *acute cardiac tamponade*. In this the increased pressure within the pericardial sac hinders venous filling of the atria, and this in turn reduces the cardiac output and coronary blood flow. Hypotension, a state of shock, and finally death can follow rapidly unless the fluid is promptly drained by the insertion of a needle (*pericardiocentesis*).

Acute Pericarditis.   Acute serous or serofibrinous pericarditis occurs as a benign condition in young adults. Fever, sudden onset of sharp retrosternal pain that alters with the position of a patient, and a pericardial rub are the main clinical features. Coxsackie viruses and others have been isolated from a few cases, but the majority remain idiopathic.

A sterile pericarditis is a feature of acute rheumatic fever (page 383), systemic lupus erythematosus (Chapter 27), and uremia (Chapter 35). It also occurs over an acute myocardial infarct (page 390). A typical acute pericarditis may occur weeks or even months after a myocardial infarct. This is called *postmyocardial infarction pericarditis,* or Dressler's syndrome. The pathogenesis is not known, but an autoimmune reaction to damaged tissue has been suggested. Some support for this is the occurrence of a similar acute pericarditis following cardiac surgery. This *postpericardiotomy syndrome* has been estimated to occur in about 10 per cent of patients who undergo cardiac surgery. It may occur weeks after the surgical event and must be distinguished from a bacterial infection.

Suppurative pericarditis is generally bacterial in origin and is caused by spreading of infection from an adjacent site such as pneumonia or an empyema (see Fig. 5–5). Occasionally, acute suppurative pericarditis occurs as an isolated event, and spread from some inapparent focus of infection via the blood stream is presumed to be the pathogenesis.

The end-result of acute pericarditis is generally resolution, perhaps with the formation of a few unimportant fibrous adhesions. Occasionally these adhesions are extensive, and two syndromes are recognized.

Adhesive Mediastinopericarditis.   There is massive fibrosis with obliteration of the pericardial sac and adhesion to adjacent structures. This mass of fibrous tissue surrounds the heart, greatly increases the work load of the myocardium, and leads to cardiac hypertrophy and dilatation.

DISEASES OF THE PERICARDIUM

Constrictive Pericarditis. Sometimes dense fibrous tissue with foci of calcification surrounds the heart and by encasing it impedes venous filling and constricts the venae cavae. The thickened pericardium is not attached to adjacent mediastinal structures and the heart remains of normal size. In constrictive pericarditis there is heart failure and prominent venous congestion affecting liver, spleen, and elsewhere. Ascites is a striking feature.

Both adhesive mediastinopericarditis and constrictive pericarditis may be the end-result of a suppurative or a tuberculous pericarditis, but often the condition appears to be idiopathic because no evidence of a preceding infection can be found.

Review Questions

1. Describe the signs and symptoms leading you to suspect that a child might have a developmental heart lesion.

2. Compare *central cyanosis* with *peripheral cyanosis*.

3. Compare the effects of the emboli found in the following conditions:
    (a) nonbacterial thrombotic endocarditis
    (b) acute endocarditis
    (c) *Streptococcus viridans* endocarditis

4. Where may thrombi be found in the heart? List the causes.

5. Describe the necropsy changes that would be expected in the heart of patients who had had the following:
    (a) angina pectoris
    (b) a myocardial infarct six months prior to examination
    (c) a myocardial infarct seven days prior to examination

6. Describe the structural and functional effects of stenosis of the cornary arteries.

7. A patient who has had a recent myocardial infarct is being nursed in a coronary care unit. Pulse rate, blood pressure, ECG, respiration rate, and fluid balance are being carefully monitored. Discuss the signs or symptoms that would indicate that the patient's condition was deteriorating and that he might die.

8. Examine Figure 28–10A. What is the ventricular rate before carotid sinus pressure was applied? It is known that exercise has no influence on the rate of the fluttering atria, but that it does decrease vagal activity. Predict the effect of exercise on the ventricular rate of contraction in this patient.

9. Give an account of those types of pericarditis that are not caused directly by bacterial infection of the pericardial sac.

10. Describe the possible end-results of pericarditis.

Selected Readings

Abelmann, W. H.: The cardiomyopathies. Hospital Practice, 6(3):101–112, 1971.
Braunwald, E.: Heart failure. *In* Isselbacher, K. J., et al. (Eds.): Harrison's Principles of Internal Medicine. 9th ed. New York, McGraw-Hill Book Company, 1980, Chapter 236.
Brod, J.: Pathogenesis of cardiac oedema. British Medical Journal, 1:222–228, 1972.
Buja, L. M., Hillis, L. D., and Petty, C. S.: The role of coronary artery spasm in ischemic heart disease. Archives of Pathology and Laboratory Medicine, 105:221–226, 1981.
Campbell, E. J. M., Dickinson, C. J., and Slater, J. D. H.: Clinical Physiology. 4th ed. Oxford, Blackwell Scientific Publications Ltd., 1974. See Chapter 2, "The Heart and Circulation."
Davis, J. O.: The mechanisms of salt and water retention in cardiac failure. Hospital Practice, 5(9):43–50, 1970.
Leading Article: Hot spots of the heart. Lancet, 2:299–300, 1978.
Mathewson, M. A.: Prolapsed mitral valve syndrome. American Journal of Nursing, 80:1431–1432, 1980.
Myerburg, R. J.: Electrocardiography. *In* Isselbacher, K. J., et al. (Eds.): Harrison's Principles of Internal Medicine. 9th ed. New York, McGraw-Hill Book Company, 1980, Chapter 232.
Perloff, J. K.: The clinical manifestations of cardiac failure in adults. Hospital Practice, 5(9):43–50, 1970.
Scully, R. E. (Ed.): Case records of the Massachusetts General Hospital. New England Journal of Medicine, 292:255–260, 1975. A case of staphylococcal endocarditis.
Stallones, R. A.: The rise and fall of ischemic heart disease. Scientific American, 243:53–59, 1980.
Vaz, D.: Recognizing common cardiac arrhythmias. American Journal of Nursing, 79:1971–1975, 1979.

Diseases of Blood Vessels

After studying this chapter the student should be able to:

- Describe the three layers of the arterial wall.
- Describe the changes that occur in Mönckeberg's sclerosis.
- List the causes of arteriolar sclerosis.
- Describe atherosclerosis with respect to the following factors:
    - (a) early lesions
    - (b) late and complicated lesions
    - (c) vessels affected
    - (d) etiology and pathogenesis
    - (e) complications
- Classify the inflammatory diseases of arteries.
- List the causes of small-vessel obstruction.
- Describe the causes of acute vasculitis.
- Detail the pathological lesions that can cause peripheral vascular disease of a limb.
- Classify aneurysms according to their cause.
- List the ways in which aneurysms can produce damage.
- Describe the outstanding clinical and pathological effects of a dissecting aneurysm of the aorta.
- Give an account of the cause and effects of varicose veins of the leg.

DISEASES OF ARTERIES

Arterial disease and its complications are responsible for about 40 per cent of all deaths. Arteritis forms a distinct group, but the degenerative diseases (arteriosclerosis) are by far the most important. A knowledge of the structure of arteries is necessary in order to understand their diseases.

Structure of Arteries

Arteries have three coats, which are described below:

The Intima (Tunica Intima). This layer consists of endothelium together with a small quantity of underlying connective tissue — collagen, occasional fibroblasts, and muscle cells.

The Media (Tunica Media). The media is the thickest layer and contains elastic fibers and smooth muscle cells, the proportion of each depending on the type of artery.

The Adventitia (Tunica Adventitia). This outer coat consists of loose connective tissue and small vessels (the *vasa vasorum*) that penetrate the media and supply it with blood.

Arteriosclerosis

Arteriosclerosis, or *hardening of the arteries,* is a term applied to a group of disorders that appear to be degenerative in nature. Three conditions are included:

Mönckeberg's Medial Sclerosis. *This disease affects the muscular vessels, particularly those of the lower limbs.* The muscle coat becomes replaced by fibrous tissue, which subsequently calcifies and even ossifies. The thickened, pipe-stem arteries produce characteristic radiological findings; since the lumen of the affected vessels is not appreciably narrowed, however, the disease causes no ill effects and is unimportant.

Arteriolar Sclerosis (Arteriosclerosis). This condition involves *widespread thickening of the walls of small arteries and arterioles. It is an invariable accompaniment of systemic hypertension.* One effect is that the muscle coat shows hypertrophy, but the most striking change is fibrous thickening of the intima. The changes are most marked in the kidney, and the resultant ischemia leads to patchy degeneration followed by scarring. This is the pathogenesis of *nephrosclerosis* (Fig. 29–4).

Similar changes with intimal thickening of small vessels may occur as a localized event; such changes are not related to hypertension. It is found in the small vessels of the ovaries in postmenopausal women, where it is a component of the aging process. It is common in mature scar tissue, is found in areas of chronic inflammation (*e.g.,* in the base of a chronic peptic ulcer), and is particularly marked in the fibrosis induced by ionizing radiation. Under these conditions the name *endarteritis obliterans* is applied.

Atherosclerosis. This is the most important component of arteriosclerosis and will be considered in detail in the following section.

Atherosclerosis

Atherosclerosis is the commonest killing disease of all highly advanced communities; its lesions are present to some extent in every adult of such societies. *The disease characteristically affects the large elastic arteries such as the aorta and its major branches. Of the medium-sized vessels, the coronary and cerebral arteries are the most commonly involved.* This is particularly unfortunate, since the tissues supplied by these vessels are vital to life. Indeed, it is the involvement of these arteries that accounts for the lethal effects of atherosclerosis. The disease may be considered as consisting of two types of lesion: type I and type II.

Basic Lesions of Atherosclerosis

Type I: Superficial Yellow Plaques in the Intima. Lipid-containing cells (probably muscle cells) accumulate in the subendothelial layer of the vessel and later break down to release their fatty content into the tunica intima. In this way are produced the yellow streaks that are a common necropsy finding in the aorta (Fig. 29–1). When the fatty deposits occur in small arteries, they do not produce appreciable narrowing of the lumen. These early yellow plaques are sometimes referred to as *atheroma.*

Type II: Accumulation of Fatty Material in the Intima with Additional Fibrosis. This is the common type of lesion seen in middle age and old age (Fig. 29–2). The lesions consist of intimal plaques and contain a central mass of fatty, yellow, porridgelike material (from the Greek *athere,* meaning "porridge") consisting predominantly of cholesterol and its esters. This material is covered by dense fibrous tissue, which gives the plaque a white, pearly appearance.

Advanced and Complicated Lesions of Atherosclerosis

Four further changes may be seen in the plaques as they progress:

1. Hemorrhage. Proliferation of vessels from the vasa vasorum produces increased vascularity in the connective tissue surrounding the atheromatous plaque. Rupture of one of these vessels leads to bleeding into the plaque. In a small vessel such as the coronary artery, this bleeding produces acute obstruction.

2. Thrombosis. Eddy currents around the plaque can lead to superadded thrombosis.

3. Ulceration. Sometimes the fibrous covering of the plaque becomes detached so that ulceration is combined with thrombosis (Fig. 29–3).

Figure 29–1. Atheroma of the aorta.
The abdominal aorta has been opened from behind to expose the initial surface. The early lesions of atheroma are the bright, stippled areas and streaks that are seen in the lower part of the specimen. In the fresh state the lesions were bright yellow in color.

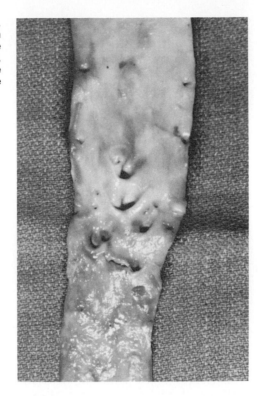

4. Calcification. The fatty material in the atheromatous plaque undergoes dystrophic calcification.

The cause of atherosclerosis is not yet known. The disease commences in childhood and progresses with age. Women are less affected than men until the menopause, but after that the number of women with the disease increases rapidly. Atherosclerosis is more common in patients with systemic hypertension. Heavy cigarette smoking also predisposes to the development of atherosclerosis, particularly that of the coronary arteries. Genetic factors

Etiology and Pathogenesis

Figure 29–2. Atherosclerosis of aorta.
In addition to yellow streaks, the intimal surface shows raised plaques of fibrous tissue overlying the fatty atheromatous material.

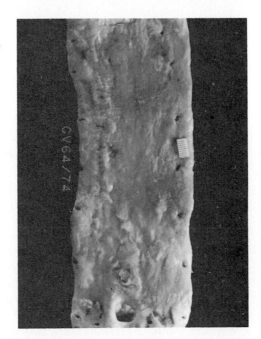

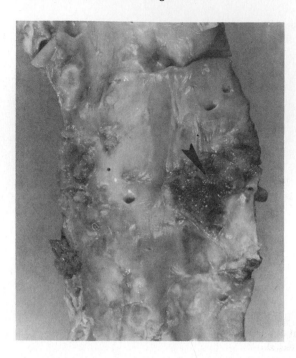

Figure 29–3. Atherosclerosis of the aorta. This aorta shows severe atherosclerosis. The arrow points to an area of ulceration that is covered by a thrombus.

seem to play a part, since the disease sometimes appears in many members of a family. In some instances there are clues to the pathogenesis. Thus, atherosclerosis is more common in persons having diabetes, which is itself a familial disease. Likewise, there are some inherited conditions of abnormal lipid metabolism in which high blood lipid levels are associated with the early development of atheroma.

It is not known whether the lesions of type I atheroma progress to those of type II, or whether the two types are independent diseases. Experimentally, lesions resembling the human fatty streaks can be produced in animals by feeding them with an abnormal diet — usually one containing a high content of cholesterol. It is believed that certain types of diet predispose human beings to develop atheroma. Much of the cholesterol in the body is produced endogenously, but the level of plasma cholesterol is related to the types of lipid that are eaten. A diet high in saturated animal fats appears to predispose a person to atheroma, and as noted previously, the rare inherited disorders of the lipid metabolism associated with hypercholesterolemia are associated with premature development of atherosclerosis. These observations have led to the *lipid infiltration or insudation theory* of the etiology of atherosclerosis. Some factor is assumed to render the endothelium more permeable to the plasma lipoproteins.

Lesions resembling type II atherosclerosis can occur after the arterial wall has been injured. A thrombus forms, and its subsequent degeneration and partial organization produce an atheromatous plaque. This is the *encrustation or thrombotic theory* of the etiology of atherosclerosis.

It is evident that either lipid deposition or thrombosis could be involved in the pathogenesis of human atheroma, and there is currently much controversy as to the relative importance of these two mechanisms. Furthermore, they are not mutually exclusive. Initial lipid lesions produced by dietary imbalance could progress by additional thrombosis. Injury and superadded thrombosis release chemicals (*e.g.*, histamine and 5-hydroxytryptamine) that could alter the endothelial permeability and allow plasma lipoproteins to enter the intima. Degradation of the lipoprotein together with failure to remove the lipid component is believed to be the mechanism of lipid accumulation in atheroma.

Recent investigations have laid stress on the role of the smooth muscle cells of the intima. It has been found that platelets release a factor that causes these cells to proliferate. Thus, injury to the vessel wall (*e.g.,* by hypertension, local trauma, abnormal lipoproteins, or hyperlipidemia) could lead to the formation of a platelet thrombus. Smooth muscle cells of the intima could proliferate, and as lipoproteins enter the vessel wall they could be taken up by the cells and the lipid component retained. In this way the early fatty streaks (type I lesions) could be produced. Some support for this theory has come from the discovery that, using the X chromosome as a marker (see Lyon hypothesis, Chapter 3), the cells of each atheromatous plaque are monoclonal as if each were a separate "tumor."

It is evident that the pathogenesis of atherosclerosis is very complex indeed. The increase in the incidence of the disease has now reached pandemic proportions, and this is a reflection of our ignorance.

Gradual Obstruction.   Atherosclerosis of small vessels such as the coronary or cerebral arteries produces intimal thickening and progressive occlusion of the lumen. This leads to ischemia of the area supplied (Chapter 20).

Thrombosis.   This leads to sudden complete obstruction and often to infarction (Chapter 20).

Dilatation and Aneurysm Formation.   The presence of an atherosclerotic plaque causes atrophy of the adjacent media. The wall consequently weakens, and the artery involved may show either a diffuse enlargement, termed *ectasia,* or a localized dilatation, termed an *aneurysm* (Fig. 29–4). These effects are seen most often in the aorta, in which the atherosclerosis is most severe. The lesions of atherosclerosis tend to be more advanced toward the more caudal regions of the aorta, and it is therefore in the abdominal portion

Effects of Atherosclerosis

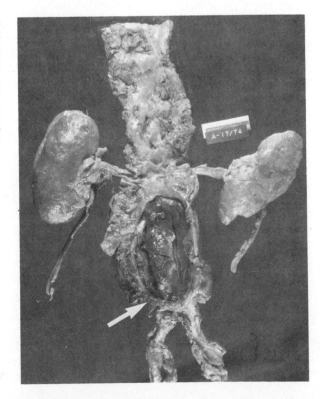

Figure 29–4. Atheromatous aneurysm of the aorta. The aorta shows severe atheroma. An aneurysm, situated below the level of the renal arteries, is filled with thrombus, but has ruptured (arrow). The kidneys are reduced in size, and their surfaces are granular. This change is due to nephrosclerosis combined with many atheromatous emboli in the renal arterioles.

that aneurysm formation is most common. The aneurysm is generally below the origin of the renal arteries, which is fortunate because surgical replacement by a plastic prosthesis is technically possible.

An aneurysm that begins to leak generally causes pain, and this is liable to be followed shortly by complete rupture with exsanguination and death.

CASE HISTORY I. (See Figure 29–4).   The patient was a 71-year-old man who had had a 15-year history of hypertension. Five years prior to the examination he had been investigated for a possible aortic aneurysm. The findings were equivocal, however, and no treatment was advised. One year prior to his present admission he had noted the onset of angina pectoris and intermittent claudication. The angina was easily relieved by nitroglycerin tablets.

The patient's present complaint was that of pain in the abdomen. His blood pressure was 220/115 mm Hg, and the blood urea nitrogen (BUN) was 50 mg/dl (normal: 10 to 20 mg/dl). A diagnosis of myocardial infarct was considered, but it was not confirmed by the electrocardiogram. The pain subsided for a few days but suddenly recurred with increased severity and was accompanied by signs of shock. The patient died before treatment for internal bleeding could be undertaken.

Necropsy revealed a ruptured aortic aneurysm, which is shown in Figure 29–4. There was extensive bleeding into the retroperitoneal tissues and into the peritoneum. The heart was enlarged (weight 850 grams, compared to 300 grams in a normal heart) owing to marked left ventricular hypertrophy. The coronary vessels showed severe atherosclerosis with narrowing.

Embolism.   It is not uncommon for atheromatous material, or overlying thrombus, to become detached and embolize distally. Usually such emboli are small and are inapparent clinically. Nevertheless, the steady occlusion of many small vessels is a contributing factor in peripheral ischemic disease of the lower leg as well as in the progressive ischemic renal disease that often accompanies atherosclerosis.

Inflammatory Diseases of Arteries

Acute Infective Arteritis

Arteritis may occur in pyogenic infections, and if the vessel wall undergoes necrosis, severe hemorrhage can result. A good example of this is the fatal hemorrhage from the lingual artery that sometimes ends the life of a patient with an ulcerating carcinoma of the tongue. Neoplastic invasion plays its part, but the major weakening effect is the result of infection. Similarly, destruction of an artery at the base of a gastric ulcer is a common cause of bleeding. Fortunately, in many chronic inflammatory lesions the artery responds by proliferation of its intimal lining so that the lumen becomes steadily occluded (*endarteritis obliterans*) and bleeding is restricted.

Syphilitic Arteritis

In tertiary syphilis an arteritis may occur, and it nearly always affects the aorta. A chronic inflammatory reaction is combined with destruction of the elastic coat and its replacement by fibrous tissue; the vessel becomes thickened, and at the same time is weakened. Either it dilates diffusely or an aneurysm (either fusiform or saccular) is formed. The thoracic part of the aorta is most severely affected; in the past, syphilis was the common cause of thoracic aortic aneurysms (Fig. 29–5). Today the disease is rare, and atheroma accounts for the majority of aortic aneurysms. Dilatation of the arch of the aorta and the aortic ring leads to separation of the aortic cusps so that in diastole they fail to meet and *aortic regurgitation* results. Syphilitic arteritis can also affect the cerebral vessels but, like syphilitic aortitis, is rarely encountered today.

Rheumatoid Aortitis

Rheumatoid aortitis, which is very similar to the aortitis of tertiary syphilis, is occasionally encountered in rheumatoid arthritis. It also leads to aortic insufficiency.

Figure 29–5. Syphilitic aneurysm of the aorta. The specimen shows part of the descending thoracic aorta from which a saccular aneurysm arises. Note the laminated thrombus in the aneurysmal sac and the wrinkled appearance of the aortic wall (arrow). This is characteristic of the syphilitic aortitis of tertiary syphilis. (Specimen from the Boyd Museum, University of Toronto.)

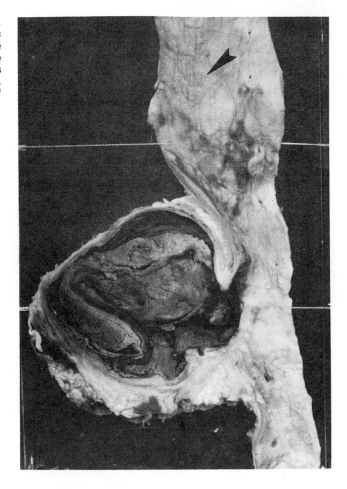

There are a number of diseases in which inflammation of the arterial wall leads to thrombosis.

Idiopathic Inflammatory Conditions

Thromboangiitis Obliterans (Buerger's Disease). This disease occurs predominantly in young men and affects the arteries and veins of the legs. Thrombosis leads to ischemia and intermittent claudication; ultimately, gangrene of the toes sets in.

Giant-Cell Arteritis. Giant-cell arteritis is a disease of elderly people. The affected artery shows thrombosis and a chronic inflammatory granulomatous reaction with many giant cells forming around disrupted elastic fibers. Since the disease commonly affects the temporal artery, it is also called *temporal arteritis*. It is characterized by pain in the region of the artery and is important because it can affect the ophthalmic artery and lead to blindness.

Polyarteritis nodosa is described in Chapter 27.

In consideration of vascular disease the capillaries and arterioles are usually forgotten. There are, nevertheless, many conditions in which so many vessels in an area are occluded that ischemia results. Because an additional effect is bleeding, petechial hemorrhages are a common feature of small vessel disease, even though the extent of the occlusion is insufficient to lead to ischemia of the total area involved. Some causes of these diseases are briefly described below:

DISEASES OF SMALL VESSELS

Frostbite. The harmful effects of cold on exposed parts are due in large measure to small vessel damage. In mild cases there is an inflammatory reaction causing large blisters to form; if the damage is severe, the vessels become completely occluded by thrombus and gangrene occurs.

Occlusion of Capillaries by Red Cells.   This response occurs in severe sludging and is a component of shock.

Occlusion by Fibrin.   This occurs in disseminated intravascular coagulation (Chapter 26). The kidney is the organ most affected.

Occlusion by Precipitated Cryoglobulins.   In cryoglobulinemia exposure of the extremities to cold leads to vascular occlusion and petechial hemorrhages.

Fat Embolism.   See Chapter 20.

Decompression Syndrome.   See Chapter 20.

External Pressure.   The best example of this is a bedsore. Continual pressure on one area produces such ischemia that necrosis of the skin and underlying tissues occurs. *It is a major duty of nurses to move nonambulatory patients often enough that no pressure sores develop.*

Occlusion by Antigen-Antibody Interaction.   This is a feature of such immune complex phenomena as the Arthus reaction (Chapter 9).

Vasculitis.   The term vasculitis is used to describe an inflammatory reaction in the wall of small vessels. Typical lesions occur in the Arthus reaction; the immune complex deposition in the vessel wall causes damage associated with a marked polymorph infiltration and thrombosis (Fig. 29–6). This type of type III hypersensitivity is thought to occur in many drug reactions as well as in some infections. The petechial hemorrhages seen in the skin in septicemia (*e.g.*, gonococcal septicemia, see Fig. 10–2) and in infective endocarditis are explained on this basis. Internal organs are affected; the

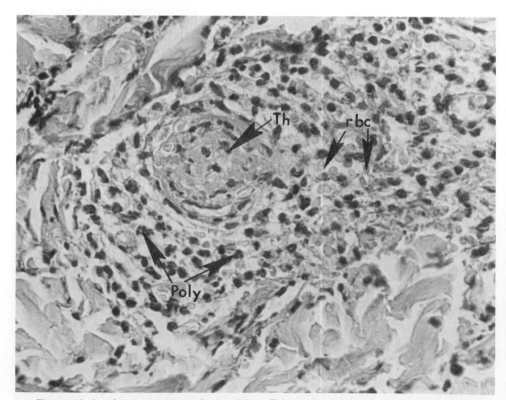

Figure 29–6.   Acute gonococcal vasculitis.   This section of dermis shows an arteriole that is obstructed by thrombus (Th). The vessel wall has undergone necrosis, and there is a heavy infiltration of polymorphs (Poly). The presence of many red cells (rbc) in the interstitial tissues indicates that the vessel has ruptured. This biopsy was taken from the patient shown in Figure 10–2.

kidney appears to be the most vulnerable. In some examples of vasculitis no cause can be found. The disease then appears to be a component of polyarteritis nodosa (Chapter 27).

"Peripheral vascular disease" is an inclusive term that is used to describe all those conditions in which the blood supply to the limbs is impaired. Usually it is the legs that suffer. The following diseases all play their part:

Peripheral Vascular Disease

1. Atherosclerosis. This tends to affect the large vessels such as the iliac and femoral arteries.

2. Thrombosis. This may be secondary to atherosclerosis.

3. Embolism. Emboli may be large thromboemboli or small clumps of atheromatous material.

4. Small Vessel Disease. Arteriolar sclerosis associated with hypertension and diabetic microangiopathy (Chapter 24) are the most important.

Effects of Peripheral Diseases. The effects are serious and disabling. The ischemia of the leg leads to atrophy of many structures, including the bones (osteoporosis) and the skin. Trivial injury can lead to chronic, persistent, and extremely painful ulceration. Ischemia of the muscle leads to pain on walking (intermittent claudication) and, ultimately, to pain at rest. Dry gangrene leading to loss of the limb is the all-too-frequent end-result.

An *aneurysm* is a local dilatation of an artery or a chamber of the heart and is due to weakening of its walls. It may be saccular or fusiform (Fig. 29–7).

Aneurysms

Weakening of the wall may be due to any of the following:

Causes of Aneurysms

1. Congenital Deficiency. A good example is a berry aneurysm of the circle of Willis (Chapter 44).

2. Trauma. Sometimes an injury can damage not only an artery but also an adjacent vein, thereby establishing a connection. This formation is termed an *arteriovenous aneurysm,* or fistula. It is important, because so much blood can be diverted from the peripheral tissues that heart failure ensues.

3. Inflammation. Syphilitic aortitis is a good example.

4. Degeneration. Atheromatous degeneration is by far the most common cause of aortic aneurysm.

An aneurysm can produce its effect in a number of ways:

Effects of Aneurysms

1. Pressure. An aneurysm of the thoracic aorta may press on the esophagus and cause difficulty in swallowing, or it may press on the recurrent laryngeal nerve and lead to changes of voice.

2. Thrombosis. The sac and aneurysm soon become filled by laminated thrombus. This effect is due in part to damage of the endothelial lining, but it is mostly the result of local stasis and eddy-current formation.

3. Hemorrhage. Rupture of an aneurysm leads to bleeding; for a while this can be quite trivial because of the plugging effect of the thrombus lining the sac. Nevertheless, when an aneurysm, such as one of the abdominal aorta, has begun to bleed, it is not long before massive hemorrhage follows and the patient dies of exsanguination.

4. Ischemia. This is due to blockage of the branches of the artery at the site of the aneurysm, an effect produced either by local pressure or by thrombotic occlusion.

The basic defect in this condition is a degeneration of the media (medionecrosis), the cause of which is unknown. The pathogenesis is described in Figure 29–7. The condition is quite common and is usually

Dissecting Aneurysm of the Aorta

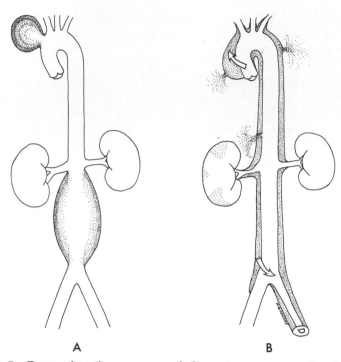

A   B

Figure 29–7.   Types of aortic aneurysm.   *A,* Shows two aneurysms. One is saccular and has arisen from the ascending aorta. It is filled with laminated thrombus. Fifty years ago this type of aneurysm invariably was due to tertiary syphilis, but today this form of the disease is so uncommon that atheroma is the usual cause. The abdominal aorta shows a fusiform aneurysm that is lined by thrombus. This type of aneurysm is usually due to atheroma and invariably affects the aorta below the origins of the renal arteries. *B,* Shows a dissecting aneurysm. It is thought to arise as a result of bleeding into the media of a weakened aortic wall. An intramural hematoma is formed, and this ruptures into the lumen of the aorta, usually in the ascending portion. Blood is then forced into the tear, and dissection occurs into the media. A false aneurysmal sac encases the aorta and can involve the entire length of the vessel as well as extending along some of its branches. Some branches are obstructed, and the effects of this account for the clinical signs and symptoms. Thus, in the aneurysm illustrated, the left femoral pulse would be weaker than the right and the ischemia of the right kidney has led to infarction. A dissecting aneurysm usually terminates by rupture of the external coat; bleeding into the pericardium, mediastinum, or retroperitoneal space causes death. Very occasionally the aneurysm ruptures internally into the aortic lumen, and the patient survives with no treatment. This accounts for the double-barreled aorta that is occasionally found as an unexpected necropsy finding. (Drawing by Margot Mackay, Department of Art as Applied to Medicine, University of Toronto.)

heralded by the sudden onset of severe chest pain. As blood is forced into the wall of the aorta, there is blockage of the ostia of important branches. The consequences vary considerably from case to case. Thus, the coronary arteries may be occluded, and myocardial infarction results. There is a varying degree of obstruction to the arteries supplying the upper limbs, so that the pulses at the wrist are often either weak or unequal. Blockage of the renal arteries leads to infarction and anuria. The outer coat of the aneurysm usually ruptures, causing fatal hemorrhage into the pericardium, the mediastinum, the retroperitoneal space, or the peritoneal cavity.

DISEASES OF VEINS

Phlebothrombosis and its important complications of embolism and pulmonary infarction are described in Chapter 20. Inflammation of veins (phlebitis) is a common event in any inflammatory process. The overlying thrombosis that accompanies it is not important as a source of embolism, since the thrombus is firmly adherent to the wall of the damaged vessel. Only if the thrombus is invaded by pyogenic organisms is embolism a hazard. Under these circumstances emboli containing bacteria are thrown off and pyemia results (Chapter 20).

Elongation and irregular dilatation of veins is known as *varicosity*. It is generally assumed that persistent increase in pressure is a cause of this; esophageal varices can certainly be explained in this manner (Chapter 33). Nevertheless, the common condition of varicose veins of the legs is not well understood. An inherited defect of the venous walls or valves has been postulated. There also seems to be a familial factor in the incidence of this common disease. Other suggested causes are the standing for long periods over many years that is required in some occupations and the lack of support for the walls of the veins that is seen in fat people. Because pregnancy seems to initiate varicose vein formation, the disease is more common at an earlier age in women. Once varicose veins have formed, their valves become incompetent, so that on standing the full hydrostatic pressure of blood is applied to the vessel wall and further dilatation ensues. Particularly important is incompetence of valves in the perforating veins that communicate between superficial veins and deep vessels. The extremely sluggish blood flow through the veins can predispose a person to thrombus formation, but embolism from this is extremely rare. The major effect of varicose veins is to produce venous stasis. The increased hydrostatic pressure leads to edema, and the skin exhibits *stasis dermatitis*. Trivial injuries lead to persistent ulcerations that characteristically overlie the medial malleoli. Even though these ulcers can enlarge, they are not painful. In this respect they contrast with the ulceration caused by arterial disease (ischemic ulcers).

Varicose Veins

Two particular circumstances under which venous thrombosis occurs are worthy of special note:

1. Thrombophlebitis Migrans.   Migratory thrombophlebitis is described in Chapter 20.

2. Painful White Leg (Phlegmasia Alba Dolens).   The painful white leg that is seen in pregnant women in the third trimester — or more often immediately following delivery—is due to ileofemoral venous thrombosis. It is thought that inflammation also involves lymphatics and that this contributes to the formation of such massive edema.

1. Describe the complications of atherosclerosis with particular reference to the changes encountered in the coronary arteries and in the aorta.

Review Questions

2. Give examples of the relationship between lipid metabolism and the development of human atherosclerosis.

3. Describe the role of the smooth muscle cell in the development of atherosclerosis.

4. List the inflammatory lesions that may affect the following:
   (a) the aorta
   (b) medium-sized arteries
   (c) arterioles

5. Describe briefly the diseases that may contribute to intermittent claudication.

6. Classify the causes of aneurysm formation.

7. Compare cutaneous stasis ulcers with ischemic ulcers with respect to these factors:
   (a) cause
   (b) site
   (c) symptoms

Leading Article: Monoclonal theory of atheroma. British Medical Journal, *1*:1371–1372, 1977.

Robbins, S. L., and Cotran, R. S.: Pathologic Basis of Disease. 2nd ed. Philadelphia, W. B. Saunders Company, 1979. See Chapter 14, "Blood Vessels."

Ross, R., and Glomset, J. A.: The pathogenesis of atherosclerosis. New England Journal of Medicine, 295:369–377; 420–425, 1976.

Spaet, T. H.: Optimism in the control of atherosclerosis. New England Journal of Medicine, *291*:576–577, 1974.

Selected Readings

**Diseases of the
Respiratory Tract**

After studying this chapter the student should be able to:

- Define the acinus of the lung.
- Define surfactant and indicate its importance in normal lung function and in the pathogenesis of lung disease.
- Define respiratory failure.
- Compare the causes and effects of ventilatory failure with those of impaired alveolar-arterial gas exchange.
- Discuss the causes of dyspnea.
- Give an account of the pathogenesis, clinical features, and pathological findings of lobar pneumonia.
- Classify the causes of bronchopneumonia.
- Give an account of the respiratory distress syndrome of the newborn.
- Give an account of legionnaires' disease.
- Describe interstitial pneumonia with respect to:
    (a) cause and pathogenesis
    (b) morphological changes in the lungs
    (c) end-results
- Describe the acute adult respiratory insufficiency syndrome.
- Define chronic obstructive lung disease and indicate its common causes.
- Give an account of chronic bronchitis.
- Describe pulmonary emphysema with respect to:
    (a) definition
    (b) pathological types and their known causes
    (c) clinical effects
- Describe the two classical clinicopathological syndromes of COLD.
- Describe the outstanding features of:
    (a) intrinsic asthma
    (b) extrinsic asthma
    (c) extrinsic allergic alveolitis
- Compare bronchial asthma with cardiac asthma.
- Describe the causes and effects of bronchial obstruction.
- Give an account of bronchial carcinoid tumor.
- Describe carcinoma of the lung with respect to the following factors:
    (a) known causes
    (b) gross appearance and types
    (c) diagnosis
    (d) histological types
    (e) spread
- Distinguish between a transudate and an exudate with reference to hydrothorax.
- Describe the types and common causes of pleuritis.
- Define empyema and pneumothorax. Give at least one cause of each.

***Development
and Structure of
the Lung***

The lung develops from a central outpouching from the primitive foregut. This develops into the trachea, and by repeated branching the bronchi and bronchioles are formed. These act as conducting tubes, and the last passage to perform only this function is defined as a *terminal bronchiole.* The part of the

Figure 30–1. This diagrammatic representation of an acinus shows a terminal bronchiole (TB), respiratory bronchioles of the first (RB₁), second (RB₂), and third (RB₃) orders, an alveolar duct (AD), and an alveolar sac (AS). The acinus is the part of the lung distal to a terminal bronchiole. (From Thurlbeck, W. M.: Chronic obstructive lung disease. *In* Sommers, S. C. (Ed.): Pathology Annual, Vol. 3. New York, Appleton-Century-Crofts, 1968.)

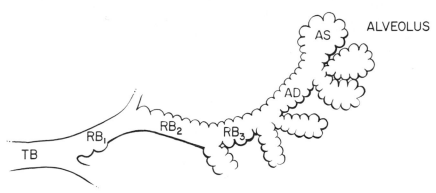

COMPONENT PARTS OF ACINUS

lung distal to a terminal bronchiole is termed the *acinus* of the lung, and it in turn consists of a number of generations of respiratory bronchioles and alveolar ducts, from the walls of which bud the alveoli, in which gas exchange takes place (Fig. 30–1). The alveoli are packed together like a mass of soap bubbles, and are themselves lined by flattened pneumocytes, of which there are two types. *Type I pneumocytes* are the most abundant and line most of the alveolar surface. *Type II pneumocytes* secrete *surfactant,* a phospholipid, surface-active compound that has the very important function of lowering surface tension at the air-liquid interface in the lung. Hence, surfactant aids inspiration by lessening the work needed to inflate the alveoli, and it also prevents alveoli from collapsing following expiration. It should be noted that the acini of the lung are not visible as entities to the naked eye, but a group of acini together form the lobules, the outline of which is often visible by the fact that carbon is deposited in the septa that separate one lobule from the next.

Normal Function

The function of the respiratory system is to enable gaseous exchange to occur between the blood and the atmosphere. The upper respiratory tract functions as an air conditioner for the lungs, the inspired air being filtered and humidified as it passes through the nose, nasopharynx, larynx, and trachea. Air eventually reaches the small air sacs, or alveoli, of the lung, where it comes into close contact with blood in the capillaries and where conditions for gaseous exchange are ideal (Fig. 30–2). Oxygen is added to the blood, and the carbon dioxide that is removed is exhaled. The gas in the alveoli is maintained at a fairly constant composition by the act of breathing, a process that has two components: *ventilation* and *distribution*.

Ventilation.   This is the bellowslike action of the chest, by which fresh air is inspired and stale air is expired. The volume is approximately 7.5 liters per minute in the adult at rest.

Distribution.   The inspired air is distributed in such a way in relation to the volume of blood perfusing the lung that the composition of the alveolar gas is maintained at a constant level. Since the arterial blood, as it leaves the lung, is in equilibrium with the alveolar gas, it follows that the gaseous tensions of oxygen and carbon dioxide in the arterial blood are also maintained at this same constant level (Fig. 30–3).

RESPIRATORY FAILURE

If through dysfunction of the lungs there is lack of oxygen or retention of CO_2 the condition is called *respiratory failure*. In the arterial blood under normal conditions, the partial pressure of oxygen, usually written Po_2, is about 100 mm Hg, and the partial pressure of carbon dioxide, written Pco_2, is

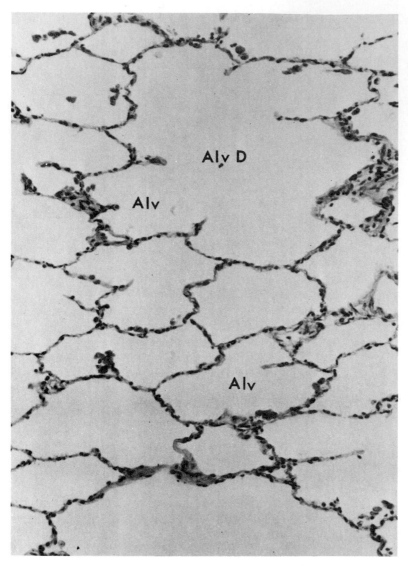

Figure 30–2. Normal lung. This section shows a number of alveoli (Alv) and an alveolar duct (Alv D) from which some of them have arisen. Note how thin the alveolar walls are (× 60).

about 40 mm Hg. In respiratory failure the P_{O_2} is under 60 mm Hg (*hypoxemia*), and the P_{CO_2} is over 49 mm Hg (*hypercapnia*).

Types of Respiratory Failure.   Two main types can be recognized:

1. *Ventilatory failure*, which is due to an inadequate volume of inspired air available for exchange.

2. *Impaired alveolar-arterial gas exchange*, which is due to failure of distribution or diffusion.

Ventilatory Failure (Hypoxia with Hypercapnia)

This condition is caused by the following factors:

1. Airways obstruction, which is considered later in this chapter.

2. Restriction of thoracic movement, such as that resulting from the presence of a pneumothorax or a large pleural effusion.

3. Neuromuscular impairment, such as that found in infantile paralysis.

4. Disturbance of the brain, such as that due to injury or to overdose of a depressant drug (*e.g.*, a barbiturate).

Effects.   Since

$$P_{CO_2} \text{ (arterial)} \propto \frac{CO_2 \text{ Production}}{\text{Alveolar Ventilation}}$$

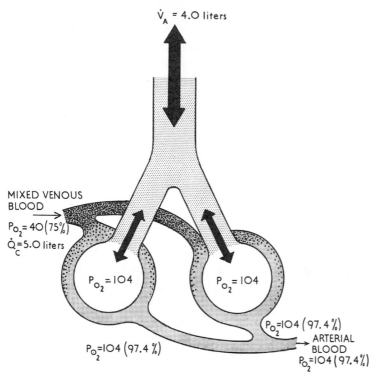

$\dot{V}_A$ = 4.0 liters

MIXED VENOUS BLOOD
P_{O_2} = 40 (75%)
$\dot{Q}_C$ = 5.0 liters

P_{O_2} = 104

P_{O_2} = 104

P_{O_2} = 104 (97.4%)

ARTERIAL BLOOD
P_{O_2} = 104 (97.4%)

P_{O_2} = 104 (97.4%)

Figure 30–3. Physiological relationships within lung. Diagrammatic representation of the lung, showing two alveoli with ideal $\dfrac{\text{Ventilation}}{\text{Blood Flow}}$ relationships. This relationship is generally written $\dfrac{\dot{V}_A}{\dot{Q}_C}$, the dot indicating that the volumes of alveolar ventilation (V_A) and capillary blood flow (Q_C) are in unit time. Thus, for the lung as a whole in a normal subject at rest:

$$\frac{\dot{V}_A}{\dot{Q}_C} = \frac{4 \text{ liters per minute}}{5 \text{ liters per minute}} = 0.8$$

In the diagram, the oxygen tensions are in mm Hg, and the figures in brackets are the percentage of the saturation level of oxygen in the blood.

The partial pressure of a gas in a mixture is the contribution that the gas makes toward the total pressure. Thus, for moist air at sea level the total pressure is about 760 mm Hg. Water vapor contributes about 24 mm Hg, and the remaining 736 mm Hg is contributed by oxygen (about 20 per cent) and nitrogen (about 80 per cent). Hence, the partial pressure of oxygen (P_{O_2}) is 20 per cent of 736 mm Hg or about 147 mm Hg. As fresh air is drawn into the lungs, it mixes with expired gases. Under normal conditions the gas in the alveoli has an oxygen tension of about 100 mm Hg. (After Comroe, J. H., et al.: The Lung: Clinical Physiology and Pulmonary Function Tests. 2nd ed. Chicago, Year Book Medical Publishers, 1963.)

and at rest the CO_2 production is constant, it follows that when alveolar ventilation is reduced, there is an increase in the arterial P_{CO_2} and an arithmetically equivalent decrease in P_{O_2}. Thus, if the P_{CO_2} rises from 40 to 60 mm Hg, then the P_{O_2} falls from 100 to 80 mm Hg. A drop of this magnitude in the P_{O_2} does not greatly affect the amount of oxygen present in arterial blood, since hemoglobin has great affinity for oxygen. Desaturation of blood with subsequent cyanosis is a late event in ventilatory failure.

The main effect is a raised arterial P_{CO_2} (*hypercapnia*), and symptoms are related to this response. The pulse is rapid, and the hands are moist and warm. The pupils are small, and the blood pressure is raised. If there is severe CO_2 retention, then confusion, drowsiness, tremors, and coma may ensue. Carbon dioxide is a vasodilator, and severe CO_2 retention causes cerebral edema, which is the explanation of the nervous phenomena and which can be detected clinically by the occurrence of papilledema. Finally, the plasma bicarbonate level is high and the patient has respiratory acidosis (Chapter 19).

***Impaired
Alveolar-Arterial
Gas Exchange
(Hypoxia Without
Hypercapnia)***

In this type of respiratory failure there is a reduction of alveolar-capillary surface available for gas exchange. This reduction may occur as a result of lung destruction, but more commonly it is due to an imbalance in the distribution of perfusion and ventilation. Frequently, these factors are combined; of the two, however, maldistribution is much more important, and it becomes prominent in all progressive lung disease.

Impaired alveolar-arterial gas exchange occurs in emphysema and severe chronic bronchitis, especially postoperatively, when there is mucous plugging of bronchi. It is a feature of pulmonary embolism.

Effects.   Oxygen uptake is interfered with, and the venous blood becomes more desaturated during exercise; increasing arterial desaturation also occurs. The patient develops central cyanosis.

Although impaired alveolar-arterial gas exchange leads to a severe interference with O_2 uptake, it interferes little with CO_2 elimination. In the distribution failure group some alveoli are underventilated relative to alveolar perfusion with blood. This situation is remedied by overventilation of the remaining lung. Overventilation serves to eliminate more CO_2 from the blood, but it cannot compensate for any unequal oxygen uptake, because it does not produce an appreciable increase above the normal level in the amount of oxygen taken up by the blood (Fig. 30–4).

DYSPNEA

In a healthy person, the rate and depth of respiration are so regulated that the individual is unaware of the movements involved in breathing. *Tachypnea* is an increased rate of respiration. Rapid, shallow breathing is seen when pain restricts respiratory movement, as in pleurisy or in increasing rigidity of the lungs, as in congestion or fibrosis. Tachypnea is sometimes accompanied by an increase in depth of breathing; the term *hyperpnea* includes both conditions. *Dyspnea* is a state in which the act of breathing causes distress. It occurs under two main circumstances:

1. *When tachypnea or hyperpnea is excessive.*

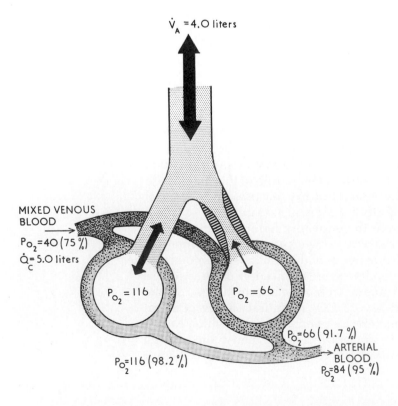

Figure 30–4.   Ventilation and perfusion within lung. Diagrammatic representation of the lung showing two alveoli that are unevenly ventilated but uniformly perfused. Note how the overventilation of one alveolus does not compensate for the underventilation of the other, with the result that some arterial desaturation occurs and the P_{O_2} is considerably reduced. (After Comroe, J. H., et al.: The Lung: Clinical Physiology and Pulmonary Function Tests. 2nd ed. Chicago, Year Book Medical Publishers, 1963.)

2. *When the movement of the chest on inspiration is small in comparison with the muscular effort needed to produce it.* This occurs in any disease interfering with the respiratory excursions of the lung, such as fibrosis or congestion. Obstruction to the major air passages — whether due to pulmonary disease like chronic bronchitis or to strangulation — has a similar effect and produces intense dyspnea. Psychological factors also play a part. Thus, the sudden blockage of a tube through which a person is breathing can cause intense dyspnea. However, if the subject is asked to block the tube himself the maneuver causes no immediate discomfort.

The respiratory distress syndrome of the newborn is a clinical state that may have one of many causes, both extrapulmonary (*e.g.,* heart failure) and pulmonary; by far the most important cause is *hyaline membrane disease,* which is responsible for approximately 30 per cent of all neonatal deaths in North America.

RESPIRATORY DISTRESS SYNDROME OF THE NEWBORN

Clinical Features. Respiratory distress generally occurs within one hour of birth and is invariably present by six hours. It is characterized by rapid grunting respiration, cyanosis, and obvious retraction of the intercostal muscles on inspiration. The overall mortality is about 50 per cent.

Predisposing Factors. The respiratory distress syndrome is more common in infants delivered by cesarean section, in infants subjected to perinatal asphyxia, and in those whose mothers have diabetes mellitus. However, by far the most important predisposing factor is prematurity, and the more premature the infant is, the more likely is the syndrome to be fatal.

Pathogenesis and Morphology. Fetal adaptation from intrauterine life to breathing air depends upon orderly and unimpaired lung development. The type II pneumocytes first develop at about 24 weeks' gestation, and at this time surfactant also begins to appear. A deficiency in surfactant activity at birth is the main direct cause of the syndrome. As would be expected, this is most likely to occur in premature infants. The infant who lacks surfactant has difficulty in expanding the lungs because the work of inflating the alveoli is increased. Characteristically at death the lungs are airless and dark red and have a liverlike consistency. Microscopically, the developing alveoli are collapsed, and the larger air passages are dilated and lined by a pink eosinophilic hyaline membrane (see Fig. 30–9).

Prediction and Treatment. Treatment is at present entirely supportive, but the possibility that hyaline membrane disease might occur can be predicted by examining the amniotic fluid. The amniotic sphingomyelin content remains constant throughout gestation, whereas amniotic lecithin levels reflect the development and function of type II pneumocytes. Hence, the ratio of lecithin to sphingomyelin is a good indicator of fetal lung development. If the ratio is greater than 2, it indicates that there is adequate surfactant and that hyaline membrane disease is unlikely to develop. If the ratio is less than 1.5, significant surfactant deficiency exists and hyaline membrane disease should be anticipated.

Pneumonia is defined as an inflammation in the alveolar parenchyma of the lung. The following causes may be listed:

PNEUMONIA

1. Infection. This is generally bacterial, mycoplasmal, or viral.

2. Physicochemical. The agent may be inhaled (toxic gases, irritant particles, or irritant fluids such as gastric juice), or it may reach the lung via the blood stream (*e.g.,* bleomycin, an anticancer agent). Ionizing radiations form a separate variety of damaging agents.

Two patterns of reaction may be found:

1. Pneumonia with Exudation into Air Spaces. The unequalified term "pneumonia" is commonly used to refer to this type. Inflammatory exudate fills the alveoli, which are thereby rendered airless and solid. This is called *consolidation,* and a portion of lung obtained at necropsy showing this will sink when placed in a beaker of water.

2. Pneumonia with Interstitial Exudate.   The terms *interstitial pneumonia* and *pneumonitis* are commonly applied to this type.

Pneumonia with Exudation into Alveolar Spaces

This type of pneumonia is invariably caused by an infectious agent. The clinical presentation is extremely variable, depending on the properties of the causative organism, the amount of lung affected, and the state of the host's defenses. The clinical course can be greatly modified by antibiotic therapy, and indeed many patients that formerly were admitted to the hospital can now be managed at home by their family practitioners. Nevertheless, it has been estimated that pneumonia accounts for approximately 10 per cent of admissions to the hospital in the United States.

In spite of the changing pattern of pneumonia that has occurred since 1940, two main types can be distinguished — *lobar pneumonia* and *bronchopneumonia.* They differ in their pathogenesis and causative organism and in the gross appearance of the lesions that result.

Lobar Pneumonia

Healthy individuals are often affected by this disease, but an underlying debilitating disease, particularly chronic alcoholism, predisposes one to it. The infecting organism is invariably a highly virulent pneumococcus that is acquired by inhalation from another victim or a convalescent carrier. The disease has a sudden onset and is accompanied by rigors, fever, and pain in the chest. The organisms that reach the lung produce a rapidly spreading inflammatory edema that soon implicates a whole lobe or, at times, several lobes (Fig. 30–5).

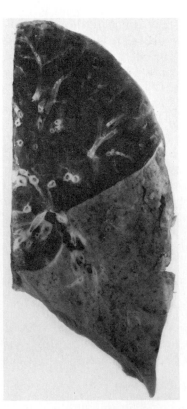

Figure 30–5. Lobar pneumonia. The lower lobe is completely consolidated, whereas the upper lobe is unaffected. Note the sharp division between the two lobes. (R30.2, Reproduced by permission of the President and Council of the Royal College of Surgeons of England.)

Pathogenesis.   The fact that infection spreads so rapidly in a gigantic wave of edematous exudate suggests that allergy is involved in the process. Perhaps the patient has already had a minor pneumococcal infection sufficient to produce an immune response. When having a second attack, the patient experiences a hypersensitivity reaction that accompanies the inflammatory response and renders it more intense. An alternative explanation is that lobar pneumonia is a primary infection. When the organisms reach the lungs, they pass on rapidly to the blood stream, proliferate in the reticuloendothelial system, and then escape into the blood to produce a septicemia. When they reach the lungs again, an allergic response occurs because of their interaction with recently formed local antibodies. This mechanism would be analogous to that described in typhoid fever and in syphilis.

Whatever the mechanism, there is no doubt that during the initial stage of the disease there is a septicemia. Sometimes the pneumococci may become localized not only in the lungs but also in the meninges, peritoneum, joints, and elsewhere. During the first few days of illness the patient is desperately ill and may die; the lobe of lung affected is *congested* and shows *inflammatory edema.* It is teeming with pneumococci.

In the next stage the lung shows complete consolidation and has a solid appearance that has been likened to that of a liver. Hence, it is sometimes called *hepatization.* The alveoli are filled with typical inflammatory exudate, with fibrin and polymorphs abounding.

The last stage of the disease is that of *resolution.* Macrophages replace the polymorphs, the inflammatory exudate is removed, and the lung returns to normal. This is an excellent example of complete resolution following acute inflammation.

During the acute stage of lobar pneumonia the overlying pleura shows acute inflammation *(pleurisy)* and is covered with a fibrinous exudate. This exudate is responsible for the creaking *pleural rub,* which may be heard with a stethoscope, and for the severe pain that occurs on inspiration.

Clinical Course.   Following the acute onset, the patient remains seriously ill for 7 to 10 days with high fever. Death may occur during this stage. As suddenly as the disease started, it terminates. Sweating occurs, the temperature drops, and there is a sense of well-being. This is termed the *crisis.* In practice these stages are rarely seen today, since antibiotics rapidly terminate the course of the disease.

Complications.   Lung abscess, pulmonary fibrosis, and empyema may occur but are uncommon, even in the untreated patient.

In bronchopneumonia, unlike lobar pneumonia, there are discrete foci of inflammation around terminal bronchioles. Patches of consolidation are scattered throughout several lobes of the lung, and the condition is usually bilateral (Fig. 30–6). The wildfire spread seen in lobar pneumonia is not present. There are many varieties of bronchopneumonia. They are best considered under two headings:

Endogenous Bronchopneumonia.   The organisms are derived from the normal flora of the upper respiratory tract.

Exogenous bronchopneumonia.   The organisms are derived from the exterior.

Bronchopneumonia

This type of bronchopneumonia is due to infection by commensal organisms normally resident in the upper respiratory passages. Of these organisms, the commensal pneumococci of low-grade virulence are by far the most important. *They cause infection whenever the defense mechanisms of*

Endogenous Bronchopneumonia

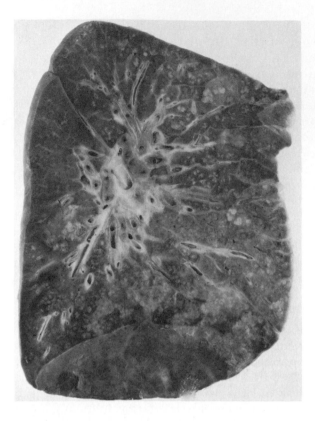

Figure 30–6. Staphylococcal bronchopneumonia. There are many discrete foci of consolidation scattered throughout the lung. Compare this with Figure 30–5, which shows lobar pneumonia. (R29.3, Reproduced by permission of the President and Council of the Royal College of Surgeons of England.)

the host are impaired. The antagonists are therefore a weakly virulent endogenous organism and an enfeebled host. This situation contrasts sharply with lobar pneumonia, in which the contending parties are a highly virulent organism and a relatively healthy host.

Causes. The conditions leading to endogenous bronchopneumonia may be classified as either general or local factors.

General Factors

Extremes of Age. Bronchopneumonia is commonest in infancy and old age.

General Debilitating Illness. It is a common terminal event in cancer, cerebrovascular accidents, and uremia.

Impaired Immune Response. It may occur with agammaglobulinemia or agranulocytosis or as a complication of glucocorticoid therapy.

Local Factors

Any local condition interfering with ciliary action and the upward movement of mucus is liable to be followed by bronchopneumonia. Possible causes are listed below:

Pre-existing Acute Upper Respiratory Disease. Bronchopneumonia often complicates influenza, measles, and whooping cough. In these infections the ciliated bronchial epithelium is shed, and organisms that gain access to the lung cannot be removed.

Local Obstruction. The trapped secretions form an admirable medium for bacterial growth, and bronchopneumonia is localized to the segment distal to the obstruction. Foreign bodies and tumors of the bronchi are good examples.

Chronic Bronchitis and Bronchiectasis. These are important predisposing causes of bronchopneumonia. Two factors are involved. First, the ciliated epithelium may be replaced by goblet cells or squamous cells, thereby impeding the upward flow of mucus. Second, the mucus itself is often of viscid consistency, and it cannot easily be removed. An excessive secretion of mucus accompanies the chronic venous congestion of heart failure because of the additional fluid contributed by transudation.

Pulmonary Edema.   In edematous lung tissue the alveolar macrophages are unable to perform their normal protective function. Bronchopneumonia is a common terminal event in congestive heart failure and indeed is a common sequel to edema from whatever cause. The basal edema that occurs in debilitated, bedridden patients, in those who are unconscious, and in those who have just undergone surgery often progresses to pneumonia; this is called *hypostatic pneumonia.* Good nursing and physical therapy can do much to prevent this complication.

Bronchopneumonia is of much longer duration than lobar pneumonia. If the primary condition is incurable, the pneumonia is merely a welcome terminal event, and obviously little attempt is made at healing. Even in the childhood bronchopneumonias that follow measles and whooping cough, a prolonged course is the rule. The course of the disease is often punctuated by relapses and remissions, depending upon whether the organism or the host is gaining the upper hand. Both the onset and the termination of the disease are gradual.

Lesions of Bronchopneumonia

The disease is usually basal, posterior in distribution, and bilateral. If an area of bronchopneumonia is examined microscopically, it is found to consist of acutely inflamed bronchioles full of pus (Fig. 30–7). Some of the surrounding alveoli contain edema fluid in which there are macrophages and polymorphs, whereas others contain a dense, fibrinous exudate in which there are innumerable polymorphs. Some are collapsed as the result of the absorption

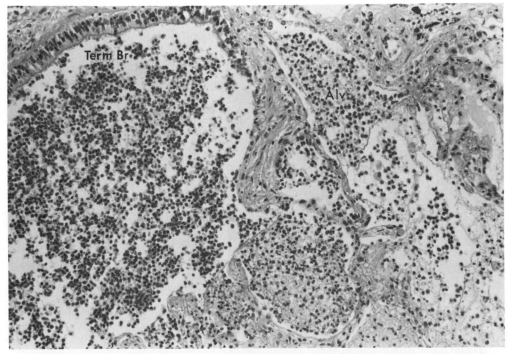

Figure 30–7. Bronchopneumonia.   Part of a terminal bronchiole (Term Br) is shown with its lining of ciliated columnar epithelium. The bronchiole contains a mass of inflammatory cells, the majority of which are polymorphs. Alveoli (Alv) adjacent to the bronchiole also contain inflammatory exudate with polymorphs and fibrin. An alveolus further away from the bronchiole contains merely edema fluid.

of air distal to the blocked bronchioles, whereas neighboring alveoli are empty and distended because of compensatory dilatation. In contrast to lobar pneumonia, in which all alveoli in a lobe are at about the same stage of the inflammatory process, in bronchopneumonia there is a very varied picture.

Sequelae of Bronchopneumonia

Resolution.   This is much less frequent than in lobar pneumonia.

Progressive Fibrosis of the Lung.   This is correspondingly more frequent. The fibrosis is due to organization of the inflammatory exudate in the alveoli. In addition, there is often a continuance of the inflammatory process, so that more and more lung tissue is destroyed and converted into fibrous tissue. This is, of course, the condition of chronic inflammation, and bronchopneumonia often becomes chronic. In due course the infection spreads, and the muscle and elastic tissue of the adjacent bronchi are destroyed and replaced by granulation tissue. Consequently there is widening of the lumina, and eventually the dilatation becomes extensive. This is the pathogenesis of *bronchiectasis,* which is both a sequel of bronchopneumonia and a predisposing cause of further attacks (Fig. 30–8).

Suppuration.   Abscess formation is not uncommon, particularly when the host's resistance is exceptionally poor and the causal organism is *Staphylococcus aureus.*

Exogenous Bronchopneumonia

When inhaled, a variety of virulent organisms may lead to severe bronchopneumonia. The host may be either healthy or enfeebled as a result of a previous disease. Examples of virulent organisms causing exogenous bronchopneumonia are listed below:

Staphylococcus aureus. The bronchopneumonia may come as a result of hospital cross-infection.

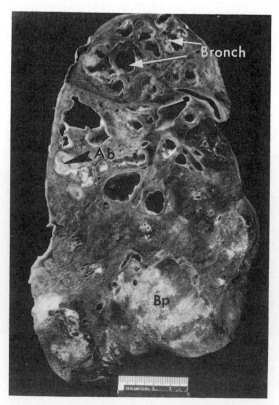

Figure 30–8. Bronchiectasis with chronic lung infection.   Since the age of 7 years, this patient had had repeated attacks of pneumonia. When he was 24 years of age, a diagnosis of cystic fibrosis of the pancreas was made. He was treated with vitamins and pancreatic enzymes by mouth but continued to be plagued by repeated lung infections. The terminal event was an overwhelming infection with *Pseudomonas aeruginosa.* The patient died at the age of 32 years. This specimen shows the effects of repeated bronchopneumonia. Toward the base of the lung there are several areas of bronchopneumonia (Bp), and the discrete areas of consolidation have fused together to become confluent. Nevertheless, the appearances are not those of lobar pneumonia. In another area the pneumonia has progressed to abscess formation (Ab). Toward the upper part of the lung there is tremendous dilatation of bronchi, and the upper lobe shows the typical appearances of advanced bronchiectasis (Bronch). Much of the intervening lung tissue has been destroyed.

Streptococcus pyogenes. Bronchopneumonia from this source was particularly common in the 1918 influenza pandemic.

Legionella pneumophila. Legionnaires' disease is a newly described type of pneumonia that first attracted widespread attention when an outbreak occurred among delegates to a state convention of the American Legion in Philadelphia in July 1976. The incubation period was about one week. The main features of the disease were fever; myalgia; a spreading type of pneumonia, sometimes with cavitation; pleural effusion; chest pain; dyspnea; vomiting and diarrhea; renal failure; thrombocytopenia with purpuric rashes; and occasionally encephalopathy. This epidemic had a mortality of about 15 per cent, and although it appeared to be due to an infection (probably airborne), no causative organism could at first be identified. Intensive study finally isolated a previously unrecognized bacterium, named *Legionella pneumophila*, that was pathogenic to guinea pigs and would grow in the yolk sacs of embryonated eggs. The yolk sac antigen is used in a serological test for the detection of antibodies in convalescent patients. Although the organism cannot be visualized in tissues by conventional staining, special silver impregnation techniques can demonstrate it. Also, it can now be grown on special media *in vitro*.

In retrospect it has become apparent that other outbreaks of this disease had occurred previously (*e.g.*, "Pontiac fever" in 1968), and outbreaks of the disease have now been reported from many parts of the world. The diagnosis of the disease is most easily substantiated by obtaining a titer of antibodies of at least 1 in 128 or obtaining a fourfold increase in the titer of antibodies during convalescence. There are at least six distinct serotypes of *L. pneumophila*. Atypical variants of this fastidious bacterium have also been encountered (atypical Legionella-like organisms [ALLO]).

Mycobacterium tuberculosis and the deep-seated fungus diseases. This type of disease is quite distinct, since the lesions produced are characteristically chronic. They are described in Chapter 10.

Mycoplasma pneumoniae. See Chapter 11.

Viruses. Many types of viruses can cause pneumonia, *e.g.*, coxsackieviruses, echoviruses, and myxoviruses (Chapter 12). The histology of this group of pneumonias is poorly defined, since death from the uncomplicated disease is rare. There is usually an acute interstitial pneumonia, often with hyaline membrane formation (page 426).

Interstitial Pneumonia (Alveolitis)

The predictable course of the bacterial pneumonias to antibiotics has highlighted a second type of pneumonia. This was originally called "primary atypical pneumonia" or "viral pneumonia," but these terms are no longer used in this context. The inflammation is most marked in the interstitial tissues of the lung (particularly in the alveolar walls) and *interstitial pneumonia* is now the accepted term for the condition in North America. The term *alveolitis* is preferred in the United Kingdom. Unless otherwise stated, when either term is used it is assumed that the condition referred to is diffuse.

Interstitial pneumonia may be acute or chronic and has a variety of clinicopathological presentations. In some instances the cause is known, but in the majority of cases neither cause nor pathogenesis is understood. It is convenient first to describe the various morphological changes that are found, and then to relate these to known causes and mechanisms.

Pathology

Interstitial pneumonia appears to be initiated by damage to the alveolar lining cells (particularly the type I pneumocytes) and also to the alveolar vascular endothelial cells. Acute and chronic variants of interstitial pneumonia are recognized.

Acute Interstitial Pneumonia (Acute Alveolitis).   Damage to the vascular walls leads to the formation of an exudate in the interstitium of the lung, *i.e.*, in the alveolar walls, in the interlobar septae, in the connective tissue sheaths around blood vessels and bronchioles, and beneath the pleura.

The exudate consists of fluid and a variable number of mononuclear blood cells. Although this exudate is initially interstitial, damage to the type I pneumocytes and their subsequent loss allows a protein-rich fluid to exude into the alveoli and alveolar ducts. The air spaces are still ventilated, and the plasma proteins, fibrin, and cellular debris are thrown onto the air space walls, where they coagulate to form an *eosinophilic hyaline membrane* (Fig. 30–9). The morphological term for this condition is *alveolitis with hyaline membrane formation.*

Acute interstitial pneumonia may terminate in death or complete recovery, or it may progress to one of the chronic forms of interstitial pneumonia.

Chronic Interstitial Pneumonia.   This condition remains a major problem in chest medicine. In a few cases a potentially removable extrinsic cause can be identified, but there remains a large group of patients in whom irreparable lung damage ultimately leads to pulmonary fibrosis and death. The disease may progress rapidly to a fatal termination within a few months, but more often the onset is insidious with progressive dyspnea and relatively little by way of other symptoms; often there is neither fever nor cough. The chest radiograph shows subtle interstitial changes. The rigidity and the swelling of the alveolar walls render the lungs stiff, so that ineffective alveolar

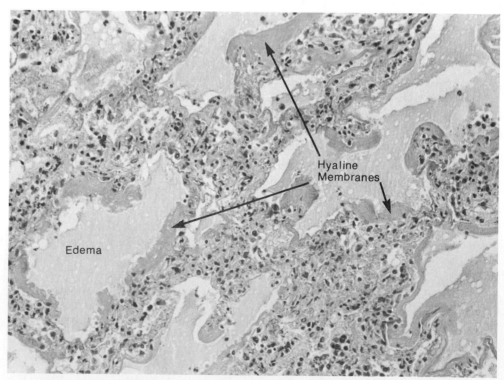

Hyaline
Membranes

Edema

Figure 30–9.   Adult hyaline membrane disease.   The alveolar walls are thickened owing to edema, congestion, and a sparse infiltration by inflammatory cells, which are mostly mononuclear. A striking feature is the lining of the airway spaces by a hyaline membrane, which stains deep red with eosin. The alveoli and alveolar ducts are also filled by a pale staining material, and in this section they are virtually airless. The material is coagulated edema fluid (×120).

ventilation in relation to arterial profusion increases the alveolar-arterial oxygen pressure difference. The mean survival time is about 4 years from diagnosis. Two main patterns of reaction can be recognized:*

1. Desquamative Alveolitis. This is also called *desquamative interstitial pneumonia,* or *DIP.* The distinguishing feature of this type is the filling of alveoli by mononuclear cells that were originally thought to be desquamated pneumocytes. It is now thought that these cells are macrophages.

2. Fibrosing Alveolitis. This is also called *usual interstitial pneumonia (UIP)* because it accounts for over 80 per cent of the cases. Alveolar fibrin is organized, and the alveolar walls show fibrosis together with a sparse mononuclear cell infiltrate. Alveoli are lined by prominent type II pneumocytes.

A number of agents or circumstances have been incriminated as the cause of interstitial pneumonia:

1. Infectious agents. Many types of viruses are thought to cause acute interstitial pneumonia, *e.g.,* coxsackieviruses, echoviruses, and myxoviruses. These examples may truly be called viral pneumonia.

2. Pneumoconioses, particularly asbestosis.

3. Collagen vascular diseases, particularly systemic sclerosis and rheumatoid arthritis.

4. Ionizing radiation, generally as a result of treatment of an adjacent carcinoma, *e.g.,* of breast, esophagus, or lung.

5. Drugs, in particular bleomycin, cyclophosphamide, methotrexate, busulfan, and chlorambucil — all drugs used in the treatment of malignant disease.

6. Severe trauma. This has certain distinctive features and is described below under the heading of *"Acute Adult Respiratory Insufficiency Syndrome."*

In spite of this impressive list, it must be confessed that in over 50 per cent of cases of acute and chronic alveolitis no cause can be identified. The term *cryptogenic fibrosing alveolitis* is used to cover our ignorance with respect to the chronic cases of unknown etiology. In some patients IgG deposits have been demonstrated in the alveolar walls, and the damage is presumably immunologically mediated. Desquamative alveolitis tends to respond to glucocorticoid therapy and has a better prognosis than the fibrosing types. This raises the important question of the relationship between the various types of alveolitis. It would be logical to assume that the desquamative type progresses to fibrosing alveolitis and ultimately terminates in pulmonary fibrosis. At present there is much contradictory evidence on this point, and future research may clarify the issue.

For the time being, it seems logical to regard the interstitial pneumonias as reaction patterns to many diverse agents. In some cases several etiological factors may be involved, and the reaction may well be determined as much by the host's response as by the nature of the agent concerned. The possible relationship between the types of interstitial pneumonia is indicated in Figure 30–10.

It should be noted in passing that it is in this area of chronic lung disease that open lung biopsy has been found to be of considerable value in determining the nature of the lesion and predicting the prognosis.

Etiology and Pathogenesis of Interstitial Pneumonia

---

*Other types have also been described but are uncommon and will not be discussed here.

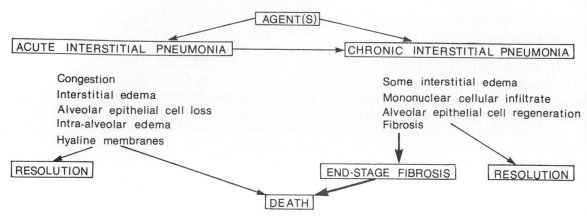

Figure 30–10. Diagram illustrating the course of and interrelationship between the types of interstitial pneumonia. It is suggested that acute interstitial pneumonia may undergo resolution, cause death, or progress to a chronic state. Chronic interstitial pneumonia may or may not be preceded by an acute pneumonia. The histological "types" of chronic interstitial pneumonia depend on the type and extent of the cellular infiltrate, combined with the magnitude of the epithelial regeneration and the extent of the fibrosis. Resolution is still possible, but more often there is progressive fibrosis that ends in death.

Acute Adult Respiratory Insufficiency Syndrome

It is well recognized that severe trauma is often followed by pulmonary complications that closely resemble acute interstitial pneumonia (acute alveolitis) due to medical causes. This state has been called the *shock lung syndrome,* but the term *acute adult respiratory insufficiency syndrome* is now more commonly used. It follows complicated surgery, such as that involving cardiopulmonary bypass procedures; trauma of any sort, particularly if associated with shock; burns; narcotic overdose; inhalation of irritants such as smoke in a fire, hemorrhagic pancreatitis; and severe sepsis. The common denominator among these very diverse events is not known, but the initial lesion appears to be an increased permeability of the alveolar capillaries to plasma proteins such that interstitial edema develops. Initially this leads to reflex tachycardia and hyperventilation due to stimulation of interstitial pressure stretch receptors. Respiratory alkalosis results. The lung becomes stiff, and this combined with peribronchiolar edema reduces alveolar ventilation, so that some degree of hypoxemia results. The cause of the altered vascular permeability is not known and indeed probably varies under different circumstances. It may be the direct effect of inhaled irritants or hypoxia or the effect of a circulating toxin. A factor that has gained prominence recently is the *toxic effect of oxygen.* Prolonged breathing of gas containing over 50 per cent oxygen can cause this syndrome. Following the formation of interstitial edema in the lung there appears to be damage to the type I pneumocytes, so that a similar high–protein-content fluid accumulates in the alveoli. Alveolar hypoventilation increases, and arterial PO_2 decreases even more. If the patient dies in this acute stage, the lungs are heavy, plum-colored, wet, and bulging. Collapse of the lung is not a feature.

Subsequent Changes. If the changes are insufficient to cause death, further changes occur in the lung. In those air spaces still ventilated, the alveolar high–protein-content fluid is thrown into the alveolar walls and condenses to form a fibrin-rich hyaline membrane. This is particularly well seen in the alveolar ducts, and the picture is that of the *adult hyaline membrane disease.* The type II pneumocytes proliferate, and some are desquamated into the alveoli, which become filled with cells, including macrophages, giving the picture of desquamative alveolitis. The type II pneumocytes eventually differentiate to replace the lost type I pneumocytes.

In many cases after about 2 weeks both interstitial and intra-alveolar fibrosis occur, so that the picture of chronic interstitial pneumonitis is mimicked and the lung is converted into a mass of fibrous tissue containing dilated spaces lined by bronchiolar epithelium, giving a honeycomb appearance *(honey-comb lung)*. These later complications of the acute respiratory insufficiency syndrome that lead to death 2 to 6 weeks after the initial insult have become more common since the establishment of aggressive pulmonary intensive care units that commenced around 1963. Positive pressure ventilatory support methods can force gas into fluid-filled air spaces and lead to hyaline membrane formation. The excessive use of oxygen leads to the additional effect of oxygen toxicity, and indeed some authorities feel that this is the most important factor in the pathogenesis of the condition. Thus, by prolonging life the modern pulmonary intensive care unit has made more obvious and more common the late results of the acute pulmonary complications of severe injury.

CHRONIC OBSTRUCTIVE LUNG DISEASE (COLD)

Chronic obstructive lung disease, also called chronic obstructive pulmonary disease (COPD), chronic airflow obstruction, and chronic nonspecific lung disease, is a clinical syndrome that comprises those conditions that are accompanied by *chronic or recurrent reduction in expiratory airflow within the lung*. The traditional teaching is that most cases of COLD are due to chronic bronchitis, pulmonary emphysema, or bronchial asthma. Chronic bronchitis and pulmonary emphysema often occur in the same individual and have many features in common, including a strong etiological association with cigarette smoking and the associated presence of *small airways disease*. Bronchial asthma has significant differences from these three conditions and will be described separately.

Chronic Bronchitis

Chronic bronchitis is defined in clinical terms and is present in any patient who has persistent cough with sputum production occurring on most days for at least 3 months of the year for at least 2 successive years. Sputum production due to localized bronchopulmonary disease is excluded from this definition. At first the expectoration in chronic bronchitis is intermittent and worse on rising in the morning, and eventually it becomes continuous. Chronic inflammation of the bronchi is not a constant feature, and Laennec's term bronchial catarrh is particularly apt.

The most constant morphological change in chronic bronchitis is an increased mass of mucous glands, reflected by an increase in the thickness of the bronchial mucosa. The surface epithelium of the bronchi shows metaplasia with replacement of ciliated cells by mucus-secreting goblet cells. Nevertheless, the mucus contributed by these cells is trivial compared with that produced by the large mucosal glands.

Etiology of Chronic Bronchitis. The major cause of chronic bronchitis is the inhalation of irritant chemicals. Atmospheric pollution contributes to this, but by far *the most important cause is cigarette smoking*. Heavy smokers have up to ten times the incidence of chronic bronchitis as compared with nonsmokers. In the initial stages the sputum is mucoid, but periodically there are exacerbations of the disease due to infection — the sputum increases in amount and becomes purulent, and features of airway obstruction increase. Specific viral infections may produce similar exacerbations, but more frequently the culprit is a bacterial infection, often by one of the normal commensal inhabitants of the upper respiratory tract. *Hemophilus influenzae* and the pneumococci are particularly common causes. Bronchopneumonia may follow and indeed can be a terminal event of this disease.

Symptoms.   Persistent cough with the production of mucoid or muco-purulent sputum is the outstanding symptom. Dyspnea, cyanosis, and right-sided heart failure develop later and are probably associated with the development of small airways disease.

Pulmonary Emphysema

Pulmonary emphysema is best defined as a condition in which there is an abnormal permanent increase in size of the air spaces distal to the terminal bronchioles accompanied by destructive changes of the alveolar walls. The definition is therefore a morphological one, and two types can be recognized.

1. Centriacinar Emphysema (Centrilobular Emphysema).   In this type of emphysema the central parts of the acini, *i.e.*, those formed by respiratory bronchioles, are most severely affected (Fig. 30–11). Hence, the enlarged spaces that are formed by the destructive process are readily visible in the center of the lobules of the lung and are surrounded by relatively unaffected areas in which the alveolar ducts and peripheral alveoli reside (Figs. 30–12 and 30–13). Centrilobular emphysema tends to affect the upper parts of the lung fields more severely than the bases, and as the disease advances there can be extensive destruction of all areas of lung with the production of large bullae, *i.e.*, spaces over 1 cm in diameter.

2. Panacinar Emphysema (Panlobular Emphysema).   In this type of emphysema the destructive process in the alveolar walls involves the acinus uniformly (Fig. 30–14). Hence, the process is more diffuse. This disease, in contrast to centrilobular emphysema, tends to affect the bases of the lungs rather than the upper fields.

Etiology of Pulmonary Emphysema.   The major cause of symptomatic pulmonary emphysema appears to be cigarette smoking. Since the salient feature of emphysema is destruction of lung tissue with its elastic fibers, much attention is being paid to mechanisms by which this elastic tissue could be removed. It is known that macrophages and neutrophils contain enzymes that will digest elastin (elastase), and it seems likely that the irritant properties of atmospheric pollutants, particularly tobacco smoke, lead to sufficient inflammatory changes that continual formation of elastase steadily destroys the lung. The fact that the upper lung fields are more regularly inflated during quiet breathing explains why centrilobular emphysema usually affects this part of the lung. There is some evidence that cadmium present in tobacco smoke

CENTRILOBULAR EMPHYSEMA

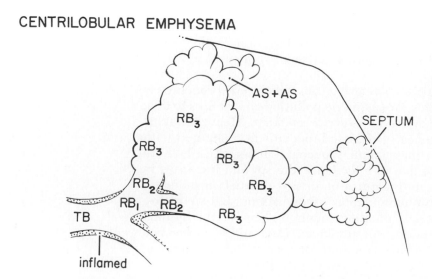

Figure **30–11.** In centrilobular (proximal acinar) emphysema, respiratory bronchioles are selectively and dominantly involved. (Abbreviations are as in Figure 30–1.) (From Thurlbeck, W. M.: Chronic obstructive lung disease. *In* Sommers, S. C. (Ed.): Pathology Annual, Vol. 3. New York, Appleton-Century-Crofts, 1968.)

Figure 30–12. Pulmonary emphysema. This thin section of a whole lung shows severe destructive emphysema. The lesions are so severe in the upper parts of the lung that light can be transmitted through the slice where there are bullae. (From Heard, B. E.: Pathology of Chronic Bronchitis and Emphysema. London, Churchill Livingstone, 1969. Reproduced by permission.)

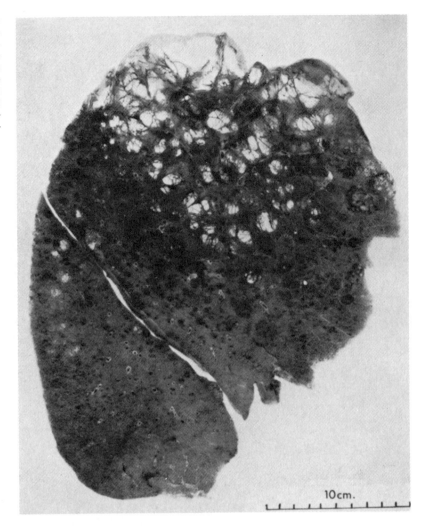

10cm.

plays an etiological role by acting as an irritant. In the case of panacinar emphysema the situation is less clear, for although this condition is also associated with cigarette smoking, it is also a feature of patients who lack an enzyme termed alpha-1-antitrypsin. This is an enzyme produced in the liver that circulates in the blood and has the property of inhibiting elastase activity. Precisely why patients with this deficiency tend to develop panacinar emphysema affecting the bases is not clear. It is reasonable that inflammatory changes due to infection or chemical irritants could be a factor in excess elastase production, but this is hardly likely to be the whole answer, since emphysema is not an obvious complication of bacterial infections of the lung such as lobar pneumonia or bronchopneumonia.

Small Airways Disease

This is defined as disease affecting airways less than 2 mm in diameter. There may be goblet metaplasia of the epithelium, mucous plugging, inflammatory changes, and scarring.

Airways Obstruction: Pathophysiology

Obstruction of the airways and therefore also to airflow can be demonstrated by a variety of techniques. The simplest is to ask the patient to take a deep inspiration and follow it by a maximum expiration. The total amount of gas expired is termed the forced expiratory volume (FEV), and by suitable measurement the amount of gas expired in one second (FEV1) can be

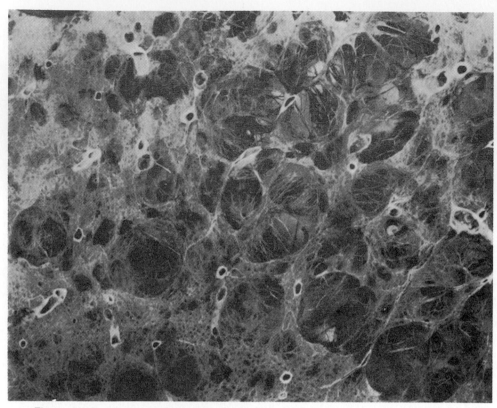

Figure 30–13. Pulmonary emphysema. Higher magnification of the center of the upper lobe of the specimen shown in Figure 30–12. Note the tremendous destruction of alveolar tissue. (From Heard, B. E.: Pathology of Chronic Bronchitis and Emphysema. London, Churchill Livingstone, 1969. Reproduced by permission.)

measured. A decrease in FEV1 indicates airflow obstruction and is therefore a feature of COLD.

In the past it has generally been considered that airflow obstruction in COLD resulted either from bronchial narrowing in chronic bronchitis or a loss of elastic recoil in emphysema. Although there is some truth in these concepts, it is now felt that chronic bronchitis alone does not produce

PANLOBULAR EMPHYSEMA

Figure 30–14. In panacinar (panlobular) emphysema, the enlargement and destruction of air spaces involve the acinus more or less uniformly. (A, alveolus; other abbreviations are as in Figure 30–1.) (From Thurlbeck, W. M.: Chronic obstructive lung disease. *In* Sommers, S. C. (Ed.): Pathology Annual, Vol. 3. New York, Appleton-Century-Crofts, 1968.)

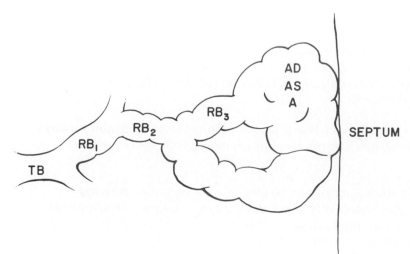

appreciable obstruction and that small airways disease and emphysema are more important. Usually they occur together in the same patient. As noted above, the small airways can be obstructed by mucus in the lumen or by inflammatory disease in the wall, possibly with fibrosis. Furthermore, the loss of elastic tissue in emphysema can allow the small airways to collapse by loss of radial support. Although it is possible to define and describe chronic bronchitis, emphysema, and small airways disease separately, in practice they often occur together and indeed seem to share many etiological factors.

Two types of this clinical syndrome can be recognized:
Type A — Pink Puffers. Typically the patient is middle-aged and complains of increasing shortness of breath and negligible cough with little sputum. On examination the chest appears to be overexpanded, and the chest radiograph may exhibit hypertranslucency. The effect of the emphysema is to reduce the total area available for blood-gas interchange, so that the patient must breath more rapidly in order to maintain the blood gases at normal levels. These patients therefore develop progressive, unrelenting dyspnea and yet remain pink. Hence, the term "pink puffers" is applied.

Type B — Blue Bloaters. Typically this patient presents at an earlier age with chronic bronchitis and increasing shortness of breath. Chest auscultation reveals scattered rales due to mucous plugging of some bronchi. Pathologically, there is chronic bronchitis and small airways disease. In spite of airways obstruction there is little dyspnea, and some areas of lung are hypoventilated. This unequal distribution of ventilation in relation to blood supply causes desaturation of the arterial blood, and the patient is therefore cyanosed. The hypoxemia stimulates the bone marrow, so that secondary polycythemia results. The low alveolar PO_2 causes vasoconstriction, and this leads to pulmonary hypertension, itself a forerunner of chronic cor pulmonale and heart failure. The poor ventilation of the lungs results in carbon dioxide retention, so that the PCO_2 rises. This causes peripheral vasodilation and accentuates the cyanosis of the skin.

Patients with chronic bronchitis, having a raised arterial PCO_2 and lowered PO_2, often tolerate these abnormal blood gas tensions remarkably well, and any sudden change can lead to serious consequences. Thus, if the hypoxemia (low PO_2) is relieved by oxygen therapy, ventilation can become so depressed that CO_2 retention with coma ensues. Alternatively, vigorous artificial ventilation can relieve the hypercapnia to the extent that the low arterial PCO_2 causes vasoconstriction and cerebral ischemia.

The administration of general anesthetics to chronic bronchitics is particularly hazardous, since any further increase in mucus production or spasm of the bronchi is liable to precipitate respiratory failure.

Patients with this syndrome can often be tided over acute attacks with antibiotics and other treatment. They therefore differ from the pink puffers, who progress relentlessly and are resistant to treatment.

Although two types of clinical syndrome have been described, these must be regarded as the two ends of a clinical spectrum, and patients will be encountered who have features intermediate between type A and type B.

Classical Clinico-pathological Syndromes of COLD

Asthma is a condition of widespread narrowing of the bronchial airways that *changes in severity over short periods of time*, either spontaneously or under treatment, and is not due to cardiovascular disease. It is characterized by *paroxysms of wheezing and dyspnea*. The bronchial obstruction is caused partly by spasm of the bronchial muscle and partly by the presence of viscid mucus (Fig. 30–15). Rarely an attack fails to remit and the patient dies (*status*

Bronchial Asthma

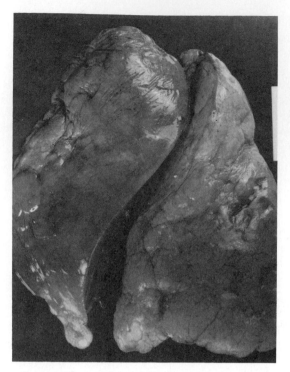

Figure 30–15. Bronchial asthma. This specimen is from a 28-year-old woman who had had a long history of bronchial asthma. She had an acute attack that became progressively more severe as dyspnea developed. She became cyanosed and finally unconscious. Despite vigorous resuscitation attempts she had a cardiac arrest and died 9 hours after the onset of the attack. The specimen shows the lung to be greatly overinflated. This is because bronchi are plugged with thick, tenacious mucus. In life this allows some air to enter the lung because on inspiration the bronchi dilate. However, the patient could not expel air so easily, and the lungs became overinflated.

asthmaticus). Many examples of asthma (usually termed *extrinsic asthma)* have a hereditary basis, and the disease is one manifestation of atopy. Attacks are brought on by the inhalation of an antigen to which the subject is sensitive. This sensitivity can be detected by skin tests. A small quantity of antigen is scratched into the skin, and if the patient is sensitive there is an immediate response with a wheal and flare. This is an example of a type I hypersensitivity reaction and is mediated by IgE.

Some types of asthma (often termed *intrinsic asthma)* appear to be related to respiratory infections, and other types are triggered by taking aspirin by mouth or by the inhalation of chemicals. The latter are usually of industrial origin, such as epoxy resins, plastics, and other chemical dusts and gases. This group may be termed *industrial asthma.*

An uncommon type of asthma is associated with pulmonary infiltrates and blood eosinophilia. In this group there is combined type I and type III hypersensitivity, and probably many types of this syndrome exist. Some may be manifestations of parasitic infections in which the worms are migrating through the lungs. Another type is due to colonization of bronchi or lung cavities by the fungus *Aspergillus fumigatus.* It is evident that bronchial asthma is a condition in which the bronchi are unduly sensitive to a variety of agents derived from either some immunological reaction or a physical stimulus. Examples of the latter are asthmatic attacks in response to exercise, cold, or psychological stress.

ALLERGIC LUNG DISEASE

Lung tissue is continually confronted with airborne antigens, and it is not surprising that allergic disease is common. Many of the types of bronchial asthma discussed above fall under this heading. In addition, there is a group of interesting diseases termed *extrinsic allergic alveolitis.* Clinically, patients experience sudden onset of fever, headache, dyspnea, and cough coming on 4 to 6 hours after exposure to fine particles of organic material to which the patient is sensitive. It is believed that sensitizing IgG antibodies are involved, and this is an example of type III hypersensitivity occurring in the alveoli.

Many known external antigens are described. Perhaps best known is the antigen derived from fungal spores in moldy hay. Breathing in dust containing these spores causes *farmer's lung*. Likewise, inhalation of antigens from maple bark, pigeon excreta, or mushrooms produces a similar picture *(e.g., bird fancier's lung)*.

The systolic pressure in the pulmonary artery is 15 to 25 mm Hg; being much lower than that in the systemic vessels, it follows that there is less tendency to edema formation (see Fig. 5–1).

PULMONARY EDEMA

The osmotic effect of the plasma proteins is relatively unopposed, and in the initial stages edema fluid accumulates in the interstitial tissues of the lung. It is drained away by the lymphatic vessels, but when this defense mechanism becomes overloaded the fluid passes into the alveolar spaces and the lung becomes solid. There are two factors that tend to ensure that pulmonary edema persists and even spreads:

1. The loose nature of the lung prevents any immediate appreciable rise in tissue tension, a fact that in most tissues limits the extent of edema formation.

2. When the lungs have become edematous the alveoli become filled with fluid, ventilation ceases, the vessel walls become hypoxic, and their permeability to protein increases. It follows that in all examples of pulmonary edema, the fluid has a high protein content. Therefore, it is more difficult to distinguish between transudates and exudates in the lungs than in other tissues.

The acute adult respiratory insufficiency syndrome may be regarded as a special type of pulmonary edema and has been considered earlier in this chapter. Therefore, an account will now be given of other types of pulmonary edema in which the alveolar spaces are airless owing to an accumulation of fluid.

Acute Inflammation. Edema occurs in the early stages of pneumonia; it is particularly marked in acute lobar pneumonia. It was a prominent feature in the bronchopneumonia that complicated the influenza of the 1918 pandemic. The lungs were described as showing acute hemorrhagic edema rather than bronchopneumonia of the classical type. Such a picture is also encountered in poisoning with certain gases, *e.g.*, phosgene, chlorine, and nitrogen peroxide. Acute pulmonary edema also follows the inhalation of gastric juice, such as may occur if a patient vomits during the inexpert administration of a general anesthetic.

Causes of Pulmonary Edema

Heart Failure. Acute pulmonary edema is a frequent complication of left ventricular failure and mitral stenosis. Although increased pulmonary venous pressure is the usual explanation offered for this complication, it is unlikely that this is the major cause of pulmonary edema in heart failure. More important is the effect of a *redistribution of the blood volume;* attacks of acute pulmonary edema *(cardiac asthma)* occur quite suddenly (sometimes at night), and they are probably initiated by peripheral vasoconstriction. The amount of blood in the peripheral circulation is thus diminished, and the excess volume is displaced into the pulmonary circulation, in which it appears as edema fluid. Support for this contention is the observation that acute pulmonary edema is a well-known hazard of epinephrine administration. This drug causes peripheral vasoconstriction. It must never be given to patients with acute pulmonary edema of cardiac origin. In bronchial asthma this drug is beneficial, but in cardiac asthma it can be lethal.

The terms *cardiac asthma* and *paroxysmal nocturnal dyspnea* are often applied to these attacks of acute pulmonary edema. The patient wakes up gasping for breath, with a sense of oppression in the chest. He sits up, but the dyspnea increases. Mounting restlessness drives him out of bed to seek the fresh air at the window. The sense of suffocation becomes intense, and with it there is profound distress. The skin has an ashen color because of the vasoconstriction combined with cyanosis, and there is also profuse sweating. The patient may cough up copious blood-stained sputum owing to a rapidly spreading pulmonary edema. In severe cases death ensues.

Overloading the Circulation.   If an excessive volume of fluid is administered intravenously, some of the excess is accommodated in the great veins, but the remainder is diverted to the pulmonary circulation and leads to edema formation. It is obvious that patients already undergoing heart failure are particularly prone to this complication (Chapter 26).

Cerebral Damage.   Acute pulmonary edema sometimes complicates damage to the brain, *e.g.,* trauma or cerebral hemorrhage. The most likely explanation is that increased sympathetic nervous impulses from the brain lead to peripheral vasoconstriction and cause diversion of the circulating fluid to the lungs, as described above.

BRONCHIAL OBSTRUCTION   **Causes.**   The common causes of bronchial obstruction are the following: (1) *tenacious mucus,* which is not expelled from the respiratory passages, as in asthma; (2) *chronic bronchitis;* (3) *inhaled foreign bodies,* such as roots of teeth or peas; and (4) *tumors,* usually carcinoma.

Effects.   The effects of obstruction depend on whether the obstruction is partial or complete.

Partial Obstruction.   The partial obstruction of a bronchus impedes the ventilation of the lung distal to the obstruction. It therefore follows that the blood perfusing that part of the lung is inadequately oxygenated, and that in effect a quantity of venous blood is shunted directly into the pulmonary veins and from there to the left side of the heart. Since the blood leaving the lungs is normally fully saturated with oxygen, it follows that no amount of overventilation of the unaffected lung can compensate for this shunt effect (Fig. 30–3). The arterial P_{O_2} is therefore lowered *(hypoxemia).* A very important example of partial obstruction of the bronchi occurs in chronic bronchitis, especially after a surgical operation requiring general anesthesia.

Widespread partial bronchial obstruction leads to overinflation of the lungs in asthma (see Fig. 30–15).

Infection commonly follows persistent bronchial obstruction. Organisms that are inhaled into the affected lung segment become trapped in the mucus, their expulsion is impaired, and bronchopneumonia follows. The infection also involves the bronchial walls; chronic infection will destroy the muscular and cartilaginous components of the walls, so that they are weakened and dilatation ensues *(bronchiectasis).* This effect is frequently seen distal to the obstruction caused by a carcinoma or a foreign body. Quite often, bronchiectasis occurs in several parts of the lung as an idiopathic condition; it might be the result of obstruction by mucus during some previous infection, such as measles or whooping cough. This type of bronchiectasis causes a chronic cough with expectoration of sputum. Recurrent attacks of pneumonia are common, and progressive lung destruction follows. Bronchiectasis is a common cause of hemoptysis, but if it is localized to one segment of the lung — particularly in an adult — the possibility of an underlying carcinoma must always be considered.

Complete Obstruction.   Where there is complete obstruction of a large bronchus, the lung distal to it shows a progressive absorption of its gas content until it becomes completely airless or collapses (*i.e.,* a *collapsed* lung). A plug of mucus sometimes causes this postoperative complication. Physical therapists can help to prevent this by encouraging the patient to breathe deeply and bring up sputum.

This group of diseases, produced by the *inhalation of dust,* is mostly occupational in origin. The most important condition is *silicosis,* which occurs in miners and in those whose work entails exposure to silica dust. Following the inhalation of this dust, the silica particles are taken up by macrophages and, being toxic, kill these cells. Fibrogenic factors that stimulate the formation of collagen are liberated. The particles themselves are once again phagocytosed by macrophages, and the process is repeated many times. Hence, numerous *silicotic nodules* of dense fibrous tissue are formed that are readily demonstrable on a radiograph (Fig. 30–16). Silicosis predisposes one to pulmonary tuberculosis.

Asbestosis is another important pneumoconiosis. It affects workers who fabricate asbestos fibers; it does not affect the miners who quarry it. Asbestosis is characterized by a diffuse interstitial fibrosis and the formation of pleural plaques of fibrous tissue. The disease is important in predisposing the subject to *cancer of the lung* and to *mesothelioma of the pleura.* It has been estimated that subjects with asbestosis have a tenfold likelihood of developing cancer of the lung. If in addition they smoke cigarettes, the incidence is about 90 times the normal. Asbestos is widely used as an insulating fire-resistant material and in car brake linings, so that many city dwellers are bound to inhale the fibers. Their presence in the lung does not alone constitute asbestosis, but how great a health hazard they constitute is not known.

Anthracosis, which is due to the inhalation of carbon, is the most common of the dust diseases, because to some extent it affects all city dwellers. The disease often severely affects coal miners, but since carbon induces little inflammatory reaction or fibrosis, the miners experience no ill effects unless the carbon accumulations are massive. Usually this occurs in association with tuberculosis or silicosis.

THE PNEUMO-CONIOSES

Figure 30–16. Silicosis. This radiograph shows numerous dense silicotic nodules scattered throughout the lung fields. Since there is a tendency to spare the bases of the lung, in this respect silicosis resembles the other pneumoconioses. Asbestosis is the only exception to this rule, because the large heavy asbestos fibers tend to gravitate to the bases of the lungs. (Courtesy of Dr. D. E. Sanders.)

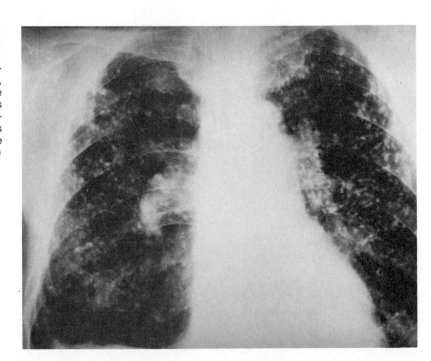

PULMONARY NEOPLASMS

The vast majority of lung tumors are epithelial in origin.

Bronchial Carcinoid Tumor

The bronchial carcinoid is of APUD cell origin (Chapter 39), and is of intermediate type since it invades locally, is of slow growth, and rarely metastasizes. Hence, lobectomy or pneumonectomy is usually curative. The tumor generally arises in the wall of a large bronchus and causes partial, and finally complete, obstruction. Distal *bronchopneumonia* and bronchiectasis, often with hemoptysis, are frequent (Fig. 30–17).

True benign tumors of the bronchi (adenomas) are rare; it should be noted that the term "adenoma of the bronchus" has often been used in the past to describe the carcinoid tumors — a practice that should be abandoned.

Carcinoma of Lung

Cancer of the lung now ranks as the commonest lethal cancer in males, and it is also prevalent in females. Cigarette smoking is a major cause. Atmospheric pollution and asbestosis are other etiological factors.

Gross Appearance. Two common types of tumor may be recognized:

Peripheral Lung Cancers. These tumors presumably arise in one of the small bronchi or bronchioles and appear as fairly discrete tumor masses in the lung parenchyma. Symptoms are often absent until the pleura and chest wall are invaded, or until distant metastases appear.

Central Lung Cancers. These tumors arise in one of the major bronchi and therefore cause early obstruction with resulting collapse, bronchopneumonia, and bronchiectasis (Fig. 30–18). Frequently, the patient presents with fever and symptoms of pneumonia. Hemoptysis is common, the bleeding being either from the ulcerated tumor itself or — more often — from the inflamed dilated bronchi beyond.

Diagnosis. *Hemoptysis, recurrent or "unresolved" pneumonia, or a persistent shadow on the radiograph should always lead to thorough inves-*

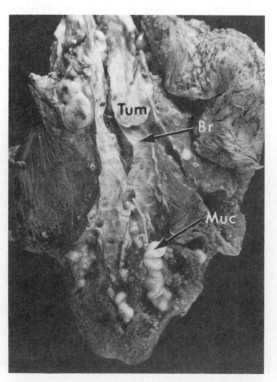

Figure 30–17. Carcinoid tumor of bronchus. This patient developed a patch of bronchopneumonia that did not clear completely with chemotherapy. Bronchoscopy revealed a tumor obstructing a bronchus in the lower lobe. Biopsy showed that it was a carcinoid type of tumor. A lobectomy was performed, and the patient made a satisfactory recovery. The specimen shows the tumor (Tum), which is growing into and obstructing a bronchus (Br). Distal to the tumor the bronchus is widely dilated and contains thick mucopurulent material (Muc). Bronchiectasis distal to an obstructing tumor is characteristic.

Figure 30–18. Carcinoma of the lung. This section through lung shows a large carcinomatous mass (Carc) in which an obstructed bronchus is embedded. The main effect of this is seen in the middle lobe (ML), where much of the lung substance has been destroyed and replaced by fibrous tissue. Bronchiectasis (Bronch) is well developed. Tumor is seen to be extending into the lower lobe (LL), but the upper lobe (UL) is unaffected. Several hilar lymph nodes (Ly N) are invaded by growth and have fused with the tumor to form one large mass. The black material in the lymph nodes is carbon. This degree of anthracosis is common in city dwellers.

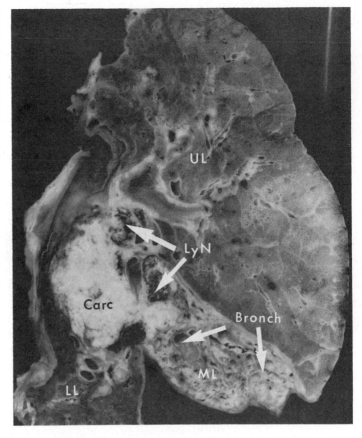

tigation, *particularly if the patient is a smoker* (Fig. 30–19). *Sputum examination* may reveal malignant cells. The tumor may be seen and biopsied at the time of *bronchoscopy.* Even if the tumor is beyond the range of the bronchoscope, mucus or pus may be aspirated from individual bronchi. The finding of malignant cells in a specimen will then localize the tumor. *Mediastinoscopy* is a useful procedure in which the mediastinum is examined

Figure 30–19. Carcinoma of the lung. This radiograph shows a hilar mass (arrow) that is produced by the tumor. The linear shadow extending outward toward the chest wall is due to secondary changes — namely, collapse, infection, and bronchiectasis. This portion of the lung might well appear like the middle lobe in Figure 30–18. (Courtesy of Dr. D. E. Sanders.)

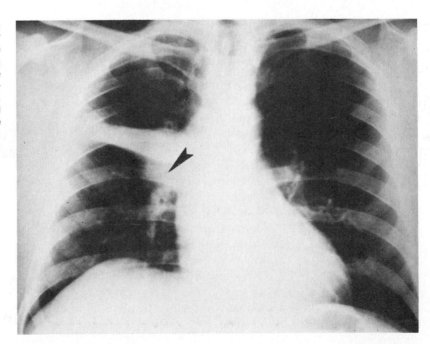

with an instrument that is inserted through a small incision in the neck. Enlarged lymph nodes may be detected and biopsied. This investigation also gives the surgeon an indication of whether the tumor is operable. If these investigations are negative, thoracotomy and direct biopsy may be necessary, since a policy of "wait and see" is rarely justifiable.

Spread.   Lung cancer spreads by all the classic routes:

Local Spread.   This can involve lung parenchyma, pleura, bronchi, arteries, and veins.

Lymphatic Spread.   The hilar and mediastinal nodes can be involved. This usually occurs early and is most marked with the oat-cell tumors. Supraclavicular and other lymph nodes are involved as the disease progresses.

Blood-Borne Metastases.   Secondary tumors are common in the *liver, bones, adrenals,* and *brain.* Even the spleen and bowel (organs not commonly the site of metastases from other tumors) may be involved. It is the frequency of distant spread that makes the prognosis so poor.

Histological Types.   Although arising from a mucus-secreting epithelium, cancers of the lung are remarkable for their histological variations.

Squamous-Cell Carcinoma.   Microscopically this resembles squamous-cell carcinoma arising elsewhere, except that well-differentiated examples are not common. The tumor arises from bronchial or bronchiolar epithelium. Prior to the development of invasive tumor the epithelium shows increasing atypia (dysplasia), with the dysplastic cells taking on some features of keratinizing squamous cells. Ultimately the in-situ carcinoma becomes invasive in a manner reminiscent of that encountered in the cervix uteri. These tumors may be either central or peripheral, and they have the most favorable prognosis.

Adenocarcinoma.   These tumors are almost always peripheral and tend to be more frequent in females. Areas of squamous metaplasia are common.

Anaplastic Carcinoma.   These tumors show little or no differentiation; two variants are recognized.

Small-Cell, or Oat-Cell, Carcinoma.   Oat-cell carcinoma of the lung appears to be a distinct tumor, which is probably derived from neurosecretory cells of the bronchial mucosa that are akin to the argentaffin cells of the intestine. In this respect it shares a common origin with the carcinoid tumor. The tumor is composed of small, darkly staining cells, which may form small rosettes and may be round or oat-shaped (Fig. 30–20). Frequently the tumors are large, and their origin is difficult to determine. They metastasize early and widely. An enormous mediastinal mass may be produced that can impede the heart's action by directly invading the pericardium and myocardium and by compressing the great vessels. Although the tumors are very radiosensitive, the prognosis is extremely bad.

THE PLEURA   The pleural cavities are normally potential spaces situated between the visceral and parietal pleura, each lined by flattened mesothelial cells. An accumulation of fluid in the pleural space is termed a *hydrothorax,* or *pleural effusion.* There are two types, which are described as follows:

A Transudate.   The fluid has a low protein content and few cells. The most common causes are congestive heart failure and the nephrotic syndrome.

An Exudate.   An exudate is formed as a result of inflammation or neoplasia involving the pleura. The protein content approximates that of plasma; inflammatory or neoplastic cells are present in the fluid.

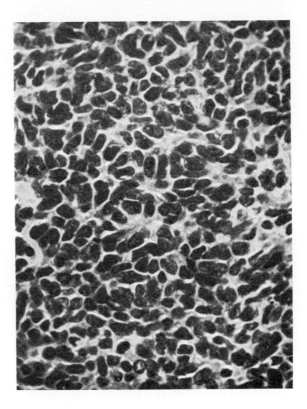

Figure 30–20.   Oat-cell carcinoma of lung. The constituent cells are small and fusiform in shape and have prominent darkly staining nuclei. Their shape has given rise to the descriptive term "oat cell" (× 500).

Pleurisy

Inflammation of the pleura (pleurisy or pleuritis) is usually secondary to underlying inflammatory or neoplastic lung disease. This may be apparent, as in acute lobar pneumonia or in a large area of infarction, or it may be inapparent, as in the pleurisy that accompanies a small tuberculous lesion. Occasionally, the cause of pleurisy is to be found below the diaphragm, *e.g.*, a subphrenic abscess.

Fibrinous Pleurisy. "Dry pleurisy" is associated with an audible friction rub and can be extremely painful, particularly when the affected person takes a deep breath. Organization of the exudate leads to the formation of fibrous pleural adhesions.

Serous or Serofibrinous Pleurisy. "Pleurisy with effusion" can lead to the accumulation of so much fluid that the affected lung is collapsed. Persistent pleural effusion should always be adequately investigated. Fluid can be withdrawn through a needle and sent for bacteriological and cytological examination. Tuberculosis and carcinoma (primary or metastatic) are two causes that must be considered.

Empyema

The presence of pus in the pleural cavity is termed an "empyema." It is generally formed as an extension of infection from a contiguous structure, *e.g.*, a lung abscess or subphrenic abscess (Fig. 30–21).

Pneumothorax

The presence of air in the pleural cavity is termed a "pneumothorax." It may arise suddenly in an apparently healthy person (spontaneous pneumothorax), and it is usually due to rupture of a small subpleural emphysematous bulla. The onset is sudden, with severe pain in one side of the chest. Dyspnea and cyanosis follow, and their severity depends on the amount of air that escapes into the pleural cavity. The condition tends to recur.

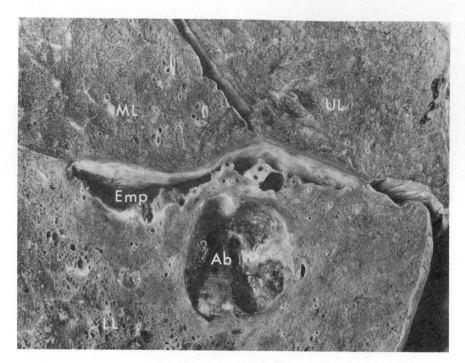

Figure 30–21. Empyema and chronic lung abscess. This section of lung shows the meeting point between the upper lobe (UL), the middle lobe (ML), and the lower lobe (LL). The lower lobe shows a chronic lung abscess (Ab), and infection has evidently spread through the pleura to involve the pleural cavity. The space (Emp) was filled with pus, and this lesion is therefore a localized form of empyema.

Pleural Tumors

The only common primary malignant tumor of the pleura is the mesothelioma. This tumor, which is related to asbestosis, forms an encasing mass around the lung.

Metastatic tumors, particularly from carcinoma of the breast and lung, are frequent in the pleural cavity.

Review Questions

1. Compare the pathogenesis and lesions of lobar pneumonia with those of a bronchopneumonia due to a pneumococcus of low virulence.

2. Give an account of the causes and pathogenesis of bronchiectasis.

3. A 30-year-old patient complains of asthmatic symptoms. Suggest the possible causes and indicate the investigations that might be useful in arriving at a diagnosis.

4. Explain why patients with chronic bronchitis may develop respiratory failure after being administered a general anesthetic.

5. A patient is involved in a car accident and develops severe respiratory symptoms. Indicate the possible causes of these symptoms and the end-results of the conditions you describe.

6. Describe the lung lesions in which the inhalation of asbestos fibers is believed to be an etiological factor.

7. Following a surgical operation performed under general anesthesia, a patient's radiograph shows areas of abnormal density that were not present before the procedure. Discuss the possible nature of these lesions.

8. A 56-year-old man states that he has coughed up blood-stained sputum on several occasions during the past four weeks. Indicate the investigations that are required to arrive at a diagnosis.

9. Describe the possible effects of a head injury on the lungs and on respiratory function.

10. Describe the signs and symptoms that would indicate a person might have cancer of the lung.

11. What lung lesions could cause an acute pain in the chest?

Ashley, D. J., and Davies, H. D.: Cancer of the lung. Histology and biological behavior. Cancer, 20:165–174, 1967.

Bourbonnais, F.: Adult respiratory distress syndrome. The Canadian Nurse, 76:51–54, 1980.

Comroe, J. H., Jr., et al.: The Lung: Clinical Physiology and Pulmonary Function Tests. 2nd ed. Chicago, Year Book Medical Publishers, Inc., 1962.

Devereau, P. M., and Goldstein, E. J. C.: Legionnaires' disease: finding answers to the etiologic riddle. American Journal of Nursing, 80:81–85, 1980.

Ingram, R. H.: Chronic bronchitis, emphysema and chronic airways obstruction. *In* Isselbacher, K. J., et al. (Eds.): Harrison's Principles of Internal Medicine. 9th ed. New York, McGraw-Hill Book Company, 1980, Chapter 263.

Ingram, R. H., and Braunwald, E.: Dyspnea and pulmonary edema. *In* Isselbacher, K. J., et al. (Eds.): Harrison's Principles of Internal Medicine. 9th ed. New York, McGraw-Hill Book Company, 1980, Chapter 27.

Kreyberg, L., Liebow, A. A., and Uehlinger, E. A.: Histological Typing of Lung Tumours. International Histological Classification of Tumours. No. 1. Geneva, World Health Organization, 1967.

Leading Article: Cancer and asbestos. British Medical Journal, 3:448–449, 1968.

Leading Article: Enzymes and emphysema. British Medical Journal, 1:1–2, 1973.

Leading Article: Diagnosing allergic bronchopulmonary aspergillosis. British Medical Journal, 4:1439–1440, 1977.

Leading Article: A sequence of pneumonia. British Medical Journal, 1:591–592, 1980. An account of Legionnaires' disease.

Ochsner, A.: Bronchogenic carcinoma, a largely preventable lesion assuming epidemic proportions. Chest, 59:358–359, 1971.

Sanford, J. P.: Legionnaires' disease — the first thousand days. New England Journal of Medicine, 300:654–656, 1979.

Spencer, H.: The Lung. 2nd ed. New York, The Macmillan Company, 1968. A detailed reference book.

Staub, N. C.: The pathophysiology of pulmonary edema. Human Pathology, 1:419–432, 1970.

Thurlbeck, W. M.: Chronic Airflow Obstruction in Lung Disease. Philadelphia, W. B. Saunders Company, 1976.

Thurlbeck, W. M.: Editorial: Smoking, airflow limitation, and the pulmonary circulation. American Review of Respiratory Disease, 122:183–186, 1980.

Wyatt, J. P.: Occupational lung diseases and inferential relationships to general population hazards. American Journal of Pathology, 64:197–216, 1971.

Selected Readings

Diseases of the Upper Alimentary Tract

After studying this chapter the student should be able to:

- Describe the mechanism of swallowing.
- Define dysphagia, classify its causes, and give a brief account of each.
- Distinguish between oropharyngeal dysphagia and esophageal dysphagia.
- List the causes of ulceration in the mouth and describe aphthous ulceration in detail.
- Describe the types of white lesions (leukoplakia) sometimes found in the mouth.
- State the clinical features, differential diagnosis, and complications of acute streptococcal sore throat.
- Compare and contrast carcinoma of the lips, carcinoma of the tongue, and carcinoma of the pharynx.
- Describe the pathogenesis and complications of dental caries.
- Describe the structures that constitute the periodontium.
- Give an account of the pathogenesis and complications of periodontitis.
- Describe the types and complications of hiatus hernia.
- Outline the main features of carcinoma of the esophagus with respect to the following:
    - (a) known predisposing causes
    - (b) site of occurrence
    - (c) symptoms
    - (d) prognosis
- Give two examples of acute sialoadenitis.
- Describe pleomorphic salivary gland tumors with respect to these factors:
    - (a) common site of occurrence
    - (b) microscopic appearance
    - (c) invasive properties
    - (d) prognosis

The alimentary tract is usually regarded as being within the body, but it is, in fact, a long tube exposed at each end to the exterior. Its contents, ranging from food in the mouth to feces in the rectum, are never within the body proper. This is an ideal arrangement, because within the lumen the chemical changes necessary for the digestion of food can occur under conditions that could not be tolerated inside the body itself. One effect of this arrangement is that many liters of digestive fluids are poured into the alimentary tract each day. Most of this is reabsorbed, but it can readily be appreciated that if much escapes to the exterior, the volume of fluid lost could reach alarming proportions. Diarrhea and vomiting are indeed potent causes of water and electrolyte loss.

The Mouth and Pharynx

In the mouth, food is masticated and mixed with saliva. By virtue of its mucus content, saliva performs a lubricating action in addition to initiating carbohydrate digestion by the enzyme ptyalin.

Swallowing (*deglutition*) is triggered by the voluntary contraction of the pharyngeal and buccal muscles. By raising the larynx and tongue, the process of swallowing throws the bolus of food against the posterior pharyngeal wall. Thereafter, an involuntary wave of peristalsis sweeps the bolus down the muscular eosophagus, and as the cardiac sphincter relaxes, the bolus enters the stomach. Difficulty in swallowing (*dysphagia*) is described later in this chapter.

The mucosa of the mouth is keratinized (like epidermis) over the hard palate and the attached gingiva. In these areas it is adherent to the periosteum of the underlying bone to form a *mucoperiosteum*. Elsewhere, the mucosa is mobile, and the epithelium is not keratinized, for it lacks the outer horny layer. This distinction is important in explaining the distribution of herpetic and aphthous ulcers in the mouth (see below).

The oral mucosa shares many diseases with the skin. In *lichen planus** a white lacy appearance of the buccal mucosa is characteristic and may be the first — or, indeed, the only — manifestation of the disease. Likewise, *pemphigus vulgaris* may first appear in the mouth. Bullous pemphigoid also affects the mouth, but less frequently than pemphigus. The severe ulcerations of the oral mucous membranes seen in the *Stevens-Johnson syndrome* are described in Chapter 41.

Lesions of the Oral Mucosa

The rash of some acute systemic *viral infections* affects the mucosa, where it is called the *enanthem*, before becoming clinically apparent on the skin, where it is called the *exanthem*. Thus, the vesicles of chickenpox may first appear on the palate. The *Koplik's spots* of measles, which occur during the prodromal stage of the disease, are reliable forerunners of the skin rash that appears within a day or two. Koplik's spots are minute white ulcers with an erythematous base and can be described as resembling small grains of salt, each having a red halo.

The primary infection with herpes simplex virus can occur in the mouth, particularly in children. There is acute inflammation of the oral mucosa (including the hard palate) and the gingivae. This acute *gingivostomatitis* is vesticular, but the blisters soon ulcerate, and the disease is characterized by multiple shallow and painful ulcers. The patient feels unwell and may have a fever. Healing occurs within about two weeks, and recurrent oral ulceration is not a complication (Chapter 12).

The common *aphthous ulcers,* or canker sores, are not due to a viral infection. They have been estimated to affect between 20 and 50 per cent of the population and are invariably recurrent. Sometimes a single ulcer is present, but often several appear either at the same time or shortly after one another. The ulcers affect the mobile oral mucosa (*i.e.*, tongue and inside of lips and cheeks) but not the hard palate or attached gingivae, since these areas are keratinized. They appear as very painful, shallow ulcers covered by necrotic slough and are surrounded by a bright erythematous zone. Healing generally occurs within a week or two, but in a few patients the lesions enlarge and persist. These may be accompanied by similar ulcerations of the genital mucosa and by recurrent uveitis (*Behçet's syndrome*). It is evident that an examination of the oral cavity can provide essential clues in the diagnosis of other diseases; such a procedure should never be neglected.

Leukoplakia. This term is applied by some authorities to any white patch of the oral mucosa. It includes the following entities:

Simple Keratoses. Keratinization of the mobile mucosa or hyperkerato-

---

*Lichen planus is a generalized papulosquamous skin disease of unknown cause. The characteristic lesions are flat-topped, violaceous papules, which are extremely itchy.

sis of the hard palate or attached gingivae is generally due to the irritation of smoking or chronic trauma — such as that produced by persistent biting of the buccal mucosa or by the rubbing of an ill-fitting denture. Microscopically the oral epithelium closely resembles the epidermis of skin. A lesion of this type is not precancerous.

Lichen Planus. The lesions of lichen planus show some tendency to become malignant, but this is less of a threat than with dysplastic leukoplakia.

Dysplasia of the Oral Epithelium. The lesions appear as white patches that microscopically show dysplasia, either mild or sufficiently severe to warrant the term carcinoma-in-situ. It is this type of "leukoplakia" that is premalignant and must be regarded seriously. Obviously, any persistent white patch of the oral mucosa should be biopsied to determine its nature and malignant potentiality.

Acute Streptococcal Sore Throat

This is an acute infection of the tonsils and adjacent pharynx by *Streptococcus pyogenes*. The onset is sudden, and the sore throat is accompanied by fever, leukocytosis, and malaise. The tonsils and adjacent pharynx are swollen and red, and a white inflammatory exudate is seen on the surface. The regional lymph nodes are enlarged and tender (*acute nonsuppurative lymphadenitis*). If the strain of streptococcus produces abundant erythrogenic exotoxin, and if the patient has no immunity to this toxin, the sore throat is shortly followed by an erythematous skin rash. At that stage the disease is called *scarlet fever.*

Streptococcal sore throat is an important disease, because in a number of patients it is followed by *acute glomerulonephritis* or *acute rheumatic fever* — conditions that are considered elsewhere in this book.

It should not be assumed that every sore throat, even if accompanied by tonsillar exudate, is due to the streptococcus. Viral infections, for instance those caused by adenovirus or the causative agent of infectious mononucleosis, can have a very similar clinical appearance, although their onset is generally more insidious. In the past it was essential to consider diphtheria in the differential diagnosis; now, however, the disease is extremely uncommon in the Western world. The diagnosis of diphtheria is confirmed by obtaining a positive culture from a throat swab.

Tumors of the Oral Cavity

Benign tumors (*e.g.*, papilloma and fibroma) of the oral cavity are not uncommon; since they are usually small and unimportant, however, they will not be considered further. The important tumor is carcinoma, which varies in character according to its site of origin.

Carcinoma of the Lips. Squamous-cell carcinoma of the lips nearly always affects the lower lip and is more common in men than in women. Predisposing causes are thought to be pipe and cigarette smoking, often combined with exposure to sunlight. The tumor usually starts as a nonhealing crack in the lower lip to one side of the midline. Provided treatment is undertaken reasonably early, the prognosis for this tumor is good, since the growth is well differentiated and lymph node metastases are late in appearing (see Fig. 17–5).

Carcinoma of the Tongue. This is the most frequent intraoral malignant tumor. Although it is more common in men, the tumor also affects women, particularly in association with the Plummer-Vinson syndrome, described later in this chapter. Cancer of the tongue appears as a nodule that soon ulcerates. Any nonhealing ulcer of the tongue, particularly if its edges are indurated, must be biopsied. Even with early treatment, cancer of the tongue has a less favorable prognosis than cancer of the lips. Approximately 60 per cent of patients live for five years following surgery or radiotherapy. If lymph node metastases are already present, the figure is reduced to about 30 per cent.

Squamous-cell carcinoma can occur in other parts of the mouth and oral pharynx. The floor of the mouth is a common site, and it is therefore very important to inspect this area when carrying out a routine examination. Too often the dorsal surface of the tongue is scrutinized with care but the carcinoma in the floor of the mouth goes unnoticed. Squamous-cell carcinoma of the pharynx is often poorly differentiated and highly malignant. Even though the primary tumor is quite small, the lesion first manifests itself as enlargement of cervical lymph nodes due to metastasis. The prognosis is poor.

The Teeth

Caries

Dental caries, commonly known as tooth decay or "cavities," is the most common affliction of mankind. Although it has been recognized since prehistoric times, the precise cause is not known. It is principally a disease of childhood, adolescence, and young adult life, affecting deciduous and permanent teeth alike. Tooth decay is particularly frequent in the Western world, where it is presumed to be due to dietary factors. Poor oral hygiene and a diet containing much refined carbohydrate appear to be the major factors.

Caries usually starts in pits, fissures, and other areas, such as the cervical parts of the tooth that are not self-cleansing. Bacterial colonies growing on the tooth surface (and forming *dental plaque*) combine with food debris to form a suitable focus for further bacterial growth. Organisms enter the small fissures in the enamel of the teeth and ferment the carbohydrate, thus leading to the production of acid. This process steadily erodes the calcific material of the enamel and later of the dentine so that a deep cavity appears; this cavity is often much larger than would be suspected from an examination of the external appearance of the fissure. When a cavity has formed, infection can spread to involve the pulp (*pulpitis*). Pulpitis can be acute and extremely painful; chronic pulpitis, on the other hand, can lead to the formation of a chronic apical abscess that is often remarkably silent clinically. It is believed that the abscess can act as a focus (or *nidus*) of infection and can lead to periodic episodes of bacteremia. This mechanism is an important factor in the pathogenesis of bacterial endocarditis.

Although dental caries appears to be related to infection, no one particular organism has been incriminated, since the bacteria that have been isolated from lesions are those constituting the normal flora of the mouth.

Periodontal Disease

Inflammation of the periodontium (*periodontitis*) is a widespread disease affecting many children and almost the total adult world population. It causes halitosis and is second to caries as a cause of tooth loss. A knowledge of the normal anatomy of the periodontium is essential for a proper understanding of the disease (Figs. 31–1 to 31–3).

Periodontitis. Unless meticulous dental hygiene is practiced, colonies of bacteria become attached to the surface of the teeth and form *dental plaque*. If this is allowed to remain, it calcifies to form *dental calculus* ("tartar"). Food debris, plaque, and calculus in the region of the gingival crevice predispose the gingiva to inflammation. This *gingivitis* is the first stage in the pathogenesis of periodontitis. With this condition the gingivae become red and swollen and tend to bleed, particularly after the teeth have been brushed. The inflammation leads to resorption of the alveolar bone (Figs. 31–3C, 31–4, and

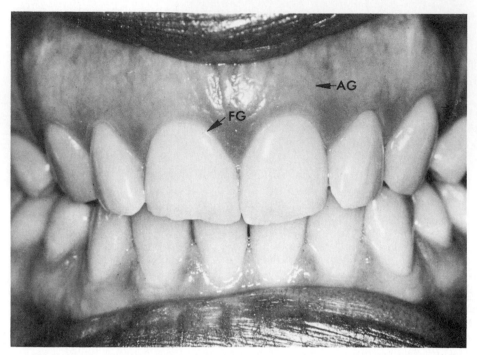

Figure 31–1.   Normal gingiva. This photograph of the anterior part of the mouth shows a normal, healthy gingival condition. The free gingiva (FG) is not attached to the underlying enamel but is separated from it by the gingival crevice. The attached gingiva (AG) is firmly adherent to the underlying alveolar bone. (Courtesy of H. D. Glenwright, M.D.S., and the Department of Clinical Illustration, Birmingham Dental School, England.)

31–5). The fibers of the periodontal membrane are also destroyed. Although the precise mechanism of this destruction is not understood, the process does lead to the formation of a pocket between the gingiva and the cementum of the tooth. Further accumulation of calculus and debris helps to perpetuate the inflammation, and the pocket deepens. At the same time, gingival epithelium migrates into the pocket, and the process extends as more and more of the alveolar bone is destroyed. The teeth become loose and rock, even when they are subjected to normal forces during eating. The excessive movement further damages the attachments that remain, and loss of the teeth — one by one — is merely a matter of time.

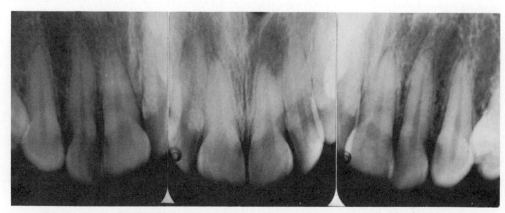

Figure 31–2.   Radiograph of a normal mouth. Note how the teeth are deeply embedded in their bony sockets. (Courtesy of H. D. Glenwright, M.D.S., and the Department of Clinical Illustration, Birmingham Dental School, England.)

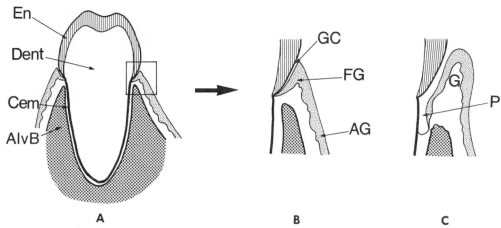

Figure 31–3. Diagrams illustrating the normal periodontium and the changes in chronic periodontitis. *A* and *B* illustrate the normal periodontium, which consists of (1) alveolar bone (Alv B); (2) cementum (Cem); (3) the periodontal membrane, consisting of fibers running between bone and cementum; and (4) the gingiva, including the free gingiva (FG) and the attached gingiva (AG). Note how the gingival crevice (GC) is the space between the free gingiva and the enamel of the tooth (En). Note: Dent = dentine. *C,* The changes in chronic periodontitis. There is loss of alveolar bone and the associated periodontal membrane. Extension of the gingival crevice has resulted in the formation of a pocket (P), and this is partially lined by gingival epithelium that has grown in. The gingiva (G) is inflamed and swollen.

The Esophagus

The esophagus, or gullet, is a muscular tube through which food is propelled to the stomach by peristalsis. Although there is some debate about the existence of an anatomical sphincter at its lower end (the cardiac sphincter), from a functional point of view there is little doubt that a working sphincter exists, because the contents of the stomach do not readily re-enter the esophagus. This phenomenon can be attested to by witnessing the gyrations of the acrobat and by noting that the bat (which has a structurally similar esophagus) can spend half its life upside down with no ill effect.

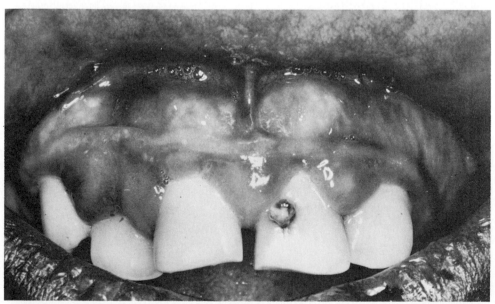

Figure 31–4. Chronic periodontal disease. The gingiva is inflamed and swollen and has lost its normal granular surface. The changes are most marked between the teeth. Deep pockets are present, because a probe can be passed between the gingivae and the roots of the teeth. One tooth is obviously carious. (Courtesy of H. G. Glenwright, M.D.S., and the Department of Clinical Illustration, Birmingham Dental School, England.)

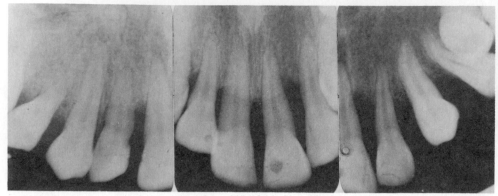

Figure 31-5. Chronic periodontal disease. This radiograph shows marked resorption of the alveolar bone. Some teeth have lost most of their bony support and are loose. They will be shed shortly. (Courtesy of H. G. Glenwright, M.D.S., and the Department of Clinical Illustration, Birmingham Dental School, England.)

Achalasia of the Cardia

In this condition there is degeneration of the ganglion nerve cells of the lower esophagus, resulting in disturbed peristalsis and a failure of relaxation of the cardiac sphincter. The patients are generally middle-aged and complain of a sensation of food sticking beneath the lower end of the sternum. Often pain is a prominent symptom. The obstruction leads to great dilatation of the esophagus.

Esophageal Webs

Folds or webs of the esophageal mucosa are quite frequently demonstrated by radiologists, but their significance as a cause of dysphagia is debatable. Often the lesions cannot be detected at necropsy. Webs of the upper part of the esophagus are found in the *Plummer-Vinson syndrome*, in which there is the triad of *iron deficiency anemia, dysphagia,* and atrophy of the mucosa covering the tongue (*atrophic glossitis*). The disease is virtually confined to women and is associated with an increased incidence of carcinoma of the oral cavity and upper esophagus.

Hiatus Hernia

The two types of hiatus hernia are illustrated in Figure 31-6. Impaired function of the cardiac sphincter leads to regurgitation of gastric contents; in turn, this leads to an associated esophagitis and peptic ulceration of the lower esophagus. The fibrosis that is associated with the healing of these ulcers can culminate in the formation of a benign stricture.

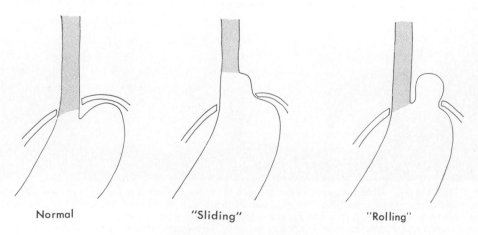

Normal   "Sliding"   "Rolling"

Figure 31-6. Hiatus hernia.

Inflammation of the lower esophagus can be due to regurgitation of gastric contents, which causes pain (heartburn). Esophagitis can result from the ingestion of irritating foods, such as hot, spicy meals and strong alcoholic beverages. The deliberate or accidental ingestion of corrosive acids and alkalies (*e.g.*, lye) can lead to severe esophagitis. If the patient survives, marked fibrosis with cicatrization results in an incapacitating stenosis.

Esophagitis

An important cause of hematemesis, esophageal varices are described in Chapter 33.

Esophageal Varices

The most important tumor of the esophagus is carcinoma. It is more frequent in males and in those who smoke excessively or who ingest alcohol to excess. Squamous-cell carcinoma is the most common type and generally arises in the lower or middle third of the esophagus. Adenocarcinoma can occur at the lower end of the esophagus and is thought to originate from either esophageal mucous glands or areas of ectopic gastric epithelium. The tumor steadily obstructs the esophagus, causing the patient to experience increasing difficulty in swallowing — at first of solid foods and later of liquids. The onset is insidious, and although the tumor tends to invade locally and to metastasize late, by the time the diagnosis has been achieved, resection is difficult, since the stomach must be brought up into the chest and anastomosed with the upper esophagus or pharynx, or alternatively a new passage must be reconstructed using a portion of colon or a tube of skin. Often resection of the cancer is impossible. Hence, the prognosis for this tumor is bad. The end stages of this disease are particularly unpleasant, since the patient is unable to swallow anything, including saliva. Constant regurgitation from the mouth, inhalation of saliva and food, and starvation combine to terminate the illness. Bronchopneumonia generally relieves the patient of his misery.

Tumors of the Esophagus

This condition is caused by a great variety of lesions, as follows:
   1. Painful Conditions. These inhibit the voluntary initiation of swallowing. Aphthous ulceration and acute tonsillitis may be cited as examples.
   2. Mechanical Interference with Swallowing. Infiltration of the tongue or pharynx by scirrhous carcinoma is an example of this type of lesion.
   3. Mechanical Obstruction. This usually occurs in the esophagus and is caused by a stricture that is either benign or carcinomatous. Dysphagia of the Plummer-Vinson syndrome, for example, is associated with obstruction of the upper end of the esophagus.
   4. Paralysis of the Muscles of Deglutition. This occurs in poliomyelitis when it affects the brain stem, as well as in pseudobulbar palsy (Chapter 44).
   5. Neuromuscular Incoordination. In elderly persons incoordination of peristalsis combined with muscular spasm may produce a sensation of obstruction and severe pain. Achalasia of the cardia has already been described.
   6. Psychosomatic Response. Difficulty in swallowing and a sensation of a foreign body in the throat are familiar accompaniments of fear and anxiety.

Difficulty in Swallowing (Dysphagia)

Clinical Classification of Dysphagia
For clinical purposes dysphagia may be divided into two types:
   Oropharyngeal Dysphagia. In this type attempted swallowing leads to the inhalation of food or its regurgitation through the nose.
   Esophageal Dysphagia. The common symptom of this type is a sensation of obstruction in the chest during swallowing. Carcinoma of the espha-

gus is the lesion most to be feared, especially if the symptoms are progressive and difficulty in swallowing affects solids and finally liquids.

The Salivary Glands

The three pairs of major salivary glands (parotid, submaxillary, and sublingual) can be afflicted by many diseases. With the exception of certain inflammations and one tumor, however, they are uncommon.

Inflammation (Sialoadenitis)

Mumps. A painful swelling at the angle of the jaw is often the first indication of *mumps*, which is due to inflammation of the parotid gland (*acute nonsuppurative parotitis*). The disease is caused by a myxovirus, has a long incubation period (18 to 21 days), and becomes bilateral in about two thirds of cases. Fever and mild malaise accompany the parotitis, and resolution occurs within one week. The most common complication of the disease in adult men is an acute orchitis (Chapter 36). Acute pancreatitis, meningitis, and encephalitis are occasionally encountered.

Acute Suppurative Inflammation. This condition is characterized by sudden swelling of the parotid gland, followed by abscess formation. Such an inflammation is encountered in patients who are either dehydrated or in shock and whose level of consciousness is decreased. Poor oral hygiene and a decreased flow of saliva combine to aid the migration of bacteria from the mouth, up the excretory duct, and finally to the parotid gland. It is to prevent this complication that careful cleansing of the mouth is an important component of the nursing care of severely ill patients.

Chronic Sialoadenitis. Recurrent attacks of acute sialoadenitis and chronic inflammation are generally encountered in a submaxillary gland and are often related to obstruction of the duct by a stone (sialolithiasis).

Tumors of the Salivary Gland

Pleomorphic Adenoma. The common tumor of the salivary gland is a pleomorphic tumor of the parotid. This tumor grows slowly to produce a painless mass in front of the external ear. Microscopically it consists of two elements. There are obvious epithelial components showing glandular differentiation with tubule formation (Fig. 31–7). Also, there are less cellular areas consisting of scattered cells with a background of material that may resemble extravasated mucus, myxomatous tissue (*"myxoid areas"*), or hyaline cartilage matrix. On the supposition that the myxoid or cartilaginous areas are of connective tissue (mesenchymal) origin, the tumor has been called a "mixed parotid tumor," since it appears to contain epithelial and connective tissue neoplastic elements. The current belief is that the tumor is purely epithelial, with the secreting epithelial cells producing the glandular elements of the tumor and the myoepithelial cells* forming the myxoid or pseudocartilaginous areas. Pleomorphic adenoma is the current name for the tumor, but "mixed salivary gland tumor" is commonly used in conversation.

Although the tumor may appear to be encapsulated, small outgrowths are present. It is from these that growth recurs following a simple enucleation of the tumor. The current treatment is to excise not only the tumor but also the surrounding parotid gland. The recurrence rate is low, and the prognosis is good. Unfortunately, the facial nerve travels through this gland, and damage to the nerve sometimes follows. Rarely pleomorphic salivary gland tumors show local invasion, and in a few instances there is metastasis to lymph nodes or to the blood stream. Hence, whereas the majority of tumors can be classified as benign, a few fall into the intermediate group.

---

*Many glands have two epithelial components. The inner secreting cells are either cubical or columnar, in contrast to the outer flattened myoepithelial cells, which by their contraction help to express secretions from the gland.

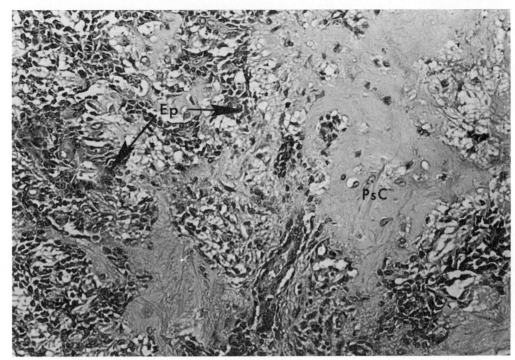

Figure 31–7. Pleomorphic salivary gland tumor. The tumor shows many clumps of obvious epithelial cells (Ep). In some areas mucin has accumulated in the stroma to produce a pseudocartilaginous appearance (PsC) (× 300).

Pleomorphic tumors occur in the other salivary glands but are much less common than those in the parotid gland.

Papillary Cystadenoma Lymphomatosum. This benign tumor is also known as adenolymphoma or Warthin's tumor. It constitutes about 10 per cent of all parotid tumors. Microscopically it is a well-differentiated tumor with glandular spaces, many of which contain papillary projections. An outstanding feature is an abundant lymphoid stroma that includes germinal centers —from this characteristic it derives its curious name.

1. A 22-year-old nurse complains of recurrent painful ulcers in the mouth. The ulcers developed over a 5-day period and then healed within 2 weeks. Discuss the diagnosis.

2. Describe how an examination of the mouth can help in the diagnosis of systemic diseases. In particular, refer to those diseases that affect the skin or the blood.

3. List the causes of esophageal obstruction.

4. Give an account of the complications of poor oral hygiene.

5. Describe the causes of enlargement of a salivary gland and indicate the features by which each condition may be recognized.

6. Explain why the terms "mixed parotid tumor" and "adenoma of the salivary gland" have been abandoned in favor of "pleomorphic salivary gland tumor."

Review Questions

Leading Article: Recurrent oral ulceration. British Medical Journal, 2:757–758, 1974.
Macphee, T., and Cowley, G.: Essentials of Periodontology and Periodontics. Oxford, Blackwell Scientific Publications Ltd., 1972. See, in particular, Chapters 1 to 4.
Morson, B. C., and Dawson, I. M. P.: Gastrointestinal Pathology. 2nd ed. Oxford, Blackwell Scientific Publications Ltd., 1979. See section 1, "Oesophagus."
Shklar, G.: The oral cavity, jaws, and salivary glands. In Robbins, S. L., and Cotran, R. S. (Eds.): Pathologic Basis of Disease. 2nd ed. Philadelphia, W. B. Saunders Company, 1979, Chapter 19. See also Chapter 20, "The Gastrointestinal Tract."

Selected Readings

CHAPTER 32 Diseases of the Gastrointestinal Tract

After studying this chapter the student should be able to:

- List the factors that stimulate the secretion of gastric juice.
- Describe chronic peptic ulceration with respect to the following:
  - (a) symptoms
  - (b) site of occurrence
  - (c) pathogenesis
  - (d) complications
- Give an account of acute gastroduodenal ulcers and their complications.
- Describe carcinoma of the stomach and indicate its prognosis.
- List the complications of partial or complete gastrectomy and indicate how each is brought about.
- Classify the mechanisms involved in the production of diarrhea.
- List the causes of acute gastroenterocolitis.
- Describe the effects of infection with:
  - (a) *Escherichia coli*
  - (b) *Vibrio cholerae*
  - (c) Salmonella
  - (d) Shigella
- Describe the manifestations of ischemic bowel disease.
- Describe the lesions and complications of Crohn's disease.
- List the features of the carcinoid syndrome.
- Classify the causes and effects of the malabsorption syndrome.
- Describe the causes, pathological findings, and clinical features of bacillary dysentery.
- Describe the lesions, effects, and complications of
  - (a) idiopathic ulcerative colitis
  - (b) diverticular disease of the colon
  - (c) ischemic colitis
- Outline the incidence and pathological effects of carcinoma of the colon.
- Describe acute appendicitis with respect to the following factors:
  - (a) incidence
  - (b) pathological findings
  - (c) clinical features
  - (d) complications
- Outline the causes of peritonitis.
- Distinguish a volvulus from an intussusception.
- List the common sites for a hernia and describe the complications.
- Distinguish between the mechanical and the nonmechanical types of intestinal obstruction. Describe the main causes and effects of each.
- Outline the common causes of an "acute abdomen."

The lower alimentary, or gastrointestinal, tract consists of the stomach, the small intestine, and the large intestine. Its functions are concerned mainly with digestion and absorption. Each region will be considered separately.

THE STOMACH

In the stomach the masticated food is softened, moistened, lubricated, and partially digested by the gastric juice. The food is kneaded by strong muscular contractions into a semiliquid mass called *chyme*, which passes steadily into the duodenum.

The gastric juice has four major active components:

1. *Mucus*, which has a lubricating action.
2. *Intrinsic factor*, which is necessary for the absorption of vitamin B$_{12}$.
3. *Pepsin*, which commences protein digestion.
4. *Hydrochloric acid*, which has an important bactericidal action and also provides the correct pH for the action of pepsin. Its presence is important in the pathogenesis of one of the common disabling human afflictions — peptic ulceration.

Whenever gastric juice comes into contact with non–acid-secreting mucosa, peptic ulceration is liable to occur. It is seen therefore at the pyloric end of the stomach, along the lesser curvature of the stomach, in the first part of the duodenum, at the lower end of the esophagus, and at the site of anastomosis between the stomach and small intestine following the operation of gastroenterostomy.

Chronic Peptic Ulcer

Chronic peptic ulcers are usually solitary and present a characteristic appearance (Fig. 32–1). Not only is the mucosa lost but also the underlying muscle layers are often destroyed, thereby producing a deep round or oval, punched-out ulcer with straight edges. For reasons that are not yet known, regeneration of the mucosal epithelium is inhibited, and chronic inflammation ensues. The floor of the ulcer consists of inflamed vascular granulation tissue covered by necrotic material that forms a slough. Bleeding is common, therefore. Deeper in the base of the ulcer the granulation tissue matures to form dense scar tissue that ultimately replaces the muscular walls.

Clinical Features.   Pain in the epigastrium is common and is related to the gastric acidity and muscle spasm. With a duodenal ulcer the pain comes on 1½ to 3 hours after a meal and frequently is severe enough to awaken the patient at night. It is usually relieved by eating food or, in particular, by the

Figure 32–1. Chronic gastric ulcer. The stomach has been opened along its greater curvature to show the mucosal surface. There is a typical chronic peptic ulcer on the lesser curvature about 2 cm from the cardioesophageal junction. Note the folds of mucosa (rugae) that are normal.

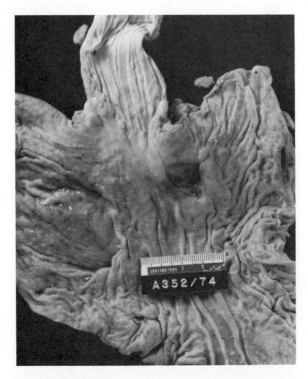

administration of alkali. With gastric ulcers the occurrence of pain is more erratic, and it may not be relieved by food or alkali. Indeed, eating may actually make the pain worse. It should be stressed that peptic ulceration can be present in the absence of any symptoms (Figs. 32–2 and 32–3).

Complications

Hemorrhage.　Repeated bleeding is a common cause of iron-deficiency anemia. Sometimes the ulcer penetrates adjacent structures, particularly the pancreas, and a large artery is eroded. When this occurs, there is massive hematemesis and melena (altered blood in the feces, with the stools appearing black and tarry).

Penetration and Perforation.　When the ulcer penetrates the peritoneal surface, it produces a localized fibrinous inflammation that may cause adjacent structures to adhere to it. In this way a chronic duodenal ulcer may penetrate into the substance of the pancreas. If adhesions do not form, the ulcer may perforate, and the gastric or duodenal contents may then be poured into the peritoneal cavity (Figs. 32–2 and 32–3). The patient immediately experiences severe pain, and generalized peritonitis soon develops.

Cicatrization.　As an ulcer heals, scar tissue tends to cicatrize and cause stenosis. Pyloric ulcers are particularly susceptible to this complication;

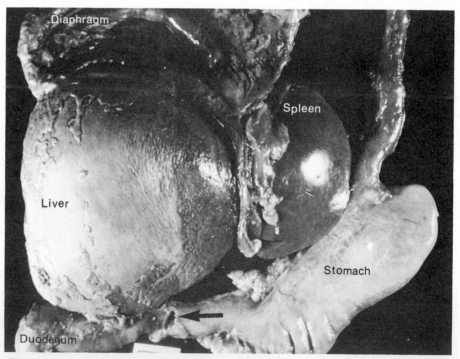

Figure 32–2.　Perforated duodenal ulcer.　The patient was a 65-year-old woman who was diagnosed as having a tumor involving the cerebellum and adjacent medulla oblongata. At surgery removal was not possible, but a biopsy was performed. It showed an uncommon tumor called a hemangioendothelioma. The patient never fully regained consciousness and died 13 days later. Cerebral edema secondary to surgical trauma was considered to be the underlying problem. There was a past history of duodenal ulcer, but no details were available because the patient was too ill to give a good history.

At necropsy a large perforated duodenal ulcer was found (arrow). Peritonitis involving the adjacent area was present and was particularly well marked on the upper surface of the liver. Between the liver and the diaphragm there was a large collection of pus. This constituted a subphrenic abscess.

This case illustrates how trauma can precipitate the perforation of a peptic ulcer — administration of prednisone can have a similar effect. In a seriously ill patient the perforation can be silent, and a subphrenic abscess can develop and be missed completely. (Courtesy of Dr. J. B. Cullen.)

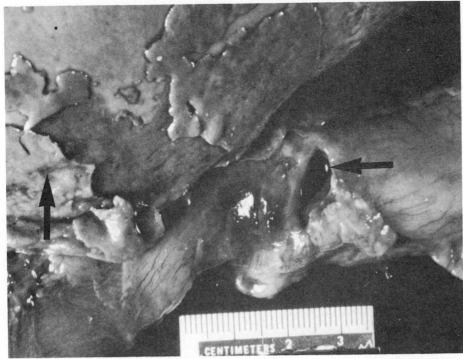

Figure 32–3. Perforated duodenal ulcer. This is a close-up of the ulcer (right arrow) shown in Figure 32–2. Note the loosely adherent purulent exudate on the surface of the liver (left arrow). (Courtesy of Dr. J. B. Cullen.)

the resulting *pyloric stenosis* causes persistent severe vomiting. This can lead to dehydration, starvation, and metabolic alkalosis resulting from loss of acid gastric juices.

Etiology and Pathogenesis. Although the pathogenesis of chronic peptic ulceration is poorly understood, it is evident that one essential factor is the presence of gastric juice containing hydrochloric acid and pepsin. It is therefore appropriate to review briefly the factors that control gastric secretion.

Acid gastric secretion is directly stimulated by four factors:

1. *Acetylcholine*, which is released at vagal nerve endings.

2. *Gastrin*, a group of polypeptide hormones produced in the antral pyloric glands. Local stimulating factors (such as digested protein in the gastric chyme) and vagal stimulation lead to gastrin release.

3. *Histamine.* The precise role of this powerful stimulant is not known, but it may be the final common mediator for cholinergic and gastrin stimulation.*

4. *Polypeptide hormones,* a variety of which are released from the small intestine. Some of these stimulate, but others inhibit, gastric secretion.

Traditionally, three phases of gastric secretion are described:

1. *Cephalic phase.* The sight and taste of food stimulate gastric secretion via the vagi. Emotions such as anger have a similar effect.

2. *Gastric phase.* Distension of the stomach and an alkaline content are stimulating.

3. *Intestinal phase.* This is both stimulatory (*e.g.*, peptides in the duo-

---

*The powerful stimulating action of histamine on gastric secretion is due to the effect of the drug on H_2 receptors. The action of the drug on bronchial and blood vessel smooth muscle is due to an effect on H_1 receptors. The commonly used "antihistamines" are H_1 receptor blockers.

denal lumen) and inhibitory (acid and fatty material in the intestinal lumen).

The medical treatment of peptic ulcers has been based on efforts to inhibit gastric secretion of hydrochloric acid and pepsin. They include:

1. Avoidance of worry. Attempts are made to give the patient mental and physical rest.

2. Antihistamine drugs, especially H_2 blocking agents such as cimetidine.

3. Anticholinergic drugs, which block the action of acetylcholine.

4. Frequent small meals.

5. Administration of antacids, including milk. The fat content of milk may also be helpful.

These measures are sometimes helpful, but it is evident from the many failures that factors other than abnormal gastric secretion are involved in the pathogenesis of peptic ulcer. The mucosal cells themselves appear to provide a barrier, but the nature of this is obscure. Irritants such as tobacco smoking, alcohol consumption, and the taking of drugs such as aspirin and phenylbutazone can cause a break in the mucosa and expose the subepithelial tissues to the effects of gastric juice. Medical treatment for peptic ulcers therefore includes avoidance of these known irritants.

That hypersecretion of gastric juice is not of overriding importance in the genesis of peptic ulceration is indicated by the observation that most patients with gastric ulcers have normal or even low gastric acidity. It has therefore been suggested that an abnormality of the pylorus is important. Bile reflux is known to occur, and it may be postulated that sudden influx of alkaline duodenal contents could damage the non–acid-secreting pyloric mucosa. Once the mucosa is damaged, acid gastric juice could continue the destructive action. Likewise, if pyloric sphincter function is abnormal, it is possible that acid gastric contents could suddenly be allowed to enter the duodenum and damage its mucosa. This is consistent with the observation that most patients with duodenal ulcers do have high gastric acidity. Also, duodenal ulcers are usually confined to the first and second part of the organ proximal to the entrance of the pancreatic duct, which pours in alkaline bile and pancreatic secretion.

It must be admitted, therefore, that the precise etiology of peptic ulceration is not known, but it seems that mucosal damage and exposure to gastric juice can combine in some individuals and lead to chronic ulceration. Genetic factors play some role in this mechanism, for duodenal ulcers are more common in those of blood group O, whereas stomach ulcers are more common in those of blood group A.

Surgical Treatment. When medical treatment fails, a variety of surgical procedures may be practiced. These include sections of the vagi (vagotomy) and operations on the pylorus and antrum (antrectomy and pyloroplasty). Another procedure is partial gastrectomy with anastomosis of the remaining stomach to the jejunum. The results of surgical treatment are sometimes satisfactory, but a number of complications must be expected. Recurrent ulceration can occur and may involve the small intestine adjacent to the enterostomy (*stomal ulcer*).

Effects of Gastrectomy. The gastric juice is not essential for digestion, apart from the secretion of intrinsic factor and its vital role in the absorption of vitamin B_{12}. Nevertheless, even partial gastric resection leads to a degree of malabsorption, because the stomach provides a place of temporary arrest that allows food to be admitted into the intestine in a slow, controlled manner. After gastrectomy there is more hurried passage of chyme through the intestine, so that digestion is rendered less complete. Furthermore, the disinfectant activity of hydrochloric acid is lost, and thus the bacterial flora of the intestine is changed. This may be accentuated by various blind loops created by the surgeon. The overall effect of these changes is to impair digestion of protein and fat, so that considerable weight loss can ensue. Furthermore, an iron-deficiency anemia is common. Two specific effects of gastrectomy should also be noted.

The Dumping Syndrome.   This occurs shortly after each meal; there is a feeling of epigastric distension and pain, accompanied by pallor, sweating, dizziness, and possibly collapse. The cause is thought to be related to the rapid entrance into the jejunum of the hypertonic chyme from the stomach. Fluid is drawn into the lumen of the bowel, and this leads to intestinal distension. Of greater importance is the passage of fluid into the intestinal lumen with a resultant sudden fall in plasma volume.

Hypoglycemic Attacks.   These attacks occur 2½ to 3 hours after a meal and consist of sweating, tremor, tachycardia, and faintness. Following a meal there is rapid absorption of glucose from the bowel, so that initially there is a high blood-sugar level. This stimulates insulin secretion, which is of such magnitude that the initial hyperglycemia is followed by a phase of hypoglycemia. The symptoms of this syndrome are therefore similar to those of insulin overdose.

Acute shallow ulcers, commonly called *erosions*, often occur in the stomach (Fig. 32–4). They are usually multiple and appear to be caused by dietary indiscretion, alcohol, and the action of irritant drugs, particularly aspirin. The ulcers are shallow and involve little more than the covering epithelium. Slight bleeding is common, but occasionally severe hematemesis may occur. Healing is generally rapid and complete.

Acute Ulceration

Acute ulceration of the stomach or duodenum is also a complication of burns and any severe injury. The ulcers are usually multiple and generally heal rapidly with minimal scarring. Occasionally they erode a large vessel or

Figure 32–4. Acute erosions of the stomach. The mucosal surface of the stomach shows many shallow erosions up to 1 cm in diameter (arrows). The patient had cirrhosis of the liver and died of bleeding from esophageal varices. Multiple erosions are a common complication of any severe stress (*e.g.,* major surgery) or in this case, severe bleeding.

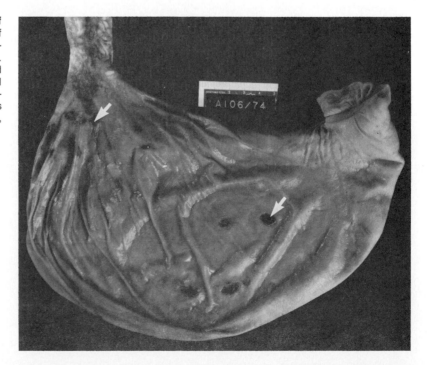

perforate into the peritoneal cavity, giving rise to severe hemorrhage or peritonitis. Sometimes severe bleeding occurs from the stomach, and no actual point of ulceration can be found. It appears that the entire stomach mucosa is congested and oozes blood. This condition is generally encountered as a complication of a severe injury or a major surgical operation.

Carcinoma of the Stomach

Gastric carcinoma is not uncommon in Northern European communities, but its incidence is now lower than that of colonic carcinoma. It is a common tumor in the Japanese, and in European communities it is more frequent in the lower social echelons than in the social elite. The tumor appears either as a fungating, cauliflower type of growth (Figs. 32–5 and 32–6) or as a typical malignant ulceration. In some instances the tumor cells invade the stomach wall so diffusely that no definite mass exists. Instead, the entire stomach wall is diffusely thickened by tumor cells and by the dense fibrous stroma that develops in response to them. This formation is called a diffuse infiltrating carcinoma of the stomach, or *linitis plastica*.

The symptoms of carcinoma of the stomach are often vague: they include indigestion, pain not relieved by food or alkalis, and weight loss. Bleeding that causes an obscure anemia is common. Blood may be present in altered form in the vomitus ("coffee-ground vomit"), and melena may occur.

Histologically, cancer of the stomach is a poorly differentiated adenocarcinoma. The prognosis is extremely bad, and even with early excision few patients survive for more than 5 years. Metastasis is to the regional lymph nodes and by blood spread to the liver and elsewhere.

THE SMALL INTESTINE

The small intestine consists of the duodenum, the jejunum, and the ileum and, in all, is about 6 meters long. The chyme that leaves the stomach is acted upon by bile, the pancreatic enzymes, and the intestinal secretion (*succus entericus*). The last contains few enzymes; the most important of these is *enterokinase*, which converts trypsinogen to trypsin — a conversion that is an essential step in the activation of pancreatic enzymes. The function of the small intestine is therefore the final breakdown of fat, carbohydrate, and

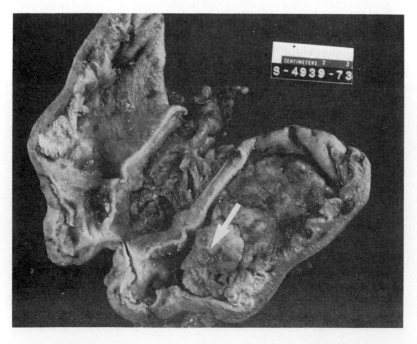

Figure 32–5. Carcinoma of the stomach. The stomach has been bisected, and both halves are shown. The wall is thickened, partly by tumor invasion and partly by the muscular hypertrophy that the tumor has caused. The mucosa is obviously invaded (compare with Figures 32–1 and 32–4) and a polypoid mass of growth is present (arrow). This is shown more clearly in Figure 32–6.

Figure 32–6. Carcinoma of the stomach. Note the cauliflowerlike mass of tumor. This is the same case as in Figure 32–5. Microscopically the tumor is a poorly differentiated adeno-carcinoma.

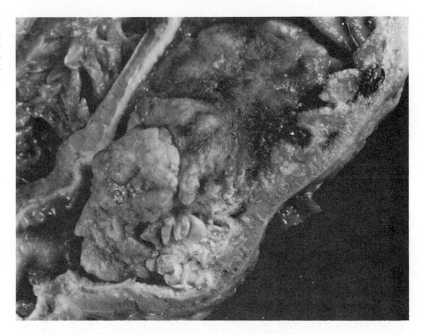

protein, as well as the absorption of the products formed. The complex structure of the mucosa with its numerous villi is well adapted to this function (Fig. 32–7A). Likewise, the microvilli of each luminal cell are designed for absorption of the products of digestion. The glycocalyx (Fig. 2–4) is thought to contain enzymes, including the important disaccharidases. These are responsible for splitting disaccharides (*e.g.*, sucrose and lactose) into mono-saccharides (*e.g.*, fructose and glucose); in this form these sugars can be absorbed.

About 8 liters of fluid enters the duodenum each day, but only 1 to 1.5 liters leaves the ileum to enter the colon. One hundred to 200 ml is passed in the feces. The driving force for the absorption of this large volume of water is mainly the osmotic pressure gradient that follows the active absorption of solutes (*i.e.*, the products of digestion of food). In particular, the absorption of glucose and amino acids induces a flow of water and sodium in the same direction. This is termed *solvent drag*. This phenomenon has been used to great advantage in the treatment of cholera. Even though there is a tremendous outpouring of fluid and electrolytes in the "rice water" stools of this disease, the administration of suitable solutions of glucose and electrolytes *by mouth* is effective treatment. Intravenous therapy is therefore not obligatory in the treatment of cholera, an observation that can save thousands of lives in the event of an epidemic involving an underprivileged area of the world in which intravenous equipment is not available on a mass scale.

Electrolyte absorption in the ileum and colon involves specific transport mechanisms. An important component of this involves cyclic AMP (see below). Before describing the disorders of intestinal absorption it is convenient to summarize the mechanisms involved in the production of diarrhea.

Osmotic Diarrhea.   The presence within the lumen of the gut of unabsorbed solutes results in water retention within the lumen. This is the mechanism by which sodium and magnesium sulfates act as purgatives. It is also a factor in the diarrhea that accompanies defects of intestinal absorption, *e.g.*, celiac disease.

Defective Permeability.   Decreased permeability of diseased bowel to

Pathogenesis of Diarrhea

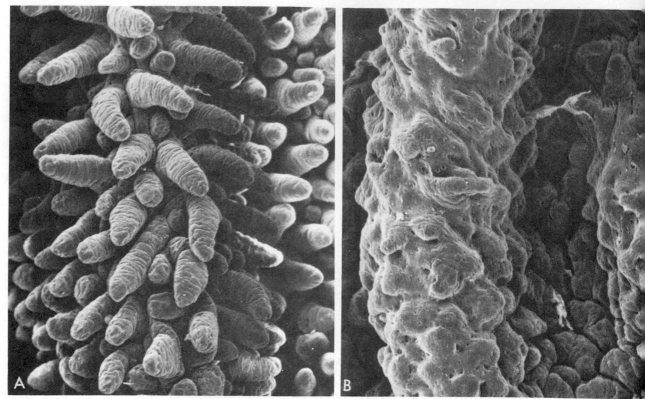

Figure 32–7.   Scanning electron micrographs of small intestine.   Both specimens are from piglet small intestine. *A* is normal and shows slender fingerlike villi; compare this with Figure 2–2. *B* is from an animal infected with transmissible gastroenteritis virus, which produces an illness similar to human rotavirus enteritis. Note that the mucosa is flattened owing to partial villous atrophy. The loss of villi is complete over the folds. Surface openings of crypts appear as pits on the irregular surface. (× 40.) (Photographs courtesy of Dr. E. Cutz, from Figure 4 in Shepherd, R. W., Butler, D. G., Cutz, E., Gall, D. G., and Hamilton, J. R.: The mucosal lesion in viral enteritis: extent and dynamics of the epithelial response to virus invasion in transmissible gastroenteritis of piglets. Gastroenterology, *76*:770–777, 1979.)

water has been demonstrated in the small intestine in celiac disease and in the colon in chronic inflammatory disease. This is also a contributing mechanism to the diarrhea of many other intestinal diseases.

Inflammation and Ulceration of the Mucosa.   An outpouring of inflammatory exudate, often with blood and mucus, causes diarrhea. This is seen in typhoid fever when there is ulceration of the ileum and in the various forms of colitis. Rectal involvement leads to straining at stool, which is termed *tenesmus.*

Intestinal Secretory Diarrhea.   Cholera toxin stimulates adenyl cyclase and leads to the formation of cyclic AMP (Chapter 2). This induces such an outpouring of salt and water into the small intestine that the colon is unable to absorb the load, and a severe watery diarrhea results. A similar mechanism is believed to explain the diarrhea caused by enterotoxigenic *Escherichia coli, Staphylococcus aureus,* and *Shigella dysenteriae.*

Endogenous agents may also increase intestinal secretion, possibly by activating the adenyl cyclase–cyclic AMP mechanism. Thus, vasoactive intestinal peptides (VIP) produced by certain tumors of the islets of Langerhans of the pancreas produce cyclic AMP and are associated with a cholera-like diarrhea. 5-Hydroxytryptamine produced by carcinoid tumors also causes diarrhea, but the precise mechanism is not known.

Increased Intestinal Motility.   This is an ill-defined mechanism and has not as yet been well documented.

From this account of the functions of the small intestine it is evident that any derangement caused by disease can easily be accompanied either by malabsorption or by the loss of large quantities of fluid and electrolytes.

Many agents cause acute inflammation of the small intestine (*acute enteritis*). Often this is accompanied by gastritis (*acute gastroenteritis*) or colitis (*acute enterocolitis*). It is convenient therefore to consider this group of intestinal diseases as a whole.

Acute Inflammation of the Intestine

Many causes of gastroenteritis and enterocolitis can be recognized. These include (1) chemicals, (2) preformed bacterial toxins, (3) bacterial infections, and (4) viral infections. In addition, some cases of intestinal inflammation are classified as idiopathic.

Etiology

Chemicals.   Poisoning may be deliberate (e.g., by ingestion of inorganic arsenic) or accidental (*e.g.*, by ingestion of poisonous mushrooms and spoiled potatoes).

Bacterial Toxins.   *S. aureus* or *Clostridium perfringens* allowed to grow in food such as a meat pie produces toxins that cause acute gastroenteritis when ingested.

Bacterial Infection.   A large number of different species of bacteria cause diarrhea by acting on the intestine in various ways.

Pathogenesis of Bacterial Diarrhea.   Three mechanisms are involved:

1. *Local Toxin Production.*   *Vibrio cholerae*, enterotoxigenic *E. coli*, *S. aureus*, and some strains of Clostridium and Salmonella adhere to the small intestinal mucosa and elaborate a toxin that causes an intestinal secretory type of diarrhea by activating adenyl cyclase as described previously. The intestinal mucosa is not invaded and there is no true infection as this term is strictly defined.

2. *Invasion of the Intestinal Mucosa.*   Pathogens invade the mucosa, damage it, and cause an acute inflammation. This results in frequent small-volume blood motions. Infections with *E. coli*, *Vibrio parahaemolyticus*, *Campylobacter jejuni*, *C. coli*, Shigella, *Yersinia enterocolitica*, and some species of Salmonella fall into this group.

3. *Damage Following Widespread Bacterial Invasion.*   The pathogens invade the mucosa but damage it days later after a preliminary phase of bacterial multiplication in some other tissue followed by septicemia. Typhoid fever is a typical example and is described in Chapter 6.

Specific Types of Bacterial Infection of the Intestine

E. coli Infections.   It should be noted that although most strains of *E. coli* are normal, harmless inhabitants of the bowel, there are a few well-recognized strains that cause enterocolitis. Three types may be recognized:

1. *Enteropathic E. coli.*   These strains cause serious infantile diarrhea (cholera infanticum). Classically the organism causes "summer diarrhea," but in recent years epidemics tend to occur in the winter among infants in hospitals or day nurseries. The organisms proliferate in the duodenum and upper jejunum, where they cause a great outpouring of fluid through a mechanism that is at present unknown.

2. *Enterotoxigenic E. coli.*   These pathogenic strains activate adenyl cyclase and produce a choleraic type of diarrhea. The organisms are responsible for outbreaks of infantile enteritis in developed countries and affect all age groups in developing countries. They are an important cause of traveller's diarrhea.

3. *Enteroinvasive E. coli.*   This group of organisms invade the colonic mucosa and cause a dysentery-like illness. Outbreaks have affected adults in many parts of the world.

Cholera.   Cholera, which is caused by *Vibrio cholerae*, has been responsible in the past for several pandemics that have originated in the Bengal basin. The disease is characterized by the sudden onset of intense vomiting and watery diarrhea, which rapidly leads to dehydration and hypovolemic shock, followed in about one third of the cases by death within 2 or 3 days. With efficient treatment by fluid and electrolyte administration, the mortality can be reduced to under 1 per cent. At a time when the disease appeared to be declining in the world, a new strain became prominent (the *El Tor* type); this appeared to have originated in Indonesia in 1961. It subsequently spread to involve large areas of the Far East, India, and Africa.

Cholera is acquired by ingesting the organisms in food or water contaminated by human excreta. The organism produces a secretory type of diarrhea by the action of its toxin on the intestinal wall; there is neither tissue invasion nor a true enteritis.

Salmonella Infections (Salmonellosis).   Over 2000 serotypes of *Salmonella* are responsible for human infection. The enteric fever organisms — *Salmonella typhi* and *Salmonella paratyphi* A, B, and C — are exclusively human pathogens, and the disease that they cause has been described in Chapter 6. The remainder of the salmonellae are predominantly parasites of animals and cause food poisoning in humans. Common types are *S. typhimurium, S. hadar, S. virchow,* and *S. enteritidis*. Infection occurs by eating undercooked infected poultry or meat, or by contamination of other food by raw meat or poultry or by human carrier. The incubation period is 12 to 24 hours, and the disease is characterized by an abrupt onset of diarrhea, abdominal pain, and vomiting. The stools may be watery (due to a toxin-induced enteropathy), or they may contain blood and mucus (due to an invasive colitis). Recovery generally occurs within a few days, and a convalescent carrier state lasting several weeks is common.

Campylobacter Infections (Campylobacteriosis).   Infection with Campylobacter produces a similar type of food poisoning to that caused by Salmonella. Animals generally provide the source of infection, and transmission is via milk or water.

Shigellosis (Bacillary Dysentery).   After an incubation period of 1 to 4 days there is an abrupt onset of fever, abdominal pain, and watery diarrhea. This phase lasts 1 to 3 days and is associated with colonization of the jejunum and a secretory type of diarrhea similar to that described in cholera. There then ensues a prolonged second phase of *colitis* as the stool volume decreases but the mucus and blood content increase. Tenesmus is often severe. This type of diarrhea is the classical feature of dysentery (the bloody flux of Hippocrates), and untreated it can last for weeks and lead to great debility and weight loss. The severity of the disease depends on the causative organism. *Shigella dysenteriae* (Shiga bacillus) is the most virulent and is the least common in North America. *S. flexneri* is intermediate in virulence and frequency, whereas *S. sonnei* produces the mildest disease and is the most common. As with other types of dysentery, it occurs in epidemic form and often occurs in custodial institutions, particularly those that care for the mentally retarded.

Pathologically, bacillary dysentery is characterized by colitis with ulceration and inflammation of the mucosa.

Other bacterial causes of gastroenteritis include infection by *Y. enterocolitica, V. parahaemolyticus,* and others. Differentiation among these various types of infection is largely a bacteriological problem.

Viral Infections.   Many viruses are known to cause diarrhea. The rotaviruses are a cause of gastroenteritis in children under 6 years old, and indeed under 2 years of age they are the commonest cause (Fig. 32–7*B*).

The *winter vomiting disease* is probably viral in origin, and various virus particles have been demonstrated in the feces of affected individuals. The disease is not uncommon and has a sudden onset of severe vomiting and diarrhea after an incubation period of 24 to 48 hours. Fever, vomiting, abdominal pain, and diarrhea generally last 2 to 3 days and are followed by complete recovery.

Other Clinical Types of Gastroenteritis

Traveller's Diarrhea. It is a common experience to develop acute gastroenteritis when travelling in hot climates, particularly in countries with inadequate sanitation. Colloquial terms such as "Delhi belly" and "Montezuma's revenge" bear witness to the widespread nature of the problem. The irritant effects of local exotic foods are now discounted as a cause, and epidemiology suggests an infective cause. Enterotoxigenic *E. coli* and Campylobacter are probably the most common causes. Other causes include infection by Shigella, Salmonella, and Giardia. Often no cause can be recognized.

Acute Infantile Gastroenteritis. In developing countries acute gastroenteritis is an important cause of infant mortality and morbidity; even in the Western world it is among the ten leading causes of death in children under 5 years of age. The disease is less common in breast-fed infants, partly because they are protected by IgA in the milk, and partly because there is less chance of contamination of the food. Rotavirus infection is the commonest cause, but *E. coli*, Yersinia, Campylobacter, Shigella, Salmonella, Giardia, and Strongyloides are other causes.

Food Poisoning. The term "food poisoning" is used to describe a wide range of conditions with presenting symptoms of diarrhea and vomiting due to gastroenteritis that develop up to 48 hours after the consumption of food or drink. It is customary to exclude the enteric fevers (typhoid), dysentery, and cholera. The causes include the infections described previously, the effects of ingested preformed bacterial toxin, chemical poisons, and probably some examples of food allergies.

Ischemic Bowel Disease

Although massive infarction of the bowel has been recognized for many years, the existence of less dramatic, more subtle lesions due to ischemia has not attracted attention until comparatively recently.

Causes. Ischemia of the bowel can result from the following causes:

1. *Arterial Occlusion.* Atherosclerosis, with or without thrombosis, and embolism are common causes. Dissecting aneurysm of the aorta and polyarteritis are less frequently encountered causes.

2. *Venous Occlusion.* Thrombosis of the mesenteric vein may arise as a complication of abdominal surgery, cirrhosis of the liver with portal hypertension, or ingestion of birth control pills.

3. *Nonocclusive Underperfusion.* This may be due to hypotension complicating shock.

Effects. The effects of ischemia depend on its degree and duration. Mild cases lead to edema, hemorrhage in the bowel wall, and superficial mucosal necrosis. Such effects cause no permanent damage, and healing occurs with minimal scarring. In more severe cases, necrosis involves the whole mucosa and perhaps the submucosa. Such a lesion may heal, but with scarring that may lead to stricture formation. The most severe cases cause full-thickness necrosis of the bowel wall, resulting in the classical picture of infarction. The wall becomes gangrenous and ruptures, leading to peritonitis, shock, and death unless emergency surgery intervenes.

Examples of Ischemic Bowel Disease. Sudden complete vascular occlusion generally leads to infarction of the whole thickness of the gut wall. Examples include mesenteric artery thrombosis or embolism, mesenteric vein thrombosis, volvulus, and a strangulated hernia.

Gradual occlusion of the superior mesenteric artery due to atherosclerosis may cause *intestinal angina,* a syndrome in which abdominal pain occurs shortly after meals owing to the increased peristalsis, which accentuates the effects of the pre-existing ischemia. Diarrhea, weight loss, and a frank malabsorption syndrome can ensue. The condition may terminate in bowel infarction.

Nonocclusive ischemia is generally a feature of shock and is therefore a complication of major trauma and surgery. Underperfusion of the bowel is accentuated by any pre-existing organic arterial occlusion such as atherosclerosis. Older patients are therefore at greater risk than the young. Any part of the bowel can be affected, and the type of lesion and the extent of the damage vary from case to case. There may be scattered areas of superficial mucosal hemorrhage and ulceration, which may heal or lead to scarring if the patient survives the primary disease. In severe cases there is widespread hemorrhage and extensive mucosal loss. If the colon is affected, the appearance closely resembles acute ulcerative colitis (page 471). Clinically, abdominal pain, cramps, and bloody diarrhea are added to the patient's other problems.

Severe ischemic bowel disease is believed to be the explanation of many cases of *pseudomembranous enterocolitis.* In this condition the bowel wall is congested and edematous, and the mucosa undergoes necrosis and hangs from the wall as a characteristic white or greenish membrane (Fig. 32–8). The lesions are patchy and affect both small and large intestine, but the rectum is

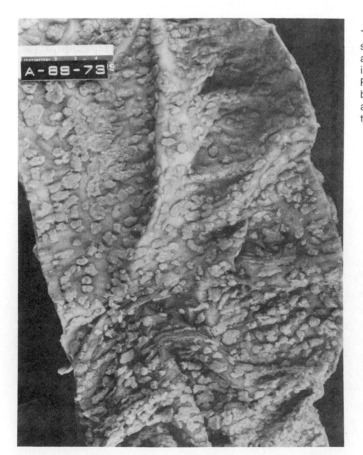

Figure 32–8. Pseudomembranous colitis. The colon has been opened to show the necrosis of the mucosa. In some areas there is ulceration, and between these denuded areas necrotic mucosa is loosely attached as isolated islands of tissue. Pseudomembranous colitis is not a disease entity but a reaction of this part of the gut to a variety of agents, including ischemia and antibiotics. (Courtesy of Dr. J. B. Cullen.)

usually spared, presumably because of its good blood supply. In some cases factors other than simple ischemia are involved. Pseudomembranous entero-colitis is a rare complication of antibiotic therapy, occurring most often with oral clindamycin. A superinfection with *Staphylococcus aureus* may play a part in a few cases, but an overgrowth of *Clostridium difficile* is believed to be a more important factor (Chapter 10).

Crohn's disease is a chronic inflammatory disease that can affect any part of the bowel but is usually most obvious in the lower small intestine (see Case History I). The bowel shows chronic inflammation that involves its entire wall. The lumen becomes narrowed, causing the patient to develop intestinal obstruction (Fig. 32–9). Constipation alternates with diarrhea. An outstanding feature of the disease is that small abscesses form on the mucosal surface; since these penetrate the muscularis, the serosa is affected. The inflammatory reaction leads to local peritonitis and to adhesions between the abdominal organs (Fig. 32–10). Sinuses and fistula develop, so that communication is established between adjacent loops of intestine, the colon, the bladder, and the skin surface. The cause of this disease, which tends to affect young adults, is still unknown. Treatment by resection of the affected bowel is sometimes successful, but recurrence in other areas is quite common. The course is therefore protracted and presents great problems to both patient and attendants.

Crohn's Disease (Regional Enteritis)

CASE HISTORY I. (See Figure 32–10.) The patient was a 30-year-old male who was admitted to a hospital with a complaint of abdominal pain and frequency of stool discharge for one year. The pain, which was colicky in nature, began between 1 and 2 hours after meals. It was relieved by having a bowel movement, which showed stools that were bulky, light brown, and foul-smelling. They floated in the toilet bowl because of their fat and gas content. Pathological examination of the feces showed the presence of pus cells, blood, and an increased amount of fat. A barium meal showed narrowing and irregularity of the bowel wall involving two or three loops of ileum. Such findings were suggestive of Crohn's disease. Since the patient was thought to have signs of subacute intestinal obstruction, a laparotomy was performed. About 50 cm of small gut was resected. The disease started about 20 cm from the ileocecal junction and extended upward. Two skip areas were noted between the lesions. The

Figure 32–9. Crohn's disease of the small intestine. The mucosa of the affected area is thickened and presents a hyperemic cobblestone appearance. Note the thickening of the intestinal wall (arrow); when marked, this can cause stenosis of the lumen. Note the sharp line of demarcation between the diseased bowel and the normal intestine. In this patient other areas of small intestine were affected; it is characteristic of the disease for there to be normal "skip areas" between them.

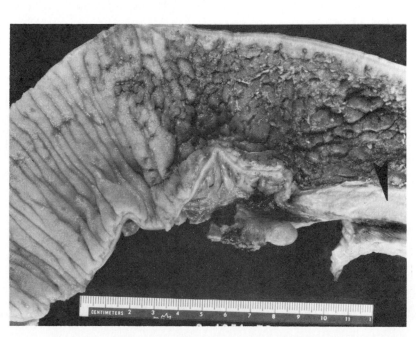

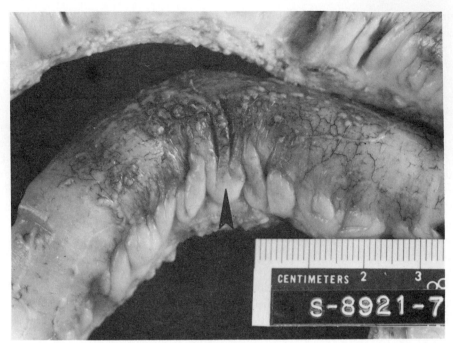

Figure 32–10. Crohn's disease of the small intestine. This portion of small intestine shows hyperemia and thickening of the peritoneal surface. Focal white areas of inflammation are present, and this loop of intestine has become adherent to adjacent structures. The fat at the mesenteric border of the intestine (arrow) is prominent and is "creeping" over the gut wall. (See Case History I for additional clinical details.)

sigmoid colon also showed thickening, which was interpreted as Crohn's disease, but since there was no sign of obstruction, the colon was not resected. The postoperative course was uneventful. Part of the resected specimen is shown in Figure 32–10. Postoperatively, the patient continued to have three or four bowel movements daily, but he felt reasonably well in spite of the occasional passage of blood. It was felt that his Crohn's disease was still present but stable.

Tuberculosis of the Intestine

This disease is now extremely uncommon.

Tumors of the Small Intestine

Small leiomyomas are not uncommon but rarely produce symptoms; carcinomas are rare. The most frequently encountered malignant tumor is the *carcinoid*. This tumor is characterized by the development of a considerable stromal reaction that causes a stricture to develop. The tumor grows slowly, but it ultimately metastasizes to lymph nodes and liver. These metastases sometimes lead to the *carcinoid syndrome* — diarrhea, valvular lesions of the right side of the heart, asthmatic attacks, and periodic flushing of the face. The pathogenesis of this syndrome is not clear, but the release of 5-hydroxytryptamine by the tumor, the activation of plasma kinin, and the deposition of platelets on the heart valves are all involved. Carcinoid tumors also occur in other parts of the intestine — the appendix, in particular. In the latter situation the tumor is usually small and does not spread.

The Malabsorption Syndrome

If the functions of the small intestine are impaired, a state of severe undernutrition results; this condition is called the *malabsorption syndrome*.

Causes. Common causes appear below:

Lack of Bile Salts or Digestive Enzymes. Obstructive jaundice and pancreatic disease, such as chronic pancreatitis, are examples of diseases causing these deficiencies.

Lack of Absorptive Area.   This problem usually follows extensive intestinal resecttons such as those performed following gunshot wounds to the abdomen or for Crohn's disease.

The Blind Loop Syndrome.   Multiple diverticulae of the small intestine (which is a very uncommon condition), fistulae between adjacent loops, and blind loops caused by surgical procedures sometimes lead to the malabsorption syndrome. The precise mechanism of this syndrome is not clearly understood, but it is believed to be related to an upset in the intestinal flora.

Intrinsic Disease of the Intestine Itself.   A good example of an intestinal disease that leads to severe malabsorption is *sprue*. The intestinal villi show atrophy, but the cause is not known (Fig. 32–11). Two types of sprue, listed below, can be recognized:

1. *Tropical sprue*
2. *Gluten-induced enteropathy*

In children, gluten-induced enteropathy is called *celiac disease;* in adults it is known as *nontropical sprue*. The intestinal lesions and the symptoms can be relieved by a diet that is low in gluten. The way in which gluten (a protein contained in flour) produces the disease is not understood. Since there is a marked familial incidence, the disease is probably inherited as an autosomal dominant trait with incomplete penetrance.

Effects of Malabsorption.   The lack of absorption produces some effects that are similar to those of starvation, *e.g.*, the effects following the dysphagia of esophageal cancer. Thus, there is a loss of weight and generalized body atrophy.

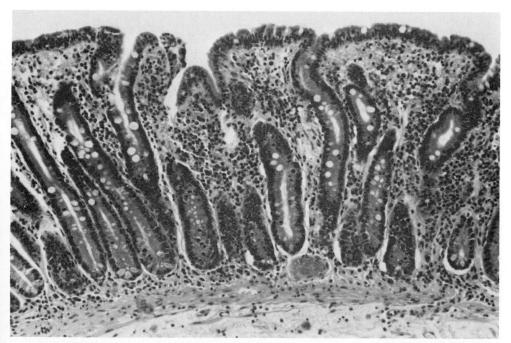

Figure 32–11. Gluten-induced enteropathy. This section is from a jejunal biopsy. Note the flat surface and absence of villi (compare this with normal intestine illustrated in Chapter 2). The lamina propria is heavily infiltrated with lymphocytes and plasma cells. Under the scanning electron microscope the appearance would resemble that demonstrated in Figure 32–7B. (× 250.)

Fat absorption is usually severely affected; therefore much fat — some of it undigested — is passed in the feces, which are pale and bulky. Excess fat in the stools is termed *steatorrhea*. There is often poor carbohydrate absorption, and the excess carbohydrate is fermented by bacteria in the bowel. The resulting gas causes the stools to be frothy and offensive.

In addition to the generalized wasting, there are the effects of specific dietary deficiencies (*e.g.*, deficiencies of the vitamin B complex, the fat-soluble vitamins A and D, and calcium). Calcium is poorly absorbed because it is bound by the fatty acids in the bowel. This results in a negative calcium balance with mild hypocalcemia and a tendency to develop tetany. A deficiency of vitamin D aggravates matters, causing osteomalacia to develop (Chapter 40). A deficiency of vitamin K leads to a low plasma prothrombin and a bleeding tendency (Chapter 26). Dermatitis, peripheral neuropathy, and inflammation of the tongue (glossitis) may all be found and may be attributable to vitamin deficiencies. A failure to absorb iron, vitamin B_{12}, and folic acid leads to severe anemia. The effects of malabsorption from the small intestine are both widespread and serious, and their occurrence is a reflection of the importance of this part of the digestive tract.

THE COLON

The colon has two main functions: (1) absorbing water and electrolytes, and (2) providing a convenient receptacle for feces, so that they may be discharged at the individual's convenience. Acute inflammation of the colon results in a derangement of its functions, and the diarrhea that results causes great inconvenience as well as a considerable loss of water and electrolytes. Infection of the colon leading to ulceration and causing diarrhea with pus, mucus, and blood in the feces is called *dysentery*. *Bacillary dysentery* has been described earlier in this chapter, and *amebic dysentery* is discussed in Chapter 15.

Ischemic colitis has been described earlier in this chapter, and *uremic colitis* is noted in Chapter 35.

Idiopathic Ulcerative Colitis

Now the commonest cause of serious bowel disease in North America, idiopathic ulcerative colitis affects all age groups and often starts in young adult life.

The disease generally commences with an acute attack of colicky abdominal pain accompanied by diarrhea and the passage of blood, mucus, and pus in the feces. Fever and malaise are also present. The acute attack generally subsides and is followed by chronic ulcerative colitis with recurrent exacerbation of symptoms. Pain, diarrhea, and the passage of blood, mucus, and pus are intermittent.

The disease generally affects the rectum and distal colon most severely, and in the acute phase it is characterized by intense hyperemia of the mucosa. On proctoscopy the mucosa bleeds at the slightest touch. In due course, mucosal ulcers develop, and these tend to undermine the mucous membrane, so that tags or pseudopolyps are formed. The ulcers are covered by a slough. Deep to this is an inflammatory reaction from which the blood and pus are derived.

In chronic ulcerative colitis the disease tends to remain confined to the mucosa. Because the muscle coat itself and the peritoneal surface of the colon are not generally affected, adhesions do not form between adjacent viscera and there is usually no perforation or fistula formation. In this respect the disease differs markedly from Crohn's disease, which can also affect the colon.

Ulcerative colitis generally pursues a chronic intermittent course, producing misery to the patient and leading to anemia, general debility, and loss of weight. A further complication is the development of carcinoma. It has been estimated that about one third of the patients who suffer from the disease for more than 12 years develop cancer. For this reason, and because of the symptoms of the disease, total colectomy is sometimes performed, and the patient is left with a permanent ileostomy. The ileum is brought to the surface of the anterior abdominal wall, a permanent opening is created, and a suitable container is attached.

Ulcerative colitis is occasionally very acute, either at its inception or at some stage in its development. The colon becomes acutely congested, its muscle becomes atonic, and the bowel dilates enormously. This type of disease follows a fulminating course; generally, the transverse colon is involved, and the patient becomes extremely ill. Multiple perforations develop, and the patient dies of toxemia associated with peritonitis. This variant of ulcerative colitis is called *acute toxic megacolon.*

Diverticular Disease of the Colon

The current Western diet, which contains inadequate cellulose (roughage), is believed by some authorities to be responsible for the high frequency of colonic diverticula. This disease is most frequent in the distal part of the colon — particularly the sigmoid part. Apart from the presence of numerous diverticula, the most striking change is muscular hypertrophy and shortening of the colon — presumably due to the muscular overactivity that is necessary to propel the small, hard feces. The diverticula themselves consist of outpouches of the mucosa that penetrate weak points in the muscular coat (Figs. 32–12 and 32–13). Often they are covered by merely a thin layer of peritoneum. Sometimes the orifices of the diverticula become obstructed by fecal material and inflammation ensues. Overlying peritonitis develops, with the formation of adhesions, pericolic abscesses, and fistulae. The condition is then called *diverticulitis.* Sometimes a mass of chronic inflammatory tissue

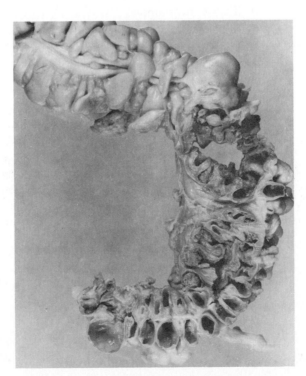

Figure 32–12. Diverticular disease of the colon. Part of this portion of descending and sigmoid colon has been opened. Numerous diverticula are present. There is no evidence of inflammation, and the condition can be labeled *diverticulosis.*

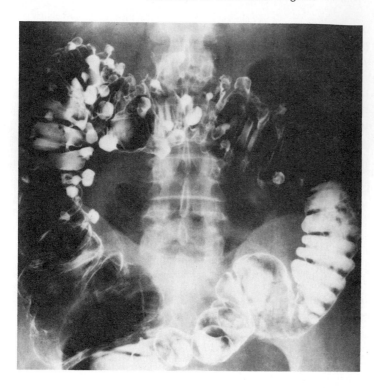

Figure 32–13. Colonic diverticula. This radiograph following a barium enema shows numerous diverticula that are outlined by the radiopaque barium. (Courtesy of Dr. D. E. Sanders.)

forming in the bowel wall is sufficient to cause obstruction and to simulate carcinoma. Occasionally diverticular disease can cause massive bleeding, which is life-threatening.

Neoplasms of the Large Intestine

Adenoma. Adenomas are common and sometimes multiple (Fig. 32–14). They tend to become pedunculated and bleed. Malignant change can occur but it is not inevitable. Nevertheless, in the hereditary condition of *polyposis coli,* there are so many tumors that one invariably becomes malignant and the patient dies of carcinoma.

Carcinoma. The large bowel ranks with the lung and the breast as the most common site of fatal malignant disease in Europeans. The rectum and sigmoid colon are most frequently involved. The tumor is usually a well-differentiated adenocarcinoma (Figs. 17–10 and 17–11). Initially it may produce a polypoid growth protruding into the lumen, but it generally soon breaks down to produce a typical carcinomatous ulcer (Fig. 32–15). The tumor tends to encircle the gut, and the fibrous stromal reaction that accompanies it produces a stricture (Figs. 32–16 and 32–17). This obstruction produces constipation, but overgrowth of organisms above this soon liquefies the feces so that diarrhea follows. *Alternate constipation and diarrhea are characteristic of partial intestinal obstruction.* When combined with the passage of blood and mucus in the stools, the diagnosis of carcinoma is almost certain. The tumor invades locally, metastasizes to the regional lymph nodes, and finally invades the blood stream to cause metastases in the liver and, later, elsewhere. Growth is often relatively slow, so that the prognosis following resection is good if the tumor is detected in the early stages of development and correspondingly poor if the tumor is detected in the later stages.

THE APPENDIX

The importance of the appendix as a site of intra-abdominal mischief is not proportional to its size or apparent uselessness. The organ is a hollow cul-de-sac opening into the cecum, and it is seldom more than 7 cm in length. Its major disease is acute inflammation.

Figure 32–14. Familial polyposis coli.
The mucosal surface of the colon shows
numerous adenomas, many of which are pedun-
culated and may therefore be labeled *polyps*.
(Specimen from the Boyd Museum, University of
Toronto.)

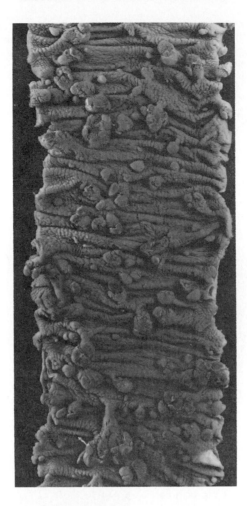

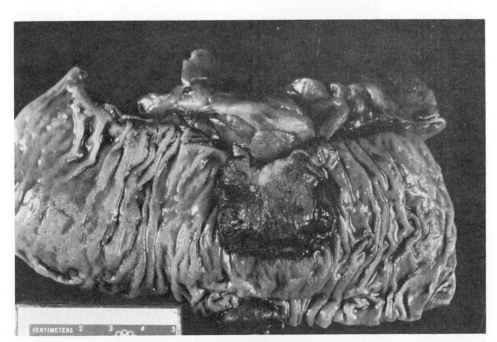

Figure 32–15. Carcinoma of the colon. The specimen shows a typical ulcerating carcinoma. It has a rolled edge where tumor is actively extending.

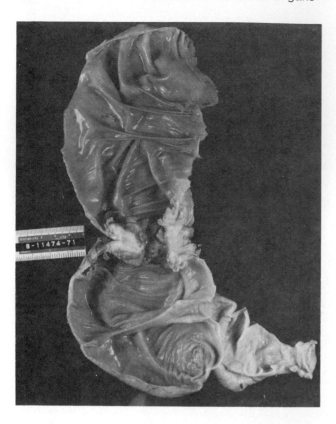

Figure 32–16. Carcinoma of the colon. This surgically removed colon has been distended with 4 per cent formaldehyde solution before being opened. Note how the carcinoma encircles the gut and has produced stenosis.

Figure 32–17. Carcinoma of the colon. This radiograph following a barium enema shows obvious obstruction in the descending colon. The lesion proved to be a carcinoma similar to that depicted in Figure 32–16. (Courtesy of Dr. D. E. Sanders.)

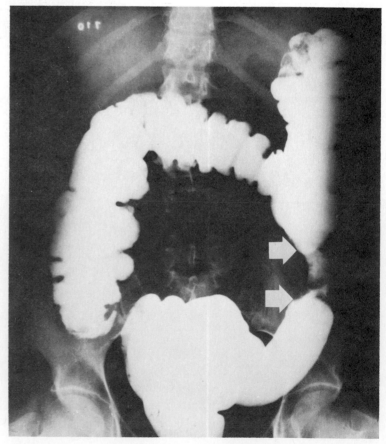

Incidence. Acute appendicitis is common in persons living in highly civilized societies, but spares the inhabitants of poor and undeveloped areas of the world. The reason for this is not precisely known, but it is presumed to be related to diet — a low roughage/high meat diet apparently predisposing to the disease. Appendicitis is rare in children under 2 years of age and has its maximum incidence in young adults between the ages of 20 and 30 years.

Pathology and Pathogenesis. No specific infective agent can be isolated from an acutely inflamed appendix; the organisms present are those normally found in the feces — in particular, *Escherichia coli*. The inflamed organ is red and swollen (Fig. 32–18); its peritoneal coat is dulled by a fibrinous exudate, and the mucosa is ulcerated. Often found blocking the lumen is a hard mass of feces (called a *fecalith*), which may play some part in initiating the disease.

Complications. Acute appendicitis may resolve spontaneously, but often the wall undergoes necrosis, becomes gangrenous, and *perforates*. Pus and fecal material pour into the peritoneal cavity. This material may become walled off by adhesions to produce a *localized abscess*, but often *generalized peritonitis* ensues, and the outlook is poor. It is impossible to predict the course of an individual case, and early removal of the appendix (appendectomy) is the treatment of choice in all cases. If the patient is seen later in the course of the disease when a localized abscess mass is present, it is best to allow the inflammation to subside and to treat the person surgically at a later date. Suppurative thrombophlebitis with portal pyemia is an occasional complication.

Symptoms. The inflamed turgid appendix causes *pain* that is referred to the midline of the abdomen at about the level of the umbilicus. *Nausea* and sometimes *vomiting* follow. As the parietal peritoneum becomes inflamed, the periumbilical pain shifts to the right iliac fossa, and local tenderness can be detected.

If each case of acute appendicitis had this typical history, the disease would present no diagnostic problems. Unfortunately, atypical cases are common, particularly in the very young and the very old, and even the most astute physician can be mistaken and misled. In view of the seriousness of perforation, it is a wise policy to operate if there is a reasonable suspicion of

Figure 32–18. Acute appendicitis. The appendix in *A* shows acute inflammation. The organ is turgid and deeply congested. The mottled appearance seen in some areas is due to underlying suppuration. This appendix would almost certainly have ruptured had it not been removed. Specimen *B* is a normal appendix for comparison; it is slender and thin. Note the fat in the mesentery of the appendix. This is normal. (Courtesy of Dr. J. B. Cullen.)

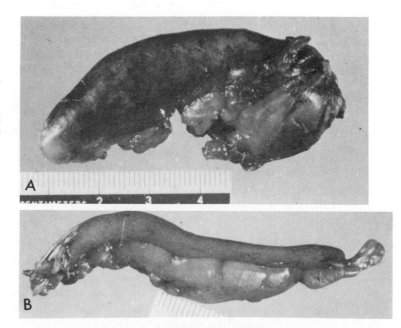

acute appendicitis. Inevitably, some unnecessary operations will be performed and normal appendices will be removed, but the operative mortality is very low. The alternative policy is to risk allowing an acute appendicitis to rupture and to go undetected. In such cases the mortality is high.

Mucocele of the Appendix. Following an attack of appendicitis, the lumen becomes blocked, and the appendix distally becomes distended with mucus. A similar appearance can occur as a result of a low-grade carcinoma of the mucosa. In the latter type of mucocele, the organ may rupture and lead to pseudomyxoma peritonei (Chapter 37).

DISEASES OF THE ABDOMINAL CAVITY AS A WHOLE

The abdominal cavity is lined by a layer of flattened cells that are sometimes classified as epithelial but are actually *modified connective tissue fibroblasts.* Following surgical procedures that have left raw areas of peritoneum, the exposed connective tissues rapidly differentiate into new peritoneal cells; hence, it is unnecessary to attempt to cover these raw areas. To cover them is detrimental, because the required sutures lead to inflammation and the formation of adhesions.

Peritonitis

Localized Peritonitis. This condition occurs over an inflamed abdominal organ. Examples, which have been described elsewhere in this chapter, include acute appendicitis, Crohn's disease, diverticulitis, and peptic ulceration. Localized pelvic peritonitis in the female is generally secondary to salpingitis, often gonococcal salpingitis. The fibrinous component of the exudate tends to wall-off the inflammation and to localize any infection. Aiding in this process is the *greater omentum,* the fibrovascular fatty apron that hangs from the stomach. This structure has been called the "policeman of the abdomen," for it tends to wrap itself around any area of inflammation; by becoming inflamed itself, the greater omentum adds its fibrinous exudate to the adhesions that limit the spread of infection.

Generalized Peritonitis. This occasionally occurs as a primary disease without evidence of infection elsewhere. The route of infection is presumed to be either via the blood stream, from a pulmonary infection, or, in young women, via the fallopian tubes. More commonly, generalized peritonitis is the result of rupture of a part of the gastrointestinal tract, *e.g.,* perforated peptic ulcer, appendicitis, toxic megacolon, volvulus, and penetrating injuries to the abdomen.

In generalized peritonitis the large area of peritoneum forms an admirable absorptive area for toxins; the patient rapidly becomes ill, develops paralytic ileus, and goes into shock. Even if the person is treated and survives, he may have localized pockets of infection that can form peritoneal abscesses. One such site is the pelvis, owing no doubt to the effects of gravity. Another is the space between the diaphragm and the liver. Indeed, an abscess in the latter situation *(subphrenic abscess)* is of great importance and should always be suspected if the patient develops signs of infection *(e.g.,* malaise, fever, leukocytosis) following an abdominal event *(e.g.,* appendicitis, laparotomy) and the site of infection is not apparent. The old adage "pus somewhere, pus under the diaphragm" is all too often forgotten (see Fig. 32–2).

Peritoneal Adhesions

Following acute peritonitis the fibrinous adhesions can organize to fibrous adhesions. Hence, these are not uncommon overlying an appendix or adjacent to a peptic ulcer. Surgery alone can produce adhesions; the irritant talc or starch used as glove powder is an important factor in their production. The gloves used by the surgeon and assistants should be well rinsed before entering the abdomen. Endometriosis as a cause of adhesion formation is described in Chapter 37.

Adhesions can cause intestinal obstruction either directly or as a complication of internal hernia formation. Extensive adhesions (*e.g.,* following pelvic irradiation for carcinoma of the cervix) render subsequent surgery difficult and hazardous, for the bowel can easily be opened inadvertently.

Much of the small intestine and parts of the colon are suspended from the abdominal wall by means of a mesentery. The twisting of a loop of bowel about its mesenteric base is called a *volvulus* and is yet another cause of the "acute abdomen." Twisting of the mesentery soon produces venous obstruction, causing the gut to become rapidly congested and edematous. Soon the arterial supply is cut off and infarction results. Urgent surgical intervention is required for volvulus. Sometimes the twist can be undone, but usually the affected gut must be resected.

Volvulus

In this condition a segment of gut becomes telescoped into the gut immediately distal to it. The trapped portion is pulled in by peristaltic motions, so that the segment of gut and its mesentery are steadily advanced towards the anus. The condition is most common in children and appears to arise spontaneously — perhaps being precipitated by an acute enteritis. In adults intussusception is sometimes caused by a benign tumor that is caught by the peristaltic motions of the gut distal to it. Symptoms of intussusception include intestinal obstruction and the sequelae of infarction of the affected bowel. Passage of blood *per rectum* is characteristic.

Intussusception

A hernia is an outpouching of an abdominal viscus through a weak point of the abdominal wall. An outpouching of parietal peritoneum occurs first. This forms the lining of the hernial sac. Into this sac pass various mobile abdominal viscera — omentum, small intestine, and, less commonly, colon, fallopian tube, and ovary.

Hernias

In the early stages of development the contents of the hernial sac can be reduced by pressure and returned to the abdomen. The formation of adhesions may later result in the intestinal loops being permanently trapped or *incarcerated*. The hernia cannot then be reduced.

An occasional complication of a hernia is that the venous return from its contents is impaired by twisting or kinking at its neck; venous congestion causes edema, with the swelling further endangering the circulation until the arterial supply is finally cut off and the contents of the sac become infarcted and gangrenous. The hernia is then said to be *strangulated*. A strangulated hernia is a serious condition, since if bowel is involved (as it usually is) it results in intestinal obstruction and is rapidly followed by generalized peritonitis. Immediate surgical treatment is imperative. The detailed anatomy of the various types of hernias is therefore of great importance to the surgeon who is called upon to operate on them.

The most common site for a hernia is the inguinal region. Two types of *inguinal hernia* are encountered. In the *indirect* type the sac follows the previous path of the descending testis. In the *direct* type the hernial sac bulges directly through weakened muscles in the inguinal region. Both types of hernia must be distinguished by the surgeon from a *femoral hernia,* which passes through the femoral canal.

Other types of hernia include the *umbilical hernia,* which is usually present at birth and may close spontaneously. In a *ventral hernia* the bowel herniates through a weak area in a laparotomy scar. Paraesophageal or *hiatus hernias* have been described in Chapter 31.

The opening of the lesser sac and the various fossae around the duodenum present potential orifices through which loops of bowel can pass to form *internal hernias.* Likewise, a hernia can form in relation to fibrous bands or adhesions.

Intestinal Obstruction

Intestinal obstruction (or *ileus,* as it is sometimes called) is a serious condition because if it is complete and it is not relieved, it terminates in death. Two types, described below, can be recognized:

Mechanical Intestinal Obstruction.   There are many causes of intestinal obstruction: strictures, tumors, hernias, volvuli, and intussusceptions are some forms of mechanical obstruction that have already been described. The obstruction may develop gradually, or it may be complete and sudden, resulting in more severe effects. The higher in the intestinal tract the obstruction occurs, the more profound are its effects and the greater is the threat to life.

Features of Mechanical Intestinal Obstruction

Pain.   The intestine above the obstruction exhibits increased peristalsis; such effects can be heard with the aid of a stethoscope. The obstruction causes pain that is diffuse, poorly localized, and cramping or colicky.

Failure to Pass Feces or Gas per Rectum.   Constipation, which becomes complete, is an important feature of intestinal obstruction.

Vomiting.   Vomiting is a prominent feature of high intestinal obstruction. The vomitus soon becomes green in color and eventually has a foul, fecal odor.

Abdominal Distention.   The gut above the obstruction ultimately becomes distended with fluid and gas, causing abdominal distention. A radiograph taken with the patient in the standing position has a characteristic appearance with many fluid levels. Abdominal distention is a late event if the site of the obstruction is low in the intestinal tract.

Nonmechanical Intestinal Obstruction.   In the absence of a mechanical obstruction, a failure of the intestinal muscle to propel the gut contents forward is commonly called *ileus.* (Strictly speaking, "ileus," from the Greek *eilos,* meaning "intestinal colic," can be applied to any type of obstruction.) Three types are recognized:

Adynamic or Paralytic Ileus.   Peritonitis is the most important cause of paralytic ileus. To a minor degree it occurs after every abdominal operation, but in such cases it does not last more than 3 days. The fully developed syndrome occurs in acute peritonitis, such as that complicating acute appendicitis or a perforated peptic ulcer. The gut dilates, vomiting occurs, peristalsis is absent, and the abdomen is silent — a silence that leads to the grave. Paralytic ileus sometimes complicates painful conditions, such as renal colic, and it is also a feature of severe hypokalemia (Chapter 19).

Ileus Due to Vascular Occlusion.   Mesenteric arterial occlusion or mesenteric venous thrombosis leads to focal intestinal paralysis and obstruction. Gangrene often follows.

Spastic Ileus.   Spasm is an uncommon cause of obstruction. It is occasionally encountered in uremia.

The Acute Abdomen

The sudden onset of acute abdominal pain, often combined with vomiting and fever, is commonly referred to as "acute abdomen." It is usually caused by peritoneal infection derived from a perforated abdominal organ. The task of diagnosis and treatment, which usually falls to the surgeon, is a subject dealt with in texts of surgery. Only a few of the common causes will be listed here: acute appendicitis, acute cholecystitis, perforated peptic ulcer, ulcerative colitis, diverticulitis, mesenteric thrombosis, volvulus, and strangulated hernia. Each of these conditions demands prompt surgical treatment.

However, there are a number of other causes for which surgery is not required and, in fact, is often contraindicated. Acute pancreatitis, acute enteritis, basal pneumonia, and acute myocardial infarction are good examples of this group. It is evident that the management of the "acute abdomen" requires great skill and considerable experience.

Review Questions

1. A 25-year-old woman is found to be anemic and complains of weight loss, diarrhea, and offensive frothy stools. Her sister had required a special diet from the age of 3 years because of a failure to thrive. Discuss the diagnosis.

2. What are the causes of diarrhea with the passage of blood and mucus in the feces? Indicate how information in the case history could give a clue to the most likely diagnosis in an individual patient, particularly with respect to the following:
   (a) age
   (b) duration of symptoms
   (c) travel abroad

3. Describe the condition known as pseudomembranous enterocolitis and give examples of the circumstances under which it develops.

4. Compare Crohn's disease with ulcerative colitis in terms of these factors:
   (a) site of disease
   (b) pathological lesions
   (c) complications

5. Describe the pathogenesis and effects of intestinal secretory diarrhea, and give examples of the circumstances under which it occurs.

6. Compare the following diseases: bacillary dysentery, amebic dysentery, and cholera.

7. A man with an inguinal hernia complains of sudden pain over the swelling. He is constipated and his abdominal region is producing loud gurgling noises (borborygmi). The patient begins to vomit; his condition deteriorates; he develops a fever and passes into shock. His abdomen is distended, tense, and silent. He dies. Give an account of the probable events that led to this man's death.

8. Under what conditions is an abnormal amount of fat found in the feces? What are the effects of this excess?

9. Describe the complications of a chronic gastric or duodenal ulcer.

10. Compare the effects of carcinoma of the stomach with those of carcinoma of the colon.

Selected Readings

Christie, A. B.: Infectious Diseases: Epidemiology and Clinical Practice. 3rd ed. Edinburgh, Churchill Livingstone, 1980. See, in particular, Chapters 2–7.

Colcock, B. P.: Benign ulcerative and granulomatous lesions of the bowel. Surgery Annual, 4:285–303, 1972.

Lambert, H. P. (Ed.): Infections of the gastrointestinal tract. Clinics in Gastroenterology, 8:547–802, 1979. This volume contains many excellent articles devoted to the pathogenesis of diarrhea and specific types of gastroenteritis, including traveller's diarrhea and antibiotic-associated colitis.

Leading Article: Erosive gastritis. British Medical Journal, 3:211–212, 1974

Morson, B. C., and Dawson, I. M. P.: Gastrointestinal Pathology. 2nd ed. Oxford, Blackwell Scientific Publications Ltd., 1979. A reference book.

Sawyers, J. L., and Herrington, J. L.: Short gut syndrome, Surgery Annual, 4:273–284, 1972.

Schwartz, S. I., and Storer, E. H.: Manifestations of gastrointestinal disease. In Schwartz, S. I., Lillehei, R. C., Shires, G. T., Spencer, F. C., and Storer, E. H. (Eds.): Principles of Surgery, 2nd ed. New York, McGraw-Hill Book Company, 1974.

Thomas, W. E. G.: Duodeno-gastric reflux—a common factor in pathogenesis of gastric and duodenal ulcer. Lancet 2:1166–1168, 1980.

CHAPTER 33 Diseases of the Liver

After studying this chapter the student should be able to:

- Describe the structure of the normal liver and distinguish between the classic liver lobule and the acinus of Rappaport.
- Indicate the circumstances under which infarction of the liver may occur.
- Indicate how the pressure in the portal vein can be measured.
- Describe the effects of portal hypertension.
- Describe the main pathways of the metabolism of bilirubin.
- List the types of jaundice and describe the main features of each.
- Relate the effects of hepatocellular failure to the normal functions of the liver.
- Define the following terms and indicate the circumstances under which the conditions are found:
    - (a) zonal hepatic necrosis
    - (b) focal hepatic necrosis
    - (c) bridging hepatic necrosis
    - (d) massive hepatic necrosis
- Outline the main features of viral hepatitis with respect to:
    - (a) causative agent and mode of infection
    - (b) changes in the liver
    - (c) clinical manifestations
    - (d) prognosis
- Distinguish among chronic lobular hepatitis, chronic persistent hepatitis, and chronic active hepatitis.
- Define cirrhosis of the liver. Discuss the causes, main pathological lesions, and outstanding clinical features of the following:
    - (a) micronodular cirrhosis
    - (b) macronodular cirrhosis
    - (c) biliary cirrhosis
- Classify the primary tumors of the liver.

The liver is the largest organ in the body and performs many vital functions. Its blood supply is unique; in addition to receiving arterial blood via the hepatic artery, nearly all the venous blood draining the gastrointestinal tract passes to it via the portal vein. It is therefore not surprising that the liver occupies a key position in relation to the digestive tract and that it performs many metabolic functions — particularly in relation to fat, carbohydrate, and protein metabolism. The secretion of bile is another important function of the liver. Bile contains the bile acids, which aid digestion, as well as the end products of hemoglobin catabolism. The size of the liver is therefore well matched by the multiplicity of its functions. In disease, each aspect of liver function can be disturbed — either separately or, more commonly, in combination.

The Liver in Relation to Its Vascular Supply; Portal Hypertension

The liver has a dual blood supply. Oxygenated blood from the radicles of the hepatic artery as well as blood from the portal vein enters the liver sinusoids; the mixed blood is then collected into tributaries of the hepatic vein. The region supplied by one terminal branch of the hepatic artery has been named an *acinus* by Rappaport (Fig. 33–1). This functional unit differs from the classic hexagonal *liver lobule,* which is pictured as centered on a

Figure 33–1.   The liver acinus. The liver acinus is depicted as an area supplied by a terminal branch °of the hepatic artery arising in a portal triad (labeled P.S.). The cells in zone 1 are closest to their blood supply, whereas those in zone 3 are most remote. Note that the acinus contains cells belonging to two adjacent classical hexagonal lobules. The latter are pictured as being centered on a terminal hepatic venule (T.h.V.). When the blood supply of the liver is impaired (as in congestive heart failure), the cells in zone 3 first undergo necrosis. The damaged area therefore assumes the shape of a sea star (designated by heavy crosshatching). (Courtesy of Dr. A. M. Rappaport. From Rappaport, A. M.: The microcirculatory acinar concept of normal and pathological hepatic structure. Beitraege Pathologie (Stuttgart), *157*:215, 1976.)

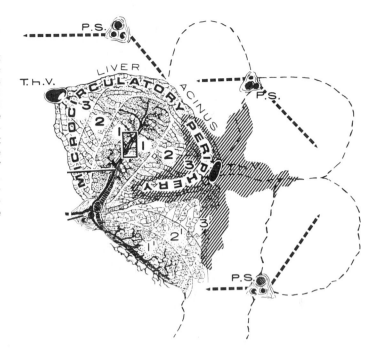

hepatic venule (Figs. 33–2, 33–6, 33–7, and 33–8). The liver receives much of its oxygen from the hepatic arterial blood; a deficiency of this supply results in necrosis in the peripheral part of Rappaport's acinus (zone 3; see Fig. 33–1). Such a response is seen in heart failure ("nutmeg liver"; see Fig. 28–12). Likewise, extensive necrosis is not uncommon in shock and septicemia. Ischemic necrosis involving the whole of many acini to produce an *infarct* is rare because of the dual blood supply, but it is occasionally encountered following obstruction to the hepatic artery or one of its major branches. Hepatic vein thrombosis (*e.g.*, secondary to invasion by a tumor) is another occasional cause.

The normal portal blood is of low pressure (3 to 13 mm Hg) but of large volume (some 1000 to 1200 ml enter the liver from this source per minute). The portal pressure can be measured in several ways. If a catheter is passed through an arm vein and past the right atrium of the heart and then wedged

Figure 33–2.   Normal liver. The cut surface shows the characteristic lobular pattern that is slightly accentuated by congestion. Each lobule has a dark center around a hepatic venule and is surrounded by a pale zone. The arrow points to a small subcapsular angiomatous hamartoma ("cavernous hemangioma").

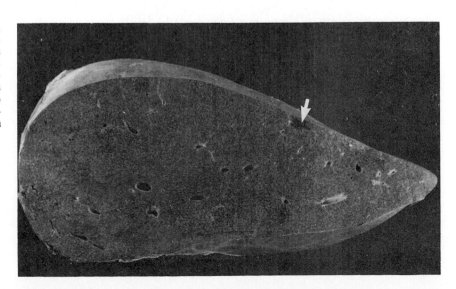

into one of the tributaries of the hepatic vein, the pressure measured in the catheter gives a good indication of the pressure in the terminal part of the hepatic sinuses. This reading is called the *postsinusoidal pressure*.

If a needle connected to a manometer is passed through the skin into the spleen, the intrasplenic pressure measured is closely related to that of blood in the portal vein itself. This is called the *presinusoidal pressure*. Splenic puncture may usefully be followed by injection of a radiopaque substance, the course of which can be followed by radiography. This is one method of demonstrating esophageal varices, a subject discussed later in this chapter.

Portal Hypertension   Obstruction of the blood flow through the liver is a common event in chronic liver disease and leads to portal hypertension. The effects, described in the following sections, are serious.

Development of Portal-Systemic Anastomoses.   There are many areas where small tributaries of the portal vein anastomose with those of the systemic circulation. When there is portal hypertension, these anastomoses enlarge and become varicose. Around the colon these varicosities are of little consequence. On the other hand, when they are around the lower end of the esophagus, the thin-walled dilated veins project into the esophageal lumen, and the overlying mucosa is liable to ulcerate following the trauma of swallowing food or as a result of esophagitis (Figs. 33–3 and 33–4). Massive bleeding is the result, and a pint or more of blood can be vomited *(hematemesis)*.

Portal-Systemic Shunting of Blood.   Portal blood destined for the liver is shunted directly into the systemic circulation. Toxic substances from the intestine pass into the systemic circulation and contribute to the neuropsychi-

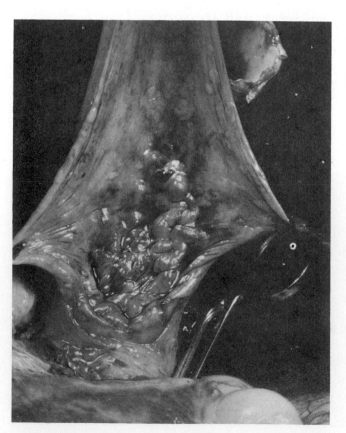

Figure 33–3. Esophageal varices. The esophagus has been opened longitudinally and the lower part held apart to show widely dilated, tortuous varicose veins. Esophageal varices are not usually seen this well at necropsy because the vessels collapse. In this instance, the veins were thrombosed.

Figure 33–4. Radiograph showing esophageal varices. The patient was given a suspension of barium sulfate to swallow; the radiograph shows the outline of the esophageal lumen. Instead of appearing as a simple tube, the esophagus shows numerous indentations that are due to bulging veins. This patient had advanced cirrhosis of the liver. (Courtesy of Dr. D. E. Sanders.)

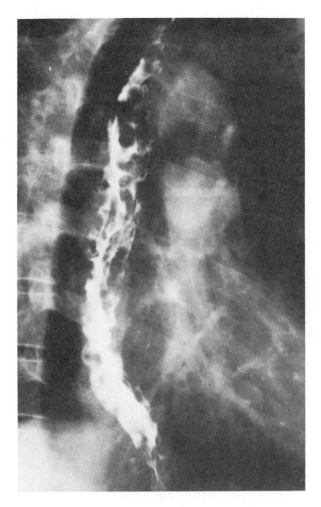

atric manifestations described later. Ammonia is believed to be one of these substances. Others are less well defined, but they may be responsible for the fecal odor of the breath noted in patients with chronic liver disease. Organisms from the gut can also gain access to the general circulation and can cause septicemia. Gram-negative endotoxic shock is sometimes seen as a terminal manifestation of liver disease.

The reduction in hepatic blood flow due to shunting can lead to hepatocellular necrosis but usually only as a terminal event when combined with systemic hypotension.

Congestive Splenomegaly.   Chronic venous congestion leads to splenic enlargement, an important diagnostic clinical sign of portal hypertension. Occasionally, hypersplenism occurs (Chapter 26).

Ascites.   This condition is considered later.

Bilirubin Metabolism and Jaundice

Of all the symptoms of liver disease, jaundice, or *icterus,* is the most immediately apparent. It is due to an excessive amount of bilirubin in the plasma and tissues. Virtually all the tissues of the body become a bright yellow; this coloration is apparent in the skin when the plasma bilirubin level reaches about 3 mg/dl (50 μmol/L). A sign of early jaundice is yellow discoloration of the sclera. This is a particularly useful sign in dark-skinned individuals, in whom jaundice in the skin is less apparent. Jaundice can be understood only in relation to bilirubin metabolism (Fig. 33–5).

When red cells are broken down, the porphyrin moiety of the hemoglobin molecule is converted into bilirubin in the cells of the reticuloendothelial

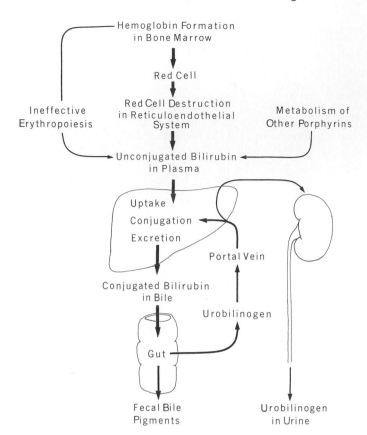

Figure 33–5. Metabolic pathways in the formation and excretion of bilirubin.

system. Bilirubin is insoluble in water; following its release from the reticuloendothelial cells, it is carried in the blood via attachment to albumin. The liver has three important functions in regard to bilirubin:

1. *The liver extracts bilirubin from the blood.*

2. *The liver conjugates bilirubin with glucuronic acid to form bilirubin diglucuronide.* The level of the conjugating enzyme is low in the newborn but can be increased by giving phenobarbital (page 54).

3. *The liver excretes the conjugated bilirubin into the bile.*

Under normal conditions 15 to 20 per cent of the bilirubin content of bile is derived from sources other than red-cell destruction. Much of this originates from the bone marrow during the *formation* of hemoglobulin *(ineffective erythropoiesis)*. The amount of bilirubin formed in this way may be increased in disease, such as in thalassemia and pernicious anemia, and this increase contributes to jaundice. A small amount of bilirubin results from the metabolism of other porphyrins present in enzymes such as oxidases and cytochromes. Figure 33–5 illustrates the main features of bilirubin metabolism. It should be noted in particular that bilirubin in the intestine is converted into urobilinogen by bacterial action; since some of this urobilinogen is reabsorbed and returned to the liver, there is a very considerable enterohepatic recirculation. A small quantity of urobilinogen is excreted in the urine.

Types of Jaundice

Obstructive Jaundice. This occurs when there is an obstruction to the passage of conjugated bilirubin from the liver cells to the intestine. Bilirubin diglucuronide is reabsorbed into the blood, and if the obstruction is complete the patient rapidly becomes deeply jaundiced. The serum bilirubin level may reach 40 mg/dl (680 μmol/L). Since the conjugated bilirubin is soluble in water and is easily excreted by the kidneys, the urine is dark, contrasting with the feces, which are clay-colored. Urobilinogen disappears from the urine.

Two major types of obstructive jaundice are recognized. In *extrahepatic cholestasis,* the bile duct is blocked mechanically. This condition is commonly caused by a gallstone in its lumen or pressure from outside by a carcinoma of the head of the pancreas. In *intrahepatic cholestasis,* the other type of obstructive jaundice, no obvious mechanical cause can be found in the major bile ducts. Instead, it is assumed that the obstruction is in the canaliculi of the liver itself. This condition can occur in a variety of situations. It is seen following the administration of certain drugs, such as chlorpromazine and other phenothiazine derivatives; it is an occasional complication of pregnancy; and it is also seen in the acute fatty alcoholic liver and sometimes during the early stages of acute viral hepatitis.

Three other characteristic features of obstructive jaundice should be noted:

1. *Pruritus.* Often severe, this condition is probably due to retention of *bile salts.*

2. *Malabsorption.* Due to the lack of bile in the intestine, this is a feature of chronic biliary obstruction.

3. *Hypercholesterolemia.* This condition is due to increased synthesis by the liver rather than to biliary obstruction. Lipid-laden macrophages accumulate in various organs and may form tumorlike masses termed *xanthomas.* These structures tend to be bright yellow because of their content of carotinoid pigments;* they are most obvious in the skin.

Hemolytic Jaundice. An excessive rate of destruction of red cells causes an increased rate of bilirubin formation; consequently, the liver is unable to deal with the increased load. Increased erythropoiesis adds to this load by contributing additional bilirubin (Fig. 33–5). The bilirubin in the blood in hemolytic jaundice is unconjugated. It is therefore insoluble in water and is not excreted in the urine. Jaundice of this type is therefore said to be *acholuric.* Increased quantities of bile pigments are excreted in the feces, and the amount of urobilinogen returned to the liver is increased.

Hemolytic jaundice rarely reaches the intensity of that seen in the obstructive variety. An exception to this is that seen in hemolytic disease of the newborn. Because unconjugated bilirubin is relatively soluble in lipids, in severe hemolytic jaundice of infancy bile pigments pass into the brain tissue and can cause severe damage to the developing central nervous system. This is called *kernicterus.*

Hepatocellular Jaundice. Jaundice due to liver cell degeneration or necrosis is the result of a number of factors. In part, there is a failure to extract bilirubin from the blood; in part, there is a failure to excrete it. The hepatocellular type of jaundice is therefore of mixed type.

Hepatocellular Failure

The main manifestations of hepatocellular dysfunction are related to the processes of protein and carbohydrate metabolism and to detoxification.

Disturbances of Protein Metabolism. The liver is responsible for the synthesis of most of the plasma proteins, with the major exception of the immunoglobulins. Progressive hepatocellular dysfunction is characterized by hypoalbuminemia. This dysfunction contributes to the formation of edema of

---

*The carotinoid pigments, or lipochromes, are exogenous lipid-soluble hydrocarbons that constitute the coloring material in beets, carrots, tomatoes, etc. They give adipose tissue and other lipid material a yellow color. This is particularly well shown in atheromatous plaques, the normal corpus luteum of the ovary, and xanthomas.

the dependent parts in addition to being a factor in the production of ascites.

The liver is responsible for the synthesis of most of the clotting factors, the only notable exception being factor VIII, which is made by endothelial cells of the blood vessels. It is hardly surprising, therefore, that liver disease is often accompanied by a tendency to bleed.

The liver is the principal site of deamination of amino acids and is probably the only organ that can convert the ammonia so produced into urea. The other site of ammonia formation is the intestine, where it is formed by bacterial decomposition of protein. Shunting of this ammonia from the portal blood into the systemic circulation has already been mentioned as a possible cause of cerebral dysfunction.

Disturbances of Carbohydrate Metabolism. Following total hepatectomy in an experimental animal there is profound hypoglycemia. The hepatic reserve is great enough that hypoglycemia is rarely a feature of human disease; occasionally, however, it is seen in acute hepatic necrosis and following an acute episode of alcoholic debauchery. Impaired gluconeogenesis is the mechanism (Chapter 23). The impaired glucose tolerance encountered in liver disease is due to portal-systemic shunting.

Failure of Detoxification.   The liver is responsible for detoxifying many agents — either by conjugating them with glucuronic or sulfuric acid, or by conjugating them with an amino acid. The conjugated products are then excreted in the bile or in the urine: conjugation of bilirubin is a classic example of this process. Many drugs are treated in a similar way, and the administration of depressant drugs such as barbiturates or morphine may induce a coma in a patient with hepatocellular dysfunction. Likewise, some steroid hormones are conjugated in the liver prior to their excretion in the urine. The failure to detoxify aldosterone is a possible factor in the formation of ascites. The gynecomastia, testicular atrophy, and loss of body hair sometimes seen in male patients with cirrhosis have been attributed to estrogen excess resulting from inadequate inactivation.

Neuropsychiatric Manifestations (Hepatic Encephalopathy). These pathological conditions assume many forms. Patients with chronic liver disease often exhibit steady deterioration in their intellect: forgetfulness and confusion can progress to stupor and finally to coma. Ataxia and a characteristic "flapping" tremor of the outstretched hands are noteworthy accompaniments. The neuropsychiatric manifestations may be chronic, with the patient exhibiting personality changes, mental deterioration, and other neurological symptoms. On the other hand, the syndrome may be acute and terminate in coma with convulsions.

Animals with a portacaval shunt, or Eck shunt,* can be maintained in a reasonable state of health if given a low-protein diet. If given a large protein meal, they develop coma and die rapidly ("meat intoxication"). It is believed that these manifestations are caused by nitrogenous substances; their precise nature is not known, however. Hepatic encephalopathy is seen in patients who have undergone a similar portacaval anastomosis as treatment for cirrhosis of the liver.

Acute encephalopathy is sometimes precipitated by bleeding esophageal varices; the explanation is that a large quantity of protein-containing blood passes into the intestine and amounts to a heavy protein meal. Since bacterial action in the intestine appears to lead to the formation of damaging nitroge-

---

*This is an artificial shunt made surgically between the portal vein and the inferior vena cava. Portal blood tends to flow directly into the vena cava rather than through the liver.

nous products, the administration of the antibiotic neomycin is currently recommended. It is also of some value in chronic liver disease with impending encephalopathy.

Terminal Manifestations of Hepatic Failure. As the patient's condition deteriorates, certain ill-understood events occur. The plasma sodium level falls, probably because of the intracellular deviation of sodium, and not because of excessive excretion, since administration of salt is not beneficial but, in fact, hastens death by producing circulatory overload and widespread edema. A terminal rise in blood urea nitrogen (BUN) is common and appears to be due to renal failure. This is common in severe hepatic failure, and the combination is known as the *hepatorenal syndrome.* It is debatable whether this is a separate entity. It probably represents renal failure occurring for a variety of reasons in a patient with terminal liver disease.

Degenerative Conditions of the Liver

The liver cells are very susceptible to the effects of many poisons. Poisonous mushrooms, carbon tetrachloride, chloroform, and many drugs (important among which is the anesthetic agent halothane) can all cause severe liver damage, either by a direct action or by some type of hypersensitivity response. Infections, in particular by the viruses of hepatitis, can also produce liver damage.

The effects of hepatotoxic agents can vary from mild, cloudy swelling and fatty change to extensive necrosis (Chapter 4). There is a variable inflammatory response, and the terms "hepatic necrosis" and "hepatitis" are often used synonymously.

Hepatic Necrosis (Hepatitis)

Types. If the liver cells are severely affected, they undergo necrosis. This usually has a *zonal distribution* — that is, the cells of a particular zone in every lobule undergo necrosis. Centrilobular necrosis (affecting Rappaport's zone 3) is the most common (Fig. 33–6). Sometimes the foci of necrosis are erratically distributed: such a response is termed *focal,* or *spotty, necrosis.* It is typical of acute viral hepatitis (Fig. 33–7).

Necrosis may be more widespread and connect central veins to each other and to portal tracts. This is termed *bridging hepatic necrosis* (subacute hepatic necrosis) (Fig. 33–7). Causes include hepatitis B infection; non A, non B hepatitis; hepatitis due to drugs; and chronic active hepatitis of unknown cause.

Occasionally the necrosis is massive and panlobular. Wide tracts of liver are destroyed. This *massive hepatic necrosis* is a feature of acute fulminant hepatitis. Causes include viral hepatitis and acute poisoning; often no cause can be identified.

Figure 33–6. Zonal hepatic necrosis. The classical liver lobules are represented as hexagons (a). The shaded areas in b depict necrosis, which in this example is centrilobular in distribution. (Drawing by Rasa Skudra, Department of Medical Photography and Art, Toronto General Hospital, Toronto.)

ZONAL NECROSIS

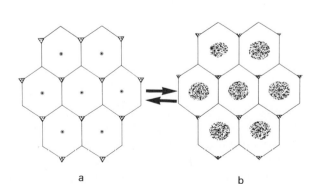

a   b

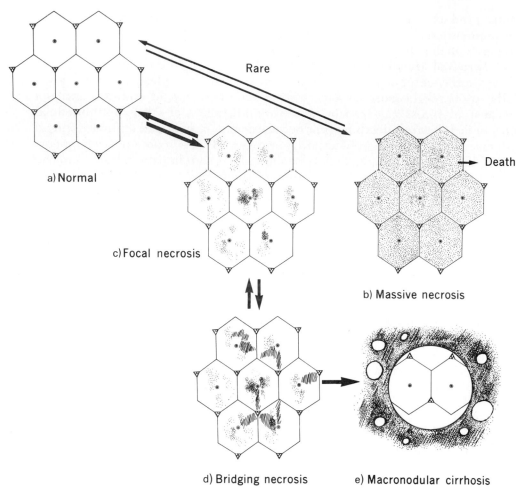

Figure 33–7. Focal and massive hepatic necrosis. Massive necrosis (*b*) generally results in death from cholemia. Occasionally the liver cells regenerate so rapidly that the liver structure returns to normal (*a*). Focal or spotty necrosis (*c*) is typical of viral hepatitis. The areas of necrosis are distributed erratically throughout the liver lobules. Usually recovery is complete, but in some cases necrosis is more extensive and connects central veins to each other and to portal tracts. This is bridging necrosis (*d*). Fibrosis often follows and a macronodular type of cirrhosis develops (*e*). Note that the regeneration nodules vary greatly in size and that in the large nodules areas of normal lobular structure remain. (Drawing by Rasa Skudra, Department of Medical Photography and Art, Toronto General Hospital, Toronto.)

Results. The outcome of necrosis depends upon the severity of the lesions and whether or not the cause persists. With *zonal and focal necrosis* the patient may have no symptoms or may suffer from an acute febrile illness with jaundice and gastrointestinal symptoms and then recover. The necrotic liver cells autolyze and are removed; since the sinusoidal structure and reticulin framework of the liver lobules remain intact, there is excellent regeneration as surviving liver cells divide to replace those that are lost. The liver returns to normal.

Bridging necrosis is a more serious affair, for although recovery is still possible, the process may pursue a chronic course; regeneration occurs from isolated groups of liver cells that remain. Since the scaffold on which these cells may be arranged has largely been destroyed or has collapsed, irregular nodules termed *regeneration nodules* are formed. The final result is one form of cirrhosis of the liver (*macronodular cirrhosis*) (Fig. 33–7).

With massive necrosis the patient often dies of acute liver failure in the initial phases. In the few patients who recover, remaining liver cells can regenerate quickly before the lobular framework collapses. The liver therefore *returns to normal*. In some cases it is probable that regeneration nodules are formed and this results in cirrhosis.

Fatty change is an important lesion and can be caused by an inappropriate diet. Starvation and overeating both cause fatty change, but an imbalanced diet results in the most severe change (see "Kwashiorkor," Chapter 23). It is also common in chronic alcoholism. *Fatty Liver*

If the cause of fatty liver is removed early enough, complete recovery is usual; such recovery is not possible if the condition is allowed to persist indefinitely and is due to alcoholism. Gradually, fibrous tissue forms around Rappaport's acinus. Hepatic cells become isolated as the lobules are split up. Some cells undergo necrosis, whereas others regenerate. This results in a finely nodular cirrhotic liver not fundamentally different from that seen after bridging hepatic necrosis (Fig. 33–8).

There can be little doubt that alcohol abuse can adversely affect the liver (Chapter 4). The liver of the chronic alcoholic often shows fatty change, and in some subjects this progresses to fibrosis and ultimately cirrhosis. Acute episodes of alcohol intake result in patchy liver cell necrosis. The cells contain alcoholic hyaline, and foci of necrosis are accompanied by a polymorph infiltration. This condition, which is called *alcoholic hepatitis*, is a phase in the evolution of alcoholic cirrhosis. *Alcohol and the Liver*

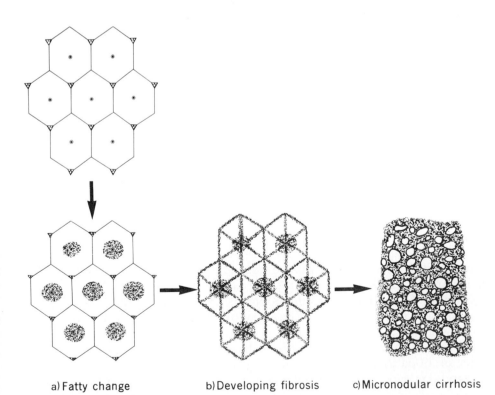

a) Fatty change   b) Developing fibrosis   c) Micronodular cirrhosis

Figure 33–8. Alcoholic liver disease. In the early stages of alcoholic liver disease fatty change develops in the centrilobular zones (*a*). Gradually liver cells undergo necrosis and fibrous tissue forms around the acini of Rappaport (*b*). In this way the lobules are split up and multiple small regenerative nodules are produced. Micronodular hepatic cirrhosis is the end-result (*c*). (Drawing by Rasa Skudra, Department of Medical Photography and Art, Toronto General Hospital, Toronto.)

Hepatitis

Acute Viral Hepatitis. Two distinct epidemiological types of acute viral hepatitis are known. Hepatitis A commonly occurs in institutions such as schools and military camps. It is contracted by the ingestion of contaminated food, has an incubation period of about 1 month, and has an excellent prognosis. Hepatitis B is usually contracted by an injection of contaminated serum; a number of patients with this type of hepatitis progress to chronic hepatitis and cirrhosis of the liver. Recently, cases of hepatitis have been described that are due neither to virus A nor to virus B (non A, non B hepatitis). The nature of the infective agents is described in Chapter 12.

Symptoms and Pathology of Viral Hepatitis. The onset is usually insidious with mild fatigue, lassitude, and sometimes fever. Nausea, vomiting, and diarrhea are not uncommon, and an aversion to both food and cigarette smoking is a curious symptom. Such a flulike illness may be the only manifestation of hepatitis, but in other patients the disease progresses and jaundice appears, evident at first in the conjunctivae and later in the skin. Some tenderness over the liver may be noticed, and enlargement of the organ may be detected.

The pathology of the usual case of acute viral hepatitis is that of *focal hepatic necrosis* with associated *lymphocytic infiltration*. Regeneration of liver cells accompanies the necrosis, and recovery is complete. Sometimes recovery is delayed and may take 3 or 4 months, or even longer. A liver biopsy performed during this period may show continuing focal hepatic necrosis (*chronic lobular hepatitis*) or merely a lymphocytic infiltrate in the portal triads (*chronic persistent hepatitis*). In either event the prognosis is excellent, and the distinction between these two types of chronic hepatitis is made on the biopsy findings. It is of academic interest only.

In some infections with virus B and in non A, non B hepatitis the liver shows more severe necrosis with bridging. Recovery may occur gradually, or the illness may progress to *chronic active hepatitis* and *cirrhosis*.

Uncommonly, viral hepatitis presents as an acute fulminant disease with a high mortality. This is least common with hepatitis A. As noted previously, if recovery does occur it is complete and the liver returns to normal.

It should be noted that in the usual case there are no clinical features by which one can distinguish among the three types of viral hepatitis. However, hepatitis A rarely if ever progresses to chronic liver damage. Approximately 10 per cent of patients with hepatitis B develop chronic hepatitis.

The pathogenesis of viral hepatitis is not understood. There appears to be an inverse relationship between the amount of virus in the liver and the severity of the disease. Thus, a great excess of HBsAg is present in the cytoplasm of the liver cells in subjects who are carriers and have minimal or no disease. Because of this it has been suggested that the liver cell damage is immunologically mediated, with the host reacting against altered liver cells rather than against the virus itself.

Chronic Hepatitis. Chronic hepatitis has been defined as "chronic inflammation of the liver continuing without improvement for at least 6 months."*

Chronic Active Hepatitis. This disease is characterized by recurrent attacks of hepatitis, ultimately developing into cirrhosis, usually of the macronodular type, which is fatal within 10 years. The disease was first

---

*Fogarty International Center Proceedings, No. 22: Diseases of the liver and biliary tract. Standardization of nomenclature, diagnostic criteria, and diagnostic methodology. Washington, DHEW Publication No. (NIH) 76–725, 1976. In practice alcoholic hepatitis and cholangitis are excluded. So also are chronic inflammations that are of obvious cause, *e.g.*, actinomycosis and tuberculosis.

described as affecting young people, 75 per cent of the patients being women. Hypergammaglobulinemia is a characteristic feature, and both antinuclear factor and rheumatoid factors are usually present. Although the disease was originally called *lupoid hepatitis*, there is no evidence that the condition is related to lupus erythematosus itself. Nevertheless, over half the patients also have arthritis. Antibodies that react with smooth muscle are present in most cases, and the disease therefore has a strong autoimmune component.

The hallmarks of chronic active hepatitis are *piecemeal necrosis*, a *lymphocytic infiltration*, and *fibrosis*. Piecemeal necrosis is defined as destruction of the liver cells at the interface between the liver parenchyma and the connective tissues of the portal triads or areas of fibrosis. There is an associated lymphocytic inflammatory reaction, and fibrosis steadily develops as the adjacent liver cells undergo necrosis. Bridging necrosis may also be present.

The syndrome of chronic active hepatitis has now been extended to include other groups of patients. Some are middle-aged women, and others are men who usually have HBsAg in their blood and are examples of patients with chronic viral hepatitis. Autoantibodies are usually present, but this autoimmune component is less striking than in the original "lupoid hepatitis." Still other cases of chronic hepatitis may be due to the effects of drugs or alcohol.

Cirrhosis of the Liver

The term "cirrhosis" (from Greek *kirrhos*, orange yellow + *nosos*, disease) was introduced by Laennec, who was impressed by the tawny color of the liver in this condition, but this is due merely to fatty change of the liver cells. The important structural features of cirrhosis are the *destruction of the liver parenchyma* and its *replacement by fibrous tissue*, thereby disrupting the normal lobular architecture. There is also active regeneration of the liver cells occurring at the same time as this fibrous reparative process. The *formation of regenerative nodules* is the third essential component of cirrhosis.

Cirrhosis is best regarded as an end-stage condition resulting from liver damage due to any cause: poisons, alcohol, inadequate diet, infection, genetic error, and others. Unfortunately, an etiological classification of cirrhosis is unsatisfactory, because the cause is unknown in many cases ("*cryptogenic cirrhosis*"). For purposes of disease classification, the condition is categorized by descriptions that are based on the gross appearance of the liver. If the nodules are small and of uniform size, the term *micronodular cirrhosis* is applied (Fig. 33–9). This condition commonly, but not always, is due to alcohol abuse. It contrasts with *macronodular cirrhosis*, in which the nodules are of varying size, many of them being large (Fig. 33–10). In practice, there is no sharp line of demarcation between these two types of cirrhosis, and many cases fall into a mixed group (Figs. 33–11 and 33–12).

Symptoms of Cirrhosis. Cirrhosis is commonly asymptomatic until some complication makes the condition obvious. The appearance of jaundice, edema of the ankles, or progressive abdominal enlargement may bring the disease to the attention of the patient. Increasing weakness, loss of weight, loss of body hair and testicular atrophy are all features that may appear. Commonly the first symptom is massive hematemesis, and this is followed by the rapid development of hepatocellular failure with coma and death.

CASE HISTORY I. (See Figure 33–9). The patient was a 62-year-old woman with a long history of chronic alcoholism. Six days before admission to a hospital, she noticed black tarry stools (melena). A few days later, she vomited about one pint of blood. On admission, her blood pressure was 95/60 mm Hg, and she was in a state of shock. Her

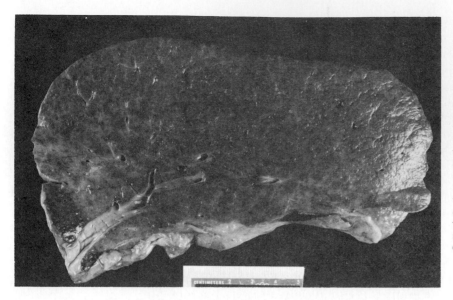

Figure 33–9.   Micronodular cirrhosis of the liver. The cut surface of the specimen shows complete loss of the normal lobular pattern (compare with Figure 33–2). The liver parenchyma now consists of poorly delineated regeneration nodules that are best seen where light is reflected from the surface of the right-hand side of the picture. In some areas, extensive fibrosis appears as obvious gray-white tissue. The specimen is from a patient who died of bleeding esophageal varices and who exhibited little clinical evidence of hepatic dysfunction until shortly before death. For a more complete description, see Case History I.

abdomen was distended because of ascites, and her spleen could not be felt. Jaundice was not evident. Laboratory investigations at this time revealed the following:

>Serum bilirubin: 1.75 mg/dl (normal, 0.3 to 1.0 mg/dl)
>Serum proteins:
>>Albumin: 1.8 g/dl (normal, 4.0 to 5.7 g/dl)
>>Globulin: 3.9 g/dl (normal, 1.5 to 3.0 g/dl)
>>Total: 5.7 g/dl (normal, 6.2 to 8.2 g/dl)
>Serum potassium: 2.5 mEq/L (normal, 3.5 to 5 mEq/L)
>Hemoglobin: 10.9 g/dl; red cells normochromic and normocytic

The hypokalemia was attributed to previous diuretic therapy (Chapter 19). Gastroscopy revealed bleeding esophageal varices, but in spite of transfusion and other supportive treatment, the blood pressure continued to fall, and the patient became more and more confused. She vomited a small quantity of blood on several occasions, but showed no obvious dramatic hemorrhage. Terminally, her urine output diminished, her blood urea nitrogen rose to 65 mg/dl, and the patient suffered a cardiac arrest. She was successfully resuscitated but had a second arrest and was pronounced dead.

Necropsy revealed bilateral pleural effusions and 1500 ml of ascites. There were multiple small acute gastric erosions, and the small hematemeses occurring in the hospital were attributed to them. The kidneys were swollen because of edema, but necrosis was not detectable microscopically (Chapter 35). The cirrhotic liver, which weighed 1900 grams (normal, about 1500 grams), is shown in Figure 33–9. Esophageal varices were present, but no definite point of bleeding could be identified; this is often difficult, since the veins are emptied of blood after death.

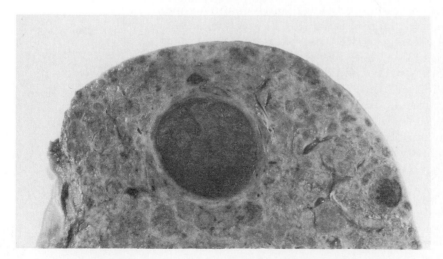

Figure 33–10.   Macronodular cirrhosis of the liver. There is replacement of liver by regeneration nodules that vary greatly in size. The two circular hemorrhagic (dark) nodules shown here consist of hepatoma.

Figure 33-11. Cirrhosis of the liver. The cut surface of the liver shows complete replacement of normal liver by regenerative nodules. Many of the nodules are small, but others are larger. See Fig. 33-12 for close-up view.

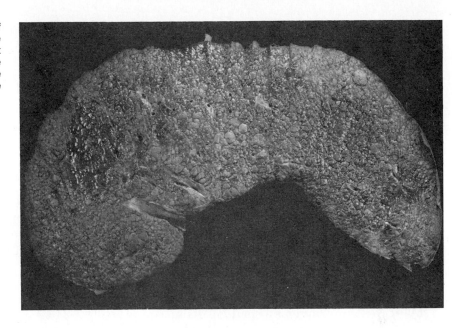

Ascites is a common manifestation of cirrhosis and has several causes. Hypoalbuminemia and aldosterone excess are contributory factors, but the main cause appears to be obstruction of the flow of blood through the liver. This obstruction is postsinusoidal and results in an increased rate of formation of lymph in the liver. Normally the lymph is drained away by lymphatics into the thoracic duct, but in cirrhosis the excess of lymph produced oozes or weeps from the liver and drips into the peritoneal cavity. A second effect of portal hypertension is an increased transudate of fluid from the surface of the viscera drained by the portal vein. This fluid presumably has a low protein content. When it is added to the lymph from the liver, the result is an ascitic fluid having a protein content of 1 to 2 g/dl. Most of this protein is albumin.

Figure 33-12. Cirrhosis of the liver. This is part of the liver shown in Fig. 33-11. Note the wide variation in the size of the nodules. Microscopically recognizable lobular structures can be identified in the large nodules. This example of cirrhosis may therefore be classified as of mixed type.

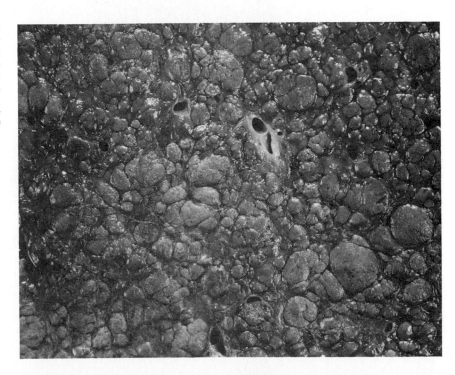

Relief of ascites by removal of the fluid also removes much albumin, often adding to the patient's problems. Also the sudden removal of a large quantity of fluid can lead to hypovolemia and shock.

The other symptoms of terminal cirrhosis — including neuropsychiatric features, coma, and a bleeding tendency — have been described under hepatocellular failure.

Biliary Cirrhosis

Obstruction to the bile duct, particularly if combined with infection (*cholangitis*) can sometimes lead to such severe liver-cell damage that cirrhosis develops. There is, in addition, a *primary form of biliary cirrhosis*. This is most frequently encountered in middle-aged women. Itching is usually the first symptom, and this is followed by the development of obstructive jaundice. The disease has an autoimmune component, for the blood contains IgM antibodies active against bile-duct components as well as IgG antimitochondrial antibodies. The detection of the latter is a useful diagnostic feature of primary biliary cirrhosis.

Tumors of the Liver

The finding of one or more *vascular hamartomas* (hemangiomas) of the liver is a common event at necropsy, but apart from the very rare occurrence of intraperitoneal bleeding, these are of no significance during life (Fig. 33–2). *Adenomas* are rare, although recently a number of cases have been reported in women on the birth-control pill. The tumors are vascular and clinically can present as a sudden intraperitoneal hemorrhage. This appears to be a rare complication of taking the birth-control pill, but since the event has only recently been recognized, its true incidence has yet to be determined.

Carcinoma of the Liver

Cancer of the liver can arise in a normal liver, but it is more often encountered in livers that are already the site of some other disease, most commonly cirrhosis (Figs. 33–10 and 33–13). Nevertheless, many other factors are involved, for although in North America and Europe it has been estimated

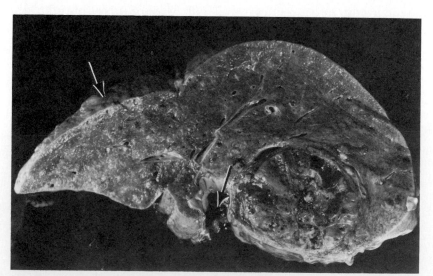

Figure 33–13.   Carcinoma of the liver. The specimen shows a large, spherical mass of tumor with several small satellite nodules. The tumor has invaded the inferior vena cava, and there is superimposed thrombosis (arrow at lower center). The remainder of the liver shows the characteristic features of micronodular cirrhosis. The nodularity can be seen best on the surface of the liver (arrow at upper left).

The patient had a 13-year history of chronic liver disease and had died following massive bleeding from ruptured esophageal varices. Necropsy revealed tumor invasion of the vena cava and the portal vein. Small pulmonary deposits were the only metastases found. Splenomegaly, ascites, edema of the legs, and testicular atrophy were other findings related to the liver disease.

that between 4 and 10 per cent of patients with cirrhosis eventually develop cancer of the liver, in some parts of Africa and the Orient the figure is closer to 60 per cent. Additional factors that seem to be involved are the ingestion of aflatoxin, an alkaloid derived from a fungus that infects peanuts, in the African diet, and the presence of HBsAg antigen, which is present in patients with hepatitis. Possibly the agents of viral hepatitis are oncogenic.

Two types of primary carcinoma of the liver are recognized:

Hepatoma. This tumor is composed of atypical hepatocytes and usually occurs in patients with cirrhosis. Quite often portal vein invasion and thrombosis lead to the sudden development of ascites in a patient known to have cirrhosis. Massive hepatomegaly is usually a feature.

Cholangiocarcinoma. About 20 per cent of primary liver tumors are derived from the bile ducts, and histologically they are scirrhous adenocarcinomas. Cirrhosis of the liver is less often a precursor to this type of cancer than it is to hepatoma.

Secondary Tumors of the Liver

It has been estimated that metastatic liver carcinoma is found in about 36 per cent of all cancer patients. It is more common in patients with cancer of the breast, stomach, and colon than in those having primary tumors of other sites. The liver is also a common site for metastatic melanoma.

Review Questions

1. The condition of a man with known chronic liver disease suddenly deteriorates, and he dies. Describe the lesions that you would expect to find at his necropsy.

2. Compare obstructive jaundice with hemolytic jaundice with particular reference to the following:
   (a) the color of the patient
   (b) the color of the urine and feces
   (c) the quantity of urobilinogen in the urine

3. Why is it dangerous to administer to a patient with advanced liver disease each of the following:
   (a) a large protein meal
   (b) morphine
   (c) intravenous saline

4. Compare hepatitis A with hepatitis B with respect to:
   (a) incubation period
   (b) mode of infection
   (c) manifestations during the acute illness
   (d) possible end-results and complications

5. Describe what is meant by bridging necrosis and indicate the circumstances under which it occurs.

6. Describe the known factors in the cause and pathogenesis of hepatic cirrhosis.

Selected Readings

Rappaport, A. M.: The microcirculatory hepatic unit. Microvascular Research, 6:212–228, 1973.

Robbins, S. L., and Cotran, R. S.: Pathologic Basis of Disease. 2nd ed. Philadelphia, W. B. Saunders Company, 1979. Note, in particular, Chapter 21, "The Liver and Biliary Tract."

Schaffner, F., Sherlock, S., and Leevy, C. M. (Eds.): The Liver and Its Diseases. New York, Intercontinental Medical Book Corporation, 1974, 353 pp. An advanced reference book covering a wide range of topics by 47 contributors.

Scheuer, P. J.: Liver Biopsy Interpretation. 3rd ed. London, Baillière Tindall, 1980, 260 pp. An excellent reference book on the morphological aspects of liver disease.

Sherlock, S.: Diseases of the Liver and Biliary System. 5th ed. Oxford, Blackwell, Scientific Publications Ltd., 1975, 821 pp.

Smetana, H. F.: Cirrhosis of the liver: principles of classification, histogenesis, and pathogenesis. Pathology Annual, 7:107–144, 1972.

Diseases of the Pancreas and the Biliary Tract

After studying this chapter the student should be able to:

- List the secretions of the pancreas.
- Describe the main features of cystic fibrosis as it affects the pancreas, the lung, the liver, and the eccrine sweat glands.
- Describe the known causes, the course, the lesions, and the complications of acute pancreatitis.
- Outline the main features of
    - (a) chronic pancreatitis
    - (b) carcinoma of the head of the pancreas
    - (c) carcinoma of the body of the pancreas
- Name the structures that constitute the biliary tract.
- List the common types of gallstones.
- Describe the factors that are thought to lead to gallstone formation.
- List the complications of cholelithiasis.
- Describe the clinical and pathological features of the following conditions:
    - (a) chronic cholecystitis
    - (b) carcinoma of the gallbladder
    - (c) carcinoma of the ampulla of Vater

THE PANCREAS

Development and Function

The pancreas is a dual organ. Its exocrine portion originates from two buds of the primitive gut. The endocrine portion forms the islets of Langerhans, which, despite their small size, are of vital importance because they secrete insulin.

The pancreas lies on the posterior abdominal wall and pours its exocrine secretions into the duodenum. These secretions contain the precursors of three important enzymes: (1) *trypsin*, which digests protein; (2) *lipase*, which splits fat; and (3) *amylase*, which splits carbohydrate. In each case the active enzyme is formed within the contents of the duodenum. The reserve capacity of the pancreas is so great that only severe atrophy of the exocrine elements or blockage of its duct leads to upsets in digestion and absorption. In practice, impairment of fat absorption is the most important disorder; steatorrhea and lack of absorption of fat-soluble vitamins are the predominant symptoms of this condition (Chapter 32).

Cystic Fibrosis (Mucoviscidosis)

This disease is inherited as a mendelian autosomal recessive trait, and unfortunately there is no way at the present time to detect heterozygote carriers. Mucoviscidosis is characterized by an abnormality of the exocrine secretory glands and is remarkable for the great variety of its presentations, depending on which glands are affected.

When the pancreas is involved, the gland secretes thick mucus that obstructs the ducts and causes them to dilate. The gland itself atrophies. If the disease develops *in utero,* the absence of pancreatic enzymes leads to such viscosity of the intestinal contents (called *meconium*) that intestinal obstruction and even perforation of the gut ensue *(meconium ileus).* In the more common type of cystic fibrosis, the infant or child develops a chronic *malabsorption syndrome,* accompanied by an excessive appetite, failure to gain weight, and often constipation.

When the lung is involved, the thick mucus together with infection produces bronchopneumonia, bronchiectasis, and lung abscesses (see Fig. 30–8). Chronic lung disease is a feature of most cases of cystic fibrosis in patients who survive for several years. Hypovitaminosis A and other effects of malabsorption complicate this clinical picture.

Occasionally the liver is affected, and chronic bile duct inflammation leads to a type of *cirrhosis.* Involvement of the cervical mucus leads to *infertility* in most female patients, and likewise most males are *sterile.* It is evident that there is involvement of many exocrine glands and that in some sites this causes symptoms. A remarkable feature of the disease is that the eccrine sweat glands secrete a sweat containing a high concentration of salt. *Chemical examination of sweat for the level of salt is a diagnostic test.*

The fundamental defect in cystic fibrosis is not yet known. The secretion of viscid mucus plays an important role in the pancreatic and lung lesions. It does not explain the abnormal sweat-gland function, because sweat contains no mucus.

Acute Pancreatitis

Acute pancreatitis can be mild and can lead to vague abdominal symptoms, but more often it is severe and of sudden onset and presents with intense pain often referred to as an "acute abdomen."

Areas of pancreas undergo necrosis, and there is an associated acute inflammatory reaction. The pathogenesis is obscure, for although in a few instances the cause is a known infectious agent (*e.g.,* mumps virus), the vast majority of cases are not so related. The disease appears to be due to the sudden release of active pancreatic enzymes within the organ itself. Blood vessels are digested, and in severe cases the whole pancreas is converted into a necrotic, hemorrhagic mass. Released lipases cause necrosis in adjacent peripancreatic fat and omentum; because of their *dystrophic calcification* these areas of fat necrosis are soon evident as chalky white areas (Fig. 34–1). So rapidly may this calcification occur that the patient actually develops symptoms of hypocalcemia (*e.g.,* tetany). The necrotic pancreatic cells release amylase, which can be detected in the blood. A blood amylase determination is a useful test for the diagnosis of acute pancreatitis.

Symptoms of acute hemorrhagic pancreatitis are sometimes difficult to distinguish from those of other causes of acute abdominal pain (*e.g.,* perforated peptic ulcer, acute cholecystitis, and acute appendicitis). Laparotomy is often performed because of the difficulty in arriving at a diagnosis; the surgeon is confronted by blood-stained ascitic fluid containing globules of fat. The detection of amylase in the fluid further confirms the diagnosis. Also characteristic is the presence of many foci of fat necrosis with calcification.

Etiology. Most patients with acute pancreatitis have chronic gallbladder disease, and attacks usually occur *after a large meal* or an *alcoholic spree.* The pathogenesis is not completely understood, but it is thought that the entry of a large quantity of acid gastric contents, particularly if it contains alcohol, can lead to excessive stimulation of the pancreas by the hormone *secretin,* which is released from the duodenal mucosa. This leads to marked secretion of pancreatic juice, but precisely how this fluid escapes into the gland substance and digests the tissues is not known. One explanation is that

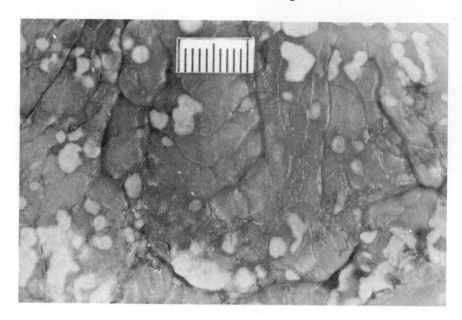

Figure 34–1. Pancreatic fat necrosis. The specimen is from the surface of the greater omentum of a patient who died of acute hemorrhagic pancreatitis. The opaque white areas are foci of fat necrosis with heterotopic calcification.

there is an obstruction produced by a stone impacted in the common channel that the common bile duct and main pancreatic duct share. This theory proposes that the bile activates the pancreatic enzymes and that the increased pressure causes rupture of the duct. This is an unlikely explanation because the bile duct and pancreatic duct do not always share a common pathway into the duodenum, and furthermore, an impacted gallstone is rarely found.

Course of Acute Pancreatitis. Up to 50 per cent of patients die in shock during the first week. Surgery can contribute to this. Complications in those who survive this period are *abscess* and *pseudocyst formation.* The latter consists of a loculated accumulation of fluid in the peritoneum adjacent to the pancreas. Such a cyst usually requires surgical drainage. Another cause of pseudocyst formation is direct injury to the pancreas by a blow to the abdomen.

Chronic Pancreatitis

Chronic pancreatitis — like the acute form of the condition — is also associated with gallbladder disease, overindulgence, and alcoholism. The clinical picture is vague; it ranges from no symptoms at all to repeated attacks of mild acute pancreatitis that are not severe enough to warrant surgical intervention. Sometimes the major complaint is one of a constant pain in the back.

In its early stages chronic pancreatitis leads to no digestive upset. Later, however, signs of malabsorption may appear, and in a few cases impaired glucose tolerance and diabetes mellitus supervene.

An important feature of chronic pancreatitis is that a surgeon may easily mistake the hard, fibrous organ for carcinoma. Even when biopsy or necropsy material is available, the distinction between a fibrosed atrophic pancreas and a scirrhous carcinoma can be very difficult.

Carcinoma of the Pancreas

Cancer of the pancreas arises from the ducts and is the most important tumor to be considered. About two thirds of the tumors arise in the head of the pancreas. Obstructive jaundice is often the first sign, and characteristically the obstruction is associated with palpable distention of the gallbladder. Carcinoma of the body or tail of the pancreas produces few symptoms until the growth is large, has invaded local structures, or has metastasized. Loss of appetite, loss of weight, vague back pain, and general malaise with depression are the symptoms of this silent killer.

The incidence of cancer of the pancreas is increasing, and the disease is now an important cause of death. Heavy tobacco smoking, a diet high in fats, and industrial exposure to aromatic amines (such as benzidine) have been suggested as possible etiological factors.

The treatment of carcinoma of the pancreas is extremely unsatisfactory. Occasionally surgical resection is possible, but the inaccessibility of the pancreas and the closeness of important anatomical structures make this disease untreatable in the majority of the cases. Anastomosis of the gallbladder to a loop of intestine relieves the obstructive jaundice with its distressing pruritus.

Diseases of the islets are considered in Chapter 24, because their major effects are on glucose metabolism.

The Islets of Langerhans

THE BILIARY TRACT

Introduction

Bile is formed continuously by the liver and passes down the *intrahepatic bile ducts* to reach the *common bile duct*. This duct empties into the duodenum, and its orifice is guarded by the *sphincter of Oddi*. Immediately above the sphincter there is a dilatation called the *ampulla of Vater*. The sphincter of Oddi is normally closed, and bile therefore flows through the *cystic duct* to reach the *gallbladder*, where it is stored and concentrated. When gastric contents — particularly those containing fat — enter the duodenum, the duodenal mucosa secretes a hormone *(cholecystokinin)* that causes the gallbladder to contract and the sphincter of Oddi to relax. Bile then enters the duodenum.

Diseases of the gallbladder are frequent. Inflammation of this organ *(cholecystitis)* ranks with appendicitis as a cause of abdominal pain requiring surgical exploration. The presence of gallstones *(cholelithiasis)* is often associated with inflammation. This topic is discussed below.

Cholelithiasis

Gallstones may be found in any part of the biliary tract, but they are most frequent in the gallbladder. They are more common in women than in men, in a ratio of about four to one. Pregnancy appears to predispose female patients to stone formation, and the typical sufferer is caricatured as being "female, fertile, fat, and forty." Nevertheless, gallstone disease often affects young adults, and any association with obesity appears to be without foundation.

Types of Gallstones. Gallstones are occasionally composed of pure cholesterol (usually solitary stones) or bile pigments (calcium bilirubinate); most gallstones are *mixed* and consist of cholesterol, bile salts, and calcium salts. Often they are multiple (Figs. 34–2 and 34–3).

Cause of Gallstones. Until recently, *infection* and *stasis* were considered to be the main factors leading to gallstone formation. It is now thought that infection and stasis are the *effects* of cholelithiasis, and that the major cause is the *secretion of an abnormal bile by the liver*. The large amount of cholesterol in bile is kept in solution by its being aggregated to form *micelles* having an outer coating of phospholipid and bile salts. A deficiency of bile salt formation appears to be the major factor in producing gallstones. Recently attempts have been made to alter the composition of bile by medical treatment. Chenodeoxycholic acid by mouth appears to lead to the dissolution of cholesterol stones, and there is every hope that in the future the treatment of cholelithiasis will be medical and not surgical.

Complications of Gallstones

Obstruction. A stone may become impacted in the neck of the gallblad-

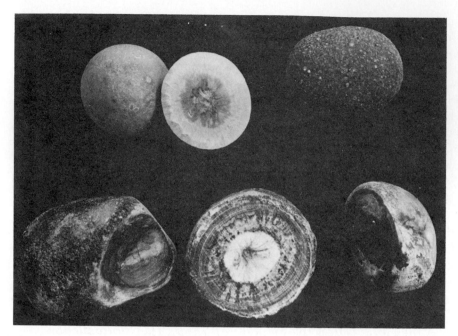

Figure 34–2. Gallstones. The three gallstones shown in the upper part of the picture were solitary stones, each being found in a separate gallbladder. They are composed mainly of cholesterol. One has been cut to show its internal structure. The appearance of lines radiating from the center is due to crystals of cholesterol.

The three faceted stones in the lower part of the picture were found in one gallbladder. One has been cut and shows a pale center of cholesterol. This is surrounded by rings that contain varying amounts of bile pigments. These stones are considered "mixed."

der or in the cystic duct. Because bile cannot enter the gallbladder, it therefore becomes distended with mucus *(mucocele).* A stone impacted in the bile duct *(e.g.,* in the ampulla of Vater) causes intermittent obstruction with *obstructive jaundice.* This condition fluctuates in intensity in contrast to the progressive jaundice of carcinoma.

If a gallstone suddenly obstructs one of the bile passages, distention of the wall causes severe pain that is felt in the midline of the abdomen. The common cause is a stone in the cystic duct. The pain is of sudden onset, persists for some hours with unremitting severity, and then abates as suddenly as it began. This is called *biliary colic* and differs from intestinal colic, in which crampy pains recur and remit at intervals.

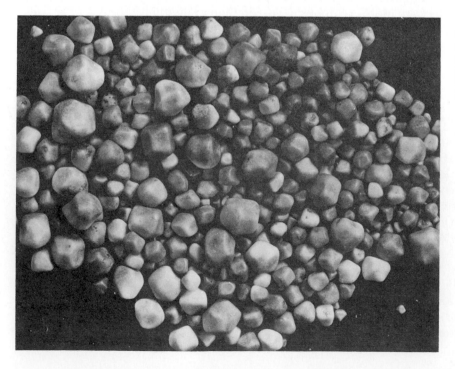

Figure 34–3. Gallstones. One gallbladder contained these small mixed stones. Note how each stone is faceted as a result of contact with its neighbors during its formation. Several "families" of stones are present.

Infection.   The presence of stones in the gallbladder predisposes the patient to the development of cholecystitis. Likewise, a stone in the common bile duct predisposes to infection in the entire intrahepatic biliary system *(ascending cholangitis)*. This can be mild and clinically inapparent, or it can cause severe symptoms. Attacks of fever with liver tenderness and jaundice indicate suppurative cholangitis with liver abscess formation.

Acute Cholecystitis.   Acute cholecystitis is characterized by the sudden onset of pain, fever, nausea, and vomiting. The pain, accompanied by tenderness, is in the right upper quadrant of the abdomen. Gallstones are present in over 90 per cent of cases, and there is often either a history of a previous attack or other symptoms attributable to the stones.

The cause and pathogenesis of acute cholecystitis are not known. Infection is not the cause, since organisms are not present in the bile in the early stages. Impaction of a stone is probably an important factor in initiating an attack. Distention of the gallbladder may imperil its blood supply so that infarction occurs.

Many cases of acute cholecystitis subside spontaneously. The mode of treatment is controversial; some surgeons delay operating until absolutely necessary. In some cases the gallbladder ruptures, leading to a severe peritonitis, which is due partly to an irritating effect of bile and partly to organisms that are found in the later stages of an acutely inflamed gallbladder.

Chronic Cholecystitis.   Repeated attacks of acute cholecystitis (either mild or severe) combined with stones results in the gallbladder's becoming greatly thickened, shrunken, and functionless. At this stage the symptoms are vague: flatulence, aversion to fatty foods, indigestion, and ill-defined pain in the upper abdomen.

Carcinoma of the Gallbladder.   This tumor is more common in women and the elderly. The prognosis is very poor, since local spread to the liver has generally occurred by the time the diagnosis has been made.

Carcinoma of the Biliary Tract

Carcinoma of the Ampulla of Vater.   This is an occasional cause of obstructive jaundice.

1. A 70-year-old man has gradually increasing jaundice. He complains of no pain. Discuss the possible causes and indicate the one that is most likely.

Review Questions

2. Describe the clinical features that one should consider in differentiating between an attack of acute pancreatitis and an attack of acute cholecystitis.

3. Courvoisier's law indicates that in obstructive jaundice due to a malignant tumor, the gallbladder is distended and can be palpated, whereas in obstructive jaundice due to gallstones the gallbladder is small and cannot be palpated. Can you suggest why this should be true?

Leading Article: Dynamics of the common duct. Lancet, *1*:236–237, 1968.
Leading Article: Vascular aspects of cholecystitis. British Medical Journal, *2*:133, 1968.
Leading Article: Abnormal bile or faulty gall bladder? British Medical Journal, *4*:571–572, 1970.
Leading Article: Cystic fibrosis in adults. British Medical Journal, *2*:1119, 1977.
Leading Article: Choosing patients for chenodeoxycholic acid therapy. British Medical Journal, *2*:626, 1979.
Robbins, S. L., and Cotran, R. S.: Pathologic Basis of Disease. 2nd ed. Philadelphia, W. B. Saunders Company, 1979. See, in particular, pp. 1071–1091 for a discussion of the biliary system as well as pp. 1092–1114, which is the chapter on the pancreas.

Selected Readings

Diseases of the Kidneys and Urinary Tract

After studying this chapter the student should be able to:

- Describe the major functions of the kidney.
- Outline the process of urine formation and indicate the relative roles of the various parts of the nephron.
- Define polyuria, polydipsia, nocturia, anuria, and retention with overflow.
- Describe the principles underlying the creatinine clearance test.
- List the methods that are used to examine urine in clinical medicine.
- List the types of casts that are found in urine and indicate their significance.
- Describe the important causes and manifestations of acute renal failure.
- Describe the important causes and manifestations of chronic renal failure.
- Describe the important causes and manifestations of the nephrotic syndrome.
- List the types of glomerulonephritis and indicate the outstanding features of each type.
- Describe the main features and known causes of interstitial nephritis.
- Discuss the pathogenesis of urinary tract infection and describe the clinical features of each of the following: acute urethritis with cystitis, acute pyelonephritis, and chronic pyelonephritis.
- Describe what is meant by the term "end-stage kidney."
- Compare clear-cell carcinoma of the kidney with carcinoma of the bladder.
- Describe the common causes and effects of urinary tract obstruction.
- Classify the types of urinary calculi and list their effects.

THE KIDNEYS

It is a popular misconception that the only major function performed by the kidneys is the excretion of the waste products of metabolism. In fact, the kidneys have many other functions, particularly in relation to maintaining a fixed internal environment. Unless these other functions are appreciated, the features of renal failure cannot be understood.

Functions of the Kidney

1. Excretion of Urea and Creatinine. These two substances are the nitrogenous end-products of protein metabolism. The normal level of blood urea is usually expressed as the blood urea nitrogen (BUN). The normal BUN is 8 to 18 mg/dl (3.0 to 6.5 mmol/L). The normal level of blood creatinine is 0.6 to 1.2 mg/dl (50 to 110 µmol/L). Renal failure results in a rise in the level of these two nitrogenous substances in the blood; the resultant condition is called *azotemia.**

2. Metabolism and Excretion of Other Substances. Insulin and many drugs are examples.

3. Regulation of Extracellular Fluids. This is accomplished by controlling the excretion of water and electrolytes — particularly sodium.

4. Regulation of Acid-Base Balance. The kidney contributes to the maintenance of a stable blood pH by the excretion of hydrogen ions. This

---

*The term is derived from *azote*, a name for nitrogen proposed by Lavoisier.

excretion takes place mainly in the distal tubule where hydrogen ions are combined either with phosphate or with ammonia. The synthesis of ammonia by the kidney and its conversion into ammonium ions is an important mechanism in acid-base homeostasis.

5. *Regulation of Blood Pressure.* The kidney is capable of forming both vasodilator and vasoconstrictor substances, but their role in the regulation of the systemic blood pressure is not understood. The vasodilators are prosta-glandins and kinins. The ischemic kidney releases renin, an enzyme that leads to the formation of the powerful vasoconstrictor angiotensin II (Chapter 20).

6. *Regulation of Erythropoiesis.* Erythropoietin is produced mainly by the kidney and acts as a stimulus to red-cell production. The precise physiological role of this process is not understood; it is known, however, that anemia is very common in renal failure. Occasionally tumors of the kidney result in excessive erythropoietin production, causing polycythemia to ensue.

7. *Vitamin D Metabolism.* See Chapter 40.

Mechanism of Urine Formation: Normal and Abnormal

The formation of urine by the normal kidney is described in textbooks of physiology; consequently, only a brief outline of the salient features will be described here.

The glomerular filtrate (approximately 180 liters per day) is derived from blood flowing through the glomerulus and has a similar composition to plasma, except that it has a very low protein content. In the proximal convoluted tubule, 80 per cent of the water and virtually all of the protein and glucose are reabsorbed. If the blood glucose level (and therefore the level in the glomerular filtrate) is high — as in diabetes mellitus — the proximal convoluted tubules are unable to reabsorb all the glucose, and this substance passes into the urine (a condition called *glycosuria*). Occasionally glycosuria occurs in the presence of a normal blood glucose level; this condition, which is known as *renal glycosuria*, is due to defective tubular function.

In many renal diseases the glomerular vessels become more permeable to protein, and the proximal convoluted tubules are unable to reabsorb the excess protein. The *proteinuria* that results is an important and common finding in renal disease.

Absorption of electrolytes in the proximal tubules is such that the luminal fluid is isotonic with plasma, and the process is therefore called "iso-osmotic absorption." Urea passes freely out of the tubules.

In the ascending limb of the loop of Henle there is considerable transfer of sodium chloride from the lumen to the interstitial fluid of the medulla. Because this part of the renal tubule is impermeable to water, it follows that the modified filtrate within the lumen becomes progressively hypotonic, while the interstitial fluid becomes hypertonic.

In the distal tubule, the pH of the filtrate and its electrolyte composition are finally adjusted. When the hypotonic fluid leaves the loop of Henle and enters the distal tubule, it becomes isotonic with plasma once more, since this part of the nephron is fully permeable to water.

Because the filtrate is surrounded by the hypertonic interstitial fluid of the medulla, in its course through the collecting tubules it tends to maintain osmotic equilibrium by transferring some of its water to the interstitial fluid. The filtrate thereby attains the final composition of urine. The permeability of the distal tubule and collecting tubules is regulated by the circulating level of antidiuretic hormone (ADH) released by the posterior lobe of the pituitary. This hormone, by rendering the tubules more permeable to water, aids the transfer of water from the tubules into the interstitial tissue. A high level of ADH, such as occurs during dehydration, results in the production of a highly concentrated urine. In the absence of antidiuretic hormone, such as occurs in *diabetes insipidus*, a large quantity of dilute urine is produced. Normally 1½ to 2 liters of urine is passed daily; if this quantity is exceeded, the condition is termed *polyuria*. Tubules damaged by hypercalcemia or hypokalemia are less responsive to the action of ADH, and this situation also leads to polyuria. Likewise, the regenerating epithelium of the tubules following tubular necrosis is unresponsive to the action of ADH, and again polyuria results.

If the fluid in the tubules contains an excess of an osmotically active substance such as glucose, water absorption is impeded. It follows that in diabetes mellitus polyuria is a characteristic feature. Since water is lost, thirst is increased, and an excessive quantity of water is drunk (*polydipsia*). A similar situation occurs in chronic renal failure. The blood urea level is high, and the amount of urea in the glomerular filtrate is also raised, hindering water absorption. Polyuria and polydipsia ensue. It is evident that one of the features of the normal kidney is its ability to produce a highly concentrated or a highly dilute urine according to circumstances. As renal function becomes impaired, this ability is lost and eventually a urine of fixed osmolality is produced.

The continuous production of urine with a specific gravity of about 1.010 regardless of the fluid intake has several important consequences. If the fluid intake is high, then water retention occurs. If the water intake of the body is low, then dehydration results. Finally the normal ability to produce a concentrated urine during sleep is lost, forcing the patient to get up to pass urine during the night, a feature described as *nocturia*.

Tests of Renal Function   *Clearance Values.* Inulin is a substance that passes freely from the plasma into the glomerular filtrate and is neither absorbed by the tubules nor secreted by them. The amount of plasma cleared of inulin per minute is equal to the glomerular filtration rate. It is evident that:

Filtered inulin = excreted inulin
Filtered inulin = Glomerular filtration rate (GFR) × plasma inulin concentration (P)
Excreted inulin = Urine inulin concentration (U) × volume of urine (V) in ml/min

$$\text{Hence} \qquad GFR \times P = U \times V$$
$$GFR = \frac{U \times V}{P}$$

This forms the basis of a useful clinical test, and the normal value for the glomerular filtration rate is about 120 ml per minute. In practice, the inulin clearance test is difficult to perform, but since creatinine is treated similarly, the *creatinine clearance* is estimated and is a good measure of the glomerular filtration rate. The required measurements are: blood creatinine level, the volume of urine passed over a 1-hour period, and the creatinine content of a sample of this urine. The normal range is 90 to 130 ml per min. The urea clearance test is also a commonly performed test, but since some urea is reabsorbed by the tubules, the urea clearance is approximately ⅝ of the normal glomerular filtration rate; *i.e.*, the normal range is 60 to 100 ml per min.

Blood Urea. The blood urea nitrogen (BUN) is related in part to the protein intake in the diet and in part to renal function. Figure 35–1 shows the relationship between glomerular filtration rate and blood urea. Note that the BUN is an insensitive indicator of renal function and that at least 50 per cent of kidney substance must be destroyed before an appreciable rise in the BUN

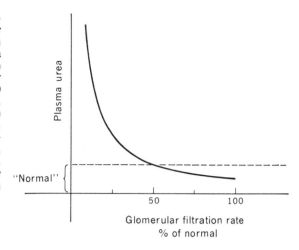

Figure'35–1.   Graph showing the relationship between the glomerular filtration rate and the plasma urea concentration. Note that the plasma urea concentration remains within normal limits until the glomerular filtration rate has fallen to less than 50 per cent of normal. (From Epstein, F. H.: Approach to the patient with renal disease. *In* Wintrobe, M. M., et al. (Eds.): Harrison's Principles of Internal Medicine. 7th ed. New York, McGraw-Hill Book Company, 1974, pp. 1367–1370. Copyright © 1974 by McGraw-Hill, Inc. Used by permission of McGraw-Hill Book Company.)

is seen. The blood creatinine level is related to muscle bulk and not to dietary intake, and the level of blood creatinine is a more useful indication of renal function.

Diseases of the kidney and urinary tract are often reflected in abnormalities in the urine and are so common that an examination of the urine (*urinalysis*) is a mandatory procedure with any patient admitted to a hospital or undergoing a routine physical examination. The following methods can be used.

Examination of Urine

Chemical Examination.   Simple tests are available for detecting protein, glucose, hemoglobin, and ketone bodies. If necessary, the amount of protein can be measured; the normal quantity excreted in 24 hours is under 150 mg. Individual proteins can be identified by electroimmunophoresis; for example, Bence Jones protein can be categorized by this method (Chapter 40).

Specific Gravity.   The normal kidney can concentrate urine such that the specific gravity reaches 1.022 or more after a period of dehydration or an injection of vasopressin. Specific gravity readings are misleading if heavy solutes such as glucose or protein are present in the urine. Under these circumstances, the freezing point method of detecting osmolarity must be used.

The normal kidney can dilute urine following a water load, but tests based on this are unreliable and are not used in practice.

Microscopic Examination.   Much can be learned by an examination of the centrifuged deposit from a sample of *fresh* urine. A scanty number of red cells, polymorphs, and epithelial cells are normally present. An excess of red cells indicates bleeding. The presence of these cells can usefully distinguish between *hematuria*, which is the presence of red cells in the urine, and *hemoglobinuria*, which is the existence of free hemoglobin in solution, as in blackwater fever. An increased number of polymorphs indicates inflammation either in the kidney or the urinary tract; generally this condition is due to infection, but it must be confirmed bacteriologically. If there is no growth on routine media a search must be made for tubercle bacilli.

Casts are cylindrical structures formed in the renal tubules and composed of a protein that is derived from the tubules themselves (Tamm-Horsfall mucoprotein). *Hyaline casts* are translucent, and a few are sometimes present in the urine of healthy people. An increased number suggests renal disease. More significant are *granular casts*, which have a specked or granular appearance due to an admixture of albumin, immunoglobulin, lipoprotein, or breakdown products of cells. When first formed, the granules are coarse (*coarsely granular casts*), but with intrarenal stasis the granules break up to produce *finely granular casts*. Ultimately the granules disappear, and highly refractile, brittle, *waxy casts* are formed. The presence of these casts is abnormal and generally indicates tubulointerstitial renal disease. Waxy casts in particular point to severe disease. *Renal tubular epithelial cell casts* contain recognizable tubular cells, and their presence indicates tubular damage. Likewise, *fatty casts* indicate tubular damage, since the fat is derived from the tubular cells. *Red cell casts* contain recognizable red cells and possibly breakdown products of hemoglobin. The red cells are usually derived from damaged glomeruli, but bleeding can also occur in acute renal tubular necrosis. Leukocyte casts indicate acute inflammation, often infective, hence, they are characteristic of pyelonephritis.

Since casts are formed in renal tubules, the diameter of the casts is an indication of the diameter of the tubule in which they are formed. Hence, large, *broad casts* are formed in dilated tubules of severely scarred kidneys, and their presence is of grave significance.

Bacteriological Examination. Urine normally contains some bacteria that are derived from the anterior urethra, but the organisms are too scanty to be seen on a stained smear of *uncentrifuged* urine. A bacterial count of over 100,000 per ml is regarded as abnormal and indicates a renal or urinary tract infection.

General Manifestations of Renal Disease

Renal disease, regardless of its cause, can terminate in renal failure. This may occur acutely or may be of a more chronic nature.

Acute Renal Failure

Acute renal failure is characterized by a sudden drop in the output of urine (*oliguria*); this may be followed in due course by complete absence of excretion of urine (*anuria*). Acute renal failure must not be confused with sudden failure to pass urine that is due to the mechanical obstruction of the urinary passages.

Causes of Acute Renal Failure

Vasomotor Nephropathy. In this condition there is a reduction in renal blood flow associated with intense renal vasoconstriction. Since this is secondary to events outside the kidney, it is sometimes called *prerenal failure*. Vasomotor nephropathy is a common event in clinical practice and is seen under the following circumstances:

1. Whenever there is a sudden decrease in blood volume, such as may occur following hemorrhage, a severe burn, and persistent vomiting or diarrhea. The pathogenesis is considered in Chapter 21, under the heading of "Shock."

2. Following the escape of free hemoglobin or myoglobin into the circulation, as after an incompatible blood transfusion or a crushing injury to the muscles of a limb.

3. Following certain complications of pregnancy — notably abruptio placentae.

Renal vasoconstriction results in a diminution in the amount of blood reaching the kidney; in addition, in shock there is a reduction in the blood pressure. Glomerular filtration is therefore severely impaired and oliguria results. The kidney at this stage shows no structural abnormality, and if the condition is adequately treated, complete recovery occurs. However, if the ischemia is not speedily reversed, the condition progresses to acute tubular necrosis.

There is evidence that the kidney can be protected from the effects of severe ischemia by the local production of vasodilator prostaglandins. Hence, if a patient with vasomotor nephropathy is given one of the nonsteroid anti-inflammatory drugs (*e.g.*, aspirin, phenacetin, etc.) that inhibit prostaglandin formation, the ischemia is potentiated and the prognosis is worsened.

Acute Renal Tubular Necrosis (ATN). Three major causes of this condition can be recognized:

Ischemia. Prolonged ischemia as described above soon results in patchy tubular necrosis affecting particularly the terminal portions of the proximal convoluted tubules and the distal convoluted tubules. Characteristically, the basement membrane is disrupted and regeneration is thereby impaired and incomplete.

Poisons. In particular, necrosis can result if poisoning is combined with prior dehydration. Mercury salts, carbon tetrachloride (used in fire extinguishers), and diethyl glycol (used in antifreeze) are important examples of these poisons.

Infections. Acute tubular necrosis is seen in Weil's disease and also in yellow fever.

In acute renal tubular necrosis, the glomerular filtrate passes from the tubules into the interstitial tissue of the kidney, which thereby becomes swollen. Little or no fluid is passed as urine. ATN is sometimes difficult to distinguish microscopically from postmortem change, but the presence of interstitial edema in ATN is one useful histological feature by which one may distinguish between the two. For reasons that are not understood, jaundice and pregnancy when combined with other conditions appear to predispose the kidney to necrosis. Sometimes in pregnancy, the ischemia leads to complete necrosis of the outer two thirds of the cortex; the condition of *bilateral renal cortical necrosis* results. This affects not only tubules but also the associated glomeruli (see Fig. 21–4).

Other less common diseases that produce acute renal failure include the following:

1. Acute renal diseases, such as acute glomerulonephritis and acute interstitial nephritis.

2. Acute tubular obstruction and subsequent necrosis are sometimes seen following the precipitation of uric acid in hyperuricemia (Chapter 24).

3. The precipitation of myeloma protein in multiple myelomatosis and the formation of sulfonamide crystals in patients who are treated with these drugs.

Effects of Acute Renal Failure. During the acute phase, oliguria with the passage of a small quantity of dark urine containing protein, blood products, and cell debris–forming casts is characteristic. In severe cases oliguria is followed by complete anuria. Uremia develops rapidly and is associated with a rise in blood urea nitrogen (BUN), blood potassium, and phosphate levels. Metabolic acidosis occurs, and there is an increase in the volume of the extracellular fluid. If the patient is overhydrated, heart failure may be precipitated, and edema develops. Death may be due to overhydration, potassium intoxication, or infection, such as bronchopneumonia. Often, however, the patient sinks steadily into a coma from which he does not emerge; presumably, this is the combined effect of many metabolic upsets.

If the patient survives, large quantities of urine are passed for a period of time because the kidneys cannot conserve electrolytes and water. At that point, the patient's life is in jeopardy because of dehydration and electrolyte loss. As the tubular epithelium regenerates, renal function is restored, but complete recovery is unusual.

Any chronic progressive disease that results in destruction of renal parenchyma leads to chronic renal failure. The diseases include glomerulonephritis, chronic pyelonephritis, nephrosclerosis, lupus erythematosus, diabet-

Chronic Renal Failure–Uremia

ic nephropathy, extensive renal tuberculosis, and radiation nephritis. Chronic obstruction of the outflow of urine, such as that caused by prostatic enlargement, is a common cause in males.

Effects of Chronic Renal Failure. The effect of chronic renal failure is uremia that is due to a failure of the kidney to regulate the internal environment. The kidneys can neither concentrate nor dilute, and the urine has a fixed specific gravity of 1.010. This leads to nocturia and easy upset in water metabolism.

Uremia is a clinical state produced by renal failure that is associated with retention of nitrogenous substances in the blood. Some of its features can be explained on the basis of known biochemical anomalies. In many instances we are ignorant of its exact pathogenesis. The features of uremia are enumerated below:

1. General. Weakness, easy fatigue, lethargy, insomnia, and malaise are common.

2. Cardiovascular Symptoms. Hypertension is common and may lead to heart failure. This contributes to edema both of the tissues in general and of the lung. A terminal sterile fibrinous pericarditis is often seen.

3. Gastrointestinal Symptoms. Anorexia, nausea, vomiting, hiccup, and diarrhea are frequent. One explanation of these symptoms is that urea present in the gastrointestinal fluids is broken down to ammonia, which is an irritant and causes *gastritis* and *colitis*. Vomiting and diarrhea can precipitate acute renal failure.

4. Neurological Manifestations. Mental clouding, inability to concentrate, and lethargy are common in advanced uremia. Convulsions and coma may occur terminally. These symptoms may be due to water intoxication and metabolic acidosis. Muscular twitching has been related to hypocalcemia. A peripheral neuropathy similar to that encountered in diabetes mellitus may occur.

5. Anemia. This is characteristic and is unresponsive to treatment. Even if the patient is transfused with red cells, the anemia soon returns.

6. Infection. Advanced renal insufficiency is commonly complicated by infection. Often this is a urinary infection and terminates in septicemia.

7. Metabolic Acidosis. This condition leads to a sighing respiration.

8. Renal Osteodystrophy. Retention of phosphate can lead to a lowering of blood calcium and hyperparathyroidism secondary to this.

9. Retention of Potassium. Hyperkalemia can lead to sudden death (Chapter 19).

The Protein-Losing Kidney (Nephrotic Syndrome)

Normally a mere trace of protein escapes into the glomerular filtrate and is almost completely reabsorbed by the proximal convoluted tubules. There are a number of conditions in which the permeability of the glomeruli is increased so that large amounts of protein (mostly albumin) escape into the filtrate and are passed in the urine because the capacity of the tubule to reabsorb protein is limited. This constant loss of albumin results in hypoalbuminemia. The complex of proteinuria, hypoalbuminemia, and edema is called the *nephrotic syndrome*. It may be a complication of many chronic diseases, such as glomerulonephritis, diabetic nephropathy, renal amyloidosis, and lupus nephritis.

The main features of the nephrotic syndrome are listed below:

1. Severe Proteinuria. Normally the 24-hour output of protein is less than 0.15 gram. In the nephrotic syndrome it can exceed 10 grams.

2. Hypoproteinemia. This affects in particular the albumin level of the plasma.

3. Generalized Edema. This condition is due in part to the hypoproteinemia and in part to an increased secretion of aldosterone by the adrenals.

4. Susceptibility to Infection. This condition is due to the loss of immunoglobulins in the urine.

5. A Raised Level of Lipoproteins in the Blood. The blood cholesterol, normally about 250 mg/dl, may exceed 1000 mg/dl. The cause of this increase is unknown.

Glomerulonephritis is a term applied to a group of diseases that are not obviously of infective nature and in which primarily the glomeruli are affected. In most types of glomerulonephritis the lesions are associated with the deposition of immune complexes in the glomeruli. Glomerulonephritis is a feature of serum sickness and chronic immune complex disease (Chapter 9). In naturally occurring glomerulonephritis similar immune-complex deposition can occur, and the antigen may be derived from a number of sources. These may be exogenous, such as infections (streptococcal infections, malaria, syphilis, or hepatitis) or drugs. In a number of cases the antigen is endogenous, and glomerulonephritis is a well-known accompaniment of tumors, particularly carcinoma of the lung. In these instances the renal damage appears to be due to the deposition of circulating immune complexes, but the reason for their deposition in the glomeruli is poorly understood. The kidney appears to be damaged as an "innocent bystander," and the pathogenesis is thought to involve the activation of complement via either the classical or the alternate pathways. In many examples of glomerulonephritis, although immune-complex deposition can be detected, the nature of the antigen is unknown. This applies to the common poststreptococcal glomerulonephritis (Fig. 35–2A). In all these examples it is assumed that the immune complexes are formed in the blood and subsequently filtered off in the glomeruli. Another proposed mechanism is that antibodies form complexes directly with antigens already present in the kidney. The antigen may be part of the normal or slightly altered glomerular structure, and this is believed to be the mechanism in the production of the lesions in Goodpasture's syndrome (page 510). In other examples it is thought that foreign antigens become localized or planted in the kidney and that subsequently antibodies form complexes with them.

Although many classifications of glomerulonephritis have been proposed, none has been found to be entirely satisfactory. The types at present recognized have been delineated on the basis of three parameters:

1. Clinical Findings. The clinical features of glomerulonephritis vary enormously. The onset may be acute or insidious. Hematuria is common but may range from insignificant to severe: the red cells present in urine may be detectable only by microscopic examination, or the urine may be "smoky" or obviously red. Albuminuria is invariable and if severe leads to the nephrotic syndrome. A patient may recover spontaneously from glomerulonephritis; occasionally the disease is fulminating and leads rapidly to death from renal failure; more often, the damage is progressive and renal failure occurs after a protracted course of many years. Associated clinical features sometimes suggest the cause of glomerulonephritis. For example, some types are associated with infection by *Streptococcus pyogenes*. For the most part, however, the origin of glomerulonephritis is unknown.

2. Immunological Findings. In many types of human glomerulonephritis, deposits of immunoglobulin (IgG or IgA) and complement can be demonstrated by immunofluorescence. The technique used is similar to that illustrated in Figure 9–15. The precise localization of the deposits varies; usually the deposits are granular and are situated in relation to the basement

Diseases of the Kidney

Glomerulo-nephritis

membrane or the mesangium. In a few types — notably the glomerulonephritis of Goodpasture's syndrome — specific antikidney antibodies can be detected in the blood and in the kidney, where they are laid down in a linear manner along the capillary basement membrane zone (Fig. 35–2B).

3. *Histopathological Findings.*   Light microscopy reveals several types of glomerular change. The glomeruli may appear normal or show the changes described as proliferative, membranous, or crescentic. These are described below. It must be stressed that the changes are purely descriptive. They are merely reaction patterns of the glomerulus to damage and are not specific for any one type of disease.

Electron microscopy has greatly added to our knowledge of the types and causes of glomerulonephritis. Deposits of material (mostly immune complexes and complement) are found in the basement membrane itself or on either side of it. Various patterns and types of deposit have been described, but these details are beyond the scope of this book. A characteristic electron microscopic finding is fusion of the foot processes of the epithelial cells of the glomeruli (Figs. 35–3 and 35–4). This appears to be an effect of an increased permeability of glomerular vessels to protein and is therefore present whenever there is proteinuria. It is thought that the processes merely become

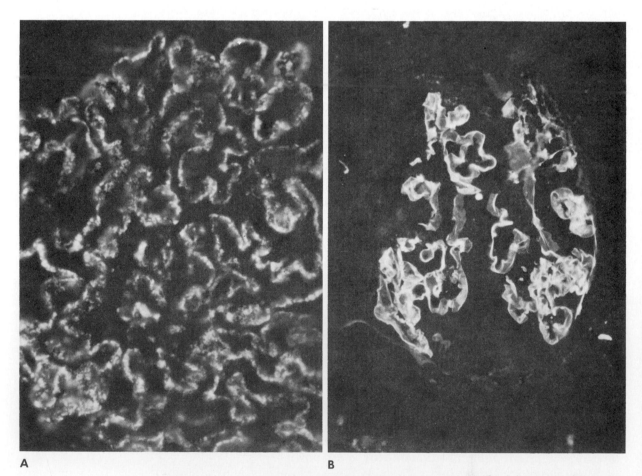

A   B

Figure 35–2.   Immunofluorescent patterns in glomerulonephritis. *A,* Part of a glomerulus in acute poststreptococcal glomerulonephritis. Note the granular deposits of IgG in the immune complexes deposited in the basement membrane zone. *B,* Goodpasture's syndrome. There is a uniform linear band of staining along the basement membrane of the vessels in the glomerulus. (Courtesy of Dr. Susan Ritchie.)

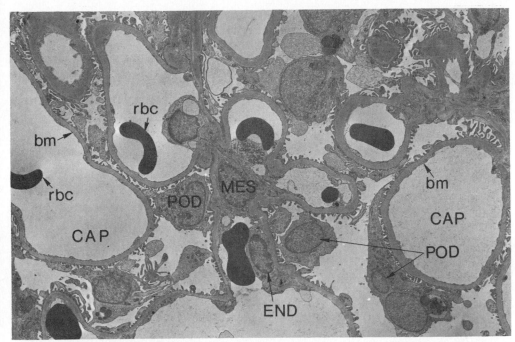

Figure 35–3.   Normal kidney. Survey electron micrograph of a portion of a normal human glomerulus. The capillaries (CAP) are lined by attenuated endothelial cells; the nucleus of one of these is labelled END. Red cells are easily identified (rbc). A mesangial cell (MES) is situated between several capillary loops. The capillaries possess a well-marked basement membrane (bm) and are covered by epithelial cells or podocytes (POD) of the visceral layer of Bowman's capsule. These cells are attached to the basement membrane of the capillaries by numerous foot processes, or *pedicles* (× 3600). (Courtesy of Dr. Susan Ritchie.)

shorter and stumpy, so that in the end the epithelial cytoplasm appears to be directly applied to the basement membrane. The processes are therefore lost, and the term "fusion of the foot processes" is inaccurate.

The technique of needle biopsy, by which a core of kidney substance can be safely removed during life, has greatly aided the investigation of glomerulonephritis in patients. The material obtained is particularly suited for immunofluorescence studies and electron microscopy as well as for routine light microscopic examination.

Types of Glomerulonephritis

1. Minimal-Change Glomerulonephritis.   The glomeruli appear normal under light microscopy, but under electron microscopy fusion of the foot processes of the epithelial cells is revealed.

The majority of the patients are children with the nephrotic syndrome. They respond well to glucocorticoid therapy.

2. Membranous Glomerulonephritis.   On light microscopy the basement membrane of the glomeruli is shown to be thickened (Fig. 35–5). Eventually this thickening causes obliteration of the vessels, and the glomeruli become functionless. The majority of patients are adults with the nephrotic syndrome. Approximately 30 per cent recover spontaneously, and the remainder continue on with their disease and ultimately die of chronic renal failure. Membranous glomerulonephritis and minimal change glomerulonephritis at one time were both classified as types of *nephrosis*. Systemic lupus erythematosus can produce an identical histological picture.

3. Proliferative Glomerulonephritis.   The glomeruli are enlarged and hypercellular because of mesangial proliferation and infiltration by polymorphs (Fig. 35–5). Poststreptococcal glomerulonephritis is the common type of proliferative glomerulonephritis. The illness occurs about 3 weeks after a

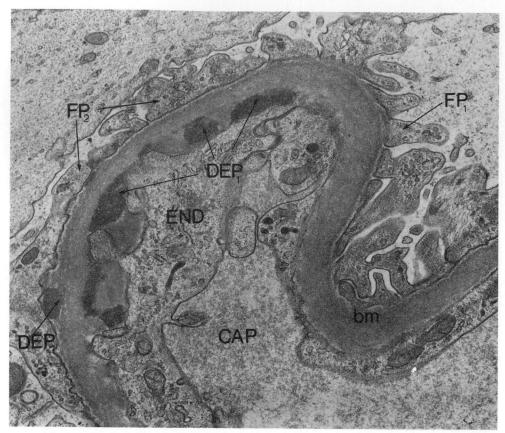

Figure 35–4.   Electron micrograph of glomerulus in lupus erythematosus. In some areas, the foot processes (FP₁) of the podocytes appear relatively normal, but elsewhere they are swollen and spread over the basement membrane (bm) of the capillary (FP₂). This change is commonly described as *fusion of the foot processes.* Prominent subendothelial deposits are present (DEP₁). Subepithelial deposits are smaller and less obvious (DEP₂). In this patient the deposits were shown by immunofluorescence to contain IgG and components of complement (× 27,500). (Courtesy of Dr. Y. Bedard.)

streptococcal infection and is characterized by hematuria and edema, particularly of the face. Certain strains of *Streptococcus pyogenes* (nephritogenic strains) are thought to share an antigen with the human glomerulus. Cross-reacting antibodies are assumed to cause the renal damage. About 80 per cent of the patients recover spontaneously, and the remainder show permanent damage and ultimately develop chronic renal failure (Fig. 35–7).

4. Membranoproliferative Glomerulonephritis (Mesangiocapillary). The glomeruli show a combination of basement membrane thickening and mesangial proliferation. Several types of membranoproliferative glomerulonephritis are recognized. One type is associated with *Streptococcus viridans* endocarditis; another is associated with a low blood complement level. The location and type of deposits found in immunofluorescent and electron microscopic studies help in delineating these types.

Clinically the patients often present with the nephrotic syndrome. The prognosis is poor.

5. Rapidly Progressive Glomerulonephritis. The glomeruli show proliferative changes and deposits of fibrin. The characteristic lesion, however, is proliferation of the epithelial cells of Bowman's capsule to produce a *crescent* (Fig. 35–5).

Clinically, rapidly progressive glomerulonephritis is associated with the rapid development of renal failure and consequent death. The disease is occasionally encountered in poststreptococcal glomerulonephritis and in polyarteritis nodosa. It is also characteristic of Goodpasture's syndrome, a condition that affects young men and is characterized by pulmonary hemorrhages, hemoptysis, and renal failure. Antibodies are present that react specifically with basement membrane material of the pulmonary and glomerular capillaries.

Focal Glomerulonephritis. Unlike the other types of glomerulonephritis described, this group affects some glomeruli but not others; indeed it may affect parts of only some glomeruli. The details relating to the various types of focal glomerulonephritis are beyond the scope of this book.

Summary. The diagnosis of glomerulonephritis is the task of the expert who has access to such sophisticated tools as electron microscopy and immunofluorescence. Precise diagnosis is of value in giving the prognosis and in suggesting the best treatment available.

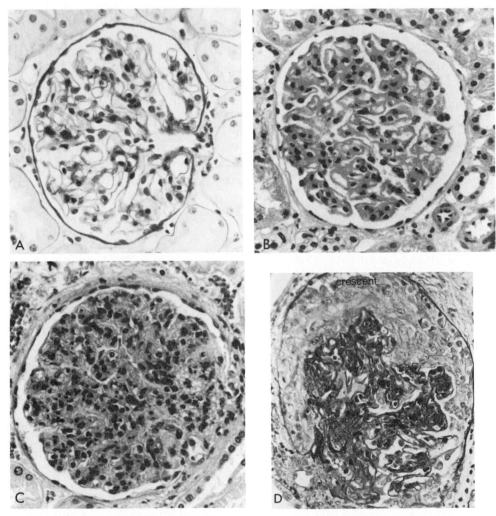

Figure 35–5. Glomerulonephritis. *A,* Normal glomerulus. The basement membrane zones of the parietal layer of Bowman's capsule and of the glomerulus are well shown. PAS stain. *B,* Membranous glomerulonephritis. Note the thickening of the basement membrane of the glomerular capillaries. H & E stain. *C,* Proliferative glomerulonephritis. The glomerulus is enlarged and shows increased cellularity that is due partly to mesangial proliferation and partly to a polymorph infiltration. *D,* Rapidly progressive glomerulonephritis. The glomerular tuft is collapsed and the deep staining of the basement membrane material is well shown. Proliferation of the epithelial cells of Bowman's capsule has produced a typical crescent. PAS stain. (*A* and *C* by courtesy of Dr. Susan Ritchie.)

Other Types of Renal Disease

Lupus Nephritis. Glomerulonephritis of either a proliferative or a membranous type is common in systemic lupus erythematosus (Fig. 35–4). Immune deposits of DNA–anti-DNA are a prominent feature. Lupus nephritis can cause a nephrotic syndrome and ultimately lead to renal failure.

Nephrosclerosis. Nephrosclerosis is a term used to describe the renal lesions of systemic hypertension (Chapter 20). In the *benign type,* the arteriosclerosis causes patchy ischemia. The affected nephrons become atrophic and are ultimately replaced by scar tissue. Hence, the kidneys in benign nephrosclerosis show thinning of the cortex and a granularity of the surface. In malignant hypertension the arteriolar necrosis causes extensive patchy foci of necrosis *(malignant nephrosclerosis)*. Renal failure is a common cause of death.

Interstitial Nephritis. Interstitial nephritis is characterized by an inflammatory reaction in the interstitial tissues. This is associated with tubular damage, but the glomeruli are spared until late in the course of the disease. *Acute interstitial nephritis* can lead to death from acute renal failure; however, the disease is usually chronic. Some cases are caused by drug intake — particularly intake of the penicillin derivative methicillin.

Another important cause of chronic interstitial nephritis is associated with prolonged intake of large doses of analgesic drugs. This condition, called *analgesic nephropathy,* is now recognized as a common cause of chronic renal disease, particularly in Australia and New Zealand. The subjects are usually women who self-administer the drugs for real or imaginary pain such as fibrositis, headache, or low back pain. Although phenacetin has been considered as the major culprit, experimentally aspirin and acetaminophen can also cause renal damage. If these drugs are combined they produce damage at a much lower dosage, particularly if combined with dehydration of the subject. This may well explain the geographic distribution of the disease.

The characteristic lesion of analgesic nephropathy is *papillary necrosis* (Fig. 35–6). The tips of one or more papillae become necrotic and may eventually calcify. The necrosis appears to be due to infarction, but the precise pathogenesis is not known. Adjacent to the necrotic papillae there is an inflammatory reaction, and sometimes the necrotic tips break off and result in hematuria and renal colic. The affected area of kidney shows an interstitial infiltration by lymphocytes. As more and more papillae become necrotic, increasing areas of renal parenchyma are destroyed, and this is associated with deterioration of renal function and ultimately uremia. It is evident that all people involved in administering health care should endeavor to dissuade patients from abusing the many analgesic mixtures that are so prominently advertised on radio and television and in the drug stores. Many cases of interstitial nephritis are idiopathic and are difficult to distinguish from chronic pyelonephritis, since the pathological findings of the two diseases are very similar. Hence, interstitial nephritis, analgesic nephropathy, and pyelonephritis are sometimes grouped together as *tubulointerstitial disease* of the kidney.

Diabetic Nephropathy. This condition is described in Chapter 24.

Renal and Urinary Tract Infection: Pyelonephritis

Bacterial infection of the urinary tract is very common and constitutes a major medical problem. The infecting organisms are usually the gram-negative intestinal bacilli, including *Escherichia coli, Pseudomonas aeruginosa,* and Proteus and Klebsiella species. Two routes of infection have been described, but their relative importance has been long debated:

Hematogenous Infection. It is believed that some infection is blood-

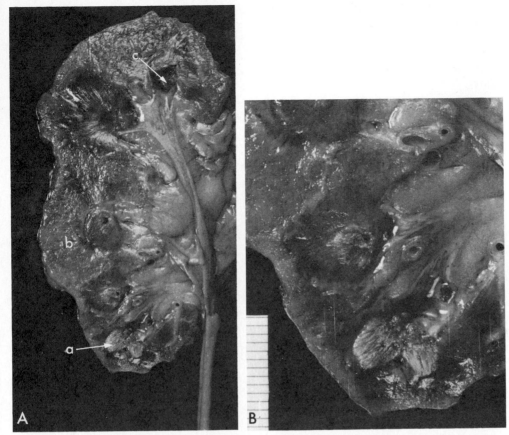

Figure 35–6.   Analgesic nephropathy. *A,* The kidney shows several necrotic papillae, seen best at *a.* Note how the cortex overlying this area is thinned compared with the more normal cortex at *b.* One papilla has become necrotic and has completely disappeared (*c*). *B,* This close-up shows necrotic papillae. The white flecking is due to dystrophic calcification.

borne from the colon. Normally organisms that avoid the reticuloendothelial cells of the liver pass into the systemic circulation; they escape into the glomerular filtrate and are expeditiously voided in the urine. If there is an obstruction to the outflow of urine, these organisms flourish and set up acute inflammation of the bladder *(cystitis),* of the renal pelvis *(pyelitis),* or of the kidney and renal pelvis *(pyelonephritis).*

Ascending Infection.   There is a rival hypothesis that infection ascends from the perineum and lower urinary tract. Acute cystitis is more common in women (particularly during pregnancy), and it is probable that this is due to the shortness of the urethra and the ease with which vulval organisms can ascend to the bladder. Likewise, urinary infection often follows repeated catheterization. Direct introduction of urethral organisms into the bladder can therefore be implicated. Following acute cystitis, "ascending infection" due to reflux of urine up into the ureters can occur. Indeed, vesicoureteral reflux (which may be familial) is an important cause of upper urinary tract infections in children; intrarenal reflux may further promote the involvement of renal parenchyma by ascending infection.

It is evident that obstruction of the urinary flow is the most important factor predisposing a person toward infection. Pyelonephritis can be unilateral if one ureter is obstructed, for example by a stone. If there has been previous blockage, the hydronephrotic kidney becomes infected to produce a sac of pus, which is known as *pyonephrosis.* Urethral obstruction, such as that due to prostatic enlargement, generally causes bilateral pyelonephritis.

The clinical features of acute urinary tract infection are those of an acute infection: rigors and an acute rise in temperature. Pain is experienced in the loins in pyelonephritis. With cystitis and urethritis the inflammation leads to urgency of micturition together with pain and burning on passing urine. The acute attack generally subsides rapidly either under treatment or spontaneously.

The urine in acute cystitis and acute pyelonephritis contains numerous pus cells; organisms can usually be seen in a stained smear of an uncentrifuged specimen. Hematuria is common.

Papillary Necrosis (Necrotizing Papillitis). This is an occasional complication of acute pyelonephritis, especially in diabetic subjects and if there is urinary obstruction. One or several papillae undergo necrosis. The lesions are similar to those encountered in analgesic nephropathy, except that the necrotic papillae are all at the same stage of evolution.

Chronic Pyelonephritis. In some cases of acute urinary tract infection there are numerous recurrences of the infection and the development of chronic pyelonephritis; this is the commonest cause of chronic renal failure. Its pathogenesis is uncertain, because in some cases there is an obvious cause such as urinary obstruction, whereas in others there is no such obstruction or other reason for urinary stasis. It may be that some intrinsic kidney damage, especially the scars of a previous infection, account for this smoldering infection. Chronic pyelonephritis is characterized by gradual destruction of the renal parenchyma and its replacement by fibrous tissue that is heavily infiltrated by lymphocytes, plasma cells, macrophages, and a varying number of polymorphs. Since the process tends to be patchy, the kidney presents an irregular scarred appearance; if bilateral, involvement is asymmetrical. Chronic pyelonephritis is often complicated by the development of hypertension, so that hypertensive vascular changes are superimposed. The ultimate result is an end-stage kidney, which is associated with chronic renal failure.

End-Stage Kidneys

Small, scarred, granular kidneys are often found at the necropsy of a patient who died of renal disease. It is difficult — or even impossible — to distinguish between the various types of kidney disease (*e.g.*, chronic glomerulonephritis, chronic pyelonephritis, analgesic nephropathy, nephrosclerosis, diabetic nephropathy, and chronic interstitial nephritis [Fig. 35–7]). It is

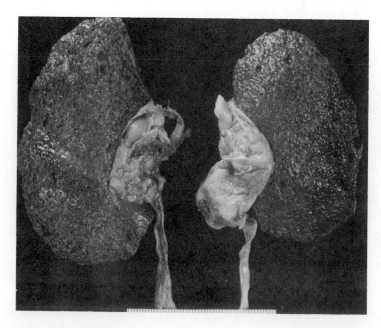

Figure 35–7. Chronic glomerulonephritis. Both kidneys are reduced in size and display a fine granular surface. The patient had developed acute glomerulonephritis following a streptococcal sore throat. Renal failure and systemic hypertension slowly evolved over the next 15 years. Death was due to cerebral hemorrhage. It is not possible to distinguish between the various types of chronic renal disease by a gross examination.

in these cases that the overall clinical course and results of previous renal biopsies are of value in arriving at a correct reconstruction of the events leading to death.

Occasionally one kidney is small (hypoplastic) or completely absent (agenesis). The kidneys may be abnormally placed either at the brim of the pelvis or in the pelvic cavity itself. In *horseshoe kidney* the two organs are fused together either at their upper or lower poles to produce a horseshoe deformity. These anomalies are of importance to the radiologist or surgeon who is investigating urinary tract disease. Horseshoe kidneys are found in approximately 0.1 per cent of the population. A more frequent malformation is *polycystic kidney*. The common adult type of this condition is inherited as an autosomal dominant trait but does not become manifest until the teens or later. Numerous cysts steadily form, so that ultimately both kidneys become enormous (Fig. 35–8). The cysts communicate with the renal tubules, so that bleeding into one of them causes hematuria, in addition to the pain due to the mechanical distension of the cyst wall. Systemic hypertension is common, and eventually renal failure ensues. In the past such patients rarely lived beyond the age of 50 years, but this gloomy outlook has been changed by the advent of renal transplantation. Berry aneurysms are present in about 15 per cent of cases, and subarachnoid hemorrhage is an additional hazard, especially as there is often high blood pressure (Chapter 44).

Congenital Diseases of the Kidney

Adenoma. The common benign renal tumor is an adenoma that is usually pinhead-sized and appears as a yellow-white nodule situated beneath the capsule. Its cells are usually arranged in a papillary cystadenomatous pattern and closely resemble those of a carcinoma.

Tumors of the Kidney

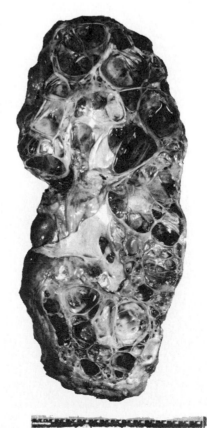

Figure 35–8. Polycystic kidney. The patient was first diagnosed as having polycystic kidneys at the age of 23 years, when he was investigated following an episode of hematuria. He remained in fairly good health until the age of 30, by which time he had developed hypertension and a BUN of 180 mg/dl. He complained of a dragging sensation in the abdomen, evidently due to the enormous enlargement of both kidneys. Peritoneal dialysis was carried out, but the patient's condition deteriorated and he died of uremia at the age of 31. This was in 1963, when renal transplantation was not as readily available as it is today.

The specimen is the left kidney, which has been sectioned to show extensive replacement of renal substance by innumerable cysts ranging in size from microscopic to over 6 cm in diameter. The kidney weighed 4000 g and its size was recorded as 35 cm × 15 cm × 8 cm.

Carcinoma of the Kidney. This is the malignant counterpart of the adenoma and usually appears as a large, soft mass at one or the other pole (see Case History I and Figure 35–9). A section shows that it has a variegated appearance, with some areas being white, others yellow or orange; elsewhere there are foci of bleeding. Microscopically it consists of large spheroidal cells with clear cytoplasm. In well-differentiated tumors these cells are arranged to form tubules. Although the cells resemble those of the normal renal tubules, it was at one time believed that the tumor arose from ectopic adrenal tissue situated on the surface of the kidney. This belief was the origin of the name *hypernephroma*, a term that is still widely used. It has since been discovered that the tumor arises from renal tubular epithelium; all grades of transition can be found between the anaplastic tumors and the benign adenoma.

The clear appearance of the cells is due to their high content of lipid and glycogen, both of which are lost during routine paraffin wax sectioning. The yellow appearance is due to the carotinoid pigments dissolved in the lipid. Probably the best name for this tumor is *clear-cell carcinoma of the kidney*.

Clinically carcinoma of the kidney is often silent for a long time. *Painless hematuria and an abdominal mass are the two common presenting features.* Distant and blood-borne metastases are common, with the liver, lungs, and bones being especially involved.

CASE HISTORY I. (See Figure 35–9).   In 1967, at the age of 57 years, the patient presented with a complaint of chronic cough. A radiograph showed ill-defined shadows in both upper lung fields; these were interpreted as being produced by fibrosis. Nineteen years previously, a radiograph was reported to have shown similar shadows, and at that time pulmonary tuberculosis had been suspected. The diagnosis had never been proved, and no treatment had been given.

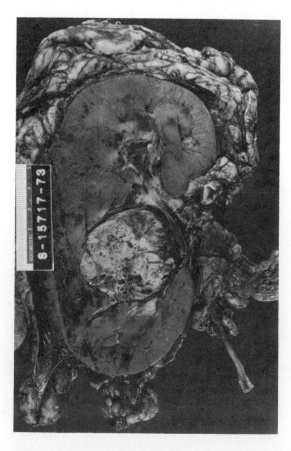

Figure 35–9.   Carcinoma of the kidney. The kidney contains a well-circumscribed tumor about 4 cm in diameter. It was yellow in color in the fresh state. Microscopy revealed a clear-cell renal carcinoma. See Case History I for clinical details.

Several samples of sputum and gastric washings were examined for tubercle bacilli without success. A lymph node biopsy taken at mediastinoscopy revealed noncaseating granulomas. No organisms could be identified in the sections. However, shortly after the procedure, a nodule was noted on the left nostril, and a biopsy again revealed a granulomatous reaction — this time fungi were detected. A repeat biopsy of the nodule was cultured and *Histoplasma capsulatum* was grown. Amphotericin B therapy was instituted, and the patient's condition improved. Nevertheless, he complained of easy fatigue and periodically had attacks of nausea and vomiting. No cause was found.

Two years later, difficulty in passing urine and nocturia led to a transurethral resection of an enlarged prostate. Histopathological studies revealed a benign prostate enlargement, but a radiograph revealed a translucent area in the first lumbar vertebral body. In spite of the pathology report a diagnosis of carcinoma of the prostate with bony metastases was made. Stilbestrol (a synthetic estrogen) therapy was initiated. Several episodes of painless hematuria were attributed to carcinoma of the prostate. Two years later, however, a cystoscopy failed to detect any bladder or prostatic lesion. Further investigations (an intravenous pyelogram and an arteriogram) showed a lesion in the left kidney. A nephrectomy was carried out for carcinoma of the kidney (see Figure 35–9). Shortly after surgery, the patient collapsed and died in shock.

Autopsy revealed no evidence of carcinoma of the prostate. Both adrenal glands showed almost complete replacement by caseous material due to histoplasmosis (see Figure 39–3). The lesion in the vertebra also showed histoplasmosis. The upper lobes of both lungs were fibrotic and contained scanty granulomas. This case illustrates several points:

1. Histoplasmosis, like tuberculosis, can become active after remaining dormant for many years.

2. Attacks of vomiting combined with weakness suggest a diagnosis of Addison's disease.

3. Major surgery in a patient with Addison's disease is hazardous unless adequate glucocorticoids are given.

4. In the absence of pathological proof it was unwise to make a clinical diagnosis of prostatic cancer. The significance of the attacks of painless hematuria was not appreciated, causing the diagnosis of carcinoma of the kidney to be delayed for over 1 year.

An interesting feature of the tumor is the phenomenon of dormancy. Bony metastases may suddenly erupt many years after the apparently successful removal of the primary growth.

Nephroblastoma, or Wilms' Tumor.   This is a tumor of infancy and is described in Chapter 17.

Ureteric Obstruction.   Sudden complete obstruction of one ureter, such as by a calculus, leads to atrophy of the affected kidney and compensatory enlargement of the other. Partial obstruction of a ureter by a stone, tumor, or pressure from an adjacent mass leads to dilatation of the ureter above the obstruction (*hydroureter*) and dilatation of the pelvis of the affected kidney (*hydronephrosis*).

Urethral Obstruction.   The following causes should be noted:

1. Carcinoma of the urethra. This is uncommon.

2. Fibrous stricture. This may follow repeated catheterization or may be an aftereffect of gonococcal urethritis.

3. Carcinoma of the prostate.

4. Benign prostatic enlargement. This is by far the most common and important cause of urethral obstruction and will be considered in detail.

Benign Prostatic Enlargement.   It has been estimated that between 30 and 50 per cent of men develop some degree of obstruction after the age of 50 from this cause. Common symptoms are difficulty in starting the act of urination (micturition), a poor stream of urine, and incomplete emptying of the bladder after micturition. This increase in the residual urine predisposes to *infection*. As the bladder refills, the urge to urinate returns and there is

THE LOWER URINARY TRACT

Urinary Tract Obstruction (Obstructive Uropathy)

frequency of micturition and nocturia. The bladder dilates and its muscular wall hypertrophies in response to the increased work needed to expel urine. Its wall becomes trabeculated (see Fig. 36–1). Protrusions of mucosa produce outpouchings, or *diverticula,* which further predispose to urinary stasis and infection.

Sudden urethral obstruction due to benign prostatic enlargement can occur at any time and is presumably due to congestion or infection. The enlarged median lobe of the prostate overlying the urethra can act like a ball valve.

Acute urethral obstruction must be distinguished from anuria. In both conditions no urine is passed through the urethra, but with obstruction the bladder becomes painfully enlarged. Ultimately, the increased pressure may force some urine through the urethra. This *retention with overflow* can deceive the unwary attendant into believing that the obstruction has been relieved.

The treatment of acute urinary obstruction requires expert attention. Either a catheter is passed through the urethra or else a needle is inserted into the bladder through the anterior abdominal wall; in either event, the obstruction is relieved. Urine must not be drained too quickly, however, or the sudden reduction in pressure will lead to bleeding. In addition, sudden decompression can cause an equally sudden diuresis, and this can cause hypovolemic shock.

Effect of Urinary Obstruction on the Kidney. Obstruction of the outflow of urine produces a back-pressure effect on the kidney that results in tubular atrophy and ultimately in destruction of renal parenchyma. The pelvis dilates and hydronephrosis results (Fig. 35–10). Evidence of chronic renal failure, such as a raised BUN, in an elderly person always suggests the likelihood of obstructive uropathy, particularly if the azotemia (excess of nitrogenous substances in the blood) fluctuates in intensity over a period of a few days.

Neurogenic Bladder

When lesions of the spinal cord damage the corticospinal tracts, there is loss of voluntary control of micturition. As the bladder dilates, local reflexes are responsible for automatic evacuation of urine. If the cord lesion is low, or if the nerves to the bladder are directly involved, even this automatic reflex is lost, and the bladder fills and finally overflows. In either event, urinary stasis — particularly when combined with repeated catheterization — predisposes the patient to urinary tract infection.

CASE HISTORY II. (See Figure 35–10). In 1948, at the age of 44 years, the patient noticed that his urine suddenly became red. Microscopic examination of the urine showed numerous red cells; tests for hemoglobin were positive. Cystoscopy revealed numerous "papillomas" in the bladder, and these were *fulgurated* (burned with an electric spark). Because of numerous recurrences the diagnosis was subsequently changed to papillary carcinoma. During the next 25 years the bladder tumors were treated on at least 34 occasions. In 1973, when the patient was 69 years of age, a mass was noted in the left side of the abdomen. This was identified as a nonfunctioning kidney and was removed. There were further recurrences of tumor, and in 1975 a partial cystectomy (removal of part of the bladder) was undertaken. A tumor similar to that shown in Figure 35–11 was found.

Ureteric Reflux

It is not uncommon to find hydroureter and hydronephrosis in the absence of any organic obstructive lesion. In such cases, it is believed that these are examples of neuromuscular incoordination. Radiographic studies indicate that in some patients urine passes up the ureter by abnormal peristaltic waves traveling in an upward direction.

Figure 35–10.   Hydronephrosis. The kidney shows dilatation of the pelvis and severe damage to the renal parenchyma such that the organ is converted into a bag of fluid. The condition resulted from intermittent ureteric obstruction by a low-grade carcinoma of the bladder. See Case History II for clinical details.

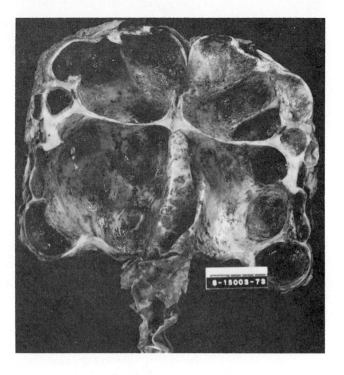

Apart from carcinoma, tumors of the urinary passages are uncommon.

Carcinoma.   Well-differentiated tumors of the transitional epithelium are often multiple and appear as noninvasive papillomatous growths with delicate fronds that give the lesions a resemblance to a sea anemone (Fig. 35–11). Histologically, these tumors are papillomatous and appear benign, but unfortunately they tend to recur even after local treatment (see Case History II). In practice it is wise to regard them as low-grade carcinomas. Neverthe-

Tumors of the Urinary Passages

Figure 35–11.   Carcinoma of the bladder. This radical cystectomy specimen was inflated with 10 per cent formalin solution before being opened. Numerous papillomatous tumors are seen attached to the bladder lining. Microscopy revealed a papillary transitional-cell carcinoma.

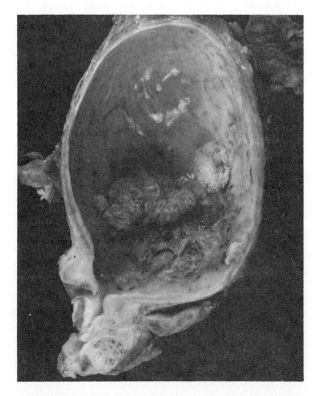

less, some authorities recognize the entity of benign papilloma of the bladder and attribute recurrence to the formation of new tumors. The less well-differentiated transitional cell tumors are the obvious carcinomas that show invasion of the wall and appear as sessile nodules or papillomatous lesions that break down into indurated malignant ulcers.

Histologically, the tumors are transitional cell carcinomas of varying degrees of differentiation. In some tumors there are areas of squamous-cell change, and not infrequently tumors are found in which the entire growth is composed of squamous-cell carcinoma. These cases tend to have a poor prognosis. Cancer of the bladder is particularly common in the Middle East and is associated with schistosomiasis. The increased incidence of bladder cancer in aniline dye workers and in those engaged in the rubber industry has been noted in Chapter 17. There is also an increased incidence in those who indulge in heavy cigarette smoking. Users of analgesic mixtures containing phenacetin are at a much higher risk of developing transitional-cell carcinoma of the renal pelvis than are nonusers. Carcinoma may therefore be a late complication of analgesic nephropathy, which is described earlier in this chapter.

Urinary Calculi   Urinary stones, or calculi, have plagued mankind for centuries; they are particularly common in the hot desert regions of the Middle East. Calculi can be divided into two main groups: primary and secondary.

1. Primary Calculi. These are presumed to occur because of a high concentration of chemicals in the urine or because of a defective mechanism for keeping these crystalloids in solution. Three common types are known:

Urate Stones. These are smooth, consist of uric acid and urates, and are common in patients who suffer from gout.

Calcium Oxalate Stones. These characteristically have a spiky surface that causes hematuria by damaging the mucosa.

Mixed Calcium Oxalate and Phosphate Stones. This type of stone occurs in the hypercalcemia that accompanies hyperparathyroidism and prolonged periods of recumbency.

2. Secondary Calculi. These stones are composed of calcium and magnesium oxalates and phosphates. They are formed around a focus of necrotic tissue, organisms, fibrin, a foreign body, or a primary stone. They are often secondary to infection. The most common type is found in the renal pelvis; as it grows, it assumes the shape of the pelvis and produces a shape that has been likened to that of a staghorn.

Effects of Urinary Calculi

1. Infection. Patients with recurrent urinary tract infection should always be investigated for the possibility of urinary stones.

2. Obstruction. This is frequently intermittent.

3. Hematuria.

4. Pain. A stone formed in the renal pelvis can pass down the ureter and cause severe colicky pain lasting for a time ranging from several minutes to several hours. This *renal colic* is usually accompanied by hematuria.

Review Questions

1. Explain why a deficiency of vasopressin (antidiuretic hormone, or ADH) causes polyuria.

2. Explain how the creatinine clearance test is carried out. What is the significance of a value of 30 ml per minute?

3. Describe the changes that occur in the blood in uremia.

4. Outline the principles involved in the classification of glomerulonephritis.

5. A 65-year-old male patient is in the hospital, having had a myocardial infarction ten days previously. His urine output suddenly diminishes. Suggest reasons for this sudden change.

6. Discuss the abnormalities that would be expected in the urine of a patient with each of the following conditions:
    (a) clear-cell carcinoma of the kidney
    (b) transitional-cell carcinoma of the bladder
    (c) acute pyelonephritis
    (d) severe chronic pyelonephritis
    (e) severe amyloidosis affecting the kidney

7. List the common causes of hematuria. How may hematuria be distinguished from hemoglobinuria? Outline the investigations that may be carried out to arrive at a correct diagnosis.

8. Describe the role of analgesic drugs in the pathogenesis of renal disease.

Selected Readings

Frazier, H. S.: Renal regulation of sodium balance. New England Journal of Medicine, 279:868–875, 1968.

Heptinstall, R. H.: Pathology of the Kidney. 2nd ed. Boston, Little, Brown and Company, 1974. A comprehensive reference work in two volumes. See, in particular, Chapters 7 to 14 for information on glomerulonephritis.

Leading Article: Vesico-ureteric reflux. Lancet, 1:1072–1074, 1968.

Leading Article: Defensive mechanisms of the bladder. British Medical Journal, 3:486, 1969.

Leading Article: Escherichia serotypes and renal infection. Lancet, 1:532–533, 1971.

Leading Article: What is chronic pyelonephritis? British Medical Journal, 2:61–62, 1971.

Merrill, J. P., and Hampers, C. L.: Uremia. New England Journal of Medicine, 282:953–961; 1014–1021; 1970.

Schumann, G. B.: Urine Sediment Examination. Baltimore, Williams and Wilkins, 1980.

CHAPTER 36 Male Reproductive Organs

After studying this chapter the student should be able to:

- Describe the development of the testis and relate this to the following:
  - (a) The occurrence of inguinal hernias
  - (b) The blood supply of the testis
  - (c) The metastatic spread of testicular tumors
  - (d) Spermatogenesis
- Describe cryptorchidism and its complications.
- Give an account of torsion of the testis.
- Classify the common causes of orchitis and epididymo-orchitis.
- Classify the tumors of the testis.
- Describe the clinical and pathological features of benign prostatic enlargement.
- Describe carcinoma of the prostate with regard to the following factors:
  - (a) Frequency
  - (b) Clinical features
  - (c) Spread

The Testes

The testes develop from a mass of mesoderm in the posterior abdominal wall. While still retaining their original blood supply, they migrate downwards and forwards, traversing the anterior abdominal wall through the inguinal canal until they finally come to lie in the scrotum. A process of peritoneum accompanies this descent, forming the tunica vaginalis, which surrounds the testis and its epididymis. The sac usually loses connection with the peritoneal cavity, but the inguinal region remains a point of weakness throughout life and is a common site for the development of a hernia. This is the price that has to be paid for having the male gonads in the scrotum, where the temperature can be maintained at a lower level than is found in the abdomen, from which the testes descended. There is evidence that this cool environment is necessary for the development of sperm (spermatogenesis).

Cryptorchidism

In *cryptorchidism* one or both testes fail to descend and reach the scrotum. The glands are then situated either within the abdomen or in the inguinal canal. Failure in spermatogenesis results in infertility if both testes are affected. An undescended testis remains immature and is liable to develop a malignant tumor, particularly a seminoma. Unless an undescended testis can be made to descend, by either medical or surgical means, it should be removed, since it remains a permanent hazard.

Torsion of the Testis

During violent exercise or following trauma the testis can rotate, causing a twist of the spermatic cord and its blood vessels. This rotation causes sudden pain; unless the testis can be untwisted soon (either by manipulation or by open surgery), first the veins and then the arteries become obstructed. The organ becomes intensely congested and subsequently infarcted. Torsion of the testis tends to occur if the testis is abnormally mobile because of a mild developmental defect, which is sometimes bilateral. Hence, following torsion of one testis, the other should be fixed to prevent a similar event occurring on the other side.

Acute infections of the epididymis (epididymitis) and testis (orchitis) generally occur secondarily to infection of the urinary tract or prostate. Acute epididymo-orchitis sometimes follows prostatitis and is a well-recognized complication of surgery on the prostate unless the vas deferens and its related lymphatics have been tied previously. Gonococcal epididymo-orchitis is an important complication of this infection. In bacterial infections, the brunt of the damage falls on the epididymis, while the testis is affected secondarily. In mumps orchitis, it is the testis that suffers most. It has been estimated that from 20 to 25 per cent of adult males who develop mumps suffer from acute orchitis about one week following enlargement of the parotid glands. With resolution of the disease some testicular atrophy takes place; if this is severe — particularly if it is bilateral — permanent sterility can result. The testis is enclosed in a dense fibrous coat, the tunica albuginea; in acute inflammation there is a rapid rise in tissue tension. Hence, severe pain is a feature of acute orchitis and epididymo-orchitis.

Infections of the Testis

Tuberculosis of the urinary tract sometimes spreads and affects the epididymis. Years ago, in tertiary syphilis a testicular gumma was not uncommon, but now this lesion is distinctly rare.

Although rare, neoplasms of the testis are the most common form of cancer to affect males between 20 and 35 years of age. The majority of the tumors are thought to arise from primitive pluripotential germ cells. As might be expected, they give rise to tumors that vary greatly in their differentiation and prognosis. Four major types, which are described below, have been recognized:

Neoplasms of the Testis

Seminoma. This is the most common tumor and occurs in a somewhat older age group than the others. It consists of uniform cells having clear cytoplasm, and it tends to produce a uniform bulky enlargement of the testis. Local invasion beyond the testis is not evident, but the tumor first metastasizes to the lymph nodes. It should be noted that the lymphatics of the testis follow the blood vessels and terminate in lymph nodes around the aorta. Seminoma of the testis, although malignant, is very responsive to radiotherapy and chemotherapy. Hence, with treatment it has a good prognosis, and a 5-year survival rate of 90 per cent of patients can be expected.

Teratoma. This neoplasm shows a mixed histological picture, having both epithelial and connective tissue elements. Occasionally, the tumor is well differentiated and cystic, and it resembles the ovarian teratoma. Nevertheless, the vast majority of testicular teratomas are solid and show areas of anaplastic growth — usually of the epithelial element. Teratomas tend to form a discrete nodule in the testis and subsequently invade the capsule. Since there is metastasis to the regional lymph nodes and via the blood stream, the prognosis is worse than that of seminoma. The 5-year mortality of patients with this tumor is approximately 30 to 50 per cent.

Embryonal Carcinoma. This unsatisfactory term is used to describe a tumor that microscopically resembles a carcinoma and also shows glandular differentiation and considerable pleomorphism. The tumor, which is often quite small, exhibits a more aggressive and lethal behavior than either seminoma or teratoma. The 5-year survival rate of patients is about 35 per cent.

Choriocarcinoma. This is the least common and most malignant type of testicular tumor. It metastasizes via the blood stream, and the primary growth is often small. In fact, the growth is sometimes of microscopic dimension, so that the patient presents clinically with multiple metastases — the primary tumor being located only at necropsy after a painstaking search. Histologically, the tumor resembles its counterpart in the female.

Combined Tumors. These tumors show a mixture of the types described above. Their existence supports the concept that these testicular tumors have a common cell type of origin. Further support for this thesis is the production of *chorionic gonadotropins* and *alpha-fetoprotein** by these tumors. As would be expected, this is most marked with choriocarcinoma, but it is also found with some cases of teratoma and embryonal carcinoma. The presence of these substances in the blood can be used as an aid to the diagnosis of testicular tumors, as well as to detect the presence of metastases following removal of the primary neoplasm.

Other rare tumors of the testis are known. The most intriguing of these is one derived from the stroma: the *interstitial cell tumor,* which, like its parent cell, secretes androgens. When this tumor occurs in children, there is precocious sexual development. When it occurs in adult males, estrogen production sometimes predominates so that feminization with gynecomastia results.

Hydrocele

An accumulation of fluid in the tunica vaginalis is called a *hydrocele.* When the tunica still communicates with the peritoneal cavity, this condition may be found in any case of ascites. Under normal conditions in which the tunica is an isolated sac, the development of a hydrocele suggests either an inflammatory condition of the testis or epididymis, or it suggests the development of a tumor. The presence of fluid can easily be detected by placing a flashlight behind the swelling and observing that it transilluminates. A mass in the scrotum produced by a solid tumor does not behave in this way. Between 25 and 50 per cent of acute hydroceles are due to trauma; in such cases there may be blood present also. Much blood in the sac is termed a *hematocele.*

The Prostate

The prostate gland is situated at the base of the bladder and is traversed by the first part of the male urethra. Its functions are largely unknown, but it contributes its secretions to the seminal ejaculate during intercourse and its enlargement is a source of considerable annoyance in old age.

Prostatitis

Acute prostatitis is generally a complication of urinary tract infection and can be a complication of gonorrhea. It is sometimes precipitated by catheterization and cystoscopy. The changes are similar to those of inflammation in other situations and therefore can terminate in suppuration.

Chronic prostatitis is extremely common as an incidental finding at necropsy. It generally accompanies urinary tract infection and may be associated with numerous calculi within the gland. Chronic prostatitis of clinical significance leads to fibrosis, which may give the gland a firmness that can be mistaken for carcinoma.

Benign Prostatic Enlargement

This is the most common disease of the prostate and is also called *prostatic hypertrophy* or *nodular hyperplasia.* The disease is extremely

---

*This is a globulin normally found in the blood during early fetal life but absent after birth. Its reappearance in the blood suggests the development of a tumor — liver and testis are the usual primary sites.

common in men over 50, and its incidence increases with age. Consequently, in men over the age of 70 years, about 95 per cent have some degree of involvement. The prostate gland becomes enlarged and nodular. This can be detected clinically by rectal examination. On cross section, cystic nodular areas are found, which can be proved microscopically to be due to foci of glandular hyperplasia. In other areas, there is overgrowth of smooth muscle or fibrous tissue. These elements give the gland a texture that is firm but not usually so hard that it mimics carcinoma. The nodular elements press on local blood vessels, so that focal areas of infarction are not uncommon. Bleeding can occur into these areas, and clinically hematuria is a frequent symptom. The other major effect of prostatic enlargement is distortion of the prostatic urethra and its obstruction (Fig. 36–1). The clinical features and secondary effects of this enlargement on the bladder and kidneys are described elsewhere (Chapter 35).

The cause of benign prostatic enlargement is not known, but it is presumed to be related to hormonal imbalance of old age. A deficiency of androgens or an excess of estrogenic substances has been suggested but not proved.

The treatment of significant benign prostatic enlargement is surgical. Prostatectomy can be performed through an abdominal incision or through the urethra using an operating endoscope. Not all patients with prostatic enlargement require treatment. It has been estimated that between 5 and 10 per cent of patients require surgical resection for relief of urinary tract obstruction or infection.

Carcinoma of the prostate is the second most frequent cause of death from carcinoma in men in the United States. It is common to find small foci of carcinoma in elderly patients dying from other causes, but the significance of these has been disputed. Progressive clinical cancer of the prostate is less common and may present with urinary obstruction or the development of symptoms due to local invasion or metastatic growth. Cancer of the prostate involves such local tissue as seminal vesicle, rectum, and bladder; it also

Carcinoma of the Prostate

Figure 36–1. Benign prostatic enlargement. This specimen of bladder and prostatic urethra has been opened from the front. The prostate is enlarged, and its nodular median lobe projects into the bladder, acting as a ball valve to obstruct the passage of urine. The bladder wall is greatly thickened. Hypertrophy of muscle bundles is responsible for the ribbed or trabeculated appearance of its lining. (Specimen from the Boyd Museum, Toronto.)

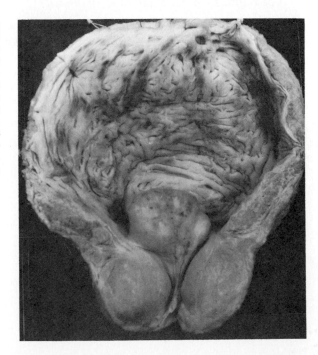

metastasizes to the regional lymph nodes. More significant is the blood-borne metastatic spread; approximately 70 per cent of cases show bony metastases, particularly of the lower spine. These lesions are noteworthy for being osteosclerotic. Metastatic spread to the liver and lungs is also common.

Microscopically, cancer of the prostate is generally a well-differentiated adenocarcinoma, and it tends to excite a considerable scirrhous reaction. A prostate with cancer is stony hard — the salient clinical feature, which can be detected by rectal examination. In any patient suspected of having malignant disease, particularly with metastatic bony spread, a rectal examination is mandatory if the patient is over 50 years of age.

The normal prostatic epithelium secretes acid phosphatase. In carcinoma, particularly if the bulk of tumor and its metastases is great, there is an elevation of the blood level of this enzyme. A test of the level of prostatic acid phosphatase is useful diagnostically, but a normal level does not exclude an early carcinoma.

Prostatic massage can express material through the urethra; malignant cells can be found in this fluid. This method is not completely reliable and has been criticized, since malignant cells appear in the blood following massage, and this could conceivably initiate the formation of metastases.

The most satisfactory method of diagnosis following clinical suspicion is a biopsy, which can generally be performed through the urethra.

The normal prostate is dependent upon androgens, and many carcinomas also are dependent upon androgenic hormones. Some degree of hormonal control of cancer of the prostate can be obtained by estrogen administration, castration, or a combination of the two. The results are sometimes quite striking; generally, they are of limited duration. The once-popular high-dosage estrogen therapy is now less favored, since it has been found that patients tend to have a much higher incidence of death from cardiovascular complications. The gynecomastia and skin pigmentation are other disadvantages of estrogen therapy.

Review Questions

1. Discuss the possible causes of a swelling that occupies one side of the scrotum and appears to involve one testis. How would the clinical history and the presence of pain influence the differential diagnosis?

2. Describe the common symptoms and signs of advanced carcinoma of the prostate. What biochemical abnormalities would be expected in the blood?

Selected Readings

Blandy, J. P.: Benign prostatic enlargement. British Medical Journal, *1*:31–35, 1971.
Leading Article: Undescended testis. British Medical Journal, 2:248–249, 1970.
Robbins, S. L., and Cotran, R. S.: Pathologic Basis of Disease. 2nd ed. Philadelphia, W. B. Saunders Company, 1979. Chapter 25, which discusses the male genital system, should be used as a source of further information and references.

Female Reproductive Organs; Pregnancy and Its Disorders

After studying this chapter the student should be able to:

- Describe the hormonal changes that are associated with the following:
    - (a) the development of the female secondary sexual characteristics
    - (b) the menstrual cycle
    - (c) pregnancy
    - (d) lactation
- Describe the Stein-Leventhal syndrome.
- Give an account of the ovarian tumors that are derived from the germinal epithelium.
- Describe the causes and important effects of salpingitis.
- Differentiate between the exocervix and the endocervix.
- Describe what is meant by a "cervical erosion".
- Give a general account of carcinoma of the cervix with regard to the following factors:
    - (a) predisposing causes
    - (b) age of onset
    - (c) mode of development
    - (d) symptoms
- Define amenorrhea, menorrhagia, metrorrhagia, and dysmenorrhea. Give at least one cause of each condition.
- Describe the outstanding features of each of the following:
    - (a) uterine fibroids
    - (b) carcinoma of the endometrium
    - (c) endometriosis
    - (d) endometrial hyperplasia
- List the features of toxemia of pregnancy.
- Describe what is meant by "ectopic pregnancy."
- Define spontaneous abortion and give one common cause of this process.
- Classify the causes of bleeding during pregnancy.
- Contrast placenta previa with abruptio placentae.
- Describe the outstanding features of hydatidiform mole and choriocarcinoma.

The hormones secreted by the ovary play a leading part in regulating the development of the female reproductive system. It is therefore appropriate to describe these before the individual organs and their abnormalities are discussed.

Childhood and Adolescence. During childhood the ovary secretes small quantities of *estrogen;* this secretion is sufficient to inhibit the hypothalamus. Hence, the release of gonadotropins from the pituitary is inhibited (Chapter 39). After the age of about 7 years, the hypothalamus becomes less sensitive to estrogen and its set-point is raised, and this leads to release of gonadotropin (chiefly *follicle-stimulating hormone,* or FSH) from the adenohypophysis.

Introduction: Hormonal Aspects of the Female Genital Tract

Ovarian estrogen production is thereby stimulated sufficiently to cause the *development of secondary sexual characteristics:* the breasts and uterus enlarge, and the subcutaneous fat is redistributed to produce the characteristic female contours. Shortly after this, the "cycling" center in the hypothalamus comes into operation and menstruation commences.* Under the influence of FSH, the ovarian follicles enlarge and secrete estrogen. At midcycle there is a surge of pituitary *luteinizing hormone* (LH) that causes ovulation. The follicular cells are converted into the corpus luteum, and *progesterone* is secreted.

Endometrial Changes in the Menstrual Cycle. During the first half of the menstrual cycle the endometrium (both glands and stroma) undergoes hyperplasia. Following ovulation, progesterone causes the glands to form secretion; the endometrium is thus suitably prepared for implantation of the developing fetus. If conception does not occur, the corpus luteum degenerates, and estrogen and progesterone levels decline; the endometrium undergoes necrosis and is passed in the menstrual flow as the cycle starts again.

Pregnancy. The fetal chorionic tissue that forms the placenta secretes *chorionic gonadotropin,*† which maintains the corpus luteum for the duration of pregnancy. In turn the corpus luteum secretes estrogen and progesterone. These inhibit the hypothalamic-hypophyseal system so that ovulation does not occur. Breast development is induced by the combined effects of placental hormones (estrogen, progesterone, and placental lactogen). During the latter part of pregnancy pituitary prolactin induces further changes.

Lactation. Following delivery, lactation is established under the influence of prolactin. The act of suckling causes release of oxytocin — this helps to express the milk by causing contraction of myoepithelial cells.

THE OVARY

Development

The ovaries develop, as do the testes, in the mesoderm of the posterior abdominal wall. Each ovary has three components: (1) a covering of *germinal epithelium* that is modified peritoneal mesothelium; (2) a *stroma* derived from mesoderm, and (3) *germ cells* that later mature into ova. Stromal cells form each *graafian follicle,* and after the release of the ovum they also form the *corpus luteum.* Both these structures manufacture sex hormones, as previously described. It should be noted that the primitive gonad is asexual, being neither male nor female. The primordial germ cells, which are sequestered early in the formation of an embryo and are probably of endodermal origin, migrate to the gonad and there develop into either ova or sperm. The stroma of the gonad has the ability to secrete hormones of either female or male type. Hence, it is not surprising that tumors of the ovary sometimes produce an excess of either male or female hormones.

Diseases of the Ovary

Cysts

Cysts derived from unruptured graafian follicles or from corpora lutei are extremely common. Since they rarely exceed 3 cm in diameter, they seldom cause trouble.

Stein-Leventhal Syndrome. This syndrome affects young women and is characterized by secondary amenorrhea, sterility, and bilateral polycystic ovaries. Several entities are included under this heading, and in some of them there is associated hirsutism (excess body hair) and obesity. The hypothalam-

---

*The rhythmic cycling center that awakens at puberty is peculiar to the female. It is responsible for the coordinated formation of releasing factors that in turn control the adenohypophysis and ultimately ovarian function. The presence of male hormones in the fetus prevents the development of a cycling center in the male.

†Human chorionic gonadotropin (HCG) is produced soon after implantation of the fertilized ovum. Its detection in the urine forms the basis for the common pregnancy tests. The test becomes positive at the time of the first missed menstrual period.

ic cycling center appears to be nonfunctional, with the result that there is a continuous release of gonadotropins. Hence, ovulation does not occur, and sterility results. Sometimes the ovarian stromal cells produce excess androgen, which is responsible for the hirsutism and occasional virilism. Surgical resection of a wedge of ovarian tissue is often curative, but the mechanism is obscure. The simple explanation that it allows the imprisoned ova to escape appears to be without foundation.

Benign Tumors of Germinal Epithelium. Benign tumors of the germinal epithelium form cystic spaces with papillary epithelial ingrowths. They are therefore called *papillary cystadenomas*. Two types of tumor should be noted: *Primary Tumors*

Mucinous Cystadenoma. These cystic tumors are usually unilateral and can reach enormous size, filling the pelvis and causing abdominal distension. The cystic spaces are filled with a mucinous fluid and are lined by an epithelium that resembles that of the lining of the endocervix. Malignant change may occur but is uncommon. A rare complication is rupture: the whole peritoneum is flooded with mucin, and multiple tumor implants take root on the peritoneal surface, with the result that all the abdominal viscera become bound together. This produces a surgeon's nightmare if a laparotomy is required for a complication such as intestinal obstruction. The condition is called *pseudomyxoma peritonei* and is generally regarded as local metastasis from a low-grade, well-differentiated carcinoma. A similar condition can complicate the neoplastic type of mucocele of the appendix.

Serous Cystadenoma. This type of tumor is more common than the mucinous variant. In about one third of patients the tumor is bilateral. The cystic spaces are lined by an epithelium that resembles that of the lining of the fallopian tubes. Malignant change is quite common.

Malignant Tumors of the Germinal Epithelium. *Papillary cystadenocarcinoma* is the most common primary malignancy of the ovary and is the malignant counterpart of the cystadenoma, usually the serous type. As with papillomatous neoplasms of the bladder, it is difficult to draw a line between benign and malignant lesions. There is a gray area between the two extremes, and in this area individual pathologists will differ in their opinions. The malignant ovarian tumors show profuse papillomatous projections both into the cystic cavities and from the surface. Since peritoneal seeding is common, the other ovary is often involved (Fig. 37–1). Abdominal swelling due to *ascites* may be a prominent and distressing clinical manifestation. The presence of malignant cells in ascitic fluid is a helpful diagnostic finding. Lymph node and widespread blood-borne metastases occur, as with other carcinomas.

Other Primary Ovarian Tumors. The benign teratoma is a germ cell neoplasm and has been described in Chapter 17 (see Fig. 17–14). Occasionally a component of this tumor becomes malignant, such as in the formation of squamous-cell carcinoma or even a choriocarcinoma.

Other ovarian tumors form a complex group, the description of which is beyond the scope of this book. Some tumors secrete estrogens; others secrete androgens. Hence, the possibility of an ovarian tumor must be considered in any woman showing definite signs of masculinization or of excessive endometrial hyperplasia.

The ovary is involved in metastatic growth more often than any other pelvic organ. The common primary sites are the large intestine, the stomach, and the breast. *Secondary Tumors*

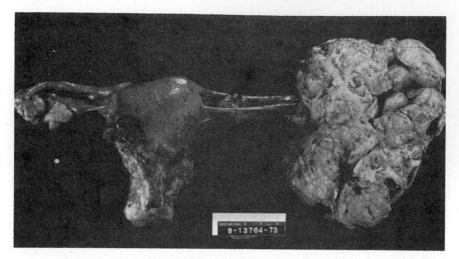

Figure 37–1. Carcinoma of the ovary. The specimen consists of the uterus with both fallopian tubes and ovaries. The left ovary is enormously enlarged by tumor; the right ovary shows a white area that also contains tumor. Numerous peritoneal nodules of metastatic growth were present in this patient. Note the asymmetry of the body of the uterus. When the organ was opened, a septum was found. It divided the cavity into two unequal parts and was the result of imperfect fusion of the two müllerian ducts.

THE FALLOPIAN TUBES

The fallopian tubes, the uterus, and most of the vagina develop from the two müllerian ducts. Normally these ducts fuse completely to form a single midline uterus and vagina, but sometimes this fusion is incomplete. The most extreme example of this is the rare anomaly of a double uterus and a double vagina. Much more frequent is an incomplete fusion of the parts of the primitive uterus, so that this organ develops with two horns or has a septum partially dividing its cavity (Fig. 37–1). The upper, or cephalic, part of the müllerian duct normally remains separate and forms the fallopian tube. Note that the lumen of the fallopian tubes remains open to the peritoneal cavity, because it is through this opening that the ova reach the lower genital tract.

Inflammatory Disease of the Fallopian Tubes

Pyogenic infections of the female genital tract tend to spare the vagina and endometrium but attack the fallopian tubes severely. The result is *acute salpingitis*. The fimbriated ends of the tubes become sealed over, and the infection enters a chronic phase. The tubes are distended with pus and assume the shape of retort tubes *(pyosalpinx)*. Ultimately the infection subsides, and the tubes remain distended with clear fluid *(hydrosalpinx)*. Sometimes the infection is not controlled, and a chronic abscess involving the fallopian tubes and ovary is formed. This *tubo-ovarian abscess* requires surgical relief.

Salpingitis is often accompanied by inflammation of the adjacent pelvic structures, including the peritoneum and bowel. It then forms a component of a more widespread *pelvic inflammatory disease (PID)*. When this disease is acute, because of the peritonitis there are manifestations of an acute abdomen. When chronic, the condition causes painful intercourse *(dyspareunia)*, painful menstrual periods *(dysmenorrhea)*, and intestinal obstruction secondary to the formation of fibrous adhesions. The *sterility* that results is due to the closure of the fimbriated ends of the fallopian tubes; partial blockage of the tubes by adhesions leads to an increased incidence of ectopic pregnancy.

The most common type of PID used to be gonorrheal, but this infection responds so well to chemotherapy that the incidence of gonococcal salpingitis has now declined. PID is more often due to other pyogenic organisms — staphylococci, streptococci, and the coliform organisms. PID is now encountered principally as a postpartum or a postabortal infection. The nongonococcal types of infection tend to involve the whole wall of the fallopian tubes rather than merely affect the mucosa as is typical of the gonococcal cases. Hence, thickening of the tubes and dense adhesions to adjacent structures are more common.

Tuberculous Salpingitis.   This was once a disease to consider as a cause of sterility. The disease, fortunately, is now rare.

The uterus consists of two parts: the *cervix* and the *body*.

THE UTERUS

The cervix (neck) of the uterus consists of two parts: the *endocervix* and the *exocervix*. The endocervix is lined by a mucus-secreting epithelium with associated glands, whereas the vaginal part, or exocervix, protrudes into the vagina and is covered by stratified squamous epithelium.

The Cervix Uteri

In women who have borne children, the cervix is often scarred and distorted. Sometimes the endocervical mucosa is everted or "turned out" and can be seen on vaginal examination. This is the common type of "cervical erosion" and was so named because it appeared as if the normal squamous epithelium of the exocervix had become eroded and covered by endocervixlike mucosa. This mechanism is not generally accepted, but the term "erosion" is still widely used. The condition is important in two connections:

Cervical Erosion

1. Cervical erosion is often accompanied by chronic cervicitis and a persistent mucoid or mucopurulent vaginal discharge *(leukorrhea)*.
2. The appearance may mimic that of a carcinoma.

Inflammatory folds, or polyps, of endocervical mucosa are very common and can protrude through the external os into the vagina. Ulceration and bleeding, particularly following intercourse, can arouse suspicion of cancer. Polyps do not, however, predispose to malignancy.

Cervical Polyps

Cancer of the cervix is a common malignant tumor of the female genital tract and now ranks sixth as a cause of cancer deaths in women (behind cancer of breast, colon, lung, ovary, and pancreas). It may grow as a cauliflowerlike tumor *(exophytic type)*, or it may invade the cervix to produce a nodular, hard mass with overlying ulceration *(endophytic type)*. The peak age of incidence is about 50 years, but the in-situ stage is present 10 to 15 years before that. Ninety-five per cent of the tumors are squamous-celled, and the remainder are adenocarcinomas. The chief symptoms are a vaginal discharge, intermenstrual bleeding, and postmenopausal bleeding. It must be appreciated, however, that these are the symptoms of advanced (and often incurable) disease. Carcinoma of the cervix spreads to involve local structures (intestine, ureters, and bladder) and later metastasizes to regional lymph nodes. Widespread metastases can occur, but death is often due to the local effects of the tumor or to radiation damage.

Carcinoma of the Cervix

Predisposing Causes.   According to statistics, cancer of the cervix is most common in low-income groups, in women who have had sexual intercourse at an early age, and in women who have had frequent intercourse and many sexual partners. It is uncommon in ethnic groups (*e.g.,* Jews and Indian Muslims) that practice male circumcision at an early age. Herpesvirus type 2 infection is more common in patients with carcinoma of the cervix than in control groups, but this may be coincidental and have no etiological relationship; both diseases are more prevalent in the promiscuous.

The Development of Cancer of the Cervix.   Cancer of the cervix is believed to develop slowly, from increasingly severe dysplasia, to carcinoma-in-situ, and finally to invasive cancer. These stages can be detected by a cytological examination of scrapings from the cervix (see the "Pap Smear," Chapter 17). Regular examination of all adult women should therefore eliminate deaths from this disease, since early lesions can be treated and cured.

When a Pap (from Papanicolaou, who originated the test) test is found to be positive for abnormal cells, it should be repeated to eliminate errors of interpretation or labeling. The precise course of action varies from one center to another. Patients with mild dysplasia can be followed for evidence indicating that their disease is progressing. Severe dysplasia and carcinoma-in-situ demand more active treatment. The experienced gynecologist can detect abnormal areas of the cervix by using the colposcope: these areas can be biopsied (to exclude invasive cancer) and treated by local destructive agents, such as extreme cold, as used in cryotherapy. Another course of action is to biopsy a large "cone" of cervical tissue and search for abnormal areas. When invasive cancer is present, the treatment of choice may be hysterectomy, radiotherapy, or a combination of both. It is evident that the management of carcinoma of the cervix involves technical skills and good judgment. There are few other areas in medicine in which collaboration among the technologist, the pathologist, and the clinical physician is so necessary to guarantee that their patients receive the best treatment. Overdiagnosis and overtreatment can result in unnecessary surgery that can prevent young women from bearing children. Underdiagnosis and undertreatment, on the other hand, can kill the patient.

The Body of the Uterus

The body of the uterus consists of a powerful muscle (the *myometrium*) and a mucosal lining (the *endometrium*).

The changes that take place in the endometrium during the normal menstrual cycle have already been described. Endometrial abnormalities often cause changes in menstruation; these will be described first.

Abnormalities of Menstruation

Some menstrual irregularity occurs in every woman's life. This section deals only with certain facets of this important and complex problem.

Amenorrhea, or absence of menstruation, is normal before the menarche, after the menopause, and during pregnancy and lactation. *Primary amenorrhea* denotes a failure to commence menstruation and is usually due to ovarian disease (*e.g.,* ovarian dysgenesis) or to hypothalamic-pituitary disorders. *Secondary amenorrhea* is usually defined as absence of menstruation for more than 12 months, excluding pregnancy and the menopause. Hormonal imbalance due to detectable disease of the ovaries, hypothalamus, or endocrine glands is an occasional cause, but amenorrhea is also a feature of numerous general illnesses, including mental disturbances such as worry, emotional disappointment, and depression. The mechanism is presumably related to nervous influences on the hypothalamic cycling center.

Menorrhagia, meaning excessive or prolonged blood loss occurring at menstruation, is extremely common. Sometimes it is due to a failure of ovulation. No corpus luteum is formed, and estrogens acting in the absence of progesterone lead to *endometrial hyperplasia.* Curettage performed during the latter half of the menstrual cycle shows *absence of secretory activity.* The procedure of curettage is therefore a useful way of diagnosing this type of anovulatory bleeding.

Metrorrhagia refers to intermenstrual bleeding or such irregularity that no periodicity is present. Sometimes this condition is due to an irregular endometrial response to normal ovarian hormonal influence. Thus, secretory and proliferative areas of endometrium exist side by side.

Abnormalities of menstruation may be symptomatic of local uterine disease — polyps, endometrial hyperplasia, endometriosis, fibroids, or carcinoma. When no obvious cause can be found, the clinical term "functional uterine bleeding" is sometimes used.

Endometrial Hyperplasia

Thickening of the endometrium is a common finding in patients with menorrhagia or metrorrhagia. It may occur in young women and is a feature of the Stein-Leventhal syndrome. Most frequently, however, it is an affliction of women at the time of the menopause. Microscopically there is glandular hyperplasia, indicating that the condition is due to the unopposed action of estrogen. The menstrual cycle is usually anovulatory. The hyperplasia may affect the whole endometrium, or its distribution may be focal.

Microscopically the hyperplastic endometrium may show focal areas of atrophy — the atrophic glands show cystic dilatation, and the appearance may be described as a "Swiss cheese" pattern. Of greater significance and importance is the presence of *epithelial atypia*. This can vary from slight atypia to carcinoma-in-situ. Hence, endometrial hyperplasia with atypia is considered to be a condition that can evolve into endometrial carcinoma, which as noted below is predominantly a disease of postmenopausal women. There is considerable evidence that prolonged exposure to estrogen is a major cause of this. The source may be exogenous in the form of medication given to treat menopausal symptoms, or it may be endogenous from an estrogen-producing tumor of the ovary. Much more frequently it is produced as a result of some hormonal dysfunction of undetermined cause.

Tumors of the Body of the Uterus

Leiomyoma. The leiomyoma is a benign tumor of smooth muscle and usually contains an admixture of fibrous tissue (Fig. 37–2). Hence, it is also called a fibroleiomyoma or "fibroid." Fibroids arise in the myometrium and are generally multiple. They vary in size from those that are scarcely visible in the gross to those weighing over 100 pounds! Some fibroids become pedunculated and appear as subserosal or submucosal nodules. Uterine fibroids are the commonest tumor to afflict women and are present in about 25 per cent of the adult female population. They may cause symptoms in various ways. Their presence may be associated with menorrhagia and irregular bleeding.

Figure 37–2. Leiomyoma of the uterus. The uterus has been opened to show one large well-circumscribed tumor. Several smaller fibroids were also present, but they are not visible in this photograph. This tumor was an incidental finding in a patient who died as a result of carcinoma of the colon. (Courtesy of Dr. A. Vayalumkal.)

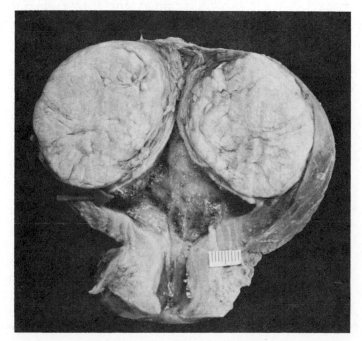

Occasionally they cause mechanical difficulties during labor. Fibroids appear to be estrogen-dependent, because they diminish in size, degenerate, and even calcify after the menopause.

Carcinoma of the Endometrium. Adenocarcinoma of the endometrium is a disease of postmenopausal women with a peak incidence in persons between 50 and 60 years of age. It is less common than carcinoma of the cervix, but the incidence is on the increase, partly because of longer life expectancy. The disease is more frequent among childless women than among multiparous ones.

Carcinoma of the endometrium is characterized by irregular vaginal bleeding accompanied by leukorrhea. The disease probably begins with the development of endometrial hyperplasia, dysplasia, and carcinoma-in-situ. Nevertheless, this orderly sequence of development is less well-documented than the stages of development of carcinoma of the cervix.

Endometriosis

Pelvic Endometriosis (Endometriosis Externa). In this type of endometriosis, ectopic endometrium is present in the pelvic region (ovaries, uterine ligaments, vagina) and in the peritoneal covering of the bladder and uterus. The pathogenesis of this remarkable state has been much debated. Endometrial tissue regurgitated through the fallopian tubes during menstruation could become implanted in the pelvic organs. Alternatively, peritoneal cells could undergo metaplasia. The occasional occurrence of endometriosis in the umbilicus — and even in the lung — has raised the possibility of lymphatic or blood-borne spread. The pathogenesis remains a mystery!

Endometriosis is a disease of women during active reproductive life; the endometrial tissue undergoes the same changes as the uterine endometrium during the menstrual cycle. Bleeding into the affected areas causes pain and often stimulates marked fibrosis. If this is extensive it can lead to the formation of dense adhesions to the pelvic organs. Chronic pelvic pain, dysmenorrhea, dyspareunia, and pain on defecation or urination are common symptoms. The effects and symptoms of endometriosis are therefore very similar to those of chronic inflammatory pelvic disease.

Adenomyosis (Endometriosis Interna). This is a common condition in which normal-appearing endometrium invades the myometrium and causes enlargement of the uterus. Menorrhagia is the most common functional effect, but patients may also complain of dysmenorrhea and dyspareunia.

COMPLICATIONS OF PREGNANCY

Hyperemesis Gravidarum

Nausea and morning sickness are common in early pregnancy, but the origin of these symptoms is not understood. Occasionally the vomiting becomes severe enough to cause dehydration, starvation, and death. Wernicke's encephalopathy can develop in fatal cases (Chapter 44).

Toxemia of Pregnancy

Although the term "toxemia" is in common use, no specific toxin has ever been identified. The condition occurs during the last three months (trimester) of pregnancy, and its early stages are characterized by three features:

1. *Hypertension.* This is the most constant feature.
2. *Albuminuria.* This occurs in severe cases.
3. *Edema.* Some degree of water and salt retention resulting in edema of the legs is common in normal pregnancy and is of no significance. However, edema of the face or arms, and any marked weight increase due to water accumulation immediately suggests toxemia.

Severe toxemia (termed *pre-eclampsia)* is characterized by headache, visual disturbances (ranging from flashes of light to blindness), abdominal pain, and vomiting. It is a serious condition, because it can be followed by *eclampsia*. This is the most severe manifestation of toxemia and is characterized by epileptiform convulsions that start with twitching of the face, are followed by a *tonic phase* lasting one to two minutes, and terminate in a *clonic phase* with violent, convulsive movements during which the pregnant woman may damage herself.

Toxemia is sometimes familial; it is associated with abruptio placentae, twin pregnancies, and the presence of a hydatidiform mole. It is most common in primigravidae (women who are pregnant for the first time). Vascular spasm appears to be the cause of the headaches, cerebral edema, visual disturbances, and convulsions. Necropsy findings include glomerular changes and liver necrosis together with evidence of disseminated intravascular coagulation. Rarely bilateral renal cortical necrosis results in renal failure (see Chapter 21 and Fig. 21–4).

These observations have done little to shed any light on the etiology of toxemia. The disease that causes an appreciable fetal and maternal mortality has no known cause other than that it is associated with pregnancy. Nevertheless, with early diagnosis the condition responds well to simple medical remedies, such as bed rest and salt restriction. For this reason, good antenatal care always includes *routine examination of the patient for hypertension, albuminuria, edema, and excessive weight gain.*

Ectopic Pregnancy

By the time the ovum, which is fertilized in the fallopian tube, reaches the uterus, it is at the correct stage for implantation. If its passage is delayed, implantation occurs in the tube; this is the most common type of ectopic pregnancy. The fetus grows for a time, but its growth usually causes the tube to rupture by the sixth week. Pain and severe intra-abdominal hemorrhage are the result. When the fetus dies, the endometrium is shed and vaginal bleeding occurs. This sign helps to distinguish a ruptured ectopic pregnancy from other abdominal catastrophes.

Abortion

The expulsion of a nonviable fetus* is termed *abortion* or *miscarriage*. Approximately 10 to 15 per cent of all pregnancies terminate in this way, usually between the ninth and the thirteenth week of gestation. Many causes, both fetal and maternal, have been described. Chief among them is fetal abnormality; spontaneous abortion is an important mechanism by which defective fetuses are eliminated, for 50 to 60 per cent of all spontaneous abortuses have a karyotypic abnormality (Chapter 3).

Bleeding During Pregnancy

Bleeding from the genital tract during pregnancy not only is alarming for the patient but also is often a warning of a serious abnormality. The types of bleeding may be divided into two groups, described below:

1. **Bleeding in Early Pregnancy** (before 28 weeks' gestation). Three important causes should be noted and are considered elsewhere in this chapter.

(a) abortion
(b) ectopic pregnancy
(c) hydatidiform mole

2. **Bleeding in the Later Months of Pregnancy.** Bleeding that occurs after the twenty-eighth week of gestation and before delivery is called *antepartum hemorrhage*. Two causes are of paramount importance:

(a) *Placenta Previa.* In this condition, part or all of the placenta is

---

*The age at which a fetus becomes viable is arbitrarily set at 20 weeks' gestation by some authorities and at 28 weeks by others.

attached to the lower uterine segment. This part of the uterus stretches and thins out in late pregnancy and especially during labor. The more rigid placenta becomes detached, and this provokes external bleeding. The initial bleeding is often slight and painless; it can be followed by massive bleeding that endangers the life of both mother and child. Urgent hospital treatment is necessary, and often cesarean section is required.

(b) *Abruptio Placentae.*   In this condition there is premature separation of a normally situated placenta. Bleeding occurs between the placenta and the uterine wall, and there may or may not be external bleeding. The condition is most common in primigravidae and in patients with toxemia. Abruptio placentae is characterized by abdominal pain, tenderness of the uterus, and the development of shock. Death sometimes results, usually because of hemorrhage shock. As with placenta previa, urgent hospital treatment is necessary.

Hydatidiform Mole

This lesion may be regarded as a benign tumor of the placenta (Fig. 37–3). No fetus develops. The chorionic villi are avascular and become swollen to produce a grapelike mass of tissue (Fig. 37–3). The mole is usually well-developed at about the seventeenth to twentieth week of gestation. There is excessive enlargement of the uterus for the stage of pregnancy, vaginal bleeding, and finally spontaneous passage of the mole per vaginam.

Chorioadenoma destruens is a type of mole that is more invasive than the ordinary type of hydatidiform mole. Part of the mole may be passed, but some remains in the uterine wall. Removal by curettage is not possible, but the tumor responds to chemotherapy.

It has been estimated that 1 to 2 per cent of hydatidiform moles become malignant (choriocarcinoma).

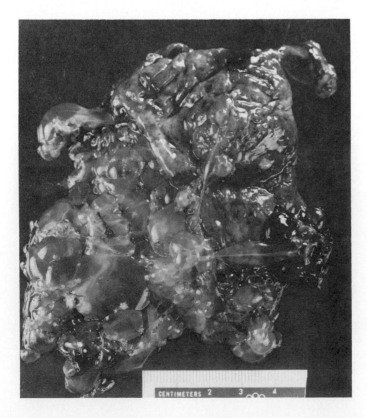

Figure 37–3. Hydatidiform mole. The normal placental tissue has been largely replaced by the mole. Note the presence of numerous fluid-filled cysts, from which the lesion gets its name. *Hydatis* is from the Greek, meaning "a drop of water."

This is a highly malignant tumor of placental tissue. It may arise in a previous hydatidiform mole, or it may follow either an abortion or a normal labor. The tumor is highly invasive and metastasizes widely. Nevertheless, some cases respond dramatically to chemotherapy with methotrexate. Both hydatidiform mole and choriocarcinoma produce large quantities of chorionic gonadotropin. Consequently the detection of chorionic gonadotropin in the urine is a useful test in these conditions, both for initial diagnosis and for the detection of recurrences or metastases. *Choriocarcinoma*

Occasionally hydatidiform moles and choriocarcinomas produce a thyrotropin-like hormone and the patients develop *thyrotoxicosis*.

Review Questions

1. An ovarian mass has been diagnosed by pelvic examination. Speculate on its possible nature. At laparotomy an ovarian tumor was found, and a biopsy revealed that it was a choriocarcinoma. Suggest how the tumor arose and how it might have been diagnosed before surgery.

2. What is the significance of finding no secretory activity in uterine curettings taken 26 days after the first day of the last menstrual period?

3. Explain why carcinoma of the cervix uteri is a preventable disease.

4. Discuss how the incidence of carcinoma of the endometrium might be decreased.

5. Describe the hormonal functions of the placenta.

6. Speculate on the causes of vaginal bleeding in each of the following women:
    (a) a 13-year-old girl
    (b) a 26-year-old married woman who has missed her last two periods
    (c) a woman who is due to give birth in 2 weeks
    (d) a pregnant woman who is under treatment for toxemia of pregnancy

Selected Readings

Leading Article: Management of eclampsia. British Medical Journal, 2:1485–1486, 1976.
Leading Article: Screening for cervical cancer. British Medical Journal, 3:659–660, 1976.
Novak, E. R., and Woodruff, J. D.: Gynecologic and Obstetric Pathology. 8th ed. Philadelphia, W. B. Saunders Company, 1979. A comprehensive reference book.
Robbins, S. L., and Cotran, R. S.: Pathologic Basis of Disease. 2nd ed. Philadelphia, W. B. Saunders Company, 1979. Chapter 26 provides a general overview of the subject.

Diseases of the Breast

After studying this chapter the student should be able to:

- Describe the structure and development of the female breast.
- Describe the main features of acute mastitis, plasma cell mastitis, fat necrosis of the breast and mammary dysplasia.
- List the groups of women who are especially liable to develop carcinoma of the breast.
- Discuss briefly the evidence suggesting that cancer of the breast is due to a viral infection.
- Classify the types of carcinoma of the breast.
- Given an account of the early detection, the prognosis, and the treatment of carcinoma of the breast.
- Describe the routes of spread of breast cancer.
- Define gynecomastia and give three examples of this condition.

Structure and Development

The human breast is not a single gland but, on the contrary, consists of about 20 separate glands or *lobes,* each with its own duct opening separately onto the surface of the nipple. The lobes develop, as do the sweat glands, by ingrowths from the surface epidermis; during infancy, they consist only of rudimentary branching ducts surrounded by cuffs of connective tissue that are an extension of the papillary dermis. In the male this state persists throughout life, but in the female during the three- to four-year period before the onset of menstruation, the breasts enlarge and the ducts and the specialized loose periductal stroma that is a characteristic feature of the breast tissue proliferate. During adolescence stromal growth continues, and buds form at the end of the ducts. These are the *lobules,* and they are the beginnings of the secretory gland structure that develops later if pregnancy occurs.

In the adult female the breast shows cyclical changes that parallel those of the endometrium during the menstrual cycle. Under the influence of estrogen there is epithelial proliferation during the first half of the cycle; this proliferation continues as progesterone is added during the second half of the cycle. During this second phase there is abortive secretory activity, and the gland enlarges and feels tense.

The breast attains its maximum development during pregnancy and lactation. The epithelial proliferation and secretory gland formation are such that the organ closely resembles other secretory glands, such as the pancreas.

In the normal resting breast the epithelial component constitutes about 15 per cent of the organ. The remainder consists of lobules of fat contained by fibrous septa that stretch from the dermis to the fascia overlying the pectoral muscles. These septa play a large part in giving the female breast its firmness and configuration. The septa also form an avenue for the spread of carcinoma to the skin and pectoral muscles.

The lymphatic drainage of the breast has been intensively studied, mainly with the aim of devising radical operations for the treatment of cancer of the breast. Lymph drains into the axillary, supraclavicular, internal mammary (within the chest), and abdominal lymph nodes. As will be explained later in this chapter, radical operations designed to remove these nodes do not seem to have influenced the prognosis of this form of cancer. Hence, a detailed knowledge of the lymphatic drainage of the breast has not proved to be of any great practical value.

Supernumerary Breast Tissue. Most mammals develop breast tissue along a milk line. In humans this extends from the anterior axillary fold to the groin; occasionally, accessory nipples are found along this line. When associated with accessory breast tissue in the female, these enlarge and cause pain at puberty and particularly during pregnancy.

Enlargement of the Breast. It is common to find some enlargement of the breasts in newborn infants in whom some secretion ("witch's milk") may be formed. This enlargement lasts for one to two weeks and is due to the action of maternal hormones. On rare occasions enlargement of one or both breasts takes place during childhood if there is excessive estrogen produced as a result of a functioning tumor of the ovary, adrenal, or pituitary.

The most common type of enlargement of the breast (generally called *hypertrophy*) is seen in girls at adolescence. One or both breasts become so enlarged that partial surgical removal *(reduction mammoplasty)* is required. This *virginal hypertrophy* of the breast is presumably due to hormonal imbalance.

Developmental Anomalies

Acute Mastitis. Acute bacterial mastitis is generally seen in the breast during the first few weeks of nursing a firstborn child. The offending organism, *Staphylococcus aureus,* gains access through a crack in the nipple. Suppuration requiring surgical drainage generally follows unless early antibiotic treatment is instituted.

Plasma Cell Mastitis. This is an uncommon condition and generally affects women about 40 years of age. There is often a history of difficult nursing due to inverted nipples, cracked nipples, or infection. In one quadrant of the breast an area of thickening is found that extends beneath the nipple to cause some distortion. There is usually pain and tenderness and sometimes a discharge from the nipple. Pathologically, there is dilatation of the associated ducts; this appears to be the prime lesion. The ducts are filled with a creamy liquid and contain many macrophages with vacuolated cytoplasm. Rupture of this inspissated material into the surrounding stroma causes a chronic inflammatory reaction with many plasma cells and sometimes with tuberculoid granulomas, causing a picture that mimics tuberculosis. Tuberculosis of the breast is, in fact, very rare.

Fat Necrosis. This condition is generally encountered in fat, pendulous breasts. In about half the patients a history of trauma is obtained. Histologically, there is necrosis of fat cells with an associated inflammatory reaction, at first acute and then progressing to chronicity with foreign body giant cells and a granulomatous reaction. The lesion presents as a lump in the breast, and the histological picture must be differentiated from that of tuberculosis.

Acquired Disease of the Breast

Inflammation

This common condition has been given many names in the past, the most common being chronic mastitis. Nevertheless, the condition is not inflammatory and appears to be the end-result of the hormonal changes that take place during women's reproductive life. As noted previously, the breast undergoes cyclic changes of hyperplasia and regression during menstruation. The combined effect of these changes over many years is to produce in some women imbalance between the amount of epithelium and the specialized fibrous tissue. The disease may affect one segment of one breast, commonly

Mammary Dysplasia (Fibrocystic Disease)

the upper and outer quadrant, and produce a relatively localized mass, or it may affect much of the tissue of both breasts, producing a widespread lumpiness. A characteristic feature that helps to distinguish these lesions from carcinoma is that the lumps tend to increase in size and to become more tender before each menstrual period. Several types of mammary dysplasia have been described, but they represent aspects of a single disease rather than constituting separate entities.

Microscopically, mammary dysplasia exhibits the following features either alone or in combination: There is *fibrosis,* which when marked gives the breast a firm, rubbery texture. *Epithelial hyperplasia* is common and particularly affects the ducts. Sometimes intraduct papillomatous ingrowths are formed. The hyperplastic epithelium may have atypical features suggesting that malignancy might develop. At times the epithelium shows metaplasia and takes on the characteristics of apocrine sweat gland epithelium. Proliferation of small ductules may be accompanied by fibrosis to produce a histological picture that can easily be mistaken by the unwary pathologist for carcinoma. This is termed *sclerosing adenosis,* and clinically it tends to affect one segment of the breast, thereby forming a mass. Finally, *cyst formation* is common and is usually bilateral.

Relationship to Carcinoma. Views on the relationship of mammary dysplasia to the subsequent development of carcinoma have varied considerably during the last few decades. At one time it was fashionable to regard the condition as premalignant. Many simple mastectomies were performed with a view to averting the development of cancer. Current belief is that although some of the hyperplastic lesions, particularly if there is atypia, may show an increased tendency to become malignant, the overall pattern is that of a disease bearing little direct relationship to cancer. Nevertheless, cancer of the breast is more common in women who also have mammary dysplasia. Since the tumor often arises in the breast not affected by the dysplasia, it is suggested that the hormonal influences leading to dysplasia also predispose to malignant change.

The importance of mammary dysplasia is that it presents as one or more lumps in the breast; these lumps must be distinguished from cancer, generally by biopsy.

Benign Neoplasms of the Breast

Fibroadenoma. Fibroadenoma is the commonest tumor of the breast, occurring in women younger than 30 years of age. Although it may be regarded as a localized form of mammary dysplasia, since it is so localized and encapsulated, it is generally classified as a benign tumor. Nevertheless, it responds to hormonal stimulation like the normal breast. The tumor enlarges during pregnancy and regresses after the menopause.

Papilloma. One or more intraductal or intracystic papillomatous growths are sometimes found in women at or shortly before the menopause. The lesions appear as raspberrylike nodules filling a duct or growing from the wall of a cyst. The lesions frequently bleed and lead to a blood-stained discharge from the nipple. The relationship to carcinoma is disputed, but undoubtedly a number of papillomas do progress to carcinoma, and their removal is a wise precaution.

Malignant Neoplasms of the Breast

Carcinoma

In North America cancer of the breast is the most common malignant tumor in women. Breast cancer is responsible for more deaths than any other single tumor. Under the age of 25 years breast cancer is rare; it attains its maximum incidence at about the menopause. The disease is much less frequent in Japan and the Far East. A number of groups in whom the disease is more frequent than in a control population can be singled out:

1. Women of high socioeconomic status
2. Jewish women
3. Women with a family history of breast cancer
4. Women with a preceding history of breast problems, *e.g.*, mammary dysplasia
5. Single women
6. Women who have had no children
7. Women whose onset of menstruation (the menarche) was early (under 12 years)
8. Women whose menopause was after the age of 50 years
9. Obese women

The explanation for these observed differences is uncertain. Genetic factors play some part, but environmental factors must be equally important, because in North America the disease is increasing in frequency.

Cause of Breast Cancer. A vast amount of research has been carried out on this subject, and three factors appear to be important.

1. Inheritance. The incidence of cancer of the breast varies greatly in different strains of mice. In humans it has been found that if a sister or mother has had cancer of the breast, a woman's chances of developing a similar tumor are increased.

2. Viruses. The Bittner virus causes cancer of the breast in female mice of suitable strains (Chapter 17). The virus is passed from mother to offspring in the milk, and the high incidence of tumors in a strain, while appearing to be hereditary, is in fact due to neonatal infection.

In an inbred Parsi community living in Bombay there is a group of women who have a very high incidence of breast cancer. Samples of their milk contain particles that resemble the Bittner virus and also contain RNA-dependent DNA polymerase. Evidence is steadily accumulating to incriminate an RNA virus as a factor in the cause of human breast cancer. Whether it is a crucial factor or merely one of many agents acting in concert to cause cancer remains to be discovered.

3. Hormones. Prolonged exposure of breast tissue to the action of estrogen may be important as a factor in causing breast cancer. This would explain the increased incidence associated with advancing age, an early menarche, a late menopause, and those who have not been pregnant.

Types of Breast Cancer. Cancer can arise either in the lobules or more frequently in the ducts.

Lobular Carcinoma. The early stage in the development of this cancer is an *in situ* carcinoma. It is only when the malignant cells invade the surrounding tissues (*infiltrating lobular carcinoma*) that a mass can be felt clinically. Lobular carcinoma accounts for about 10 per cent of the total number of patients with carcinoma; the tumor is of importance because it often arises multifocally. Since about 20 per cent of patients have a tumor in the opposite breast, it is a common practice to take blind biopsies of the other breast when the mastectomy is performed.

Ductal Carcinoma. In *in situ ductular carcinoma* the duct becomes filled with malignant cells. This lesion is difficult to feel but may be detected radiographically. In due course, tumor cells invade the surrounding connective tissues and form one of the varieties of infiltrating carcinoma:

1. Scirrhous Carcinoma. This type accounts for about 75 per cent of all cancers of the breast. The tumor is *stony hard* and nonencapsulated (Fig. 38–1). Microscopically these tumors are adenocarcinomas with varying degrees of differentiation (Fig. 38–2). An outstanding feature is the dense fibrous tissue stroma, which accounts for the hardness of the tumor. It is common to see rows of cancer cells trapped in fibrous tissue in single file. Clincally, this

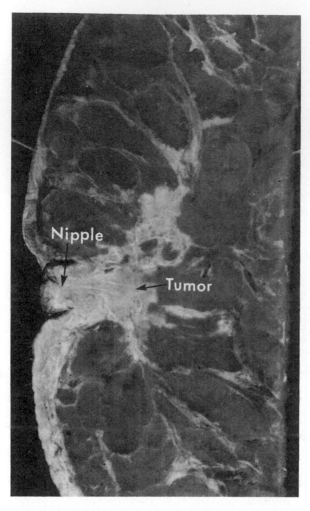

Figure 38–1.   Carcinoma of the breast. The figure shows a section through the breast. The carcinoma is deep to the nipple, to which it is firmly attached. Note how the tumor extends along the fibrous septa in the breast. The tumor is not encapsulated, and by gross examination it is impossible to tell how far the growth has extended.

This is an example of an advanced carcinoma of the breast: involvement of the nipple, skin, and axillary nodes results in a poor prognosis. In this particular case, the surgical wound became infected with *Escherichia coli* and *Streptococcus pyogenes*. The patient died as a result of hemorrhage from the wound. This case dates back to 1932; although penicillin had been discovered three years previously by Fleming, it had not yet been introduced into clinical medicine, and the sulfonamides had not yet been discovered. For a more complete description, see Case History I. (Specimen courtesy of the Boyd Museum, Banting Institute, Toronto.)

common type of cancer presents as a hard lump in the breast. As the tumor infiltrates the fibrous septa of the breast, it reaches the skin and pectoral muscle. The lump then becomes *fixed* to both these structures. Contracture of the stroma causes skin dimpling and retraction of the nipple. Invasion of lymphatics and lymphedema give the skin an orange rind appearance (peau d'orange), whereas actual invasion of the dermis converts the skin into a hard mass of tumor like a shield or cuirass *(cancer en cuirasse)*.

2. *Medullary or Encephaloid Carcinoma.*   This tumor is a very cellular adenocarcinoma with a lymphoid stromal infiltrate but little fibrous reaction. It is therefore bulky and soft. The prognosis is better than that of the usual infiltrating ductal carcinoma.

3. *Mucoid Carcinoma.*   This uncommon variant is characterized by slow growth and the formation of a bulky, gelatinous, soft tumor.

Metastatic Spread of Carcinoma.   Embolic spread is the feature that causes carcinoma of the breast to be so lethal.

Lymphatic Spread.   Lymphatic permeation and embolism are so common in cancer of the breast that lymph node metastases are present in over 50 per cent of patients when the tumor is first diagnosed. The axillary group are the nodes most frequently involved, particularly from cancers of the upper and outer quadrant. This is the commonest site for cancer. Intrathoracic nodes are involved, especially from tumors in the medial quadrants. The supraclavicular nodes are the third common site for metastases.

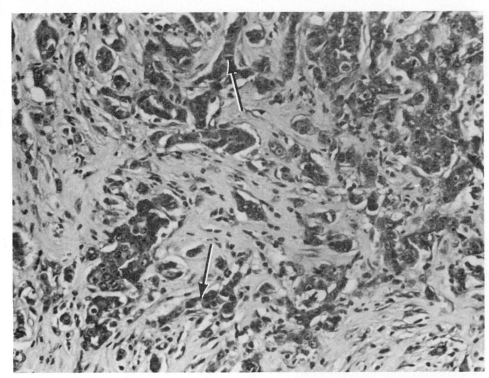

Figure 38-2. Carcinoma of the breast. This photomicrograph shows groups and columns of carcinoma cells embedded in a dense fibrous stroma. In some areas, single columns of cells can be seen (arrows); elsewhere, there is the beginning of tubule formation. The tumor is therefore classified as a poorly differentiated adenocarcinoma. The gross appearance of this tumor was that of a typical scirrhous carcinoma similar to the one depicted in Figure 38-1. The name is derived from the Greek *skirrhos,* meaning "hard" (× 300).

CASE HISTORY I. (See Figure 38-1).   The patient had noticed a lump in the right breast one year before consulting her doctor. A discharge from the nipple finally convinced her of the need to seek medical advice. On examination the right breast was found to be smaller than the left. A hard mass could be felt deep to the nipple. The nipple itself was indrawn and adherent to the mass. Mobile enlarged axillary lymph nodes contained secondary deposits of tumor.

Blood-Borne Metastases.   Hematogenous spread leads to involvement of the lungs, liver, adrenals, ovaries, and bone (Fig. 38-3). These secondary growths are not often detectable at the time of initial diagnosis, but they make their presence known sometimes years later, even after apparently successful treatment. These dormant tumors are common.

Diagnosis of Breast Cancer.   Cancer of the breast usually presents as a *painless mass in the breast* discovered by the patient herself or during a routine physical examination.

Any lump in the breast must be presumed to be malignant until proven otherwise. Usually this determination involves biopsy or local excision. It is useless to rely on detecting the classical signs of cancer — fixation to skin, retraction, and elevation of the nipple, among others. Tumors diagnosed by these signs are often already incurable.

Management of Breast Cancer.   The introduction of radical mastectomy (removal of breast, pectoral muscles, and axillary contents with lymph nodes) by Halsted did much to improve the prognosis of breast cancer. Unfortunately, the appearance of late metastases was not influenced by local surgery; alternative, less multilating procedures have thus been introduced. Radiotherapy (alone or combined with simple excision of the tumor), removal of the

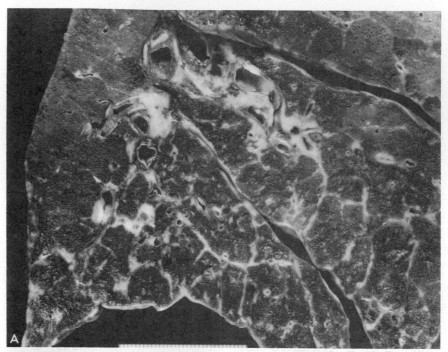

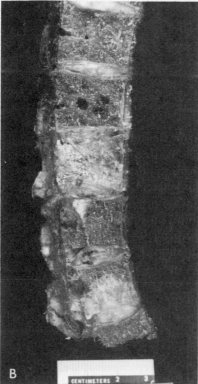

Figure 38–3. Metastatic breast cancer. At the age of 53 years the patient underwent a modified right radical mastectomy for carcinoma of the breast. Seven months later she developed shortness of breath and pain in the right side of the chest. Radiographs revealed evidence of metastases in the lungs and the spine. Nodules of tumor next appeared in the scalp, and a biopsy of one of them confirmed the diagnosis of metastatic, poorly differentiated adenocarcinoma. She died shortly afterward; necropsy disclosed metastatic tumor in the lungs, bones, adrenals, thyroid, and brain. The liver contained multiple masses of tumor similar in appearance to those depicted in Figure 17–8.

Specimen A shows the cut surface of parts of the three lobes of the right lung. Carcinoma has invaded the lymphatics of the septa as well as the region around the blood vessels and bronchi. This reticulated appearance resulting from extensive lymphatic involvement is common in metastatic breast cancer in lung, and it contrasts with the multiple nodular appearance presented by pulmonary metastases from other tumors and the deposits of growth in the liver found in this case.

Specimen B shows a segment of the bisected thoracic vertebral column. The bodies of two vertebrae show obvious white tumor.

breast alone (simple mastectomy), and simple removal of the tumor ("lumpectomy") all have their advocates. The results of treatment seem to be about the same with each of these methods, and there is no agreement as to which is the best. The present trend is to avoid the radical surgery that was once practiced, *e.g.*, radical mastectomy and radical mastectomy combined with removal of intrathoracic lymph nodes (super-radical mastectomy).

Hormone therapy has its uses as a palliative treatment of metastatic disease. It includes the removal of the ovaries, adrenals, or pituitary in premenopausal women; the administration of testosterone; and, somewhat surprisingly, the administration of estrogens in older patients. Normal breast tissue has estrogen receptors, which can be detected by their uptake of tritiated estradiol. Breast cancers also have estrogen receptors, and those tumors with the highest receptor content appear to respond more favorably to hormone treatment than those that lack such receptors.

Early Detection of Cancer of the Breast.   One would think that the ease with which the breast can be examined and removed would make early diagnosis and effective treatment easy; such is not the case. It seems that spread has often occurred by the time a lump is palpable. Routine physical examination, either by the woman herself or by a medical attendant, might improve the prognosis, but there is no proof of this. Radiography, or mammography, detection of hot spots by thermography (tumors tend to be vascular and hot), ultrasonic studies, and other methods have been introduced, but their value is unproved and their cost is considerable. Undoubtedly, small lesions can be detected, but a small lesion is not necessarily an early one. Prognosis depends on factors other than mere size.

Prognosis of Cancer of the Breast.   About two thirds of patients have lymph-node involvement at the time of initial diagnosis, and about 25 per cent are inoperable. The overall 5-year survival rate is 35 to 40 per cent, but of those treated by radical surgery, about 50 to 55 per cent are alive 5 years later. The prognosis depends on many factors, including the following:

1. Pregnancy, which sometimes adversely affects prognosis.

2. Histological grade of tumor. Poorly differentiated tumors do poorly compared with well-differentiated ones. Mucoid and medullary carcinomas have a relatively good prognosis.

3. The type of tumor in terms of the size of the primary tumor (T), the presence and extent of lymph-node involvement (N), and the presence of distant metastases (M). This is the TNM system of classification. A patient with stage-1 tumor (tumor less than 5 cm in diameter with no lymph-node or distant metastases) has an 80 per cent 5-year survival rate, and a 62 per cent 10-year survival rate, but the tumor can recur even after 10 years, even though the chances diminish with each passing year. For a stage-2 tumor, the 5- and 10-year survival rates are 36 per cent and 22 per cent, respectively, whereas for stages 3 and 4 the outlook is even worse. The overall 5-year survival rate for breast cancer is about 50 per cent, and this figure has apparently not changed for over 40 years.

The spread and prognosis of breast cancer have been described in some detail because they illustrate the difficulties in assessing the effects of therapy. There are so many types and stages of the disease that unless each medical center uses a similar and comprehensive classification, it is not possible to compare the results of different treatments, or even the same treatment at different centers.

Paget's Disease of the Breast.   This is a chronic eczematous condition involving the nipple, which microscopically shows invasion of the epidermis by large malignant Paget cells (Fig. 38–4). There is almost invariably an underlying ductal carcinoma. Opinions are divided as to whether Paget's disease represents an intraepithelial spread of a breast cancer, or whether epidermis and ductal epithelium are both involved simultaneously in a primary malignant process.

Other Malignant Tumors.   Fibrosarcoma and other malignant tumors occur, but they are rare.

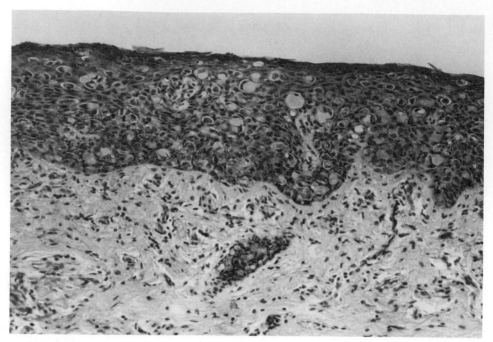

Figure 38–4. Paget's disease of the nipple. The epidermis is thickened and contains numerous round cells with cytoplasm that stain palely because of their mucin content. The appearances are typical of Paget's disease.

The 74-year-old patient had had a red, scaly area of "eczema" of the left breast for over one year. The lesion was centered on the nipple and was about 4 cm in diameter. It had failed to respond to the application of a variety of steroid creams. A simple eczema (dermatitis) should have cleared with this treatment, but Paget's disease is quite unresponsive. Under these circumstances a biopsy is essential. The photograph shown is from a 3-mm punch biopsy specimen. Palpation revealed no tumor in the breast, but mammography showed a mass highly suggestive of carcinoma. Mastectomy was performed, and the presence of carcinoma was confirmed.

The Male Breast

The diseases of the female breast can also occur in the male, but they are rare. Carcinoma is about 100 times less common in men than in women, but it has a poorer prognosis. Gynecomastia deserves separate consideration.

Gynecomastia is the name given to enlargement of the male breast. As a transient phenomenon it is not uncommon during adolescence and old age, presumably because it is related to hormonal imbalance during these periods of sexual development and decline. Other causes of gynecomastia include Klinefelter's syndrome (Chapter 3), heavy dosage of estrogens (*e.g.*, for carcinoma of the prostate), cirrhosis of the liver (Chapter 33), the effects of certain drugs (*e.g.*, digitalis), and estrogen-secreting tumors of the adrenal, the testis, or other site.

Review Questions

1. The super-radical mastectomy, which involves removal of the breast, part of the chest wall, and the axillary, supraclavicular, and internal mammary lymph nodes, was evolved with a view to increasing the cure rate of breast cancer. Explain why you think this operation was designed. Discuss the reasons it has been unsuccessful in attaining its objective.

2. Describe the changes that you would expect to find in an autopsy performed on a woman who had died of carcinoma of the breast.

3. Identify those features that would classify a woman as being at a higher-than-average risk for developing breast cancer.

4. List the conditions that can produce a localized swelling or lump in one breast.

Henderson, I. C., and Canellos, G. P.: Cancer of the breast. The past decade. New England
    Journal of Medicine, 302:17–30; 78–90; 1980.
Jensen, E. V.: Hormone dependency of breast cancer. Cancer, 47:2319–2326, 1981.
Leading Article: Paget's disease of the skin. British Medical Journal, 1:707, 1972.
Leading Article: Treatment of early breast cancer. British Medical Journal, 2:417–418, 1972.
Robbins, S. L., and Cotran, R. S.: Pathologic Basis of Disease. 2nd ed. Philadelphia, W. B.
    Saunders Company, 1979. Consult Chapter 27 for further details of breast diseases. The
    figures relating to the incidence and prognosis of cancer quoted in this chapter are derived
    from this source.

**Selected
Readings**

CHAPTER 39

Diseases of the Endocrine Glands

After studying this chapter the student should be able to:

- Describe the mode of action of hormones.
- List the hormones that are manufactured in the hypothalamus.
- Give examples of the common manifestations of hypothalamic disorders.
- Describe the components of the neurohypophysis and the adenohypophysis. Indicate how each part develops.
- Outline the features of diabetes insipidus.
- List the types of endocrine cells of the adenohypophysis, indicate how they have been identified, and list the hormones that are manufactured by each cell type.
- Describe the main actions of each of the hormones secreted by the adenohypophysis.
- Describe the common manifestations of hyperpituitarism and hypopituitarism. Give at least two causes of each condition.
- List the hormones produced by the adrenal glands.
- Describe the manifestations of Addison's disease.
- Describe the syndromes produced by adrenal cortical hypersecretion.
- Indicate the value of glucocorticoid therapy and list the important complications.
- Define goiter and give four examples of a condition that may cause it.
- Compare hyperthyroidism with hypothyroidism.
- Describe Graves' disease, Hashimoto's disease, and de Quervain's thyroiditis.
- Outline the types of thyroid carcinoma.

Introduction

Although the nervous system exerts the major controlling influence over the activities of the higher animals, there is an additional mechanism by which one type of cell can influence another — hormone secretion. By the secretion into the blood stream of potent chemicals called *hormones* cells can exert influence at a distant site. Secreting cells that perform this endocrine function may be grouped together to form one of the well-known endocrine glands, such as the thyroid gland, or they may be scattered more diffusely in the tissues. An example of the latter type is the cells in the pylorus that secrete the hormone *gastrin* when stimulated by the presence of food in the stomach. Gastrin stimulates the fundus of the stomach to secrete hydrochloric acid.

This chapter deals only with the common disorders of the major endocrine glands.

Mode of Action of Hormones

The hormones have an extremely potent and highly specific action on their target cells. This selective action is due to the binding of the hormones to specific receptor sites. The water-soluble hormones, such as epinephrine and glucagon, act on receptors on the cell membrane; cyclic AMP is formed, and it acts as a second messenger to stimulate or depress a characteristic biochemical activity (see Fig. 2–7). The lipid-soluble steroid hormones act on receptors within the cell, and the hormone-receptor complex enters the nucleus and then acts by affecting the expression of the cell's genetic material.

Although the pituitary gland has been called the "leader of the endocrine orchestra," many of its activities are themselves controlled by the hypothalamus, which, although part of the brain, also has many endocrine functions (Fig. 39–1).

THE HYPOTHALAMUS

The hypothalamus consists of a complex collection of nerve cells and fiber tracts that participate in, and help regulate, many functions of the body. These include regulation of the autonomic nervous system, temperature, blood pressure, plasma osmolality, hunger, thirst, emotions, sexual drive, and sleep. The hypothalamus controls body rhythms; a specific *cycling center* is responsible for controlling the menstrual cycle.

Hypothalamic Hormones. The hypothalamus may be regarded as an endocrine organ, because its cells synthesize two groups of hormones:

1. Oxytocin and Vasopressin. These are discussed later in this chapter.

2. Releasing and Inhibiting Factors or Hormones. These are polypeptides of low molecular weight that pass to the adenohypophysis via a short portal vein and stimulate or inhibit it.

The following releasing factors are recognized:

Corticotropin-releasing factor (CRF).

Thyrotropin-releasing factor (TRF).

Gonadotropin-releasing factors (GRF).

Growth hormone–releasing factor (GHRF).

Prolactin-releasing factor (PRF).

The action of these hormones may be understood by an examination of the action of CRF. This hormone leads to the release of corticotropin (also known as adrenocorticotropic hormone, ACTH) from the adenohypophysis. ACTH acts on the adrenal cortex to cause the release of cortisol (hydrocortisone). ACTH inhibits the release of CRF, while cortisol inhibits the release of both CRF and ACTH. This inhibition is an example of negative feedback, which is a mechanism encountered in the regulation of other hormone secretions.

The releasing factors are produced in picogram (10^{-12} gram) quantities, the pituitary hormones are produced in nanogram (10^{-9} gram) quantities, and the target cells (*e.g.*, the thyroid) produce hormone in microgram (10^{-6} gram) quantities. Thus, the chain reaction shows a considerable amplification effect.

In addition to forming releasing factors, the hypothalamus also forms *inhibiting factors*. Inhibitors of the release of thyroid-stimulating hormone (TSH), prolactin, melanocyte-stimulating hormone (MSH), and growth hormone have been described. The latter, termed growth hormone release–inhibiting factor or *somatostatin*, in addition to being a powerful inhibitor of growth hormone secretion by the pituitary, also inhibits the release of other hormones (*e.g.*, insulin) throughout the body. Indeed, the account given here of the various releasing and inhibiting factors is a simplified version of the facts. Thus, pure TRF causes release of both TSH and prolactin.

Many pathological processes (*e.g.*, encephalitis, vascular lesions, head injury, hamartoma, and tumor) can affect the hypothalamus. The effects differ widely, depending on which function is deranged the most. These effects include the following:

Diseases of the Hypothalamus

1. Obesity due to overeating.

2. Somnolence or increased restless activity.

HYPOTHALAMUS

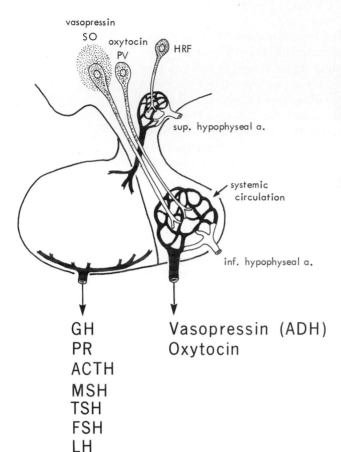

vasopressin
SO   oxytocin
PV   HRF

sup. hypophyseal a.

systemic circulation

inf. hypophyseal a.

GH
PR
ACTH
MSH
TSH
FSH
LH

Vasopressin (ADH)
Oxytocin

Figure 39–1. The relationship between the hypothalamus and the pituitary gland. Vasopressin (antidiuretic hormone, ADH) and oxytocin are manufactured in nerve cells in the supraoptic (SO) and paraventricular (PV) nuclei of the hypothalamus. These hormones are not released into the circulation until they have reached the neurohypophysis. The shaded area surrounding the SO cell body represents the "osmoreceptor" that is responsive to changes in osmolality of the fluid perfusing it. HRF represents an ill-defined group of cells that secrete a series of releasing factors into the primary capillary network of a portal vein. This vein passes in the pituitary stalk to the adenohypophysis, where cells manufacture the seven hormones of this lobe of the pituitary: growth hormone (GH), prolactin (PR), adrenocorticotropic hormone (ACTH), melanocyte-stimulating hormone (MSH), thyroid-stimulating hormone (TSH), follicle-stimulating hormone (FSH), and luteinizing hormone (LH). (Drawing by Margot Mackay, Department of Art as Applied to Medicine, University of Toronto. After a drawing by E. Blackstock in Ezrin, C., Godden, J. O., Volpé, R., and Wilson, R. (Eds.): Systematic Endocrinology, New York, Harper & Row, Publishers, 1973.)

3. Failure to maintain body temperature.

4. Diabetes insipidus that is due to lack of vasopressin, also known as the antidiuretic hormone (ADH).

5. Delayed puberty due to a failure to form gonadotropin-releasing factor. When combined with obesity this condition is known as *Fröhlich's syndrome*.

6. Precocious, or premature, puberty.

7. Visual disturbances due to pressure on the optic chiasma.

The regulation of the hypothalamic-pituitary function is complex, for apart from the gross lesions mentioned above, hypothalamic function is also influenced by impulses emanating from other parts of the brain. Some specific examples will illustrate this. Psychological stress, even mild, can lead to amenorrhea in young women. Failure to grow in childhood can be due to severe emotional trauma (*maternal deprivation syndrome*). A return of close emotional support leads to increased growth hormone secretion.

THE PITUITARY GLAND (HYPOPHYSIS)

Although small, the pituitary gland, or hypophysis, secretes an amazing variety and number of hormones. The gland and its stalk consist of two parts: the *neurohypophysis*, which develops as an outpouching from the primitive brain, and the *adenohypophysis*, which originates as a diverticulum from the primitive foregut (Fig. 39–1).

The neurohypophysis consists of the posterior lobe of the pituitary, part of the pituitary stalk (the *infundibular stem*), and part of the brain adjacent to the hypothalamus (the *median eminence of the tuber cinereum*). Two peptide hormones, oxytocin and vasopressin, are manufactured by cells in the hypothalamus and pass via the cells' axons into the neurohypophysis, where they are stored and subsequently released when needed.

The Neurohypophysis

Oxytocin.   This hormone causes uterine contraction during labor and is responsible for milk ejection when an infant is breastfed. The act of suckling initiates a reflex that causes oxytocin release.

Vasopressin (Antidiuretic Hormone).   This hormone acts on the distal and collecting tubules of the kidney and causes water to be retained. Its release is governed by the action of "osmoreceptors" in the hypothalamus. An increase in plasma osmolality associated with dehydration leads to a release of vasopressin and water retention.

Diabetes Insipidus.   This disease is caused by a failure in the development of the neurohypophysis or its destruction by a tumor or inflammation. Huge quantities of very dilute urine are passed (*polyuria*), leading to excessive thirst and drinking (*polydipsia*).

The adenohypophysis consists of the pars anterior, or anterior lobe, of the pituitary, the pars intermedia (which barely exists in humans), and the pars tuberalis in the pituitary stalk. Early attempts to delineate the types of cell present in the pituitary gland were based on staining with eosin and methyl blue. The *acidophils* stained red and the *basophils* stained blue, whereas the *chromophobes* remained unstained. More complex methods of staining, including immunostaining using the peroxidase technique (Chapter 1), have identified at least five cell types, which are named according to their secretion:

The Adenohypophysis

1. *Thyrotroph cells.* These cells secrete *thyrotropin*, which is also called *thyroid-stimulating hormone* or *TSH.*
2. *Lactotroph cells.* The secretion *prolactin* acts on the breast to initiate and maintain lactation. Before this can happen the breast must have been developed by the action of other hormones — estrogens, progesterone, and so forth.
3. *Gonadotroph cells.* These cells produce the two pituitary gonadotropins:
   (a) *Follicle-stimulating hormone* or *FSH*, which stimulates follicle development in the ovary and gametogenesis in the testis.
   (b) *Luteinizing hormone* or *LH*, which promotes the formation of the corpus luteum in the ovary. In the male it stimulates the interstitial cells of the testis to produce testosterone.
4. *Corticotroph-lipotroph cells.* These cells form a precursor compound from which are derived:
   (a) *Corticotropin* or *adrenocorticotropic hormone (ACTH).* This stimulates the adrenal cortex to produce cortisol but also acts on some other tissues directly, *e.g.*, the liver.
   (b) *β-lipotropin.*
   (c) *Melanocyte-stimulating hormone* or *MSH.* This hormone causes darkening of the skin. It is doubtful whether the human pituitary secretes MSH, but ACTH and β-lipotropin have an MSH-like action. MSH is important in amphibians because it enables them to change color rapidly.
   (d) *Endorphins*, which act as analgesics with a morphine-like action.
   (e) *Enkephalin*, which is a central nervous system neurotransmitter.

5. *Somatotroph cells.* Somatotrophs secrete *somatotropin*, or *growth hormone*. Growth hormone may act directly on cells or via intermediate compounds termed *somatomedins* that are formed outside the pituitary — probably in the liver. Growth hormone is needed for the growth of many tissues, especially the skeletal tissues.

Chromophobe cells appear to be nonsecreting cells and are probably the resting forms of other cell types — predominantly the lactotrophs.

Disorders of the Adenohypophysis

Hyperplasia or neoplasia of the anterior lobe of the pituitary gland may be associated with hypersecretion of one, or several, of the pituitary hormones. On the other hand, non–hormone-secreting tumors of the pituitary, or tumors arising in the neighborhood, may press on and destroy the parenchyma, leading to a diminished hormonal secretion. This also occurs when the pituitary is destroyed by other lesions, *e.g.*, infarction or inflammation. Because the clinical picture may be complex, only the common types will be outlined. Tumors in the pituitary region give rise to two additional characteristic effects, owing to their anatomical situation: *compression of the optic chiasma*, which causes loss of the temporal visual fields of both eyes (bitemporal hemianopsia), and *enlargement of the sella turcica*, which is detectable radiologically.

Hyperpituitarism. Adenomas of the pituitary produce varying effects, depending on the type of cell involved. The *prolactinoma* is the most common, and the excess prolactin that it secretes causes amenorrhea and sometimes inappropriate secretion of milk (*galactorrhea*). In males the effects are less striking, but impotence can occur. An *adenoma of the somatotrophs* demonstrates the effects of excess growth hormone production. If the condition arises in childhood, the result is *gigantism*: the individual is well proportioned, but huge. If the tumor arises in an adult after the epiphyses have fused, the result is *acromegaly*, in which the hands, feet, and lower jaw are enlarged. There is coarsening of the facial features (Fig. 39–2) and a high incidence of impaired glucose tolerance (see Chapter 24). Clinical diabetes occurs in 10 to 15 per cent of patients.

An *adenoma of the corticotrophs* leads to excess ACTH production and is the cause of *Cushing's disease*, which is described later in this chapter. If the disease is treated by adrenalectomy, the pituitary is stimulated to even greater activity, and the excess ACTH production leads to marked hyperpigmentation of the skin. This can mimic Addison's disease, and the condition is called Nelson's syndrome — this emphasizes the MSH-like activity of ACTH.

Adenomas of other cell types of the adenohypophysis are known but are rare. In some cases of hyperpituitarism the lesion may best be regarded as hyperplastic rather than neoplastic. Sometimes several hormones are secreted, so that mixed syndromes occur. Occasionally the pituitary lesion is frankly carcinomatous.

Hypopituitarism. In children, deficiency of growth hormone causes severe retardation of growth, resulting in midgetism. The unopposed action of insulin can lead to attacks of hypoglycemia (Chapter 24).

Hypopituitarism with lack of gonadotropins leads to lack of testicular or ovarian maturation. Puberty does not take place. Fusion of the epiphyses, normally produced by the sex hormones, is delayed. If growth hormone production is normal, these eunuchoid patients develop abnormally long limbs — their span exceeds their height (normally they are equal). Gonadotropin deficiency can occur in adults. Males exhibit testicular atrophy and loss of libido; females develop amenorrhea and regression of secondary sexual characteristics.

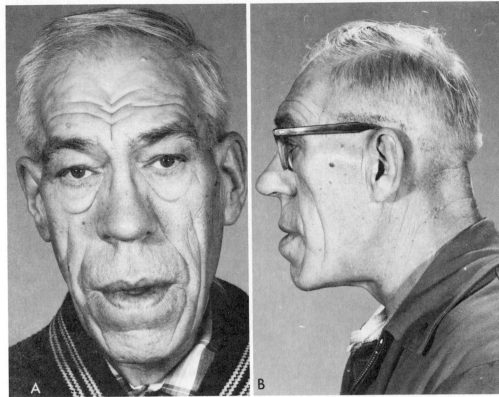

Figure 39–2. Acromegaly. Note how the thickening of the skin has exaggerated the facial wrinkles and coarsened the features. The ears, nose, and lips are prominent. Prominence of the lower jaw (termed prognathism) is particularly characteristic of acromegaly and is best seen in the lateral view (*B*). The patient died of a myocardial infarction, and at necropsy an acidophilic adenoma was found. (Photograph courtesy of Dr. L. F. W. Loach, Department of Medicine, Toronto General Hospital.)

In adults, anterior pituitary insufficiency can manifest itself as hypothyroidism; often this is combined with evidence of adrenal cortical and gonadotropic deficiency.

Acute pituitary insufficiency sometimes occurs after parturition and is due to infarction of the gland. The condition is then called *Sheehan's syndrome*. When destruction of the adenohypophysis is complete, the condition, called *Simmond's disease*, is characterized by extreme wasting. The patients are apathetic; without treatment they ultimately die of adrenal insufficiency (see discussion later in this chapter). Simmond's disease must be distinguished from *anorexia nervosa*.

Anorexia Nervosa.   This condition, often encountered in psychoneurotic adolescent girls, is the development of an obsessive aversion to food. Extreme wasting and amenorrhea are the main features and are due to starvation. The patients are restless and hostile. Although endocrine abnormalities are present, these are generally regarded as being secondary to the starvation. The precise etiology of this distressing disease is unknown. Anorexia nervosa has a 10 to 20 per cent mortality.

The adrenal medulla is derived from the neural cleft and contains both ganglion cells of the sympathetic nervous system and pheochromocytes, cells that can secrete epinephrine and norepinephrine into the blood. These hormones cause a rise in blood glucose, a rise in blood pressure, and a redistribution of blood such that the individual is better adapted for fight or flight. A rare tumor, the *pheochromocytoma*, secretes these agents in excess

THE ADRENAL GLANDS

The Adrenal Medulla

and leads to systemic hypertension. The other important tumor of the adrenal medulla is the *neuroblastoma*, which is derived from the precursor cells that normally mature to ganglion cells. The neuroblastoma is one of the common tumors of childhood and ranks with leukemia, Wilms' tumor, and medulloblastoma of the brain as a principal form of lethal cancer in the young. The tumor has some remarkable properties. When it appears at birth or in patients under one year of age the prognosis is relatively good, because either the tumor undergoes spontaneous regression or its cells differentiate into ganglion cells and then behave in a benign manner. Such a tumor is then called a *ganglioneuroma*. When the tumor occurs after the age of one year it behaves in a very malignant fashion.

The Adrenal Cortex

Three major groups of hormones (corticoids) are secreted:

Glucocorticoids, e.g., hydrocortisone (cortisol). In physiological concentrations these steroids accelerate the synthesis of glucose from noncarbohydrate precursors and inhibit the actions of insulin. These hormones also have a mild salt-retaining activity.

Mineralocorticoids, e.g, aldosterone, which primarily affects electrolyte metabolism. It causes sodium retention and increases potassium loss in the urine. Aldosterone production is stimulated by angiotensin II and is therefore regulated by the renal blood flow (Chapter 20).

Sex hormones, e.g., estrogen, androgens, and progesterone.

Adrenal Cortical Insufficiency

Primary Adrenal Cortical Insufficiency (Addison's Disease). Idiopathic atrophy, perhaps mediated by an autoimmune process, and destruction of the glands, usually by tuberculosis, are the two common causes of Addison's disease (Fig. 39–3). Extreme weakness, loss of appetite, loss of weight, a low blood pressure, and eventual death are the main features. As would be

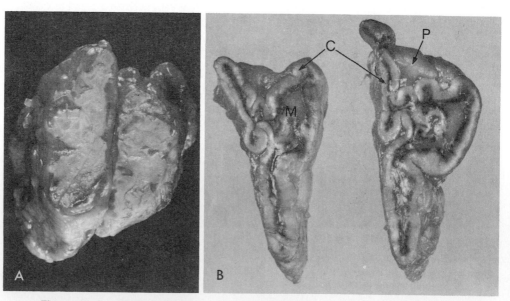

Figure 39–3. Histoplasmosis of the adrenal glands. *A,* The two adrenal glands are enlarged, and the cut surface shows complete replacement of the normal tissue by necrotic, caseous material. *Histoplasma capsulatum* was identified in this specimen. The gross appearance of these specimens is identical with that of tuberculosis, a disease that once accounted for most cases of Addison's disease (today, idiopathic atrophy is now more frequently encountered as a cause of Addison's disease). See also Figure 35–9 and Case History I, Chapter 35, for details of this case.

B, Normal adrenals for comparison. (C, cortex; M, medulla; P, periadrenal fat.)

expected, hypoglycemia, a fall in serum sodium (hyponatremia), and a rise in potassium (hyperkalemia) are among the clinical findings. The skin and mucous membranes, including the oral mucosa, show increased melanin pigmentation. This is because the low plasma hydrocortisone level stimulates the pituitary to produce excess ACTH and β-lipotropin, both of which cause a darkening of the skin by an effect on the melanocytes. Diagnosis is not easy in the early stages, but it is important to diagnose Addison's disease because substitution therapy is life-saving. The normal maintenance dose of prednisone is 7.5 mg (1½ tablets) daily. This is equivalent to the output of cortisol by the normal adrenal. An acute exacerbation of the disease (acute adrenal insufficiency or addisonian crisis) may occur at any time, particularly when the patient is subjected to any type of stress, *e.g.*, trauma or an infection. The crisis is characterized by extreme weakness, hypotension, hypoglycemia, epigastric pain, vomiting, diarrhea, coma, and death.

Secondary Adrenal Cortical Insufficiency. Adrenal cortical insufficiency may be secondary to pituitary hypofunction in which there is a decreased output of ACTH. It differs from Addison's disease in that the blood level of ACTH is low, skin hyperpigmentation is absent, and aldosterone secretion is unaffected. As in Addison's disease, acute life-threatening crises may occur if the patient is subjected to stress and is not given increased doses of glucocorticoids.

Adrenal overactivity may be secondary to pituitary hypersecretion of ACTH. Usually, however, the overproduction of corticoids is due to idiopathic adrenal hyperplasia, adenoma, or (rarely) a carcinoma. The clinical picture is often mixed, but three main patterns may be discerned.

Adrenal Cortical Hypersecretion

Adrenogenital Syndrome. In boys, puberty may occur prematurely — even as early as four years ("infantile Hercules"). In girls, male characteristics may develop. In adult women this masculinization, called *virilism,* is manifested as atrophy of the breasts, enlargement of the clitoris, cessation of menstruation, growth of a beard, and deepening of the voice.

Conn's Syndrome. Excess aldosterone secretion, usually by an adenoma, produces a low serum potassium with sodium and water retention as well as hypertension.

Cushing's Syndrome. Obesity is the most common feature and is particularly evident in the face, trunk, cervicodorsal region, and supraclavicular area. The limbs are relatively thin owing to muscular wasting. Typically there is a round "moon face" (Fig. 39–4) and a dorsal "buffalo" hump. Other features are systemic hypertension, hyperglycemia, osteoporosis, acne vulgaris, and increased growth of body hair in women. Psychiatric disturbances are common, and over 50 per cent of patients with Cushing's disease have emotional disorders, particularly of the depressive type.

Cushing's "disease" was originally described as being due to a pituitary adenoma. However, the same clinical picture (Cushing's "syndrome") is encountered under other circumstances:

1. With hypersecretion of ACTH due to hypothalamic-pituitary dysfunction.

2. With adrenal hyperplasia or neoplasia.

3. With ectopic ACTH syndrome. An ACTH-like hormone can be produced by some tumors, *e.g.*, oat-cell carcinoma of the lung.

4. With glucocorticoid therapy. The syndrome, or mild forms of it, is commonly seen when glucocorticoids are administered in massive doses. Rounding and swelling of the face ("moon face") are particularly characteristic (Fig. 39–4).

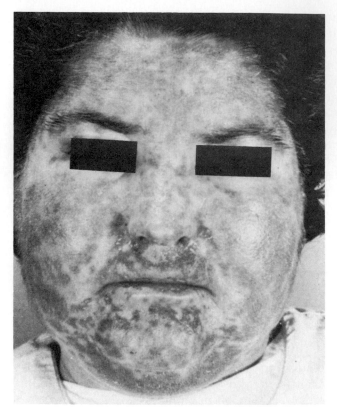

Figure 39-4. Cushing's syndrome. Note the rounded, moon-shaped appearance of the face that is characteristic of this condition. The patient first presented with a severe autoimmune hemolytic anemia. No definite cause for this was found, and it was decided to treat her with prednisone. Doses of up to 100 mg per day were needed to control the anemia, and she became markedly cushingoid. Unfortunately, she developed a widespread infection with *Cryptococcus neoformans* and subsequently died of this superinfection. The erythematous, blotchy eruption seen on the face is an unusual manifestation of generalized cryptococcosis, but it was biopsy of similar lesions on the thigh that led to the diagnosis.

Glucocorticoid Therapy

Replacement glucocorticoid therapy is logical and useful in patients with adrenal insufficiency. However, when used in massive (pharmacological) amounts, the glucocorticoids have two additional actions that can be useful:

1. Anti-inflammatory Action. The glucocorticoids (*e.g.,* prednisone) have a suppressive effect on the inflammatory reaction; for this reason they are used in many diseases, *e.g.,* rheumatoid arthritis, herpes zoster, and polyarteritis nodosa. They may be used to advantage when bacterial inflammation might produce serious damage, but antibiotics must also be administered, so that the infection does not spread.

2. Lymphoid Atrophy and Depression of the Immune Response. This may be used to advantage in treating acute lymphatic leukemia, autoimmune diseases, and hypersensitivity states, such as bronchial asthma. The immunosuppressive action of prednisone is of great use in suppressing the graft rejection reaction, such as in patients with kidney grafts.

Complications of Glucocorticoid Therapy. The administration of large doses of glucocorticoids over a prolonged period can have serious consequences. Indeed, these may be more serious than the disease for which the treatment was initiated. Important complications are:

1. Cushing's Syndrome. (See above.)

2. Susceptibility to Infection. Infections of many types are common in patients on glucocorticoid therapy, and this is related to the immunosuppressive effect of the compounds. Attacks of bronchopneumonia and urinary tract infections can be troublesome. Fungal and viral infections can be devastating (see Fig. 39-4). A quiescent tuberculous focus can be reactivated and then lead to miliary tuberculosis.

3. Osteoporosis. Severe and widespread osteoporosis can lead to fracture formation after trivial injury. Collapse of vertebrae is common.

4. Inhibition of Wound Healing.   Wound contraction, granulation tissue formation, and collagen formation are inhibited.

5. Peptic Ulcer.   Peptic ulceration, if present, is adversely affected. Complications such as perforation and bleeding may be precipitated.

6. Cataract Formation.   (See Chapter 42.)

7. Diabetes Mellitus.   (See Chapter 24.)

8. Mental Effects.   An acute mental breakdown (psychosis) may be precipitated. Suicide is an occasional cause of death during glucocorticoid drug therapy.

9. Systemic Hypertension.   The development of hypertension or the accentuation of existing disease appears to be due to the salt-retaining activity of most glucocorticoids.

10. Acute Adrenal Insufficiency.   This emergency, characterized by hypotension, shock, and sudden death, occurs if steroid therapy is suddenly withdrawn. It may also occur if a patient who is taking a steroid develops a severe infection or is subjected to severe injury such as a major surgery and does not have his dose increased. *It is vital that all patients on glucocorticoid therapy as well as their medical attendants be aware of this possibility.*

The Waterhouse-Friderichsen Syndrome.   This disorder is often cited as an example of acute adrenal cortical insufficiency. The syndrome most commonly occurs during the course of an overwhelming meningococcal septicemia and is characterized by bleeding into the skin and in internal organs. The adrenals in particular are the site of massive bleeding. Death occurs rapidly and is probably attributable to septicemia associated with disseminated intravascular coagulopathy rather than to any acute adrenal insufficiency. It should be noted that adrenal insufficiency does not occur until over 90 per cent of both glands has been destroyed. Hence, clinically apparent effects are rarely seen with tumors involving the adrenal glands, *e.g.*, the common metastatic carcinoma that is seen in cases of carcinoma of the lung and breast.

THE THYROID GLAND

The thyroid gland has the unique ability to trap iodine from the blood and incorporate it as thyroglobulin in the colloid of its vesicles (Fig. 39–5). By the action of a proteolytic enzyme on thyroglobulin the iodine-containing thyroid hormones thyroxine (T_4) and triiodothyronine (T_3) are released. This occurs when the gland is stimulated by thyroid-stimulating hormone (TSH) from the pituitary. TSH secretion is itself stimulated by a low blood level of thyroid hormone both directly and indirectly via thyrotropin-releasing hormone (TRH). Both T_3 and T_4 are carried in the blood bound to protein and in a free form, the latter being the active state. T_4 is the most avidly bound to protein, and in the peripheral tissues some is converted into T_3. The latter is the most active compound. Estimation of the serum levels of T_3 and T_4 and the total protein binding power are tests commonly employed to assess thyroid function.

The inconspicuous C cells of the thyroid secrete calcitonin. They are the cells of origin of medullary carcinoma of the thyroid. So far, no syndrome has been described in relation to an excess or deficiency of this hormone (Chapter 40).

Action of the Thyroid Hormones.   In spite of much research, the precise mode of action of the thyroid hormones is not known. However, much has been learned by comparing the normal individual (who is described as *euthyroid*) with those who suffer from excessive or diminished secretion (*hyperthyroid* and *hypothyroid*, respectively).

A *deficiency* of the thyroid hormones causes any or all of the following

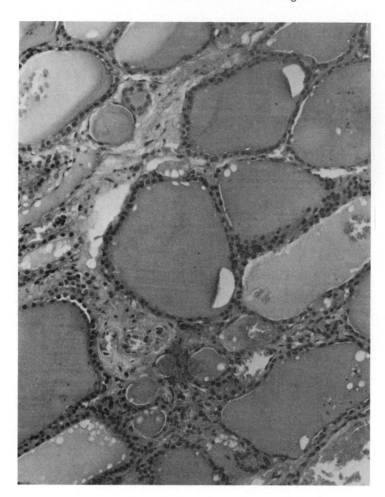

Figure 39–5. Normal thyroid. The gland consists of follicles of varying size, lined by a simple flattened or cubical epithelium and filled with homogeneous colloid. The colloid contains thyroglobulin (× 250).

conditions: a reduction in metabolic rate; impaired mental and physical growth (most marked in childhood); and anemia, which is less constant.

A hypersecretion of thyroid hormones causes an increase in the metabolic rate and the other changes encountered in thyrotoxicosis that are described later.

Goiter   Any enlargement of the thyroid is called a goiter, and to a minor extent this occurs at times of stress, *e.g.*, during puberty and pregnancy. Indeed, in ancient Egypt the rupture of a thread tied around the neck of a bride was used as an indication of pregnancy. A more potent cause is a diet deficient in iodine. The reason is that the thyroid, being unable to manufacture its hormone, cannot check the secretion of TSH that stimulates it to activity. Before iodine was added to table salt, goiters were common in many parts of the world (*e.g.*, the Great Lakes area of North America, the Andes, the Himalayas, and Derbyshire, England) because the soil carried insufficient iodine for foodstuffs to contain even minute quantities of iodine. Repeated phases of hyperplasia followed by involution led to the formation of large, nodular goiters containing many colloid-filled areas, some of which showed necrosis and dystrophic calcification (*nodular colloid goiter;* Fig. 39–6).

The goiters associated with hyperthyroidism, Hashimoto's disease, and neoplasia are described later in this chapter.

Hypothyroidism   Hypothyroidism was once frequent in areas of endemic goiter due mainly to iodine deficiency. Goitrogenic substances in the diet can also block thyroid

Figure 39–6. Nodular colloid goiter. The specimen consists of the left lobe of the thyroid and shows two nodules, both encapsulated. One is solid, whereas the other is cystic and contains dark, altered blood. Hemorrhage into this degenerate nodule accounts for the sudden swelling experienced by this patient. For further clinical data see Case History I.

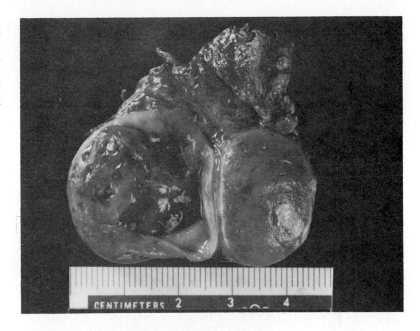

function and lead to hypothyroidism. The effects of hypothyroidism in the child differ from those in the adult.

Cretinism. An insufficiency of thyroid hormone in the infant leads to cretinism. The child has a bloated face, protruding tongue, and a vacant expression and becomes mentally defective. There is a retardation of growth, and dwarfism results (Fig. 39–7).

Endemic cretinism is usually due to a lack of iodine in the diet but is occasionally caused by a dietary goitrogenic substance. A similar effect is seen if the mother is taking a drug that blocks thyroid function, *e.g.*, thiourea or one of its derivatives. *Sporadic cretinism* occurs in non-goitrogenic regions and is caused by agenesis of the thyroid or a congenital absence of one of the enzymes necessary for T_3 and T_4 synthesis.

Myxedema. This condition is the manifestation of hypothyroidism in the adult. There is a reduction in mental and physical activity, and the patient exhibits a characteristic bloated appearance because of a curious edema of the skin. This disease is associated with an excessive accumulation of mucoprotein (Chapter 2).

Patients with myxedema are intolerant of cold and may develop hypothermia in cold climates. The patient may then pass into a coma and die (*myxedema coma*). Muscle weakness, a hoarse voice, and an increase in body weight are other features of the disease. Myxedema may occur as an end-result of toxic goiter, nodular colloid goiter, or Hashimoto's disease or following surgical removal or irradiation of the gland. Under these circumstances the serum levels of T_3 and T_4 are low, but the TSH level is high. Myxedema that accompanies pituitary or hypothalamic hypofunction also exhibits low serum T_3 and T_4 level, but the serum TSH level is also reduced.

CASE HISTORY I. (See Figure 39–6.) *Nodular colloid goiter.* The patient was a 45-year-old woman who complained of a swelling in the neck. The swelling moved when she swallowed and had the features of an enlarged thyroid (goiter). The patient had had seven pregnancies; it was during the last two that she had noticed some swelling of the neck. However, it was only after the last delivery (one year previously) that the goiter had rapidly become obvious. On examination, several nodules could be felt in the enlarged thyroid. An echogram revealed that one of them was cystic;

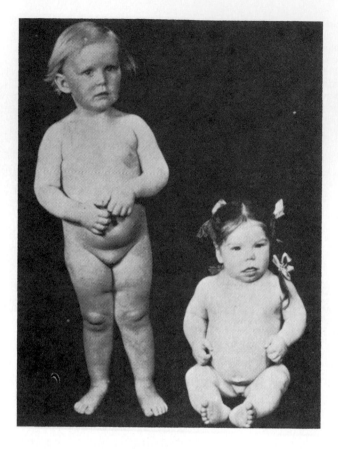

Figure 39–7.   Cretinism. Note the dwarfed appearance of the cretin as compared with a child of like age on her right. Other distinctive features are the torpid expression, round face, eyes set widely apart, enlarged protruding tongue, and umbilical hernia. (Courtesy of Mr. G. S. Hoggins.)

radioactive studies showed no uptake by this "cold" nodule. T_3 and T_4 levels in the blood were normal. Although a diagnosis of nodular colloid goiter seemed obvious, the fact that the thyroid enlargement had occurred soon after delivery rather than during the pregnancy raised the possibility of malignancy. Cold nodules should always be viewed with suspicion. The left lobe of the thyroid and one nodule in the right lobe were removed.

Hyperthyroidism   This condition is also known as *thyrotoxicosis* and occurs in two forms:

Graves' Disease (Primary Hyperthyroidism).   This disease is characterized by a diffuse enlargement of the thyroid gland (goiter) due to a marked hyperplasia of its epithelial elements (Fig. 39–8). There is a raised metabolic rate that manifests itself as a persistent increase in the heart rate; in elderly patients this may lead to atrial fibrillation and heart failure. The individual is typically jumpy, nervous, and intolerant of hot weather. The hands are warm and sweaty; they are seldom at rest and exhibit a fine tremor when the fingers are stretched out. In spite of a good appetite there is weight loss. Muscular weakness, which is a common symptom, can be severe. If left untreated, Graves' disease often terminates in heart failure. The eyes have a characteristic appearance: the eyelids are retracted, giving the patient a staring expression; in severe cases, the globe is actually pushed forward to produce *exophthalmos* (Fig. 39–9). This is produced by edema and lymphocytic infiltration of the contents of the orbit. If severe, these changes can cause loss of sight (*malignant exophthalmos*).

Patients with thyrotoxicosis may experience sudden exacerbations of their symptoms with hyperactivity, hyperpyrexia, coma, and death. This is termed a *thyroid storm* and demands rapid and energetic treatment if life is to be saved.

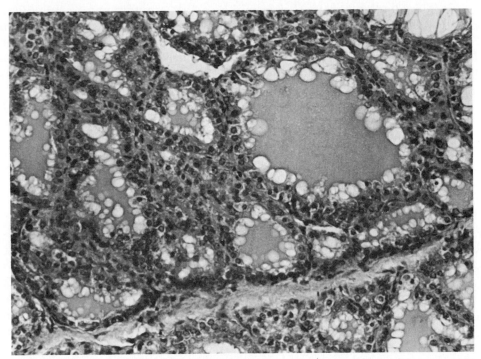

Figure 39–8. Graves' disease. This section shows that the thyroid gland is hyperplastic. The epithelium is columnar, and in some small follicles where colloid is deficient it encroaches upon the acinar spaces. In the large follicles the colloid shows vacuolation where it abuts on the epithelium (× 250).

Graves' disease is not due to overstimulation of the thyroid by TSH. Instead, there is an IgG autoantibody present in the blood that has the property of stimulating the thyroid gland into activity (thyroid-stimulating immunoglobulin or TSI).* This is thought to be an antibody directed against TSH receptors on thyroid cells, but definite proof of this hypothesis is lacking.

---

*A variety of autoantibodies have been described in the past, and these include long-acting thyroid stimulator (LATS) and long-acting thyroid stimulator protector (LATS-P). It is likely that these are either identical or closely related, and this group of autoantibodies is now termed TSI.

Figure 39–9. Ocular manifestation of Graves' disease. This patient noted the development of prominence of both eyes at the same time as the appearance of other symptoms of Graves' disease. The eyelids and periorbital tissues are swollen; the conjunctiva is congested and moist because of excessive lacrimation. The globe itself is pushed forward (*proptosis*) by an accumulation of mucoprotein in the orbital tissues. A similar change is sometimes encountered in the skin of the lower leg and is called *pretibial myxedema*. Note that this occurs in Graves' disease. (Courtesy of Dr. N. Pairaudeau.)

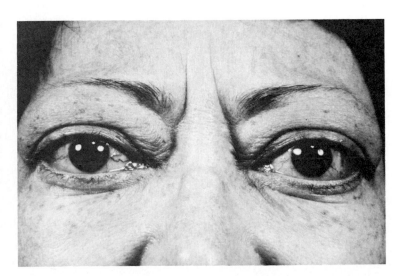

It is evident that Graves' disease has a strong autoimmune component and in this respect has much in common with Hashimoto's disease. Both diseases tend to occur in the same family and may indeed even occur in the same patient. It is therefore suggested that in both diseases there is an additional genetic component that renders the individuals susceptible to this type of autoimmune disease.

Toxic Nodular Goiter (Secondary Hyperthyroidism). This occurs as a secondary phenomenon in a patient who is already suffering from a goiter from some other cause, such as iodine deficiency. The condition is less severe than Graves' disease, and exophthalmos and other ocular manifestations do not occur. Sometimes a solitary nodule ("toxic adenoma") is present and the remainder of the gland is suppressed.

Hashimoto's Disease

Like most thyroid disease, this is more common in women than in men. The gland is diffusely enlarged, showing atrophy of its epithelial elements and a massive infiltration by lymphocytes and plasma cells (Fig. 39–10). Clinically the outstanding feature is the development of a goiter; the patient may be euthyroid, but hypothyroidism generally develops in due course. A characteristic of the disease is the presence of antithyroid antibodies in the blood; these include antibodies to thyroglobulin, to other components in thyroid colloid, and to microsomal antigen in thyroid cells. The immunoglobulins do not appear to injure thyroid cells directly, nor does complement activation appear to be involved. Nevertheless, the antibodies could lead to damage being caused by K cells by the mechanism of antibody-dependent cell-mediated cytotoxicity. There are also suggestions that T cells are involved in causing thyroid damage, probably by a direct cytotoxic activity. T helper cells could aid antibody formation or alternatively suppressor T cells

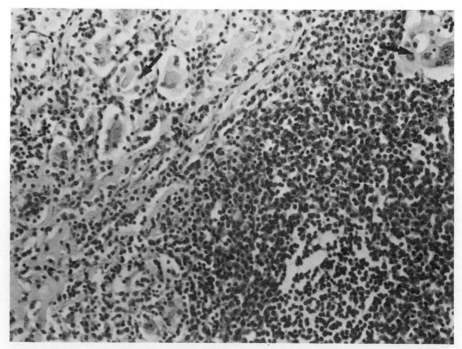

Figure 39–10. Hashimoto's disease. Much of the thyroid parenchyma has been replaced by lymphocytes; remnants of thyroid follicles can still be seen (arrows). In the early stages of Hashimoto's disease, the patient may be hyperthyroid, but by the time the gland shows the degree of destruction depicted in this figure the patient is hypothyroid ($\times$ 250).

could either aid or hinder B or T cell functions. It is evident that both Hashimoto's disease and Graves' disease are closely related, but their pathogenesis is obscure.

This is less common than Hashimoto's disease and is suspected of being a viral infection, although a specific agent has yet to be identified. The disease commonly follows 2 to 3 weeks after an upper respiratory infection. The clinical course is that of fever, tender enlargement of the thyroid gland, and spontaneous resolution within a few weeks. Microscopically the gland shows nonspecific inflammatory changes that later develop a granulomatous component with the presence of many giant cells. For this reason the disease is also sometimes called giant-cell thyroiditis.

Subacute Thyroiditis (de Quervain's Thyroiditis)

Benign encapsulated nodules in the thyroid gland are common, but the majority are probably focal areas of hyperplasia. These are usually multiple (nodular colloid goiter).

Tumors

Carcinoma was apparently not uncommon in goitrous districts, but today it is distinctly rare. Carcinoma does not usually take up radioactive iodine and appears as a "cold" nodule on a thyroid scan. The most common type of carcinoma of the thyroid gland is papillary adenocarcinoma, which has a good prognosis (Fig. 39–11). Other well-differentiated tumors more closely resemble normal thyroid tissue. Anaplastic tumors are uncommon but have a bad

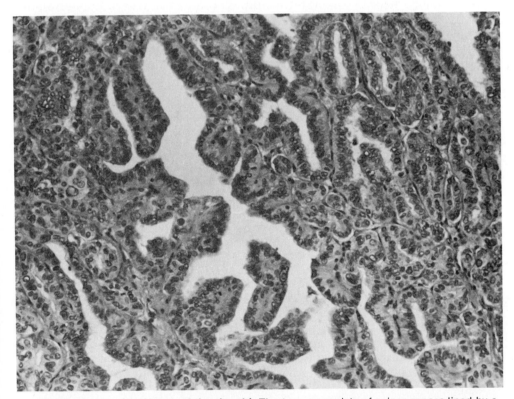

Figure 39–11. Carcinoma of the thyroid. The tumor consists of acinar spaces lined by a columnar epithelium. The spaces vary greatly in size and do not contain colloid. Papillary projections fill the larger acini, and the overall pattern differs markedly from that of the hyperplastic gland (compare with Figure 39–8). The cells of the tumor are uniform in appearance, and mitoses are not in evidence. On the basis of histological findings it is tempting to label this tumor a papillary adenoma. However, careful search will generally reveal invasion of its capsule; the tumor also regularly metastasizes to lymph nodes. Hence, it should be called a *papillary adeno-carcinoma* (× 250).

prognosis. Hence, with carcinoma of the thyroid the histological features are important when assessing the outlook for the patient. As noted previously, the uncommon *medullary carcinoma* has several features that set it apart from other neoplasms of the thyroid. Its cell of origin is the C cell, its stroma frequently contains an abundance of amyloid, and the tumor can secrete a variety of hormones (calcitonin and ACTH) as well as histamine and prostaglandins.

THE DIFFUSE NEURO- ENDOCRINE SYSTEM

The concept of a widely dispersed system of cells derived from the neural crest has recently been proposed. The term APUD cells has also been applied to this group of cells.* The cells of the diffuse neuroendocrine system are recognized on electron microscopy by the presence of characteristic dark granules in their cytoplasm. They secrete either amines or polypeptides. At present the following cells are included in the group: the chromaffin cells (*e.g.*, the pheochromocytes of the adrenal medulla), non-chromaffin paraganglia cells (*e.g.*, of the carotid body), the argentaffin cells of the intestine and elsewhere, the pancreatic islet cells, the C cells of the thyroid gland, and some cells of the adenohypophysis. Tumors of these cells have been called apudomas. These may secrete an excessive amount of their corresponding hormone, in which case they are called orthoendocrine, or they may secrete a hormone that is characteristic of some other APUD cells, in which case they are called paraendocrine.

A good example of an orthoendocrine tumor is one of the beta cells of the islets of Langerhans that secretes insulin and causes attacks of hypoglycemia. But occasionally such a tumor may secrete an ACTH-like hormone and produce Cushing's syndrome. In this case it would be a paraendocrine apudoma. Other examples of paraendocrine apudomas causing Cushing's syndrome are the oat-cell carcinoma of the lung, medullary carcinoma of the thyroid (derived from cells that normally secrete calcitonin), and bronchial carcinoid tumors. In each case an ACTH-like hormone is produced.

The tumors of the diffuse neuroendocrine system are not common but produce a great variety of syndromes, depending upon their particular secretion. Sometimes tumors of several types of cell occur together and produce the *multiple endocrine adenopathy syndromes*. The details of these rare tumors are beyond the scope of this work.

Review Questions

1. Explain why hormones have a specific action; that is, they affect only their target organs or tissues. Illustrate the answer by using as examples glucagon, insulin, and a steroid hormone.

2. Compare Simmonds' disease with anorexia nervosa.

3. A patient with Cushing's disease has both adrenal glands removed and is given hormone-replacement therapy. One year later marked hyperpigmentation of the skin is noted. Can you explain this?

4. It is proposed that a patient be treated with large doses of prednisone (a glucocorticoid). List the items in a patient's medical history and physical examination that would warn you of the possible dangers of this treatment.

5. Give an account of the endocrine disorders that affect the systemic blood pressure.

---

*The term is derived from the initial letters associated with three important properties: the high content of *a*mines, the capacity for amine *pr*ecursor *u*ptake, and the presence of amino acid *d*ecarboxylase. The original concept that all members of this group of cells are derived from the neural crest has not been accepted by all authorities. Indeed, there is good evidence that there are exceptions. The islets of Langerhans are almost certainly derived from the endodermal cells of the exocrine pancreas. Also, neurosecretory granules can be found in some tumors derived from cells that are not included in the APUD series. Hence, the term apudoma is tending to fall into disuse.

6. Give an account of the circumstances under which hypothyroidism may occur.

7. Read Case History I in Chapter 35. What investigations might have led to a diagnosis of Addison's disease in this patient?

Catt, K. J.: ABC of endocrinology. Lancet, *1*:763–765; 827–831; 933–939; 1097–1104; 1383–1389; and 2:255–257; 353–358; 1970.

Ezrin, C., Godden, J. O., Volpé, R., and Wilson, R.: Systematic Endocrinology. 2nd ed. New York, Harper & Row, Publishers, 1979. Chapters 1 to 5 and 7 should be consulted for topics covered in this chapter.

Guillemin, R., and Burgus, R.: The hormones of the hypothalamus. Scientific American, 227(5):24–33, 1972.

Hershman, J. M. (Ed.): Endocrine Pathophysiology. 2nd ed. Philadelphia, Lea and Febiger, 1982.

Leading Article: Endocrine exophthalmos. British Medical Journal, 3:68, 1972.

Selected Readings

CHAPTER 40

Diseases of the Bones, Joints, and Muscles

After studying this chapter the student should be able to:

- Describe the formation of bone in the human embryo and distinguish between membrane bone and that formed by endochondral ossification.
- Distinguish woven bone from lamellar bone.
- Give an account of the forms in which calcium occurs in the plasma; describe the actions of parathyroid hormone and calcitonin.
- Give an account of the various forms of vitamin D, their metabolism, and their actions in relation to calcium metabolism and bone formation.
- Describe the pathogenesis of acute staphylococcal osteomyelitis and chronic osteomyelitis.
- Outline the features of tuberculous infection of the spine.
- Describe the causes of localized osteoporosis.
- Classify the causes of fracture.
- Describe the stages in fracture healing, and list the causes of fibrous union, nonunion, and delayed union.
- Lists the causes of ischemic necrosis of bone.
- Give a brief account of each of the following conditions:
  - (a) osteogenesis imperfecta
  - (b) achondroplasia
  - (c) osteopetrosis
  - (d) fibrous dysplasia
- Classify the causes of hyperparathyroidism and indicate the main bony and renal lesions that ensue.
- Compare rickets with osteomalacia.
- Classify the causes of generalized osteoporosis.
- Describe the main features of Paget's disease.
- Describe the main features of hypertrophic osteoarthropathy and list the common causes of this condition.
- Give an account of the common tumors of bone.
- Describe multiple myelomatosis.
- Describe Ewing's tumor.
- Describe the structure of a synovial joint.
- Differentiate between a sprain, a subluxation, and a dislocation.
- List three organisms that commonly cause an acute suppurative arthritis and indicate the end-result.
- Contrast rheumatoid arthritis with osteoarthritis.
- Describe how ankylosing spondylitis differs from the classic form of rheumatoid arthritis.
- List the causes of muscle atrophy.
- Give a brief account of:
  - (a) muscular dystrophy
  - (b) myasthenia gravis
  - (c) malignant tumors of muscle

Introduction

During normal embryonic development, condensations of primitive mesodermal connective tissue, called *mesenchyme,* are laid down at the sites of future bone, and by the end of the second month ossification commences. In the development of some bones, notably the vault of the skull, there is a direct conversion of the membranous sheet of mesenchyme to bone. Mesenchymal cells differentiate into osteoblasts, and the bones formed in this way are therefore called *membrane bones*. The long bones develop in a different way: in these, the mesenchyme first differentiates into cartilage, which is subsequently *replaced* by bone. The cartilage cells swell up and die, and the intervening cartilaginous matrix calcifies. This acellular calcified cartilage is eroded by multinucleate osteoclasts, and at the same time osteoblasts lay down lamellar bone (see below). The osteoblasts, once they are embedded in the bone, become *osteocytes*. This process, which is called *endochondral ossification,* continues at the epiphyseal ends of the long bones until adult stature is achieved. Proliferation of cartilage at the epiphyses and its subsequent ossification is therefore the way in which the long bones grow in length.

Bone is composed of calcified osteoid tissue; the latter consists of collagen fibers embedded in a specialized ground substance. Although the precise composition of bone salts is not known, they are generally considered to be composed of hydroxyapatite, a complex molecule of calcium phosphate and calcium hydroxide. Bone also contains small quantities of magnesium, sodium, and potassium as well as carbonate and citrate ions.

Structure of Bone

Depending on the arrangement of the collagen fibers, two histological types of bone may be recognized:

Woven Bone. This type shows an irregular arrangement of collagen bundles and is the type of bone that is formed under the following three circumstances: (a) during the initial stages of the formation of membrane bones; (b) when bone forms in the midst of differentiating granulation tissue, as in fracture healing; and (c) in certain bone disorders and tumors.

Lamellar or Mature Bone. In this type of bone the collagen bundles are arranged either in parallel sheets or in concentric laminae around a central vessel, thereby forming haversian systems (Fig. 40–1).

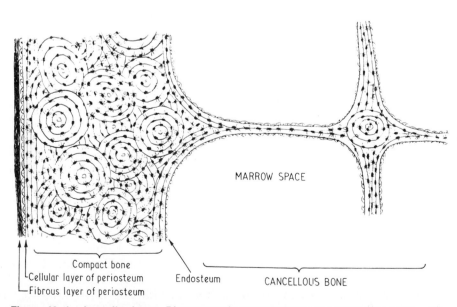

MARROW SPACE

Compact bone
Cellular layer of periosteum
Fibrous layer of periosteum
Endosteum   CANCELLOUS BONE

Figure 40–1. Lamellar bone. Diagrammatic representation of a transverse section through part of the shaft of a long bone to show the arrangement of lamellar bone. The cortex is composed mainly of haversian systems.

In the outer dense cortex of the long bones, haversian systems predominate, whereas flat plates are seen under the periosteum and endosteum. This type of bone is called *compact bone*.

The central portion of the long bones is hollowed out to form the medullary cavity, which contains marrow. Thin struts of bone remain, which are constructed of flat bundles of collagen with few haversian systems. The central trabeculated part of the bone is called *cancellous;* like compact bone, it is composed of lamellar bone.

Lamellar bone is formed when bone is laid down on a previous scaffolding. This may consist of the following: (a) calcified cartilage, as in normal endochondral ossification; (b) woven bone, as in growing membrane bones; and (c) lamellar bone itself, as in the circumferential growth of all long bones.

In the normal adult the entire skeleton is composed of lamellar bone. Although bone appears rigid and inert, it is as susceptible as the soft tissues to adverse circumstances. Indeed, the effects on bone are often more severe and permanent.

The osteocytes play an important role in bone homeostasis. If they die (as in ischemic necrosis), the bone crumbles and is removed. Osteocytes are able to demineralize the bone adjacent to them and also remove its osteoid matrix. This process is called *osteolysis* and is probably of great importance in the hour-to-hour regulation of the plasma calcium level (see below). There is a continuous process of remodeling of bone throughout life, with bone resorption not only by osteolysis but also by the action of *osteoclasts,* which are large multinucleate cells that remove both the bone salts and the protein matrix of bone. This destructive osteoclastic activity is probably of great importance in the general remodeling of bone that is continually taking place. Following the removal of bone, osteocytes differentiate into osteoblasts and lay down more osteoid, which subsequently calcifies to form bone. It is evident that the integrity of bone is maintained by the delicate balance between bone destruction and bone formation. If either predominates, osteoporosis or osteosclerosis results. *Osteoporosis*, also called *osteopenia,* is a condition in which the organic matrix *(osteoid),* although reduced in amount, is normally mineralized. Osteoporosis is therefore defined as a condition in which there is a decrease to below normal in the amount of bone tissue per unit volume of anatomical bone. Microscopically, osteoporotic bone shows normal structure and calcification, but there is too little of it; the cortex of an osteoporotic bone is thin, and the trabeculae in the cancellous portion are attenuated. Hence, as a whole the bone is fragile and liable to fracture, or in the case of a vertebra liable to crushing. The radiographic appearance of osteoporotic bone is one of rarefaction. The condition may be brought about either by excessive destruction of bone or by defective formation.

In *osteosclerosis* there is excessive formation of osteoid, which, being calcified, makes the bone appear dense on a radiograph. In spite of its density, osteoporotic bone is brittle and also liable to pathological fracture (page 575).

Osteoblasts manufacture the enzyme *alkaline phosphatase,* but the precise role of this in bone formation is not understood. Some of the enzyme escapes into the blood, and the serum level is a good index of the overall osteoblastic activity within the body. For example, in Paget's disease (page 579) it is high. The enzyme produced by bone differs from that formed in the liver. The two isoenzymes can be separated and identified. Hence, the high alkaline phosphatase level of obstructive jaundice can be differentiated from that due to excessive osteoblastic activity.

Bone serves as a reserve of both calcium and phosphate, containing 99 per cent of the total body calcium and 90 per cent of the total body phosphorus. Nevertheless, the remaining 1 per cent of calcium is a vital fraction, because it is available to the soft tissues, and it is necessary for proper neuromuscular activity, cardiac rhythm, and enzyme activities, such as in blood coagulation.

Metabolic Functions of Bone: Calcium Metabolism

Calcium in the blood exists in three forms: (1) *Ionized calcium,* which is diffusible and constitutes 65 per cent of the total plasma calcium. The normal level is about 6.4 mg/dl (1.1 mmol/L). (2) *Protein-bound calcium,* which is nondiffusible, since it is attached to albumin. (3) *Nonionized diffusible calcium,* which is the smallest fraction and exists as citrate. The ionized calcium is the most important fraction and is in equilibrium with the calcium salts in bone.

In spite of a varying diet, the amount of calcium absorbed from the intestine, the amount excreted in the urine, and the amount deposited or withdrawn from bone are so regulated that *the level of plasma ionized calcium remains constant.* The actions of parathyroid hormone, vitamin D, and calcitonin are vitally concerned in this homeostatic mechanism.

Parathyroid Hormone.   There is a continuous secretion of hormone from the parathyroid glands; the rate of secretion is influenced by the plasma ionized calcium level. A fall in calcium level stimulates parathyroid secretion, while a rise in calcium level inhibits it. The major effect of parathyroid hormone is on bone. It promotes osteolysis by osteocytes and stimulates osteoclasts, which proliferate and cause bone destruction with both removal of osteoid and release of its contained minerals. The net effect is release of calcium salts from bone, so that the plasma calcium level rises. Parathyroid hormone appears to be the major factor in regulating the level of plasma ionized calcium.

Vitamin D.   Various forms of vitamin D exist. The first apparently pure compound was called D_1 but was in fact a mixture. The radiation of ergosterol produces an active substance called D_2, and this is present in the diet containing artificially fortified foods. Natural vitamin D is produced in the skin by the ultraviolet radiation of 7-dehydrocholesterol and is called D_3 or cholecalciferol. Both vitamins D_2 and D_3 are hydroxylated in the liver to 25-hydroxy compounds ($25[OH]D_2$ and $25[OH]D_3$). These compounds are subsequently further hydroxylated in the kidney to form the final active metabolites ($1,25[OH]_2D_2$ and $1,25[OH]_2D_3$). This final hydroxylation is promoted by a number of factors, including a low blood calcium level and parathyroid hormone.

The main action of vitamin D is to aid the absorption of calcium from the gut. The vitamin also has a mild parathyroid hormone–like action on bone, but this is probably unimportant. Very high doses of the vitamin given therapeutically can, however, lead to hypercalcemia and hypercalciuria. A deficiency of vitamin D results in impaired absorption of calcium from the intestine and subsequent hypocalcemia. There is a *diminution, or even complete cessation, of calcification in cartilage and osteoid.* In the growing child this results in *rickets,* whereas in the adult there is *osteomalacia.* Both of these conditions are described later in this chapter.

Although parathyroid hormone and vitamin D both play important roles in maintaining calcium homeostasis, the action of vitamin D is the more vital. Patients with hypoparathyroidism can be maintained on vitamin D therapy and additional calcium. On the other hand, the absence of vitamin D leads to severe skeletal disease, and no substitute for the vitamin will prevent it.

Calcitonin.   This hormone is secreted by the C cells of the thyroid and has the action on bone of reducing bone absorption by inhibiting osteoclastic activity. The precise role of this hormone in calcium homeostasis has yet to be determined, but it could clearly complement parathyroid hormone since the stimulus for its secretion is hypercalcemia.

The normal plasma calcium level is 9.2 to 10.4 mg/dl (2.3 to 2.6 mmol/L) and in healthy persons is remarkably constant because of the efficiency of the regulating mechanisms. The serum calcium and phosphate together tend to maintain a reciprocal relationship. Thus, if there is a rise in the serum level of either calcium or phosphate, there is a corresponding fall in that of the other. However, if the level of one substance is low, the other does not necessarily rise.

Infections of Bone

Pyogenic Infections

The term "osteomyelitis" is applied to pyogenic infections because both bone marrow cavity and the bone itself are involved. The infection may be blood-borne or result from direct extension either from a nearby focus (*e.g.*, an ulcer of the foot in a diabetic subject) or by contamination of a compound fracture (page 576).

Acute Suppurative Osteomyelitis. This infection occurs most often in childhood; generally it develops at the end of one of the long bones of the lower limbs. The explanation for this localization is that this is an area commonly traumatized; furthermore, if an injury occurs during the course of a bacteremia associated with a skin infection, the organisms, commonly *Staphylococcus aureus,* become localized and set up a metastatic lesion. An acute inflammatory reaction ensues, and this is accompanied by rigors, fever, and acute tenderness of the region. Owing to the rigidity of the bone, the increased tension produced by the exudation leads to compression of blood vessels and ischemia. Necrosis of marrow and bone consequently follows; pus is formed, and it tracks under the periosteum, thereby further imperiling the blood supply to the cortex. In this way, quite extensive necrosis of bone can occur; indeed, the whole shaft can eventually become involved. *During the early stages,* however, no necrosis may be evident on radiography, and if a child has an illness suggestive of acute osteomyelitis, treatment is begun before enough time has passed to produce radiographic changes.

With modern therapy, acute osteomyelitis frequently resolves. This was not so in the preantibiotic days. The dead bone, called a *sequestrum,* acts as a foreign body and provides a focus for continued growth of organisms. Together with the trapped collections of pus, the conditions are ideal for the development of chronic inflammation.

Chronic Suppurative Osteomyelitis. Pus ruptures through the periosteum into the muscular and subcutaneous tissues and ultimately escapes to the skin surface through one or more sinuses. The vascular periosteum attempts to re-form the shaft of bone by producing new bone that encases the sequestrated shaft and is called an *involucrum* (Fig. 40–2). Osteoclasts slowly erode the sequestrum and detach it at each end, but this process may take many months or years to accomplish; in practice, spontaneous healing does not occur. If the condition is not treated, it may lead to death as a result of pyemia, toxemia, or amyloid disease.

Chronic suppurative osteomyelitis is fortunately very rare these days. However, a description of it is useful because it illustrates the typical features of a chronic suppurative inflammation. It demonstrates the combination of the following factors: (1) *acute inflammation* with fluid exudation and pus formation; (2) *demolition* by macrophages and osteoclasts; (3) *regeneration* of bone by osteoblasts; and (4) *repair* with granulation tissue and extensive scar tissue formation.

Figure 40-2. Osteomyelitis of the tibia. This amputation specimen shows the typical appearance of extensive chronic osteomyelitis. The dead shaft of the bone forms a sequestrum and is surrounded by thick, irregularly shaped new bone that constitutes the encasing involucrum. The sequestrum can be seen through a hole in the involucrum at the lower end of the specimen. (HS44.1, Reproduced by permission of the President and Council of the R.C.S. Eng.)

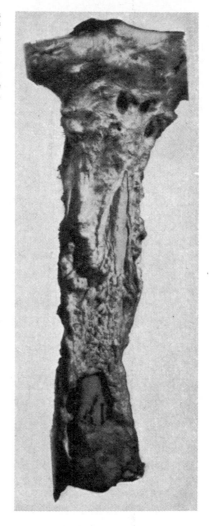

Other types of chronic osteomyelitis are known but are uncommon. *Brode's abscess* is a localized chronic suppurative lesion that causes pain and may simulate a bone tumor. *Salmonella osteomyelitis* can affect several bones simultaneously. It is most common in children, particularly those with sickle cell disease.

Tuberculosis of Bone. Unlike pyogenic osteomyelitis, tuberculosis of bone is generally insidious in its onset and is characterized by bone destruction with very little reactive new bone formation. One of the common sites of infection is the vertebral column *(Pott's disease)*. The affected vertebrae frequently collapse and produce an angulation of the spinal column; forward deviation is called a *kyphosis* and lateral deviation is called a *scoliosis*. The combination is called *kyphoscoliosis,* and if severe this can interfere with the act of breathing to the extent of causing respiratory acidosis, pulmonary hypertension, and eventually right-sided heart failure (Chapter 28). As with tuberculosis elsewhere, caseous tissue is formed. When this softens, it becomes a "cold abscess" that tracks along the line of least resistance and is ultimately discharged to the exterior. In tuberculosis of the spine, the pus tends to enter the psoas sheath, track down in it beneath the inguinal ligament, and present as a fluctuating mass that subsequently discharges to the surface. Fortunately, tuberculosis of bone is now a rarity.

Nonsuppurative Infections

Syphilis.   Syphilis of bone is now extremely uncommon. It is generally seen in the later stages of the disease, with periostitis predominating. The bone tends to become osteosclerotic, in contrast to becoming osteoporotic in tuberculosis.

Ischemic Bone Disease

The blood supply to certain bones is precarious and can easily be interrupted by traumatic damage, such as that caused by an adjacent fracture. Well-recognized sites are the head of the femur and the carpal scaphoid bone. *Ischemic necrosis* (infarction) is also called *avascular necrosis* and can occur under other circumstances:

1. *Thromboembolism,* from the heart or elsewhere.

2. *The decompression syndrome,* when nitrogen bubbles block small vessels.

3. *Sickle cell anemia,* when packed abnormal red cells occlude small vessels. The necrosis may predispose to salmonella infection (page 573).

4. *Fat embolism.* Fat emboli from a fatty liver are the suggested cause of the ischemic necrosis observed in *alcoholism* and as a complication of *glucocorticoid therapy.*

5. *Idiopathic condition.* There are a number of conditions affecting growing children in which an epiphysis undergoes ischemic necrosis without apparent cause. The best known example is *Legg-Perthes disease,* which affects the head of the femur.

Infarction of bone causes no immediate problem to the patient, and healing occurs slowly by the process of *creeping substitution* (Chapter 9). However, if the bone is subjected to pressure it may crumble, and this is particularly important in weight-bearing areas. Thus, with ischemic necrosis of the head of the femur (following fracture of the neck of the femur or in Legg-Perthes disease) the bone collapses, the head becomes flattened, the joint is distorted, and osteoarthritis later develops.

Bone Disorders Caused by Physical Disturbances

Whenever a joint is immobilized, either by a cast or by disease, the neighboring bones develop osteoporosis. This effect is a form of disuse atrophy — the greater the degree of immobility, the more marked the osteoporosis. Thus, if there is paralysis of a whole limb (*e.g.,* in poliomyelitis), osteoporosis affects all the bones of that limb.

Localized Osteoporosis

Pressure Atrophy

Any expanding lesion that exerts pressure on bone causes local ischemia and pressure atrophy. Recall that cartilage — being avascular — does not show this pressure atrophy. Thus, an aneurysm of the aorta that presses on the vertebral column causes pressure atrophy of the vertebrae, but the intervening discs remain unaffected.

Benign tumors arising in bone cause pressure atrophy; the adjacent periosteum responds by producing new bone around the lesion. Thus, a benign tumor gives the appearance of expanding the bone.

Fractures

Causes
Excessive Mechanical Force
Direct Violence.   A good example is a blow that causes a depressed fracture of the skull or a broken scapula.

Indirect Violence.   A fracture of the clavicle caused by falling on an outstretched arm is an example.

Muscular Action.   Sudden, unexpected strains during violent exercise can cause fractures in normal bones (*spontaneous fractures*).

Fractures of Abnormal Bone.   A fracture in a diseased, weakened bone that has been subjected to a normal strain is called a *pathological fracture.* Secondary carcinoma must always be borne in mind as a cause of this. Indeed, a pathological fracture may be the first indication of malignancy, *e.g.,* carcinoma of the lung.

Stages in Fracture Healing.   The stages in fracture healing are illustrated in Figure 40–3. Notice that the hematoma between the bone ends is organized and that the granulation tissue so formed matures to either woven bone or cartilage. This hard material, which initially unites the bone ends, is called *callus.* The woven bone or cartilage of which it is composed is gradually replaced by mature lamellar bone. Thus, during regeneration of bone the two embryological methods of bone formation — endochondral and intramembranous — are faithfully repeated in later life.

Abnormalities of Fracture Healing

Repair or Fibrous Union.   Although the cells of the granulation tissue of a healing fracture are called osteoblasts, they are capable of differentiation along several lines. If immobilization is not satisfactory, the cells behave like fibroblasts, and the bone ends become united by ordinary fibrous scar tissue that cannot be converted into bone.

Fibrous union is particularly common in situations in which the blood supply is impaired or immobilization is difficult. Thus, it occurs in fractures of the carpal scaphoid bone; when fibrous union has occurred, surgical intervention is necessary to remove the fibrous tissue and to create thereby a new fracture in which bone formation can occur.

Nonunion.   Complete lack of union between the fracture ends results from the interposition of soft parts. Muscle or fascia can separate the two bone ends, and because there is no continuous hematoma between them, union of

Figure 40–3.   Stages in the healing of a fracture. *a,* Hematoma formation. *b,* Acute inflammation followed by demolition. Loose fragments of bone are removed, and the bone ends show osteoporosis. *c,* Granulation-tissue formation. *d,* The bone ends are now united by woven bone, cartilage, or a mixture of the two. This hard material is called *callus. e,* Lamellar bone is laid down; calcified cartilage and woven bone are progressively removed. *f,* Final remodeling.

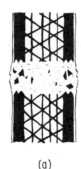
(a)

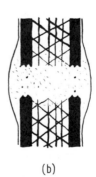
(b)

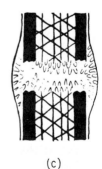
(c)

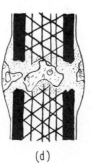
(d)

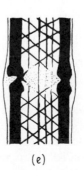
(e)

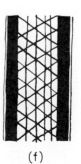
(f)

any sort is impossible. This phenomenon is sometimes utilized deliberately in order to form a new false joint.

Delayed Union.   In the presence of a continuous hematoma, any cause of delayed healing retards bone regeneration. In practice the following causes are most important:

Movement.   Movement of any sort is harmful to the healing process, because it excites an inflammatory reaction, damages the delicate granulation tissue, and inhibits the formation of bone. In surgical practice every effort is made to reduce movement to a minimum. If the bone ends are impacted, union is usually rapid; indeed, one method of treating a fracture is to bring the ends of the broken bone together under high compression. This provides rigid immobilization and speeds healing. If the bone ends are not impacted, the fracture is stabilized either by external splints or by casts. Alternatively, an operation is performed, and then screws, nails, or plates are inserted to minimize movement between the ends of the broken bone.

Infection.   Infection produces osteomyelitis and can lead to extensive ischemic necrosis with sequestrum formation. Infection is particularly liable to occur if the failure is *compound, i.e.,* if one of the bone ends has penetrated the skin and is exposed to the exterior.

Poor Blood Supply.   Whereas complete loss of blood supply results in necrosis of bone, poor blood supply leads to slow granulation-tissue formation and to slow healing. Certain sites (*e.g.,* fractures of the neck of the femur, the shaft of tibia, and the carpal scaphoid bone) are notorious for this complication. In these situations it is particularly important to avoid other possible causes of delayed healing, such as movement. For example, a pin is passed into the head of the femur so that rigid immobilization is immediately obtained. This technique is particularly useful in old people. If an elderly person falls and fractures the neck of the femur, the injury can be treated by external immobilization in a plaster cast. Unfortunately, the patient is confined to bed for many weeks and is liable to develop many complications: venous thrombosis, pulmonary embolism, bronchopneumonia, and urinary tract infection. Pinning the head, on the other hand, can allow the person to get up immediately and to escape these hazards of recumbency.

Myositis Ossificans.   If there is an extravasation of fracture hematoma into surrounding muscles, its subsequent organization and ossification results in the condition called *traumatic myositis ossificans.* Sometimes the large masses of bone formed around a joint can seriously interfere with movement.

GENERALIZED BONE DISORDERS

There is no satisfactory classification of generalized bone disorders, but in practice they can be considered under three headings:

1. *Developmental anomalies.*
2. *Abnormalities due to metabolic disorders.*
3. *Abnormalities occurring in the adult;* these are generally of unknown cause.

Developmental Abnormalities

Many developmental abnormalities of bones are known, but these are rare, for the most part. Four examples will be considered below:

Osteogenesis Imperfecta

In this condition the bones are thin and brittle. The cortex is thin, and there is a decrease in the amount of cancellous bone. The fragility results in frequent fractures that occur either spontaneously or as a result of trivial injuries. The fractures heal well, but their multiplicity generally leads to severe deformities.

Two types of the disease are known. In the *congenital type,* which is inherited as an autosomal recessive trait, multiple fractures occur *in utero* or during birth, and the prognosis is poor. In the *tarda form* the disease is less severe, and if the child survives, the tendency to sustain fractures decreases after puberty. This form is inherited as an autosomal dominant trait and is an illustration of the dictum that dominant traits tend to be less severe than recessive ones (Chapter 3).

Osteogenesis imperfecta appears to be a condition with widespread hypoplasia of the mesenchyme. Affected subjects are of short stature; have lax ligaments, leading to hypermobility of the joints; and have thin sclerae of the eyes, allowing the pigment of the choroid to give them a blue color.

Achondroplasia

This disease is also transmitted as an autosomal dominant factor. The essential feature appears to be defective endochondral bone formation, and the long bones of the limbs are therefore short. A person with this condition is called an *achondroplastic dwarf.* The trunk and head are of normal size, although the middle of the face tends to be depressed because the base of the skull is formed of cartilage and is therefore affected. The person with this condition has normal intelligence, is very muscular and agile, and is frequently seen in the circus ring.

Osteopetrosis (Albers-Schönberg Disease)

In this condition there is increased formation of bone, so that the skeleton is hard and inelastic. However, the bones are particularly liable to fracture because of their inelasticity. Bone encroaches on the marrow cavity, and this can result in leukoerythroblastic anemia (Chapter 26). As with osteogenesis imperfecta, there is a severe form of the disease that is inherited as a recessive trait, and a benign form with dominant inheritance.

Fibrous Dysplasia

Fibrous dysplasia of bone is characterized by the appearance of areas of bone resorption and their replacement by fibrous tissue in which there are thin trabeculae of woven bone. The marrow space is obliterated in the area affected. Any bone may be affected, and the etiology is unknown. In the common type of the disease young people (median age 14 years) are affected and only one bone is involved *(monostotic fibrous dysplasia).* Polyostotic fibrous dysplasia usually manifests itself in early life, is of insidious onset, and affects many bones on one side of the body only. If the skull and facial bones are involved, there is much disfigurement.

Abnormalities of Bone Due to Metabolic Disorders

Endocrine Disturbances.   Skeletal changes associated with pituitary and thyroid disease are considered elsewhere. By far, the most important hormone in relation to bone metabolism is parathyroid hormone, which is derived from the four parathyroid glands.

Hyperparathyroidism

Hyperparathyroidism can be divided into two groups:
Primary Hyperparathyroidism.   This condition is due to the excessive production of parathyroid hormone, usually by a parathyroid *adenoma,* occasionally by *idiopathic hyperplasia,* and rarely by a *carcinoma* of a parathyroid. The effects of hyperparathyroidism are to increase bone resorption by osteolysis and to promote osteoclastic proliferation and activity. The blood calcium level is raised, and there is increased urine loss of calcium (hypercalciuria). As bone is destroyed it is replaced by fibrous tissue; the end-result is osteitis fibrosa cystica (see below).
Secondary Hyperparathyroidism.   Hyperplasia and hypersecretion of the glands can be induced by a persistently *low level of serum ionized*

calcium. This is seen most frequently in two groups of conditions: (1) *rickets and osteomalacia,* which are described later in this chapter; and (2) *chronic renal disease.*

The relationship between chronic renal disease and parathyroid function is complicated. In chronic renal disease there is retention of phosphate and a raised serum level (hyperphosphatemia). There is also a depression in the level of serum calcium, which in its turn acts as a stimulus to the parathyroids, leading to their hyperplasia and hypersecretion. Calcium is mobilized from the bones, which become progressively demineralized. The calcium is excreted by the kidney, but this excretion can lead to further renal damage by metastatic calcification and stone formation. Furthermore, in chronic renal disease there is impaired hydroxylation of vitamin D to yield the active dihydroxy compound (page 571). Hence, there is in effect vitamin D deficiency and defective calcium absorption from the intestine. Chronic renal disease produces its most severe effects on the growing skeleton of children. Growth is stunted (causing renal dwarfism), and the bones show the combined changes of rickets and osteitis fibrosa cystica *(renal osteodystrophy).*

Osteitis Fibrosa Cystica* (von Recklinghausen's Disease of Bone). In the early stages of this disease there is generalized bone involvement. The outstanding features are pains in the bones and weakening of the bones that can result in bending, deformity, and spontaneous fracture. Since there is an increased excretion of calcium via the kidneys, renal stones are not uncommon and can be responsible for the initial symptoms — that is, hematuria, pain, and urinary infection. Metastatic calcification is common (see below). In the late stages of hyperparathyroidism, the bones contain tumorlike masses composed of osteoclasts together with localized blood-filled cysts. These *brown tumors,* as they are called, closely resemble histologically the giant-cell tumors of bone but are considered to be merely focal areas of hyperplasia.

Metastatic Calcification. Metastatic calcification is the deposition of calcium salts in normal tissues other than osteoid or teeth; it is due to a derangement of calcium or phosphate metabolism. The most common cause is hypercalcemia due to hyperparathyroidism or extensive destruction of bone that can occur with multiple osteolytic tumors. It is also a feature of chronic renal disease.

Calcification can occur in many sites, but in the kidney the results are the most serious, because combined with the effects of calculi, progressive renal damage leads to progressive renal failure.

Vitamin D Deficiency: Rickets and Osteomalacia   The metabolism of vitamin D has already been discussed (page 571). It will be recalled that the main effects of vitamin D deficiency are impaired absorption of calcium from the gut and defective calcification of cartilage and osteoid.

Rickets. In rickets there is a failure of the calcification of cartilage that normally occurs at the growing epiphyses. Cartilage is therefore neither removed nor replaced by osteoid. Continued growth of the cartilage causes a considerable enlargement of the bone ends. Similarly, the costochondral junctions are enlarged, producing the clinical deformity called the "rachitic rosary." Because the overall growth of bone is diminished, the child becomes dwarfed. Even the osteoid that is formed is poorly calcified, and the weakened bones are liable to bend and become deformed. Knock-knees, kyphosis, and other deformities are common.

---

*The term is a poor one, because the disease is not inflammatory and the cysts are not always present.

Osteomalacia. The counterpart of rickets in adults is osteomalacia. It is most common in women, because pregnancy imposes an additional drain on the supplies of calcium and vitamins.

The normal adult bone is continually being remodeled; as bone is removed by osteoclasts it is replaced by osteoid laid down by osteoblasts. In healthy persons the osteoid promptly calcifies, but in people with vitamin D deficiency this calcification fails to occur and the bones ultimately consist largely of osteoid. This is the condition of osteomalacia (softening of the bone): although there is an abundance of osteoid, it is poorly calcified. In osteoporosis, by contrast, the matrix is normally calcified but is reduced in quantity.

In osteomalacia all bones are affected, but it is in the weight-bearing areas that the effects are most severe. Gross pelvic distortion occurs and causes complications in subsequent pregnancies. Collapse of the vertebrae gives rise to pain resulting from compression of the spinal nerves as they leave the intervertebral foramina.

Abnormalities of Bone Occurring in the Adult

Generalized Osteoporosis

Disuse Osteoporosis. Prolonged recumbency leads to increased osteoclastic activity and resorption of bone. There is excessive mobilization of calcium, resulting in hypercalciuria and a tendency for renal stones to form. The blood calcium level remains normal, since the process is gradual.

Idiopathic Osteoporosis. Some degree of bone loss is a normal process of aging and results from a slight imbalance between bone formation and bone destruction. The process is slow and continues over many years, so that the blood levels of calcium and alkaline phosphatase are normal. In some patients the process is more marked and the condition becomes pathological. This is termed *senile osteoporosis* and affects particularly the pelvis, spine, and ribs. The vertebrae are compressed, and this causes backache, which can be severe (Fig. 40–4). There is also some diminution in height, but since the condition occurs so slowly the patient rarely notices this. Osteoporosis is particularly common in women past the menopause *(postmenopausal osteoporosis);* this has been attributed to lack of estrogens. Occasionally osteoporosis occurs in a younger age group for no obvious reason.

Other Types of Osteoporosis. Osteoporosis also occurs when collagen formation is impaired, as in:

1. Scurvy.

2. Cushing's syndrome. This includes prolonged administration of glucocorticoids, such as prednisone.

3. Impaired supply of protein, *e.g.*, in starvation and in the malabsorption syndrome.

Paget's Disease of Bone (Osteitis Deformans)

This disease is not an inflammatory one, although it was so considered by Sir James Paget in the nineteenth century. The cause is not known, and the disease seems to be more common in males, particularly those over the age of 40 years.

In the early stages of the disease the bones become softened because of osteoclastic resorption, and the weakened bones tend to bend. Since this is particularly noticeable in the weight-bearing bones, bowing of the femora is characteristic. In the later stages of the disease, irregular subperiosteal bone formation occurs, causing bones to become thicker and hardened. Serum calcium and phosphate levels remain within normal limits, but the serum alkaline phosphatase is greatly raised because of the rapid turnover of bone.

The skull is frequently affected, and as it becomes increasingly thick-

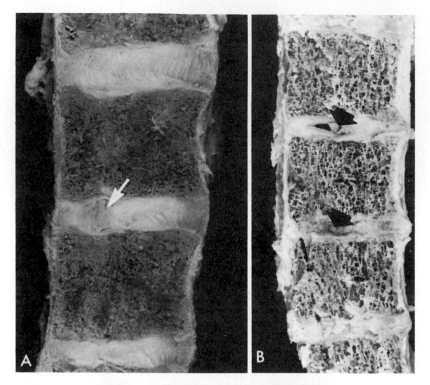

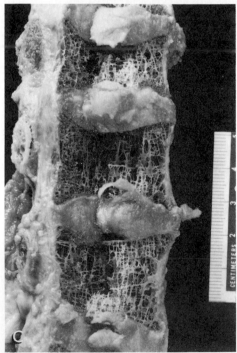

Figure 40–4.   Normal vs. osteoporotic vertebral bodies. *A,* Normal vertebral bodies. *B,* Moderate osteoporosis. *C,* Severe osteoporosis. The vertebral bodies have been sectioned to show their internal structure. Note the well-formed cancellous bone of the normal vertebral bodies in *A* as well as the structure of the intervertebral discs. One small focus of degeneration can be seen (white arrow). In *B* the specimen shows well-developed osteoporosis, but the overall shape of the vertebrae is preserved. The discs show severe degenerative changes (black arrows). In *C* the specimen shows severe osteoporosis. The vertebrae have been compressed by the bulging discs.

ened, the patient notices a need for an increased hat size. Blindness, deafness, headaches, and facial paralysis are complications that may result from compression of nerves in their bony canals. An occasional complication is the development of osteosarcoma, a tumor that is uncommon in adults except in association with this disease.

In its fully developed form this syndrome has three components:

1. *Clubbing of the Fingers and Toes.* The nails of the fingers and toes are curved, and the angle between the nail plate and nail bed is flattened to 180° or more instead of the normal 160°. The nail fold is swollen and spongy.

2. *Subperiosteal Bone Formation (Periostitis).* This affects the distal ends of the long bones.

3. *Swelling and Pain of the Joints (Polyarthritis).* This commonly affects the hands and feet and, when acute, can closely mimic early rheumatoid arthritis.

The importance of hypertrophic osteoarthropathy is that it is a complication of a wide variety of underlying diseases. Indeed, it is sometimes the presenting symptom. The common causes are carcinoma of the lung and chronic intrathoracic infection such as lung abscess, bronchiectasis, empyema, and tuberculosis. Clubbing of the nails is the most common manifestation of hypertrophic osteoarthropathy and occurs as a sole finding in cyanotic congenital heart disease, bacterial endocarditis, biliary cirrhosis, ulcerative colitis, Crohn's disease, and a number of other disorders.

The pathogenesis of hypertrophic osteoarthropathy is not understood, but if the underlying disease can be removed or cured (*e.g.*, pneumonectomy in the case of lung cancer), its manifestations abate.

Hypertrophic Osteoarthropathy

The tumors of bone form a complex group in spite of the apparent simplicity of bone structure. Indeed, the histogenesis of some of the tumors is quite obscure. The occurrence of tumors arising from the marrow and the frequency of skeletal metastases add further to the confusion.

TUMORS

Tumors of Bones

It is noteworthy that *pain is often the first symptom of a bone tumor,* and this is due no doubt to the pressure exerted by the dividing abnormal cells on the rigid, unyielding surrounding bone. It will be recalled that in most situations pain is a late symptom of neoplasia.

Benign Tumors. Osteoma, chondroma, fibroma, and other tumors all occur but are uncommon.

Intermediate Tumors

Giant-cell Tumor of Bone. This tumor characteristically occurs in the ends of the long bones in young adults. Pain is the predominant symptom, and its onset is followed by swelling. The radiograph generally shows a characteristic appearance; because the tumor destroys areas of bone, these appear as a series of translucent areas that have been likened to a mass of soap bubbles (Fig. 40–5). Microscopically, the tumor consists of fusiform cells and abundant multinucleate giant cells that resemble osteoclasts. On this account the tumor has also been called an *"osteoclastoma,"* but since the precise nature of the cells is not settled, *giant-cell tumor* is now the current name.

The behavior of giant-cell tumors is generally that of a benign tumor. Nevertheless, local invasion can occur, and between 10 and 15 per cent of the tumors metastasize.

Malignant Tumors

Chondrosarcoma. This tumor is composed of atypical cartilage cells, and it is often difficult to distinguish histologically from a benign chondroma. Local invasion and later metastasis to the lungs are the main features.

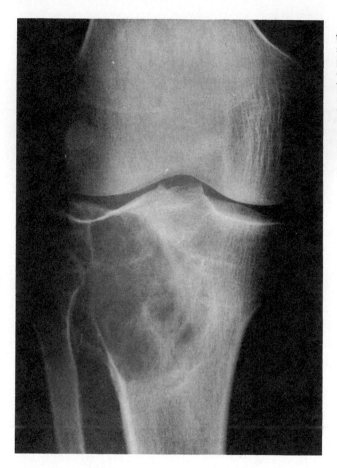

Figure 40–5.   Giant-cell tumor of bone. This radiograph shows the "soap bubble" appearance of a tumor that occupies the upper end of the tibia. Note how the joint space is not encroached upon by the growth. Cartilage cannot exhibit pressure atrophy because it is avascular. (Courtesy of Dr. D. E. Sanders.)

Osteosarcoma.   Osteosarcoma is the most common and most malignant of this rare group of primary bone tumors. It affects males more frequently than females, and it is most commonly seen in persons between the ages of 10 and 25 years. Pain is the usual presenting symptom (see Chapter 1, Case History I).

The tumor is composed of malignant osteoblasts that exhibit considerable pleomorphism; giant cells are often abundant. In well-differentiated tumors there is a considerable amount of osteoid produced, which may or may not calcify to form bone. When there is much bone formation, the tumor is described as *osteosclerotic*. Tumor spreads beneath the periosteum, elevates it, and produces a fusiform swelling. Spicules of new bone radiate from the periosteum (Fig. 40–6). On radiography this gives a characteristic "sun ray" appearance. In tumors producing little calcified material the lesion is described as *osteolytic;* the radiograph shows an irregular bony defect and a surrounding soft tissue shadow as growth elevates the periosteum and finally penetrates it.

The outlook for a patient with osteosarcoma is extremely poor, because pulmonary metastases appear early.

Tumors of Bone Marrow

Myeloma.   This tumor is derived from cells that show a marked tendency to differentiate into plasma cells. Because the neoplasia is usually multicentric, the condition is known as *multiple myelomatosis*. It occurs predominantly in persons over 40 years of age and produces multiple osteolytic, punched-out lesions of bone, particularly in the bones in which red marrow is normally found, *i.e.*, the skull, the vertebrae, and the ribs (Fig. 40–7). This widespread involvement of the skeleton can produce so much demineralization that hypercalcemia, metastatic calcification, and renal failure occur. The bony lesions often produce severe pain; a pathological fracture is sometimes the first evidence of the disease.

The tumor cells form large amounts of a homogeneous immunoglobulin called *myeloma protein*. In addition, some tumors produce an excess of light chains, and the polypeptide produced *(Bence Jones protein)*, having a molecular weight of about 22,000, is excreted by the kidney and can be recognized by heating a sample of urine. It precipitates when the urine is heated to between 60° and 80°C and redissolves on further heating or cooling. Bence Jones protein may precipitate in the tubules of the kidney, cause obstruction, and lead to renal failure. Metastatic calcification, renal stone formation, and amyloidosis add their quota to kidney damage.

Ewing's Tumor. This uncommon tumor occurs in young children and most often affects the shaft of a long bone. It is composed of small, undifferentiated round cells and is osteolytic. The raised periosteum may produce layers of new bone around the tumor, leading to an onionlike appearance radiologically. The nature of the tumor is obscure. It appears to be a distinct entity, but it can be closely mimicked by metastatic neuroblastoma—a neoplasm that also occurs at the same age. Ewing's tumor is radiosensitive, but the prognosis is bad because it usually metastasizes to other bones and viscera.

Metastatic Tumors. Secondary tumors of bone are much more common

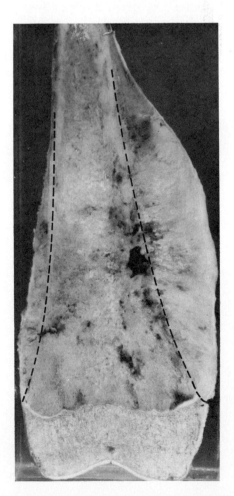

Figure 40–6. Osteosarcoma. The lower end of the femur is greatly expanded by this malignant tumor. The original cortex of the shaft, which can still be discerned, is indicated by the dotted lines. Tumor, in addition to replacing the marrow cavity, has extended beneath the periosteum.

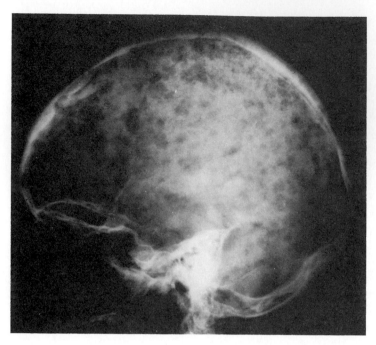

Figure 40–7. Multiple myelomatosis. This radiograph of the skull shows numerous osteolytic tumor deposits that produce a typical moth-eaten appearance resulting from numerous punched-out areas where bone has been destroyed. An appearance similar to this can sometimes be seen in secondary carcinoma. (Courtesy of Dr. D. E. Sanders, Toronto General Hospital.)

than the primary ones. They develop from blood-borne metastases of carcinoma, and the primary site is generally the prostate, breast, bronchus, kidney, stomach, or thyroid (Fig. 40–8). Metastatic tumors are generally multiple and destroy bone locally to produce rarefaction on radiography *(osteolytic secondaries)*. Exceptions to this tendency to destroy bone occur with carcinoma of the prostate and occasionally carcinoma of the breast or other site (Fig. 40–8). In these instances the tumor stimulates new bone formation, and the tumors are hard and radiopaque *(osteosclerotic)*. A pathological fracture or pain is the

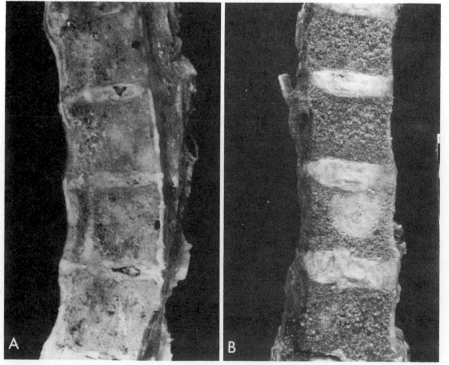

Figure 40–8. Secondary carcinoma in bone. *A,* This section of bone is from a patient who died of carcinoma of the prostate. The cancellous bone in the vertebral bodies shows patchy white tumor deposits that are densely hard because of new bone formation. *B,* Solitary osteolytic metastasis from a carcinoma of the kidney.

usual presenting symptom. In addition, if the disease is extensive, a leukoerythroblastic anemia can result.

A synovial joint consists of two or more opposing *cartilage-covered bone ends* that are united by a sleeve of connective tissue called the *capsule*, the innermost layer of which is modified into a secreting membrane called the *synovium*. The synovium consists of one or more layers of flattened or cubical cells that secrete a clear, pale, viscid fluid *(synovial fluid)* containing mucoprotein. The synovial fluid not only lubricates the joint but is also the main, if not the only, source of nourishment of the hyaline cartilage covering the bone ends.

DISEASES OF JOINTS

Arthritis is an inflammation of a joint. There is usually an increased amount of synovial fluid present because of a concomitant inflammation of the synovial membrane *(synovitis)*. Arthritis may be traumatic, as after the forcible twisting, hyperextension, or hyperflexion of a joint. Such an injury may lead to a minor tear (called a *sprain*) in the capsule, but if the injury is more severe, the capsule may rupture and allow partial or complete displacement of the bone ends to occur. A partial dispalcement is called a *subluxation*, and a complete one is called a *dislocation*. Simple sprains heal well, but the weakness that follows capsular rupture predisposes to recurrent dislocation. Arthritis may be infective in nature. It may follow a penetrating joint injury when the infection is introduced from outside. The infection may be bloodborne; thus, a suppurative (septic) arthritis may complicate gonorrhea, lobar pneumonia, or staphylococcal septicemia. Unless energetically treated in the early stages with antibiotics, infective arthritis leads to rapid destruction of the articular cartilage; the whole joint cavity fills with inflammatory exudate that organizes and obliterates the joint space. In this way the joint is destroyed, and the bone ends are united first by fibrous tissue *(fibrous ankylosis)* and later by bone *(bony ankylosis)*.

Arthritis

Tuberculous arthritis may occur as an isolated lesion or may complicate an adjacent tuberculous osteomyelitis. The disease is now uncommon.

The common types of chronic arthritis are rheumatoid arthritis and osteoarthritis.

Rheumatoid Arthritis. This disease occurs most frequently in young women and is characteristically polyarticular (affecting many joints) and symmetrical. The small joints of the hands and feet are most severely affected, but the elbows and knees also suffer badly. Rheumatoid arthritis is a systemic disease, and in its active phases there are malaise, anemia, pyrexia, weight loss, and bouts of sweating. The onset of the disease is occasionally acute, but usually it is insidious as swelling, pain, and stiffness of the joints develop.

The affected joints are swollen, tender, and painful. In the early stages the synovial membrane is acutely inflamed; later, there is proliferation of its connective tissue component together with a heavy infiltration by lymphocytes and plasma cells. The proliferating synovium steadily encroaches upon the articular margins, and a layer of inflamed granulation tissue, called a *pannus*, spreads over the cartilage of the joint surface and destroys it. The joint space is gradually obliterated by fibrous adhesions, and eventually fibrous ankylosis occurs. In this late stage there is severe disuse atrophy of the adjacent bones and muscles, and the overlying skin is smooth and shiny. The results of advanced rheumatoid arthritis are tragic to see: progressive contractures lead to flexion deformities that are found in particular in the hands, which have a characteristic ulnar deviation of the fingers (Fig. 40–9). The flexed, ankylosed larger joints render the patient immobile and bedridden.

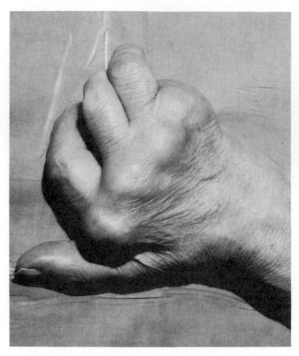

Figure 40–9. The hand in rheumatoid arthritis. This patient had had rheumatoid arthritis for many years and was severely incapacitated. The hand shows marked swelling of the metacarpophalangeal joints and extreme deviation of the fingers toward the ulnar side. Apart from movement of the thumb, very little movement was possible. The hollowed appearance between the metacarpal bones is due to atrophy of the small muscles of the hand. This patient was in a hospital because a rheumatoid nodule had developed in the sclera of her left eye. To prevent perforation of the globe and loss of the eye, a fascia lata graft was applied and was successful in saving her sight.

The nature of rheumatoid arthritis is unknown, but the basic lesion seems to be fibrinoid necrosis of collagen. It has therefore been classified as a collagen disease (Chapter 27). The widespread nature of the process is evidenced by the development of lesions in places other than the joints. The most characteristic of these is the subcutaneous nodules that develop over pressure points. They consist of a large area of necrobiotic collagen surrounded by a palisaded layer of fibroblasts and epithelioid cells. Similar nodules are encountered elsewhere; thus, in the sclera of the eye a rheumatoid nodule can break down and cause perforation of the globe. A destructive process with fibrosis can involve the aorta; the condition then has the appearance of syphilitic aortitis. Generalized enlargement of the lymph nodes and splenomegaly may also be present. Amyloidosis is an important complication; indeed, it is the only significant fatal lesion in rheumatoid arthritis, which may otherwise smolder for many years and produce complete crippling.

The sera of most patients with rheumatoid arthritis contain an autoantibody that reacts with human immunoglobulin. This antibody is called the *rheumatoid factor.* Although its detection is useful in diagnosis, its significance in the pathogenesis of the disease is not known. The rheumatoid factor is not present in psoriatic arthritis; this is a useful distinguishing point between the two diseases, which in other respects closely resemble each other.

Ankylosing Spondylitis

This condition is related to rheumatoid arthritis and is believed by some authorities to be a variant of that disease. Nevertheless, there are some rather striking differences:

1. The disease generally affects young men.

2. The vertebral joints and large peripheral joints, such as the hip, are generally affected, whereas the small distal joints are spared.

3. There is bony ankylosis of the affected joints in the later stages of the disease. The spinal ligaments and margins of the intervertebral discs undergo ossification and in due course the spinal column is converted into a composite bony mass, the so-called *bamboo spine.*

4. Subcutaneous nodules are not formed, and the rheumatoid factor is not present.

Osteoarthritis, despite its name, is not an inflammatory, but rather a degenerative, disease of joints. Osteoarthrosis is an alternative name that is sometimes used. It is one of the commonest human afflictions, because it is essentially an accentuation of the inevitable aging process of articular cartilage. The nourishment of the hyaline cartilage of joints is normally rather precarious and depends on the synovial fluid. The constant wear and tear of the joints after many years' activity leads to a gradual deterioration of the central part of the articular cartilage. This process is greatly aggravated by injury; thus, a joint injured in some athletic activity can be complicated by osteoarthritis several years later — even when the patient is still young. Nevertheless, osteoarthritis is generally a disease of later life and affects the spine and large weight-bearing joints, especially the hips.

Osteoarthritis

The smaller joints, however, do not escape entirely. Osteoarthritis, unlike rheumatoid arthritis, is not a systemic disease. The general health remains unaffected, and life is not shortened.

Osteoarthritis begins with softening and fraying of the articular cartilage, which becomes progressively thinner. Ultimately, the underlying bone is exposed, and its surface becomes hard, worn, and polished (a change called *eburnation*). Meanwhile, there is proliferation of the cartilage cells of the margin of the articular area. This new cartilage soon ossifies. The result is that the periphery of the articular cartilage is raised and bossed (a process called *lipping*); this is an important radiological finding. The projecting nodules of new bone at the margins of the joint are called *osteophytes*. These not only interfere with the range of the joint's movement but also may become nipped off to form *loose bodies* ("joint-mice"). These loose bodies are a constant nuisance, because they tend to be caught between the opposing bone ends during movement. The result is locking of the joint, which can be excruciatingly painful if a fringe of synovium is also included. A prominent site for osteophytes is the terminal interphalangeal joints of the fingers of elderly people. These painless bony swellings are extremely common and are called *Heberden's nodes*.

In osteoarthritis the joints do not become ankylosed, but the destructive process and the osteophyte formation seriously limit movement, which may become very painful. In such cases the replacement of the joint by an artificial metallic prosthesis has been most useful.

Skeletal muscle constitutes 45 per cent of the mean body weight and is afflicted by remarkably few diseases. It is composed of muscle fibers, each of which is an elongated multinucleate cell containing contractile protein in the form of myofilaments. Two types of muscle fiber are described: The *type 1* fibers (red fibers*), which contain an abundance of myoglobin and mitochondria, are adapted to slow, repetitive contractions over long periods of time. The *type 2* fibers (white fibers*) contain more myofilaments and are designed for rapid contraction; they show fatigue relatively quickly. The proportion of each type of fiber in any particular muscle depends on the age and sex of the subject, its anatomical site, and use to which the muscle has been put. Muscle is remarkably adaptable, a fact that supports the value of physical training. Exercise can increase the number of myofibrils, cause mitochondria to increase in size and number, and improve the microvascular bed so that it is

**DISEASES OF
SKELETAL
MUSCLE**

---

*The distinction between red and white fibers is obvious in birds but is not evident in humans.

more efficient in sustaining the contractile elements. The proportion of type 1 fibers to type 2 fibers can change. There is indeed a firm basis for the physical therapists' efforts to retrain and build up muscular activity and bulk. It should be noted that the number of muscle fibers present in a muscle is fixed and that any increase in size of the muscle is brought about by hypertrophy of each individual fiber only.

If muscles are not used, owing to lack of exercise, pain, or disease, disuse atrophy occurs. There is diminution in size of muscle fibers, and ultimately some are lost. Loss of motor nerve supply has a similar effect, but the atrophy tends to be in groups of fibers within the area of affected muscle. Whether the muscle as a whole becomes small or not depends on whether adjacent fibers undergo hypertrophy.

Muscular Dystrophy   Muscular dystrophy encompasses a group of uncommon inherited conditions in which there is progressive degeneration of muscle fibers. Microscopically, the fibers show varying stages of degeneration, culminating in complete destruction. The distribution of affected fibers is random, so that there is variation in size, some fibers being small and degenerate, and others enlarged owing to compensatory hypertrophy. Various types of muscular dystrophy have been described, based largely on the mode of inheritance and the clinical picture.

Duchenne Muscular Dystrophy.   This type is inherited as an X-linked trait and therefore affects males only. The disease commences at birth, initially affects the muscles of the pelvic girdle, and later spreads to the shoulder girdle. A striking feature is enlargement of the calf muscles due to an infiltration of fat cells that accompanies the degeneration of muscle fibers. The child with Duchenne muscular dystrophy has difficulty in walking, has a waddling gait, and is never able to run. He eventually becomes bedridden and dies of respiratory failure between the ages of 20 and 30 years.

Facioscapulohumeral Muscular Dystrophy.   This type is inherited as an autosomal dominant trait and, as its name implies, affects the muscles of the shoulder girdle and face. The onset is in adolescence, and the disease progresses slowly, so that life expectancy is normal.

Limb-Girdle Dystrophy.   This type of dystrophy is inherited as an autosomal recessive trait and begins in childhood or adolescence. Both pelvic and shoulder girdle muscles are involved, and ultimately all four limbs are affected. Progression of the disease is variable, and the condition may not be a separate entity but rather a group of disorders that do not fit readily into the other two types of muscle dystrophy described above.

Myotonic Muscular Dystrophy.   This type of muscular dystrophy differs in many respects from the other three described. A characteristic feature is *myotonia*, a term that describes the difficulty the patient has in relaxing his grip. Limb weakness is initially most marked distally, so that there is weakness of the hands. Facial muscles show weakness often evident as drooping of the eyelids *(ptosis)*. The disease has several other characteristic features. *Cataracts* (Chapter 42) develop sooner or later in all patients, and males suffer from *testicular atrophy* and *premature baldness*. The disease is inherited as an autosomal dominant trait.

Enzymes in the Diagnosis of Muscular Dystrophy.   Several enzymes are characteristic of muscle, and their blood level is increased when muscle fibers are degenerating. The highest levels are seen in the Duchenne type of muscular dystrophy. The most characteristic enzyme is creatine phosphokinase (CPK), but this is so sensitive a test that it may give false positive results. Other enzymes that are elevated are SGOT and LDH (Chapter 4).

Myasthenia gravis is a disease characterized by muscular weakness and pronounced muscle fatigability that is associated with the presence of a circulating antibody to acetylcholine receptors.

The disease generally starts at about the age of 20 years and affects females more frequently than males. The weakness characteristically affects the ocular and cranial muscles, leading to ptosis, double vision *(diplopia)*, and difficulty in chewing and in swallowing. The limb muscles can also be affected. The disease fluctuates in intensity, and its course is unpredictable. During crises the respiratory muscles may be affected, and the patient can die of respiratory failure. The ready fatigability of the muscles can be temporarily overcome by the administration of anticholinesterase drugs.

Pathogenesis. Skeletal muscular contraction is initiated by acetylcholine, which is released from motor nerve terminals and acts on acetylcholine receptors of the muscle motor end plates. In myasthenia gravis the number of receptors is reduced, apparently owing to the presence of an autoantibody to receptor protein. The precise relationship of the antibody to the disease is not clear, for cell-mediated immunity has also been suggested in the pathogenesis of the disease. Virtually all patients have circulating antibodies to acetylcholine receptor protein, and in about three quarters of patients there is enlargement of the thymus. Usually there is simple hyperplasia, but in older patients there may be a neoplasm *(thymoma)*. Removal of the thymus generally improves the myasthenia, and this is the common form of treatment, particularly if the gland can be demonstrated to be enlarged and if the myasthenia does not respond adequately to the administration of anticholinesterase drugs, glucocorticoids, or other immunosuppressive drugs.

Myasthenia Gravis

The myositis of dermatomyositis (Chapter 27), trichinosis (Chapter 14), and gas gangrene (Chapter 10) has been described elsewhere. Other types are uncommon.

Myositis

Primary Tumors. Most examples of benign *rhabdomyomas* occur in the heart and are probably malformations rather than neoplasms. *Rhabdomyosarcomas* are highly malignant tumors of striated muscle and fortunately are rare. They may occur at any age, and various types are described. One type is seen in children and young adults and can involve the orbit of the eye or the genitourinary tract, particularly the *vagina*.

Metastatic Tumors. In spite of the bulk of muscle present in the body, metastatic tumors are rare.

Neoplasms of Muscle

1. Describe the circumstances under which woven bone is formed.

2. Explain how a knowledge of the embryological development of bone helps to account for how a fracture can unite.

3. A patient with a persistent urinary tract infection is found to have a serum calcium of 17 mg/dl and a blood urea nitrogen (BUN) of 80 mg/dl. How may these observations be related?

4. Compare metastatic calcification with dystrophic calcification, giving examples of each type.

5. Predict the effect of a prolonged excessive intake of vitamin D.

6. Give an account of avascular necrosis of the head of the femur with respect to its causes and effects.

7. Compare generalized osteoporosis with osteomalacia.

8. Describe osteosarcoma in terms of the following factors:
   (a) known predisposing causes

Review Questions

(b) age incidence
(c) radiographic features
(d) clinical presentation
(e) prognosis

9. Explain why renal failure is common in patients with multiple myelomatosis.

10. Patients with rheumatoid arthritis sometimes have the following condition:
    (a) osteoporosis of the spine
    (b) renal failure
    (c) aortic valve insufficiency
Explain the pathogenesis of these extra-articular lesions.

11. Comment briefly on each of the following:
    (a) serum alkaline phosphatase
    (b) serum calcium
    (c) the rheumatoid factor
    (d) Bence Jones protein
    (e) brown tumors of bone

12. Compare myasthenia gravis with the muscular dystrophies with respect to their etiology, clinical features, and pathological findings.

Selected Readings

Ham, A. W.: Histology. 8th ed. Philadelphia, J. B. Lippincott Company, 1979. Note, in particular, the chapter on "Bone," for an account of the structure of bone, its growth, and the healing of a fracture.

Lichtenstein, L.: Diseases of Bone and Joints. St. Louis, The C. V. Mosby Company, 1970, 228 pp.

Lichtenstein, L.: Bone Tumors. 4th ed. St. Louis, The C. V. Mosby Company, 1972, 441 pp.

Robbins, S. L., and Cotran, R. S.: Pathologic Basis of Disease. 2nd ed. Philadelphia, W. B. Saunders Company, 1979, Chapter 30.

Walter, J. B., and Israel, M. S.: General Pathology. 5th ed. Edinburgh, Churchill Livingstone, 1979. Note especially pp. 116–119 for an account of fracture healing.

Diseases of the Skin

After studying this chapter the student should be able to:

- Define the following words: erythematous, macule, patch, papule, plaque, vesicle, bulla, pustule, squamous, telangiectasia, excoriation, and pruritic.
- Differentiate among acute, subacute, and chronic dermatitis.
- List the clinical types of dermatitis and describe the outstanding features of each type.
- Describe the main features of psoriasis, pityriasis rosea, urticaria, toxic erythema, and erythema multiforme.
- Describe the types of skin reaction that drugs can cause.
- Classify the vesiculobullous diseases and describe the main features of each type.
- Describe the pathogenesis and lesions of acne vulgaris.
- Compare acne vulgaris with rosacea.
- Describe the common melanotic and vascular hamartomas of skin.
- Classify the types of squamous-cell papilloma of skin.
- Describe the lesions that can precede the development of squamous-cell carcinoma of skin.
- Give an account of squamous-cell carcinoma of the skin and compare it with keratoacanthoma.
- Classify the types of malignant melanoma and relate the types to the prognosis.

Introduction

It has been estimated that between 15 and 20 per cent of patients who consult their doctor do so because of some skin disorder. Nevertheless, the teaching of dermatology is usually sadly neglected in medical education. Perhaps this is due to the complexity of the subject, because the number of diseases of the skin that have been described in literature far exceeds that of any other individual organ. There are several reasons for this. First, the skin is exposed to many insults from the external environment. Second, it is a complex composite organ, because in addition to having a surface epithelium called the *epidermis*, it has associated *hair follicles* with their *sebaceous glands, eccrine* and *apocrine sweat glands,* and a specialized connective tissue called the *dermis,* itself composed of dense collagenous bundles and elastic fibers. Third, the skin can be examined and biopsied easily. Fourth, throughout the ages, people have considered the appearance of skin to be very important; this fact has added to the complexity of dermatology. This chapter describes some of the common skin diseases and also a few that, although uncommon, are so serious that they must be recognized early if adequate treatment is to be given.

Terminology

There are few areas in medicine that can compete with dermatology for hiding truth with complex names. Nevertheless, with some basic facts and a minimal knowledge of Latin, it is possible to master this terminology.

An area of skin that is altered, usually red (*erythematous*), flat, and not palpable (*i.e.,* cannot be felt) is called a *macule* if it is less than 1.0 cm. in diameter; if it is larger, it is called a *patch*. Similar areas that are palpable are called *papules* if they are small (less than 1.0 cm in diameter) and *plaques* if they are over that size. A blister is called a *vesicle* if small and a *bulla* if large. *Pustules* contain pus. In due course the inflammatory fluid in a vesicle, bulla, or pustule dries to form a *crust*. If flakes of keratin are seen obviously adherent to a lesion, this lesion is called *squamous*. Since most such lesions can be felt, they are called *papulosquamous*. The presence of visible abnormally dilated vessels is called *telangiectasia*. Shallow ulcers or erosions are termed *excoriations* if they are produced by scratching. The observation and description of each individual skin lesion is important, because certain types are characteristic of certain diseases. For example, psoriasis is characteristically papulosquamous and is occasionally pustular, but is never vesicular.

The distribution of the lesions seen in any skin disease is important. A localized rash often indicates a localized cause. Thus, a dermatitis on only one wrist is probably due to sensitivity to a wrist band or a watch strap. Some diseases, *e.g.*, smallpox, characteristically affect the distal parts, such as the hands, feet, and face, whereas others, *e.g.*, chickenpox, tend to affect the trunk rather than the extremities. In a consideration of any skin disease, it is important therefore to include the distribution of the rash and the individual characteristics of its lesions.

The presence of itching is characteristic of certain skin diseases, such as scabies, neurodermatitis, and atopic dermatitis. The term *pruritus*, which is commonly used, is synonymous with itching. Note that the presence or absence of itching is as dependent upon the make-up of the individual as it is on the nature of his lesions. Some people itch easily, and others do not.

Dermatitis and Eczema

Dermatitis and *eczema* are synonymous terms used to describe a particular skin reaction pattern that primarily involves the epidermis. Based on their clinical appearances and the histological pattern of reaction, three types are recognized: acute, subacute, and chronic.

Morphological Types of Dermatitis

Acute Dermatitis. Clinically, acute dermatitis is characterized by erythema, swelling, and the formation of blisters, which can vary from small vesicles to large bullae (Figs. 41–1 and 41–3). If the vesicles rupture, the surface becomes wet or "weeping," and as the exudate dries the lesion become crusted. Histologically, the epidermis shows intercellular edema (*spongiosis*) that terminates in the separation of epidermal cells and in the formation of vesicles or bullae (Fig. 41–1). The dermis shows an acute inflammatory reaction with edema and, surprisingly enough, a perivascular lymphocytic infiltrate. The absence of polymorphs is noteworthy but is not understood.

Chronic Dermatitis. Clinically, chronic dermatitis appears as scaly papules or plaques, and the skin markings tend to be accentuated (Fig. 41–4). This latter feature is known as *lichenification*. Histologically, the epidermis is thickened; this is termed *acanthosis* and is associated with an increased mitotic activity of the epidermal cells. Keratinization is disturbed, for not only is the keratin layer increased in thickness (*hyperkeratosis*) but in places the nuclei are retained. This condition is called *parakeratosis* (Fig. 41–2). Foci of spongiosis may be present, but vesicle formation is absent.

Subacute Dermatitis. The clinical picture of subacute dermatitis has features midway between acute and chronic dermatitis. The lesions are papulosquamous, but small vesicles can be detected. Histologically, there is acanthosis and hyperkeratosis, but this is less marked than in chronic

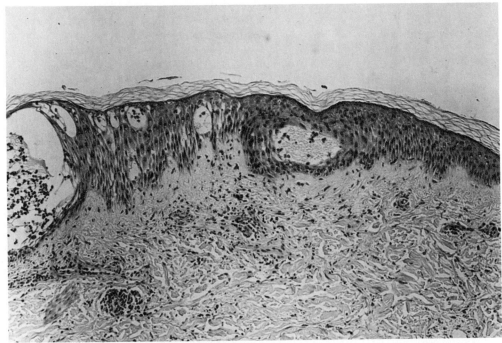

Figure 41–1. Acute dermatitis. The epidermis shows some thickening (*acanthosis*) that is due mainly to the separation of the cells by edema (*spongiosis*). In several places the cells have torn apart to produce intraepidermal vesicles. The largest of these spongiotic vesicles is on the left-hand side and contains coagulated exudate. There is a sparse infiltration of the dermis by lymphocytes. The biopsy was taken from a patient with acute allergic contact dermatitis due to exposure to poison ivy (× 240).

dermatitis. Parakeratosis and spongiosis, on the other hand, are more marked, and in places small vesicles are evident.

It should be noted that there is no sharp distinction among the three grades of dermatitis. Vesiculation is marked in acute dermatitis, inconspicuous in subacute dermatitis, and absent in chronic dermatitis. Acanthosis and hyperkeratosis are marked in chronic dermatitis, less obvious in the subacute stage, and absent in acute dermatitis.

Clinical Types of Dermatitis.   The clinical types of dermatitis are many and various. They cannot be distinguished from each other histologically but differ in their causes and clinical presentation.

Primary Irritant Dermatitis.   Externally applied chemical irritants are a frequent cause of dermatitis *(contact dermatitis):* a common example is the chronic lichenified hand eczema seen in housewives whose hands are brought repeatedly into contact with water, detergents, and other household agents. Likewise, medical and dental personnel who are involved in direct patient care and are obliged to wash their hands frequently between procedures are liable to suffer from chronic hand eczema. Alkalis, acids, and many industrial chemicals can act as primary irritants, and if applied over a long period they lead to a refractory chronic dermatitis. Laboratory technologists are particularly at risk through the use of chemicals and stains — particularly those lipid solvents, such as xylol, that remove the protective lipid covering of the skin. *Elderly individuals* with dry skin may develop a dermatitis that is due to exposure to agents such as water, soap, and detergents that would be harmless in a younger person. These agents may also affect *atopic individuals* whose skin tends to be dry, especially during the winter months in those who live in inadequately humidified houses.

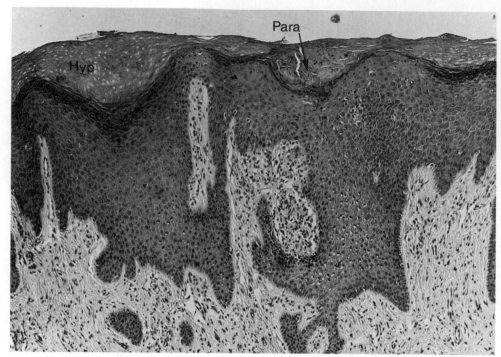

Figure 41–2. Chronic dermatitis. There is marked acanthosis and hyperkeratosis (Hyp) together with one focus of parakeratosis (Para). These changes should be compared with the normal skin present on the right-hand side of the specimen in Figure 41–1 (× 240).

Allergic Contact Dermatitis.   The development of cell-mediated sensitizing antibodies toward chemicals results in the production of *allergic contact dermatitis.* Iodine, formaldehyde, dyes, plants (*e.g.,* poison ivy), and nickel (used in costume jewelry) are among the many agents that can cause this type of allergic dermatitis (Fig. 41–3). It is noteworthy that certain parts of the skin are more sensitive to contactants than others. Thus, allergic contact dermatitis is more common on the backs of the hands than it is on the palms. Likewise, the face is particularly sensitive and may react to agents that elsewhere cause little trouble. Dermatitis around the eyes can be due to nail polish, which causes little trouble when applied to the hands or feet.

Photodermatitis.   Ultraviolet light can act on chemicals (either applied topically or taken systemically) present in the skin and so alter them that direct irritant effects *(phototoxic dermatitis)* or new antigen formation and subsequent sensitization *(photoallergic dermatitis)* result. Agents that are well known to cause this sensitizing effect when applied topically are perfumes, coal-tar derivatives, and halogenated salicylanilides (used in deodorant soap).

Many drugs taken internally can have a similar effect. Common examples are chemotherapeutic agents such as sulfonamides and tetracyclines, diuretics (*e.g.,* chlorothiazide), and tranquilizers (*e.g.,* chlorpromazine), to name a few.

Atopic Dermatitis.   Atopic dermatitis occurs in atopic (allergic) individuals, but the pathogenesis is obscure, for although the associated respiratory diseases such as hay fever and bronchial asthma appear to be caused by IgE sensitization, the skin lesions are more complex and the damage is probably cell-mediated.

The distribution of the rash varies with the age of the patient. In the *infantile phase* (3 to 18 months) the *face* and other exposed parts of the skin are commonly affected. Atopic dermatitis at this age is often called *infantile eczema*. In the *childhood phase* (over 18 months) the *elbow and knee flexures* are characteristically involved. In the *adult phase* the flexures are again involved, but the rash can be widespread and involve other areas — hands, upper limbs, and trunk. Atopic dermatitis is *intensely itchy*, so that lichenification, excoriations, and areas of crusting are common. Atopic disease has been stressed because it is extremely common, although just how common is difficult to state because estimates range from 2 to 25 per cent of the population. Probably about 5 per cent are afflicted with atopic dermatitis, and although for some it is a mere annoyance in the winter months, for others it is a lifelong illness of itching and scratching that demands constant medication and causes anguish to both patient and therapist alike. Fortunately, the disease tends to remit as age advances.

Nummular Eczema.   This condition tends to occur in atopic individuals and is characterized by the formation of localized, coin-shaped plaques of subacute or chronic dermatitis. Itching is usually marked.

Stasis Dermatitis.   Stasis dermatitis is common on the legs and is related to chronic venous stasis. It occurs following venous thrombosis in the lower limbs and in patients with varicose veins. In addition to the usual features of a dermatitis, stasis dermatitis is characterized by a brown discoloration of the skin. This is produced by hemosiderin secondary to petechial hemorrhages. The poor blood supply to the skin causes atrophy with loss of hair follicles and thinning of the epidermis. Chronic ulcers are a common complication and are usually initiated by trauma, caused either accidentally or by scratching. Such *stasis ulcers* (see Fig. 7–3) are often situated over the medial malleolus and

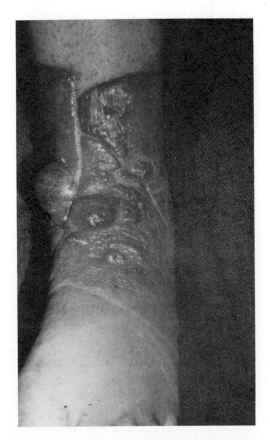

Figure 41–3. Acute dermatitis. This patient sustained a sprain of the left ankle, and adhesive tape was applied for support. Thirty-six hours later an acute vesicular dermatitis appeared and subsequently became bullous. Note how the rash is limited to the region previously covered by tape (lines of dermarcation are obvious). Areas where the skin was folded are spared.

heal slowly because of the poor blood supply to the skin. After many years of repeated ulcerations, low-grade bacterial cellulitis, and chronic edema (the result of both venous and lymphatic obstruction), there is overgrowth of the dermal connective tissues, so that the leg becomes chronically swollen and woody hard to the touch. Occasionally the tissue overgrowth, accompanied by papillomatous epidermal overgrowth, is so marked that the term *elephantiasis* is applied.

Seborrheic Dermatitis. A type of chronic dermatitis is frequently seen in the scalp and results in the formation of greasy scales or dandruff. This condition is termed *seborrheic dermatitis;* although it is extremely common, its precise nature is not understood. The dermatitis can extend beyond the scalp and affect the face. Occasionally there is involvement of the trunk, particularly the front of the chest, and the flexural regions such as the axilla or under the breasts. This type of dermatitis can be encountered in all age groups, ranging from infants (cradle cap) to old people.

Neurodermatitis. A feature of some forms of dermatitis, including the atopic variety, is marked itching. This leads to scratching and self-perpetuation because of the continued physical trauma. The condition is often referred to as *chronic neurodermatitis* (Fig. 41–4). Localized plaques of neurodermatitis, which frequently occur on the back of the neck and the front of the ankles, are called *lichen simplex chronicus.*

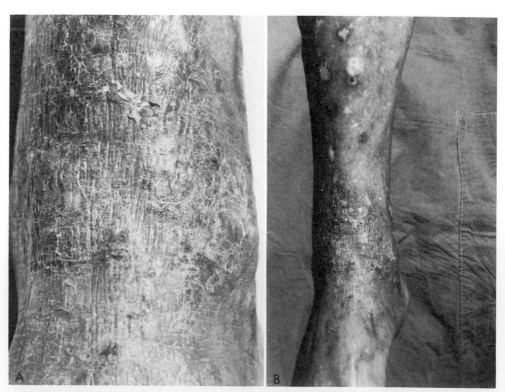

Figure 41–4. Neurodermatitis. This patient had a chronic lichenified dermatitis on the front of both ankles. *A* shows a close-up of the hyperkeratosis and accentuation of the crease lines that are typical; they are fancifully likened to lichen on a tree trunk. Constant scratching and rubbing, often with the opposite heel, perpetuated the condition. The nodules shown higher on the leg in *B* are also self-induced. They consist of dense scar tissue with overlying acanthosis and depigmentation. The lesions are called *prurigo nodularis* (from the Latin word *prurigo,* meaning "to itch") and are produced by the patient continually picking at them.

A group of diseases, of widely differing origins, is characterized by papulosquamous lesions. Common examples are chronic dermatitis, psoriasis, pityriasis rosea, secondary syphilis, and ringworm.

Psoriasis. This is a chronic disease that fluctuates in intensity both spontaneously and under the influence of treatment. It occurs as sharply demarcated erythematous plaques with a dry, silvery scale. Common sites are the elbows, knees, and other extensor surfaces. The palms, soles, and scalp are also frequently affected (Figs. 41–5 and 41–6). Psoriasis is not usually itchy, and vesicles are never formed. This distinguishes it both clinically and histologically from dermatitis. Psoriasis tends to be common in certain families, but the precise mode of inheritance is unknown.

Pityriasis Rosea. Pityriasis rosea is a common, self-limiting eruption of young adults. The first lesion to appear is an oval, sharply defined, erythematous, scaly plaque 2 to 5 cm in diameter (the *herald patch*). It may easily be misdiagnosed clinically as ringworm. About one week later a widespread eruption of pink macules or scaly papules develops; on the trunk the lesions tend to follow the lines of the ribs to give a "Christmas tree" pattern on the patient's back. The rash of pityriasis rosea can easily be confused with that of secondary syphilis, and it is a wise precaution to perform a VDRL in all cases.

Pityriasis rosea clears spontaneously in six to eight weeks and does not recur. Its cause is unknown, but the pattern of the disease suggests that it is a viral infection. To date, no virus has been isolated.

An inflammatory reaction in the dermis is present in many skin diseases, including those that affect primarily the epidermis (*e.g.*, dermatitis, psoriasis, and pityriasis rosea). A localized area of dermal inflammation is a feature of many infections (*e.g.*, tuberculosis and erysipelas), but there is a group of conditions in which the primary event is a widespread vascular inflammatory reaction within the dermis. The most mild example of this group is urticaria.

Urticaria. *Urticaria*, or *hives*, is a common disease that affects many individuals at some time or another in their life. Symptoms include an acute inflammatory reaction in the dermis that is characterized by vasodilatation, scanty polymorph accumulation, and marked edema. Clinically urticaria commences with marked itching, which is followed by the appearance of erythema and swelling. The lesions tend to develop a pale center, or *wheal*, surrounded by an erythematous edge. They thereby resemble the common mosquito bite and the triple response (Chapter 5).

Acute urticaria is sometimes a type I hypersensitivity reaction mediated by IgE, but it is also seen in immune-complex reactions. It may follow the ingestion of a particular food or drug, and as in other hypersensitivity reactions, small quantities of the agent are sufficient to induce an attack. Thus, the menthol in a cigarette or toothpaste can precipitate acute urticaria in a sensitized person.

Each urticarial lesion lasts only a few hours, but repeated attacks of urticaria may occur over a period of many months or even years (*chronic urticaria*). In patients having such attacks the cause is rarely found.

Urticaria affects the dermis. When the subcutaneous tissues are involved, the condition is termed angioedema. In both urticaria and angioedema, the mucous membranes (including that of the tongue) can be involved. In one type of hereditary angioedema there is a deficiency of C_1 esterase inhibitor. This is a serious condition, because lesions occur not only in the intestine, causing colic, but also in the larynx, in some cases leading to death from

Papulosquamous Eruptions

Diseases Characterized by a Dermal Inflammatory Reaction

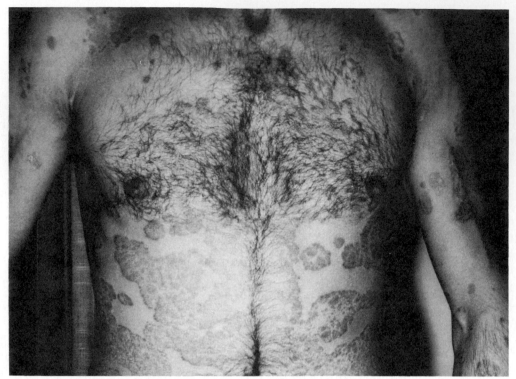

Figure 41–5.   Psoriasis. The patient has widespread psoriatic lesions. They consist of well-demarcated scaly erythematous papules that have in places joined together to form plaques.

asphyxiation (the lesions obstruct the passage). In some families many members ultimately die in this way.

Toxic Erythema.   This general term is applied to many conditions in which the epidermis is normal, at least in the early stages, but in which there is a dermal inflammatory reaction showing vasodilatation and a perivascular accumulation of cells, particularly lymphocytes. Viral exanthems (*e.g.*, measles) fall into this group. Toxic erythema is one manifestation of an adverse drug reaction.

Drug Eruptions   Drug eruptions are so common and produce such a wide variety of lesions that they must be considered in the differential diagnosis of any skin eruption. Any patient with a skin eruption must be asked what drugs are being taken — specific enquiry being directed to medications such as laxatives, headache pills, vitamin preparations, and others that are not always regarded as "drugs" by the patient. Likewise, the patient should be asked what local medications have been applied, for the original lesion may well have been overshadowed by a contact dermatitis. Some "over the counter" preparations, *e.g.*, medications for sunburn, contain potent sensitizers.

The common type of drug eruption is erythematous, papular, of widespread distribution, and very itchy (Fig. 41–7). Severe cases become vesicular and constitute one variety of erythema multiforme. Petechial lesions are not uncommon, and severe cases exhibit a definite vasculitis and lead to the formation of hemorrhagic and necrotic lesions. Sometimes the lesions closely resemble well-recognized dermatoses, such as measles and lupus erythematosus. The pathogenesis of drug eruptions varies. Those of an urticarial nature appear to be the result of a type I hypersensitivity reaction. Others are mediated by immune complexes. In most, the pathogenesis is obscure.

Figure 41–6.   Psoriasis. The characteristic psoriatic plaque is sharply delineated, red, and covered by a silvery scale. The lesions, particularly when on the soles of the feet, can easily be misdiagnosed as ringworm.

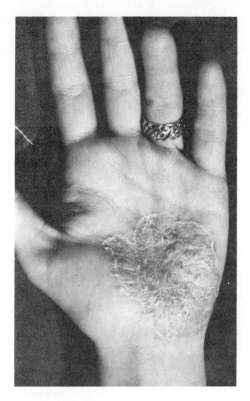

The formation of vesicles or bullae is an outstanding feature of this group of diseases. For accurate diagnosis, a biopsy of an early lesion is often necessary, because the region of origin of the vesicle is of vital importance in differential diagnosis. Some vesicles are formed within the epidermis, whereas others are formed beneath the epidermis.

Vesiculobullous Diseases

Figure 41–7.   Drug eruption. This patient developed a widespread, itchy, erythematous, maculopapular eruption as a result of taking Dilantin for her epilepsy. In places, for instance on the right arm, the lesions have become confluent.

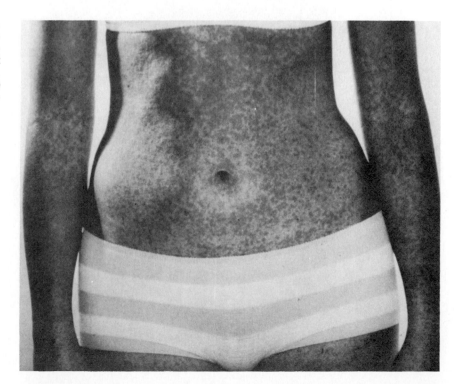

Intraepidermal Vesicles. The superficial subcorneal vesicles and pustules of impetigo and candidiasis can generally be diagnosed so easily clinically that a biopsy is not necessary. Likewise, the spongiotic vesicles of acute and subacute dermatitis rarely need pathological confirmation. There are, however, two groups of intraepidermal vesiculating diseases in which biopsy is often useful. These are pemphigus and the vesiculating viral diseases.

The Pemphigus Group of Diseases. *Pemphigus vulgaris* is a chronic blistering disease that tends to occur in middle and old age, particularly in Jews of Eastern European ancestry. Blisters frequently involve the mouth and lead to soreness, inability to eat, and great incapacity. The blisters tend to break easily, leaving eroded painful surfaces. Pathologically, the vesicles are formed by separation of the epidermal cells above the basal layer (Fig. 41–8). The cells appear to lose their cohesiveness and to become detached. This process is termed *acantholysis,* and the free or acantholytic cells are found lying in the fluid of the vesicle. The vesicles are generally flaccid, and on pressure can be made to extend laterally. Once the disease commences, it tends to progress and to be fatal after a variable course lasting, on the average, about 18 months. This poor prognosis was the rule before the advent of modern therapy. Nevertheless, even with systemic prednisone and other immunosuppressant drugs, pemphigus is still serious, because although the disease itself may not be fatal, the complications of the treatment sometimes are.

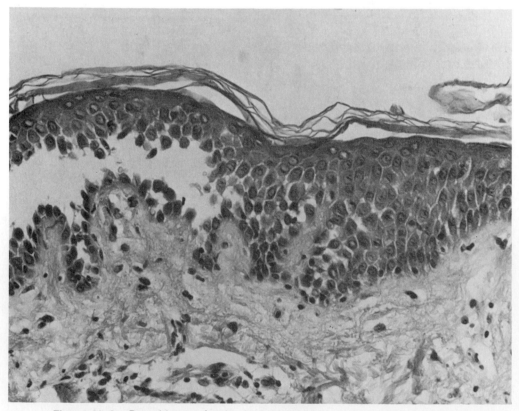

Figure 41–8. Pemphigus vulgaris. Acantholysis has produced the characteristic suprabasal blister. Note how the papillary dermis is covered by a row of basal cells, which have been likened to a row of tombstones and are still adherent to the basement membrane. Compare this acantholytic vesicle with the spongiotic vesicles of acute dermatitis ($\times$ 500).

A number of other acantholytic blistering diseases are known; some are variants of pemphigus, but others are rare and will not be considered.

The Vesicular Viral Diseases. The vesicles formed in zoster, chickenpox, and herpes simplex closely resemble each other histopathologically. The invaded epidermal cells show intranuclear inclusion bodies and swelling of the cytoplasm *(ballooning)* followed by degeneration. Some epithelial cells fuse together to form multinucleate giant cells, and as intercellular edema develops the cells show *acantholysis*. The intraepidermal vesicle so formed contains degenerate and multinucleate acantholytic cells. Smallpox and vaccinia differ from the lesions described above only by the presence of *intracytoplasmic inclusion bodies*. Distinction between the various types of virus vesicles is difficult histologically, but the clinical features combined with electron microscopy of vesicle fluid and other virological investigations can distinguish one disease from the other.

A biopsy of the lesions of a typical case of chickenpox, herpes simplex, or zoster is not generally warranted. Sometimes, however, atypical cases are encountered, and if a virological service is not available, a biopsy is useful in distinguishing such cases from other localized vesiculating diseases, such as a patch of acute contact dermatitis or a bullous drug reaction.

Subepidermal Vesicles. Subepidermal vesicles are formed in severe erythema multiforme, in certain drug eruptions, and in bullous pemphigoid.

Erythema Multiforme. This is an acute disease of unknown etiology, although in about 50 per cent of cases it may follow some precipitating factor, *e.g.,* sun exposure, herpes simplex infection (cold sore), vaccination, x-ray therapy, drug intake, pregnancy, or the presence of some malignancy of an internal organ. The onset is usually sudden, and the patient rapidly develops symmetrical lesions of varying types — urticarial, erythematous macular, papular, vesicular, or in the severe form of the disease, bullous (Fig. 41–9). The characteristic lesion is an erythematous papule with a central hemorrhagic area, so that the lesion tends to resemble a *target* or an *iris*. The dermal inflammatory reaction is sometimes so marked that fluid accumulates beneath the epidermis, and a *subepidermal vesicle* forms. The dermal reaction causes secondary degeneration of the epidermis. The severity of the dermal inflam-

Figure 41–9. Erythema multiforme. The lesions have a bright red border and a pale center produced by the subepidermal edema. In places, the papules have joined together; the lesions have an arcuate outline.

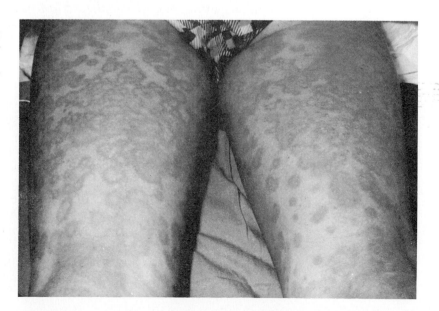

matory reaction and the degenerate appearance of the epidermal roof serve to distinguish the lesions from those of bullous pemphigoid, which is described later. The lesions of erythema multiforme may occur on any part of the body, but they tend to be most common on the extremities. Severe erythema multiforme is associated with marked constitutional upset and high fever. Bullous lesions occur not only on the skin but also on the mucous membranes, where the bullae soon rupture to form painful ulcers. This type of the disease with mucosal involvement is called the *Stevens-Johnson syndrome*. Ulcerations in the mouth and hemorrhagic crusting of the lips are characteristic. Oral feeding becomes impossible. Involvement of the conjunctiva can lead to blindness. Genital lesions can also occur in this severe form of erythema multiforme. There is no specific treatment for erythema multiforme, and recovery is the rule. However, in severe cases of the Stevens-Johnson syndrome, death can occur, generally from pneumonia.

Erythema multiforme tends to recur, particularly if the precipitating cause is itself recurrent, *e.g.*, recurrent herpes simplex.

Bullous Pemphigoid. Bullous pemphigoid is a chronic blistering disease that resembles pemphigus vulgaris clinically but has a much better prognosis. Unlike the lesions of pemphigus, the vesicles and bullae of this condition are usually tense rather than flaccid. Mucous membrane involvement is less common and less severe.

Microscopically, the vesicles are found to be subepidermal. A useful diagnostic test is the demonstration of autoantibodies to skin basement membrane, both free in the serum and fixed in the skin (see Fig. 9–15). Patients with pemphigus vulgaris also produce an autoantibody, but its specificity is directed against epidermal intercellular substance. Hence, the two diseases are quite distinct from each other both histologically and immunologically.

Acne Vulgaris   This familiar disorder of teenagers affects those areas in which sebaceous glands are plentiful — face, back, and upper chest. The primary lesions are due to the plugging of pilosebaceous follicles with adherent keratin. Oxidation of the surface of the plugs produces a dark-colored substance and results in the familiar *"blackhead,"* or *comedo.* The affected follicles dilate and become filled with the lipid secretions of sebaceous glands. In these the anaerobic saprophyte *Corynebacterium acnes* proliferates and splits the lipids to produce irritating fatty acids. When the follicle ruptures, there is an inflammatory reaction, causing papules and pustules to be formed. Tetracycline therapy, which is now so much in vogue, is designed to inhibit the growth of *C. acnes.*

Rosacea (Acne Rosacea)   This is a common disorder that affects the central area of the face and has some features in common with acne vulgaris. Three types of lesion occur:

1. *Papules, pustules,* and *cystic nodules* resembling those of the common type of acne. The pathogenesis is presumably similar in both conditions, for both respond to tetracycline therapy. Rosacea, however, occurs in an older age group, generally in persons over the age of 30 years.

2. *Periodic flushing* and finally permanent *telangiectasia.* Ingestion of alcoholic beverages and spicy foods accentuates this component of the disease.

3. *Sebaceous gland hyperplasia,* particularly of the nose, where it produces the "W. C. Fields nose" or *rhinophyma.* Plastic surgery offers the best hope to these patients.

The hamartomas of the skin are termed *nevi*. The common examples are the melanotic and angiomatous varieties.

Melanotic hamartomas are also called *nevocellular nevi* or more commonly *moles*. Almost every person has at least a dozen or more of them. The parent cell is the melanocyte, which develops from the neural crest, and migrates to the epidermis with the peripheral nerves. The melanocytes here become incorporated into the basal layer of the epidermis and appear as cells with clear cytoplasm (Fig. 41–10). A focal abnormal proliferation of these cells leads to a mass that soon invades the dermis. The proliferating cells lose their ability to produce melanin and are then termed "nevus cells." Early in the formation of a nevus, melanin-producing cells are formed at the dermoepidermal junction, and the lesion is called a *junctional nevus*. This is deeply pigmented and barely palpable. As the nevus develops, a dermal portion is formed, and ultimately a nonpigmented intradermal nevus results (Fig. 41–11). Nevi are seldom present at birth, but they develop during childhood.

Once the nevus cells have entered the dermis, they rarely show any further proliferation. The junctional element, however, can exhibit spurts of proliferation (junctional activity), and although this proliferation is of little

Figure 41–10. Melanotic nevi of skin. Sketches showing the development of melanotic nevi: The only cells drawn are melanocytes and nevus cells. *A,* Junctional nevus. Focal proliferation of melanocytes in the basal layer of the epidermis produces nests of cells that become nevus cells. *B,* Compound nevus. Some nevus cells have invaded the dermis. *C,* Intradermal nevus. The junctional activity has ceased and all the nevus cells are in the dermis. The epidermis is normal and contains scattered melanocytes that appear as clear cells in the basal layer of the epidermis. (Drawing by Margot Mackay, Department of Art as Applied to Medicine, University of Toronto.)

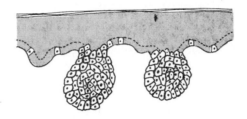

(A) Junctional Nevus

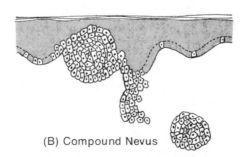

(B) Compound Nevus

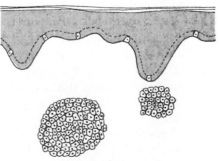

(C) Intradermal Nevus

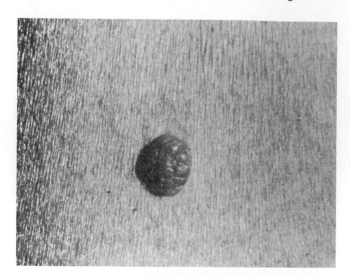

Figure 41–11. Compound nevocellular nevus. This brown lesion had been present on a 56-year-old woman's back for many years. She had detected a slight increase in size over the preceding year, and she had it excised for cosmetic reasons. The nevus has a lobulated, smooth surface, is not ulcerated, and shows no evidence of malignancy.

significance during the years of development in childhood, in adult life any marked growth is regarded with suspicion, because it may be the first indication of malignant change.

Nevocellular nevi, unlike many other hamartomas, do occasionally become malignant. *Any change, such as an increase in size, bleeding, ulceration, or change in degree of pigmentation, should suggest the possibility of malignancy.* Excision or biopsy is then indicated.

Vascular Hamartomas of Skin

Various types of vascular anomalies are encountered in the skin. Sometimes at birth or shortly afterwards a red, vascular, spongy nodule develops in the skin: this grows rapidly for a while, but regresses after a few years and leaves an area of scarring. This type of nevus is composed of capillary-sized blood spaces and is often called a *capillary hemangioma* or strawberry nevus. Another type of nevus is composed of a few dilated capillary channels. Such a lesion appears as a flat, erythematous patch that is colloquially called a *port-wine stain.* Vascular nevi are of little importance apart from their cosmetic appearance. Sometimes they are multiple, and on occasion they are associated with similar lesions in deeper organs. When vascular nevi involve the face, for instance, angiomatous lesions of the central nervous system or eye are sometimes found, and a number of characteristic syndromes can be recognized. Small hemangiomas commonly develop in elderly people and appear as bright red papules, 2 to 4 mm in diameter, on the trunk (*"cherry angiomas"*).

Benign Tumors of the Skin

Squamous-Cell Papilloma

This is used as a descriptive term that indicates a number of separate entities. The common types are described below:

Epithelial Nevus. This type of papilloma is generally present at birth and appears as a warty lesion, sometimes of linear distribution. It tends to recur after simple curettage and can then be mistaken for a malignant tumor.

Seborrheic Keratosis. Papillomas, frequently with considerable melanin pigmentation and overlying hyperkeratosis, are extremely common on the backs of the hands, on the trunk, and on the face of elderly people. The lesions seem to be stuck onto the surface of the skin and appear as flat or roughened pigmented warty nodules or plaques (Fig. 41–12). Such lesions are easily eliminated by curettage. The lesions never become malignant, but when heavily pigmented they are liable to be confused with other pigmented lesions of the skin, such as melanotic nevus, pigmented basal-cell carcinoma, or malignant melanoma.

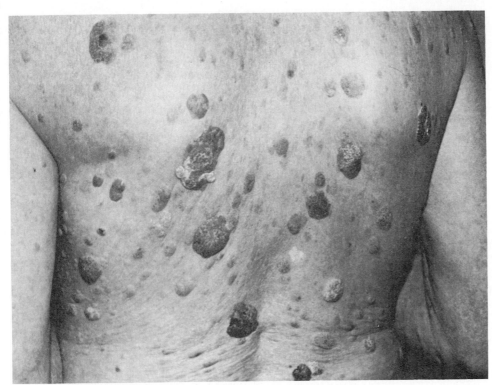

Figure 41–12. Seborrheic keratoses. The back of this elderly man is covered by numerous seborrheic keratoses, some of which are deeply pigmented with melanin. The large lesions show the characteristic stuck-on appearance, and it can be readily appreciated that these benign tumors can be easily removed by curettage. This process involves scraping the skin so as to remove the epithelial element of the tumor and leave relatively little damage to the dermis. Hence, scarring is minimal. Seborrheic keratoses should not be excised with a scalpel, since this leads to unnecessary scarring.

Verruca Vulgaris.   The *common wart* is a type of papilloma that is due to an infection by one of the papovaviruses (Fig. 17–2). Indeed, there are at least five strains of the virus, and each tends to infect different areas. Unfortunately, the virus has never been grown in tissue culture, and this has greatly hindered research. The development of a successful vaccine would be of inestimable value, for although warts are rarely serious, they are unpleasant to look at and their treatment is tedious and sometimes painful — particularly to children, who are their most frequent victims. On the soles of the feet the epidermal overgrowth and hyperkeratosis produce a painful lesion known as a *plantar wart*. Sometimes the virus produces multiple small, flat lesions called *plane warts*. In moist areas, such as on the penis and in the female genital region, pedunculated cauliflowerlike lesions are produced and are known as *condylomata acuminata*.

The most common malignant tumor of the skin in Whites is the basal-cell carcinoma. This is illustrated in Figure 41–13 and is described fully in Chapter 17. As with squamous-cell carcinoma, the major predisposing cause is prolonged exposure to ultraviolet light.

Malignant Tumors of the Skin

This tumor commonly arises on the sun-exposed skin in a pre-existing actinic keratosis (Fig. 41–14). Actinic keratoses are areas of epidermal dysplasia caused by prolonged exposure to ultraviolet light. They appear as scaly, erythematous areas on the face, ears, backs of hands, or forearms. In contradistinction to seborrheic keratoses, they must be regarded as precancerous. Squamous-cell carcinoma arising in an actinic keratosis is invasive, but

Squamous-Cell Carcinoma

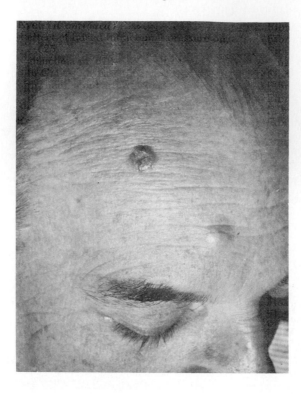

Figure 41–13. Basal-cell carcinoma. A basal-cell carcinoma of the right side of the forehead of a 56-year-old man is shown. The lesion has the typical appearance, with a depressed center and a raised, rolled edge over which dilated blood vessels can be seen traversing. The dome-shaped swelling just above the medial aspect of the right eyebrow has the features of an epidermoid cyst, commonly called a *sebaceous cyst*, or *wen*. The lesion is formed by cystic dilatation of a plugged pilosebaceous follicle.

metastases are late and the prognosis is relatively good. It should be stressed that the transition to malignancy frequently takes many years, and quite simple treatment is adequate for the cure of most actinic keratoses.

Squamous-cell carcinoma may also arise in normal skin or in persons with Bowen's disease. The latter is a type of carcinoma-in-situ that can occur on any part of the body and appears as a circumscribed, erythematous, slightly indurated, scaly patch or plaque. This type of squamous-cell carcinoma is more malignant than that arising from an actinic keratosis. It tends to metastasize to regional lymph nodes and ultimately to the blood stream.

Squamous-cell carcinoma must be differentiated both clinically and

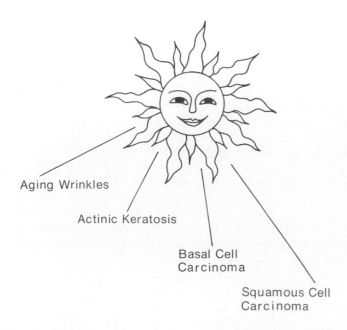

Aging Wrinkles

Actinic Keratosis

Basal Cell
Carcinoma

Squamous Cell
Carcinoma

Figure 41–14. The effect of sunlight on human skin. Although a deep suntan is regarded by many as a status symbol indicative of health, the effect of sunlight on human skin is predominantly detrimental. Prolonged exposure leads to damage to the dermal collagen fibers, and this contributes to the wrinkled appearance of the aging skin. Good advice is that if you want to look young, keep out of the sun! Epidermal damage leads to actinic keratoses and ultimately to cancer. These changes are most marked in individuals with fair skin. They have pale blue eyes and are of northern European stock (*e.g.*, Celts and Scandinavians). (Drawing by Susie Shin.)

pathologically from a keratoacanthoma, which it closely resembles and which also occurs on the sun-exposed skin.

In this lesion there is a localized exuberant overgrowth of atypical squamous epithelium that appears to invade the dermis and to surround a central keratotic plug. Around the lesion is an inflammatory reaction. Keratoacanthoma has been regarded by some as a type of self-healing carcinoma. The shape of the lesion is characteristic clinically, because it appears as a volcanolike lesion with a central keratotic depressed plug. The natural history also is quite characteristic: the lesion grows rapidly for 2 or 3 months, remains stationary, and then involutes spontaneously. Healing results in considerable scarring, and the treatment of choice is therefore simple excision, since this gives a good cosmetic result as well as providing material for pathological examination.

Keratoacanthoma

Malignant melanoma of the skin can arise in four ways (Fig. 41–15):

1. *In a pre-existing nevus.* Considering the number of nevi present in all individuals, one sees that this is a very rare event. About 20 per cent of malignant melanomas arise in this way.

Malignant Melanoma

Figure 41–15. Types of malignant melanoma. *A,* Lentigo maligna. Proliferation of atypical melanocytes in the basal layer of the epidermis is accompanied by a lymphocytic response in the dermis. After many years dermal invasion can occur. *B,* Superficial spreading melanoma. Proliferation of atypical, malignant melanocytes occurs over a wide area of the basal layer of the epidermis. The melanoma cells invade the epidermis, and in one area they also invade the dermis. *C,* Nodular melanoma. The lesion is more localized than in the case of the superficial spreading variety. Melanoma cells invade the epidermis and extend deep into the dermis. This type of tumor has the worst prognosis. (Drawing by Margot Mackay, Department of Art as Applied to Medicine, University of Toronto.)

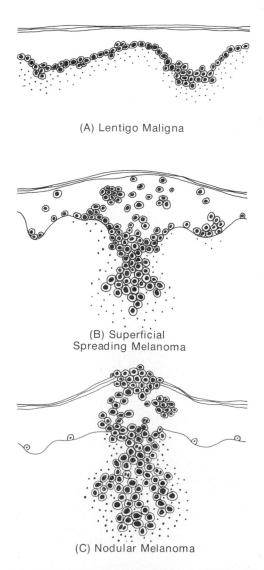

(A) Lentigo Maligna

(B) Superficial
Spreading Melanoma

(C) Nodular Melanoma

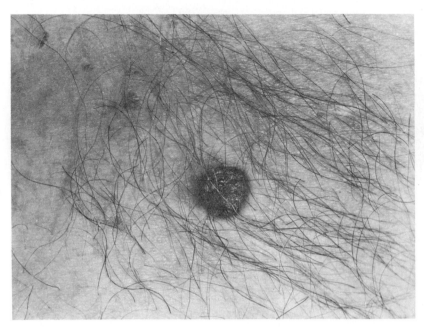

Figure 41–16. Nodular malignant melanoma. This black lesion had recently appeared and showed superficial ulceration. The clinical diagnosis was malignant melanoma. Before radical treatment of such a lesion is undertaken, it must either be biopsied or (if small enough) be completely excised locally. Histopathological diagnosis is essential before one undertakes definitive treatment of any malignant lesion. (Photograph courtesy of Dr. Wallace H. Clark, Jr.)

2. *As a nodule in previously normal skin* (Fig. 41–16). This type of tumor (*nodular melanoma*) spreads vertically into the dermis and has a very bad prognosis, since its biological tendency to early deep invasion results in early lymph node and blood-borne metastases.

3. *As a flat, variably pigmented lesion on previously normal skin* (*superficial spreading melanoma*) (Fig. 41–17). This tumor spreads horizontally for many months or even years before vertical growth results in a nodule formation. When the lesion is superficial the prognosis is good, and even when the tumor has spread into the reticular dermis the outlook is better than with a nodular melanoma.

4. *In a lentigo maligna.* A malignant lentigo is a flat, pigmented lesion that occurs on the face of elderly patients. It may be regarded as a melanoma-in-situ. After many years, dermal invasion occurs, but even then the prognosis is good.

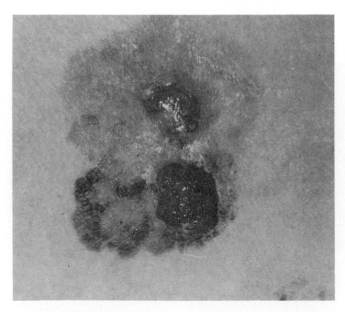

Figure 41–17. Superficial spreading type of malignant melanoma. Two black nodules of tumor are surrounded by superficial, barely palpable growth. Some areas are pigmented, whereas others show erythema. The pale areas of depigmentation are due to foci of tumor regression. Features leading to a diagnosis of melanoma in this lesion are the nodules, the irregular pigmentation, the changing clinical appearance, and the erythema. (Photograph courtesy of Dr. Wallace H. Clark. Jr.)

The types of melanomas have been described in some detail because they illustrate a very important point. Tumors that closely resemble each other microscopically sometimes have quite different prognoses. Thus, the lentigo maligna melanoma has a very good prognosis, whereas that of the nodular melanoma is appalling. This subdivision of melanoma has come about by a combined clinicopathological study of the structure and behavior of a large number of tumors.

Many different types of tumors are known, but they are described in detail in specialized texts. Their diagnosis depends on histological examination — a fact that emphasizes the necessity for submitting all excised tissue for pathological examination. The experienced clinician is not surprised to find that an occasional lesion that is "typical" of a wart or mole turns out to be something quite different. Likewise, if a lesion worries a patient, a doctor, nurse, or physical therapist is usually ill advised to reassure the person that there is nothing to worry about. The lesion should be examined carefully and treated appropriately. When there is doubt, it is better to have a small scar in six months' time than to have multiple metastases.

Other Tumors of the Skin

Review Questions

1. A young woman develops a subacute dermatitis of both earlobes, the neck, and the left wrist. Suggest the possible causes and indicate how you would confirm the diagnosis.

2. Give an account of the possible causes of a widespread vesiculobullous rash.

3. Compare pemphigus vulgaris with bullous pemphigoid.

4. Give an account of the black tumors of the skin and indicate the treatment of each.

5. Describe the development of the common mole, or melanotic hamartoma.

6. Compare and contrast basal-cell carcinoma with squamous-cell carcinoma of the skin.

Selected Readings

Behrman, H. T., Labow, T. A., and Rosen, J. H.: Common Skin Diseases. 2nd ed. New York, Grune & Stratton, Inc., 1971. A simple, well illustrated account of skin diseases.

Fitzpatrick, T. B., et al.: Dermatology in General Medicine. 2nd ed. New York, McGraw-Hill Book Company, 1979. One of the three standard texts on dermatology. A good reference.

Lever, W. F., and Schaumburg-Lever, G.: Histopathology of the Skin. 5th ed. Philadelphia, J. B. Lippincott Company, 1975. The standard reference work on skin pathology.

Milne, J. A.: An Introduction to the Diagnostic Histopathology of the Skin. London, Edward Arnold (Publishers) Ltd., 1972. An excellent introduction to the subject.

Moschella, S. L., Pillsbury, D. M., and Hurley, H. J. (Eds.): Dermatology. Philadelphia, W. B. Saunders Company, 1975. One of the three standard texts on dermatology. For reference only.

Rook, A., Wilkinson, D. S., and Ebling, F. J. G. (Eds.): Textbook of Dermatology. 3rd ed. Oxford, Blackwell Scientific Publications Ltd., 1979. One of the three standard texts on dermatology. For reference only.

Diseases of the Eye

After studying this chapter the student should be able to:

- Describe the development of the eye.
- List the common causes of conjunctivitis.
- Define cataract and give six causes of this condition.
- Classify the types of glaucoma and describe the outstanding clinical and pathological features of each type.
- Describe the pathogenesis and effects of retinal detachment and indicate the treatment.
- Classify the types of uveitis and describe the main features of acute iritis.
- Describe the important features of malignant melanoma of the choroid and retinoblastoma.

A knowledge of the complex structure of the eye and the manner of its formation is essential for a proper understanding of ocular disease. This information is summarized in Figures 42–1 and 42–2.

Many human eye disorders are poorly understood because they are difficult to investigate adequately. Because it is not practicable to take biopsies of the eye, the early morphological changes of disease cannot be examined. Sight is so valuable an asset that the eye is preserved at all costs, and its removal is considered only when there is the threat of malignant disease, or when advanced disease has destroyed all useful function.

Development of the Eye

A hollow bud of the forebrain (the primary optic vesicle) develops at the future site of the eye, and as it approaches the surface ectoderm, the vesicle becomes invaginated to form the optic cup (Fig. 42–1A and B). The outer layer of this cup remains thin and forms the pigment layer of the retina; the inner layer thickens to form the sensory layer. This complex structure contains the highly specialized rods and cones, which are sensitive to light, as well as nerve cells, whose long axons converge on the optic disc and constitute the optic nerve. It will be appreciated that the retina and the optic nerve are really part of the central nervous system, and if they are damaged in humans regeneration is impossible.

The two layers of the retina never fuse firmly; it is in the plane between these layers that separation can occur in the condition known as *retinal detachment*. The optic vesicle induces the overlying ectoderm to thicken, invaginate, and form a vesicle that matures to form the lens (Fig. 42–1B and C). Meanwhile, mesoderm around the globe differentiates to form the choroid, which is a vascular connective tissue coat containing pigmented melanocytes and helps to nourish the retina. Anteriorly, mesoderm contributes to the formation of the ciliary body and the iris. The ciliary body, the iris, and the choroid are conjointly called the *uveal tract* (Fig. 42–2). The ciliary body contains muscle that is attached via the suspensory ligaments to the lens. Contraction of this muscle changes the shape of the lens and therefore alters its focal length. The ciliary body has one other important function: its epithelium-covered processes secrete a clear fluid, the *aqueous humor*.

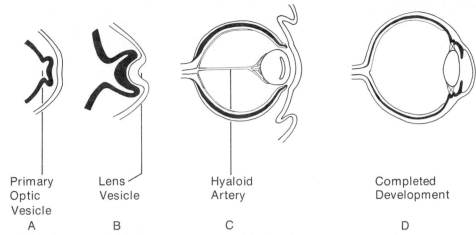

Primary   Lens   Hyaloid   Completed
Optic   Vesicle   Artery   Development
Vesicle
A   B   C   D

Figure 42–1.   Development of the human eye. See text for description. (Drawing by Margot Mackay, Department of Art as Applied to Medicine, University of Toronto.)

The ectoderm and mesoderm overlying the developing eye form the cornea. The bulk of this structure consists of orderly, parallel bundles of collagen embedded in a specialized ground substance and so arranged that the cornea is transparent. It forms the major lens component of the eye because refraction of light is greater at a tissue-air interface than at a tissue-fluid interface. The anatomical lens of the eye, surrounded by fluid, is of lesser importance in this regard. However, because the lens can change its shape under the influence of the muscles of the ciliary body, it provides a fine-adjustment mechanism by which one can focus quickly from distant to close objects. With advancing age the lens becomes more rigid and less capable of adjustment; the person with this lens rigidity finds it difficult to focus on close objects and requires a simple magnifying glass in order to read. This condition is called *presbyopia*.

The formation and disposal of aqueous humor are important because derangements of the mechanisms involved are a major cause of glaucoma and

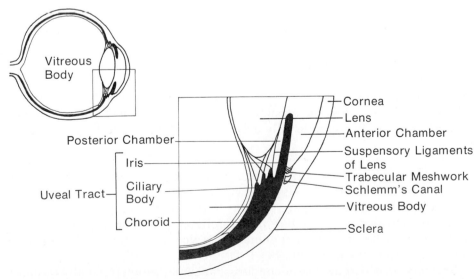

Vitreous
Body

Posterior Chamber

Iris

Uveal Tract

Ciliary
Body

Choroid

Cornea
Lens
Anterior Chamber
Suspensory Ligaments
of Lens
Trabecular Meshwork
Schlemm's Canal
Vitreous Body
Sclera

Figure 42–2.   Structure of the human eye. See text for description. (Drawing by Margot Mackay, Department of Art as Applied to Medicine, University of Toronto.)

therefore of blindness. The fluid is secreted into the posterior chamber, flows forward between the iris and the lens, and then flows through the pupil and into the anterior chamber (Fig. 42–2). This cavity is bounded anteriorly by the cornea and posteriorly by the iris. Absorption of aqueous humor occurs at the angle of the anterior chamber. Fluid passes through a meshwork of connective tissue bundles, termed the *trabecular meshwork,* and ultimately drains into the canal of Schlemm, which encircles the globe at the corneosclerotic junction. From this canal, aqueous humor passes into the venous plexuses at the corneosclerotic junction.

DISEASES OF THE EYE

Conjunctivitis

Acute conjunctivitis can occur as a result of many irritants. Dust and chemicals can cause an acute primary irritant effect. There may be an allergic reaction, such as in patients who are hypersensitive to components of eyedrops (*e.g.,* atropine). A mild conjunctivitis is commonly associated with rhinitis in patients with hay fever. Acute inflammation may be a component of the exanthem of an acute viral disease such as measles, or it may be caused by a direct infection — either bacterial, chlamydial (Chapter 11), or viral (*e.g.,* herpes simplex and zoster). Mild attacks of acute conjunctivitis show a typical catarrhal inflammation, but severe infections are purulent and more serious, because there is a constant danger of corneal involvement (keratitis), ulceration, and subsequent scarring. Infections by streptococci, staphylococci, and gonococci are usually purulent. Ophthalmia neonatorum (acute conjunctivitis occurring during the first 10 days of life) is generally gonococcal.

Injuries and ulcerations of the cornea heal by scar tissue formation, and although the scar is made of collagen, it does not resemble the normal cornea because it is not transparent. Hence, involvement of the pupil area leads to blindness. Homografts from the eyes of cadavers are useful in treating this type of blindness. Similarly, they are of value in replacing the distorted, deformed corneas that are the result of maldevelopment (*corneal dystrophy*).

Cataract

If the lens changes its physical characteristics and becomes opaque, the condition is called a *cataract*. The lens is a unique structure; it is of epithelial origin and is completely surrounded by a capsule that is in fact a basement membrane, and it has no blood supply. The hyaloid artery that nourishes it during development does not persist. Ionizing radiation, systemic administration of glucocorticoids, uveitis, trauma, hypocalcemia, galactosemia, and diabetes mellitus are among the numerous factors that can adversely affect the metabolism of the lens and result in its degeneration and opacification. Nevertheless, the most common cause of cataract formation is old age, and some degree of senile cataract is present in all persons over 70 years of age. Removal of these cataracts produces a welcome return of sight. Glasses can compensate for the loss of accommodation that an absent lens decrees. Contact lenses are also successfully used by the cataract patient following surgery.

Glaucoma

The term *glaucoma* is applied to any condition in which the intraocular pressure is increased. It is an important condition because it causes blindness. The raised intraocular pressure impairs the blood supply to the sensory retina; in particular, the sensitive nerve cells and their long processes that form the optic nerve undergo degeneration. Two major types of glaucoma are recognized: primary and secondary.

Secondary Glaucoma. In secondary glaucoma, which is usually unilateral, the increased pressure occurs as a complication of some other disease and results in mechanical obstruction of the flow of aqueous fluid from the ciliary body to the venous channels into which it ultimately drains. Generally, the obstruction is in the trabecular meshwork, which may become blocked by inflammatory exudate, fibrin, blood, or degenerate tumor. Uveitis, trauma (particularly if it is accompanied by bleeding), advanced cataracts, and tumors are causes of secondary glaucoma. Glaucoma may occur as a complication of glucocorticoid therapy, either when applied locally or when given systemically.

Primary Glaucoma.   This disease is typically bilateral and is not accompanied by any other obvious intraocular disease. Two types can be distinguished:

Open-Angle or Chronic Simple Glaucoma.   This form of glaucoma is a slowly progressive disease of the elderly and is usually painless and symptomless until late in its development. An observant patient may notice a reduction in peripheral vision, but often the person's only complaint is that of difficulty in reading. The patient probably seeks eye care simply to request a stronger pair of reading glasses. For this reason it is imperative that all patients older than middle age should have tests to detect glaucoma during the course of periodic examinations for a change in glasses. The intraocular pressure can be measured quite simply, and an ophthalmoscopic examination will often reveal another sign of glaucoma called *optic nerve cupping*. This is a name given to enlargement of the central depression normally seen in the optic disc. It is due to the pressure-induced atrophy of the optic nerve fibers. Untreated, this type of glaucoma results in blindness, whereas a patient whose glaucoma is detected early has a good prognosis for retaining vision. The pathogenesis of open-angle glaucoma is not known. The filtration angle of the anterior chamber is open, and subtle abnormalities in the trabecular meshwork have been described and are assumed to be the cause.

Angle-Closure Glaucoma.   This disease typically affects women between 40 and 60 years of age. The anterior chamber is shallow, and this anatomical variation is responsible for the obstruction of the outflow of aqueous fluid at the angle of the anterior chamber.

This form of glaucoma is characterized by a series of episodes of raised intraocular pressure. An attack can be precipitated by dilating the pupil with eyedrops containing a mydriatic drug, *e.g.,* phenylephrine hydrochloride (Neo-Synephrine). In a subacute attack there is blurring of vision and the patient sees *rainbow-colored halos around lights* because of the edema of the cornea. Later if an attack of acute glaucoma occurs, there is *pain* (so severe that it can cause vomiting), edema and congestion of the eyelids and conjunctiva, clouding of the cornea, and rapid loss of vision. Vision may be saved if an acute attack is treated early, but persistent high pressure leads to a state of absolute glaucoma, a term used to describe the end-result of any type of uncontrolled glaucoma. The eye is painful, blind, and stony hard. The eye ultimately shrinks and softens when the ciliary body stops producing aqueous fluid.

Retinal Detachment.   A retinal detachment is the result of a separation of the sensory retina from the pigmented layer; it can be produced by inflammatory exudate, hemorrhage, or tumor, *e.g.,* a malignant melanoma (Figs. 42–3 and 42–4). Nevertheless, the commonest type of retinal detachment occurs in elderly persons, particularly those who are near-sighted. Thinning of the retina leads to the formation of a hole that is usually situated anteriorly and is identified by careful ophthalmoscopic examination. Often, the first symptoms of a detachment are flashing lights and "floaters," followed by the appearance

Retinal Disease

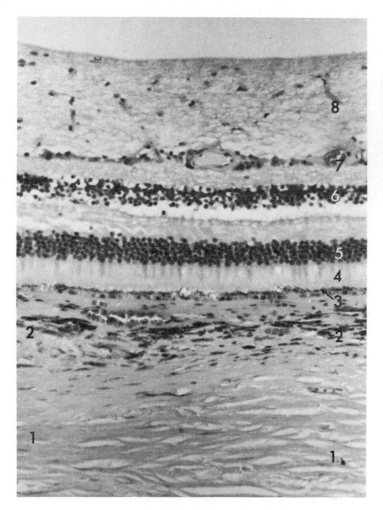

Figure 42–3.   Normal retina, choroid, and sclera. Note the following layers: (1) Sclera, composed of dense collagen. (2) Choroid, more cellular and containing blood vessels. (3) Pigment epithelium, formed from the outer layer of the optic cup. (4) Rod and cone layer consisting of processes of the photoreceptors. (5) Layer containing the nuclei of the photoreceptors. (6) Nuclei of the bipolar cells; processes of these cells connect with the photoreceptors externally and with the ganglion cells internally. (7) Ganglion cell layer; the long axons of these cells enter the layer of nerve fibers and ultimately form the optic nerve. (8) Layer of nerve fibers (× 250).

of a dark shadow in the visual field. It is essential for the physician to make a correct diagnosis, to locate the site of the tear, and subsequently to seal this tear, either by directing a photocoagulating beam into the eye or by applying diathermy to the scleral surface. If the hole is sealed, the retina reattaches and usually no further trouble occurs. However, if the hole is not sealed, the detachment will extend. Since the retina loses its blood supply from the underlying choroid, it soon undergoes degeneration and irreversible loss of function.

Retinopathy Due to Small-Vessel Disease.   The sensory retina, which is the most important functional part of the eye, derives its major blood supply from the central artery of the retina. Disease of this vessel and its branches leads to degenerative changes in the retina itself.

Hypertensive Retinopathy.   In systemic hypertension there is thickening of the small retinal arterioles. As these vessels become occluded, areas of the retina become infarcted. These lesions are called "cotton-wool spots" because of their fluffy appearance. Because the weakened vessels rupture, hemorrhages are frequent, and in the acute malignant phase of hypertension there is edema of the optic disc (*papilledema*) owing to raised intracranial pressure.

Diabetic Retinopathy.   Diabetic retinopathy is the second leading cause of adult-onset blindness in North America. This form of retinopathy, along with the renal lesions, constitutes the most important change produced by

Figure 42–4. Retinal detachment in melanoma. The sensory retina (SR) is atrophic (compare with Figure 42–3) and is separated from the pigment epithelium (Pig) by coagulated protein-containing fluid. The choroid is invaded by spindle-shaped cells of malignant melanoma (MM) (× 250).

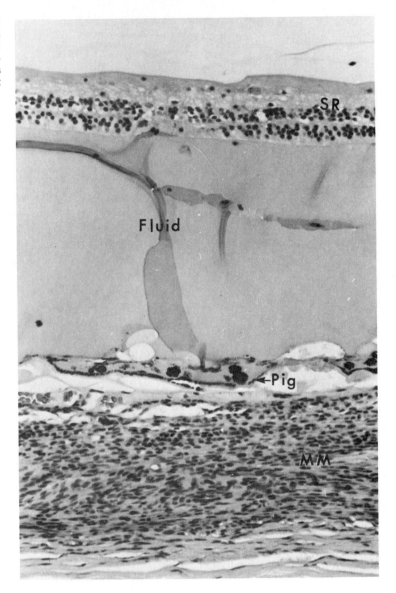

small-vessel disease in diabetes mellitus. Diabetic retinopathy usually occurs in diabetics whose disease began in youth and who have been treated for many years with insulin. Now that these diabetics are able to survive into middle age, diabetic retinopathy is becoming much more common than in the days when the patients died while still young. The characteristic finding is saclike aneurysmal dilatation of some of the capillaries. The abnormal vessels proliferate and bleed. Vision is lost because of vitreal scar tissue formation, which leads eventually to retinal detachment. As in hypertensive retinopathy, areas of infarction and inflammation also occur.

Retinoblastoma. This is the commonest intraocular tumor of childhood. It is often present at birth and invariably manifests itself before the age of four years. In some patients the disease is inherited as a mendelian dominant trait; this is one of the few human malignant tumors in which heredity has been proved to be important. Inherited cases are often bilateral.

The uveal tract, which is the principal vascular connective tissue component of the eye, is the part most severely affected by inflammatory disease.   *Uveitis*

The iris, ciliary body, or choroid may be affected separately (termed *iritis*, *cyclitis*, and *choroiditis*, respectively) or in combination. Iridocyclitis, or anterior uveitis, is a common combination. Choroiditis, or posterior uveitis, often occurs alone.

Both acute and chronic uveitis may be caused by known infective agents — bacterial, viral, protozoal, and helminthic. Nevertheless, many examples have no known cause and present a grave problem in both diagnosis and treatment.

Acute Uveitis

Acute Suppurative Iridocyclitis.   This disease is usually a complication of a penetrating injury; rarely, pyogenic organisms reach the eye during the course of a septicemia or a pyemia. The condition is serious because the infection can easily involve the entire eye (*panophthalmitis*) and can lead to loss of sight.

Acute Nonsuppurative Iridocyclitis.   This is a poorly understood condition. Probably it is not caused by simple infection but rather results from some immune mechanism. It is a complication of many systemic diseases, *e.g.*, syphilis, sarcoidosis, lupus erythematosus, rheumatoid arthritis, and particularly ankylosing spondylitis.

Effects.   In acute iritis the eye becomes painful and red, and there is hyperemia of the deep vessels of the conjunctiva. The pupil is contracted, and the iris may be difficult to see clearly because of inflammatory exudate in the anterior chamber. This response causes the aqueous fluid to become hazy or milky and to produce a "flare" in the narrow beam of light from a slit lamp. Clumps of white cells and fibrin stick to the posterior surface of the cornea as white *keratic precipitates* ("KP"). Fibrinous adhesions, which later organize to fibrous tissue, form between the iris and the lens posteriorly and between the iris and cornea anteriorly. These anterior adhesions (called *synechiae*) obliterate the filtration angle and can lead to glaucoma. To prevent these adhesions from forming and to break down any that are already present, atropine drops are used to dilate the pupil. Note that this treatment is diametrically opposite to that of angle-closure glaucoma, in which the pupil is made to constrict by the application of pilocarpine drops. Therefore, it is of vital importance to be able to distinguish between acute glaucoma and acute iridocyclitis.

Chronic Uveitis.   This is a condition that may be caused by a known infective agent, *e.g.*, *Treponema pallidum* or *Mycobacterium tuberculosis*, but it is often idiopathic. Visual defects are also a feature because with choroiditis the sensory retina undergoes degeneration.

Tumors of the Uveal Tract   The important tumor of the uveal tract is the *malignant melanoma* derived from the melanocytes that are normally present. It is a disease of white adults and is therefore rare in most parts of Africa and in the Orient.

Over 80 per cent of ocular melanomas arise in the choroid, and they are often symptomless in the early stages. Elevation and detachment of the retina occur when the tumor breaks through the pigment epithelial layer of the retina and causes subretinal fluid to accumulate (Fig. 42–4). The patient's seeing a flash of light may be the first indication of an underlying tumor. A large tumor may cause glaucoma or may bleed into the vitreous. Malignant melanoma of the choroid is known to metastasize widely, but after the eye has been removed about 60 per cent of the patients survive longer than 10 years. Even so, it is not uncommon for metastases to appear many years later. The classic, but uncommon, picture is that of a man with an artificial eye, who 30 years after enucleation presents with an enlarged liver that is due to secondary deposits from an intraocular melanoma.

1. Relate the development of the eye to the following factors:
    (a) retinal detachment
    (b) the concept of the uveal tract as a distinct entity
    (c) the ability of the optic nerve to regenerate following damage

2. Compare the symptoms, clinical findings, and treatment of acute anterior uveitis with those of acute congestive glaucoma.

3. Describe the eye changes that can complicate these conditions:
    (a) systemic hypertension
    (b) diabetes mellitus
    (c) ankylosing spondylitis
    (d) sarcoidosis treated with prednisone (a glucocorticoid)

Review Questions

Cairns, J. E.: Corneal disease. British Medical Journal, 2:33–35, 1970.

Duke-Elder, S.: Parsons' Diseases of the Eye. 15th ed. Baltimore, The Williams & Wilkins Company, 1970, 597 pp. This well-tried textbook can be consulted for clinical details of diseases of the eye.

Hogan, M. J., and Zimmerman, L. E.: Ophthalmic Pathology. 2nd ed. Philadelphia, W. B. Saunders Company, 1962, 797 pp. The standard reference book for pathology of the eye.

Leading Article: Cotton-wool spots. British Medical Journal, 4:1474, 1966.

Leading Article: The changing pattern of retinoblastoma. Lancet, 2:1016–1017, 1971.

Paton, D., and Craig, J. A.: Cataracts. Clinical Symposia (Ciba), 27:1–32, 1975.

Perkins, E. S., and Hansell, P.: An Atlas of Diseases of the Eye. 2nd ed. Edinburgh, Churchill Livingstone, 1971, 86 pp. A well-produced color atlas of eye diseases.

Vaughan, D., and Asbury, T. T.: General Ophthalmology. 9th ed. Los Altos, Cal., Lange Medical Publications, 1980.

Selected Readings

CHAPTER 43

Diseases of the Ear

After studying this chapter the student should be able to:

- List the common diseases of the external ear.
- Describe the clinical features, pathology, and complications of acute otitis media and chronic otitis media.
- Describe otosclerosis and Ménière's disease.
- Compare and contrast conductive deafness with sensorineural deafness.

The sense of hearing is comparable to the sense of sight in that it is of immense practical and psychological value to humans. The vital sensory component of the ear in the cochlea, like the retina of the eye, is highly specialized; it cannot regenerate and cannot be biopsied without irreparable damage to the sense organ. Even at necropsy the ear is technically extremely difficult to examine. Both the cochlea and the vestibular apparatus, which subserves the functions of balance and positional sense of the head, are deeply embedded in one of the hardest bones of the human body. It is therefore of little wonder that our knowledge of the pathology of these sense organs is fragmentary.

The ear is conveniently divided into three separate parts: external, middle, and internal (Fig. 43–1).

The External Ear

The external ear, with its pinna and external auditory meatus, terminates medially at the eardrum, or tympanic membrane. In general, diseases of the external ear closely resemble those of the skin. Inflammation, called *otitis externa,* is common and has many causes. It may be a component of seborrheic, atopic, or contact dermatitis. Mechanical irritation by the over-zealous use of cotton swabs, hairpins, matchsticks, and other foreign bodies introduced by the patient is a common cause, because itching is a frequent symptom. The chemical irritation produced by an accumulation of earwax is another cause; disease is sometimes perpetuated by the ill-advised use of prescription ear drops containing irritating or sensitizing chemicals (*e.g.,* neomycin). Bacterial, viral, and fungal infection, particularly by *Aspergillus* species, can sometimes be incriminated. A chronic otitis externa should also lead to the suspicion of an underlying chronic otitis media associated with a perforated drum.

The specialized ceruminous glands can produce so much secretion that the earwax blocks the auditory canal. This is a common cause of conductive deafness, and one that can be easily relieved with gratifying results.

Tumors of the External Ear

Squamous-cell carcinoma is the commonest malignant tumor of the external ear and generally begins with an actinic keratosis. Basal-cell carcinoma is not uncommon; occasionally, tumors of the ceruminous glands are encountered.

The Middle Ear

The middle ear is a cavity filled with air and lined by a flattened epithelium. The vibrations of the eardrum in its lateral wall are relayed by the

Figure 43–1. Diagrammatic section through the human ear. The ear canal, or external auditory meatus, terminates at the eardrum. From the eardrum vibrations are transmitted by the three ossicles to the oval window. The round window is covered by a membrane and is designed to equalize pressures between the middle ear and the inner ear. Thus, when the stapes is pushed inward the membrane of the round window bulges outward into the middle ear. (From Beadle, K. R.: *In* Bleck, E. E., and Nagel, D. A. (Eds.): Physically Handicapped Children. New York, Grune & Stratton, Inc., 1975, p. 93. Reproduced by permission of Grune & Stratton, Inc.)

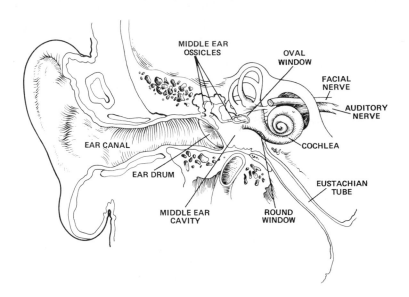

malleus and *incus* to the *stapes* (these are the three auditory ossicles), which fits into the oval window and transmits impulses to the inner ear. Anteriorly, the cavity of the middle ear communicates with the pharynx via the *auditory* (eustachian or pharyngotympanic) *tube*, whereas posteriorly there is connection with the air spaces in the mastoid process of the temporal bone.

Acute Otitis Media

Acute infections of the middle ear (acute otitis media) are usually bacterial in origin, with *Streptococcus pyogenes,* the pneumococci, *Hemophilus influenzae,* and *Staphylococcus aureus* being the common causative organisms. The disease is most frequent in children and is often a complication of an upper respiratory streptococcal or viral infection. At this age the shortness of the auditory tube and blockage produced by swelling of the nasopharyngeal lymphoid tissue ("adenoids") are factors that encourage organisms in the nasopharynx to ascend into the middle ear and cause infection. Lack of IgA in the secretions has been suggested as another predisposing factor. The disease is characterized by severe pain in the ear combined with conductive hearing loss. The inflammatory exudate that collects in the cavity of the middle ear is at first clear but can later become purulent. The eardrum becomes inflamed and may rupture. This event is often averted by surgical incision of the tympanic membrane (a procedure called *myringotomy*), because a well-placed surgical wound heals better than one produced by spontaneous perforation.

Acute otitis media usually resolves with modern chemotherapy aided by surgical drainage, but the following complications should be noted:

1. *Adhesions.* These can affect the tympanic membrane and form between the three ossicles. Fibrinous at first, they are later replaced by scar tissue.

2. *Chronic Otitis Media.*

3. *Spread of Infection.* Involvement of meninges, brain, and mastoid air cells is described later.

Chronic Otitis Media

This condition may occur insidiously or may follow an acute attack, especially if the treatment has been inadequate. Persistent ear discharge and deafness are the main features of chronic otitis media.

The chronic inflammatory reaction in the mucosa is sometimes characterized by the formation of inflammatory granulation tissue containing cholesterol crystals surrounded by foreign-body giant cells. The condition is called a *cholesterol granuloma.* Fibrous adhesions can form in the cavity of the middle ear, and by involving the eardrum and the ossicles, these adhesions can lead to conductive deafness. The lining mucosa may show metaplasia and become replaced by a respiratory type of epithelium with ciliated cells and goblet cells — the latter producing much sticky mucus. Since there is often a permanent hole in the eardrum, a persistent discharge of thick, mucoid material follows (often called the "glue ear").

Complications of Otitis Media

"Epidermoid Cholesteatoma."   This misleading name is applied to a cyst within the middle ear that is filled with keratin and lined by epidermis. The cyst is thought to be derived from squamous epithelium that migrates into the middle ear through a perforated eardrum. This condition is a serious complication of otitis media, because the cyst enlarges and produces local pressure effects as well as perpetuating a chronic infection. Surgical treatment is necessary for its cure.

Spread of Infection.   In both acute and chronic otitis media, infection can spread to involve adjacent structures. The conditions resulting are described below:

Mastoiditis.   Involvement of the mastoid air cells is a particularly serious condition, since suppuration occurs and further spread of infection is a serious hazard. The disease is characterized by generalized signs of an acute suppurative process (causing malaise and fever) together with pain, redness, and swelling of the bony mastoid prominence behind the ear.

Sigmoid Sinus Thrombosis.   The sigmoid sinus, which is one of the large venous sinuses within the skull, lies in close proximity to the mastoid air cells. Thrombosis itself is serious, but when a thrombus is invaded by pyogenic organisms, the result is *pyemia.* Infected thrombi break off and lead to pulmonary pyemic abscesses.

Meningitis.   Organisms either from the mastoid air cells or from the middle ear can penetrate the thin bone to reach the meningeal space and lead to meningitis.

Brain Abscess.   If infection reaches the meninges, adhesions may limit the spread of infection and yet allow bacteria to continue their onward march into the brain, causing either a cerebellar or a temporal-lobe abscess.

Seventh-Nerve Paralysis.   The seventh, or facial, nerve pursues a tortuous course through the middle ear and can be damaged either by otitis media or by surgery performed on a diseased ear.

Labyrinthitis.   Infection can spread to involve the inner ear.

Otosclerosis

In this disease of unknown cause, parts of the petrous temporal bone are replaced by woven bone. The disease is probably quite common, but it becomes clinically apparent only if the stapes is involved. When this bone becomes ankylosed in the oval window, deafness ensues. The disease is particularly distressing since it is generally bilateral. It has been estimated that approximately 2 per cent of all white persons suffer from deafness from this cause. The plight of these victims of otosclerosis has indeed been the inspiration for the development of microsurgery in which the surgeon operates by using a binocular microscope.

Conductive Deafness

This term is applied to any form of deafness in which there is a failure of conduction of sound impulses from the external environment to the internal sensory organ of the inner ear. Blockage of the external auditory meatus, lesions in the middle ear, and otosclerosis are the main causes. Congenital abnormalities of the middle ear are a cause of congenital deafness (see below).

This region of the ear is situated in the dense, petrous temporal bone and consists of a bony labyrinth containing the intercommunicating channels of the membranous labyrinth — the cochlea with its complex sensory auditory organ and the semicircular canals, whose main function is concerned with balance and sense of position of the head. The cochlear nerve arises from the sensory end-organs in the cochlea, joins with the vestibular nerve, and transmits to the brain stem impulses that are then relayed to the cortex.

The Inner Ear

Deafness due to a defect of the sensory organ or the cochlear nerve is termed *sensorineural*. It is beyond the scope of this chapter to describe this in any detail, but the following causes are noteworthy:

Sensorineural Deafness

Lesions in the Receptor Sensory Organ in the Labyrinth. It is well recognized that certain drugs can damage the eighth nerve; the most common are aminoglycosides, *e.g.*, streptomycin and gentamicin. Loud noise, whether from an industrial source or from pop music, is capable of causing permanent damage. Other causes are fractures, vascular occlusion, and inflammatory lesions, which may be viral, *e.g.*, mumps. Intrauterine rubella is an important cause of *congenital deafness*, other causes of which include hypoxia (associated with hemolytic disease of the newborn and difficult deliveries) and hereditary factors. The diagnosis of hereditary deafness rests on obtaining a positive family history. It is important to recognize congenital and neonatal deafness early, because otherwise the child may be misdiagnosed as being mentally retarded and appropriate education not provided.

Nerve Damage. Schwannoma of the vestibulocochlear (eighth cranial, or auditory) nerve is an important cause.

Brain Damage. Diseases that involve the nerve cells and tracts that relay impulses from the cochlear nerve to the temporal lobe cortex may produce defects in hearing. These defects are not usually noted by the patient and can be detected only by special tests.

The auditory component of the inner ear is closely connected with the organ of balance. This association is illustrated by the symptomatology of *Ménière's disease*. The disease affects the membranous labyrinth as a whole and is characterized by paroxysmal attacks of intense giddiness (*vertigo*) associated with unilateral deafness and tinnitus (buzzing in the ears). The disease is not uncommon, and Shakespeare's mention of the "falling sickness" in *Julius Caesar* is generally regarded as a reference to this disease.

Ménière's Disease

1. Describe the complications and dangers of having otitis media and a perforated eardrum.

2. A patient develops signs of an intracranial space-occupying lesion together with deafness in one ear. Discuss the possible causes of this condition and the examinations that might be performed to arrive at a diagnosis.

3. In spite of medical treatment a patient has persistent otitis externa. Suggest some reasons for this persistent inflammation.

Review Questions

Friedmann, I.: Pathology of the Ear. Oxford, Blackwell Scientific Publications Ltd., 1974, 607 pp.

Friedmann, I.: The apparently barren regions of the temporal bone. International Pathology Bulletin, *16*:9–32, 1975.

Konigsmark, B. W., and Gorlin, R. J.: Genetic and Metabolic Deafness. Philadelphia, W. B. Saunders Company, 1976, pp. 24–26, 45.

Selected Readings

Diseases of the Central Nervous System

After studying this chapter the student should be able to:

- Describe the overall structure of the central nervous system and the meninges.
- Distinguish between neurons and neuroglia.
- Describe the formation and fate of cerebrospinal fluid (CSF).
- Describe the effects of a raised intracranial pressure and list the common causes.
- Distinguish between subdural and extradural hemorrhage in terms of these factors:
    - (a) site of bleeding
    - (b) source of bleeding
    - (c) causes
    - (d) clinical effects
- Describe the cause and effects of subarachnoid hemorrhage.
- Outline the causes and effects of cerebral hemorrhage, cerebral thrombosis, and cerebral embolism; describe the differences between these three types of stroke.
- Define the following terms:
    - (a) hemiplegia
    - (b) Babinski sign
    - (c) pseudobulbar palsy
- Describe pyogenic meningitis with respect to the following factors:
    - (a) causes
    - (b) clinical effects
    - (c) CSF findings
    - (d) complications
- List the causes of cerebral abscess.
- List the agents that cause aseptic meningitis and encephalitis.
- Discuss the pathology of multiple sclerosis and describe its clinical features.
- Give examples of poisons that cause permanent central nervous system damage.
- List the neurological complications of the following conditions:
    - (a) thiamine deficiency
    - (b) pellagra
    - (c) pernicious anemia
    - (d) alcoholism and liver disease
- Outline the important features of
    - (a) Alzheimer's disease
    - (b) Parkinson's disease
    - (c) Huntington's chorea
    - (d) motor neuron disease
- Describe the outstanding features of the following:
    - (a) psychomotor epilepsy
    - (b) petit mal epilepsy
    - (c) grand mal epilepsy
    - (d) jacksonian fit
- List the causes of symptomatic epilepsy.
- Describe the types and effects of the common tumors that arise in the brain and in the meninges.

Structure and Function

The central nervous system consists of nerve cells (*neurons*) and a supporting matrix of neuroglia in which they are embedded. It is richly supplied by blood vessels and is formed as a hollow tube during development, lined on the inside by *ependyma,* and covered on the outside by a layer of *pia mater.*

The neurons are the essential cells of the nervous system. They are formed by the differentiation of primitive neuroblasts during embryonic life and are unable to divide at a later time. Neurons possess the specialized property of excitability. They may be excited by a variety of stimuli to produce an impulse that is propagated throughout the cytoplasm of the cell. Since the axon of a nerve cell is often several inches or even feet in length, the impulse is conducted from one part of the body to another. *Excitability* and *conduction* are thus two characteristic properties of the nerve cells. Under abnormal circumstances, there may be changes in their excitability and conductibility. In the case of motor neurons, the effects may be obvious enough and may take the form of paralysis or convulsions. With sensory neurons, the equivalent effects can be anesthesia or pain and paresthesia (abnormal spontaneous feeling such as tingling).

The brain cannot be regarded as a simple organ comparable to the liver. Each cell is not equivalent to its neighbor and cannot be regarded as performing a similar function. In fact, the brain acts as a series of systems, and the elaborate interrelationship between the vast number of neurons is responsible for the complex function and behavior of the nervous system of the higher animals. Not only is the nervous system responsible for receiving and transmitting all sensory stimuli from its peripheral receptor organs, but also its central organization is designed for interpreting all stimuli. At its highest level, the nervous system is responsible for consciousness, memory, and intelligence. Abnormalities in function in these areas produce diseases that at present are mainly in the realm of the psychiatrist and have no known morphological features. This aspect of the abnormalities of the nervous system cannot be dismissed lightly, since it has been estimated that approximately one half of all patients occupying hospital beds do so because of psychiatric disease.

With regard to its efferent properties, the nervous system controls or influences all muscular activities in the body, including beating of the heart, contraction of the walls of blood vessels, function of skeletal muscle, ventilation of the lungs, and motility of the gastrointestinal tract. Furthermore, much glandular secretion is influenced by the nervous system. Indeed, there is scarcely any bodily structure or function that is not in one way or another under nervous control. It is therefore of little wonder that abnormal nervous function can produce many diverse effects. When no obvious structural change is present, these effects are classified as functional diseases. Two examples of such diseases may be quoted. First, hysterical hyperventilation can be so marked that it causes respiratory alkalosis and tetany. Second, impotence in the male and frigidity in the female are most commonly related to psychological causes. Whether abnormal nervous function can produce structural abnormalities in other organs is a much debated point. Anorexia nervosa in humans and pseudocyesis (false pregnancy) in animals are good examples. In the first instance, individuals (usually young women) refuse to eat, become emaciated, and may ultimately die of starvation or one of its complications. In the second instance, the animal's hormonal balance is so changed that pregnancy is closely simulated. Whether a psychosomatic explanation is responsible for other disease states is less well substantiated.

Nevertheless, diseases such as primary thyrotoxicosis, peptic ulcer, urticaria, and psoriasis seem to be aggravated by mental stress.

To understand the behavior of the nervous system in disease, one must first have knowledge of its normal structure and function. The student is therefore advised to consult the standard texts on neuroanatomy and physiology. It is necessary to have an overall picture of the organization of the major motor tracts before many diseases can be understood.

The Motor System

The large neurons of the frontal cortex give rise to long axons that constitute the corticospinal, or pyramidal, tract. This tract crosses to the opposite side in the medulla, and its axons control the anterior horn cells of the spinal cord. Damage to the pyramidal tract results in an *upper motor neuron paralysis*. Voluntary movement is lost, but the muscles retain their tone. The arms assume a flexed position, whereas the legs are extended. The tendon reflexes are brisk, and there is a Babinski sign.* If the anterior horn cells (or their cranial equivalents) or their axons in the peripheral motor nerve are damaged, a *lower motor neuron lesion* results. There is paralysis, but the muscles are flaccid, and the reflexes are absent.

The Meninges

There are three coverings, or meninges, of the central nervous system: (1) the *pia mater*, (2) the *dura mater*, and (3) the *arachnoid*. Their functions are described briefly.

1. The *pia mater* closely envelops the brain and spinal cord.

2. The *dura mater* is closely adherent to the bony and ligamentous protective housing provided by the skull, vertebral column, and connecting ligaments. The *falx cerebri* forms an extension of the dura mater that assumes a sickle shape and separates the two cerebral hemispheres. A similar extension of the dura mater forms the *tentorium*, which separates the cerebrum above from the cerebellum below.

3. The third layer of the meninges is the *arachnoid*, which forms a thin, translucent covering like a spider's web lying between the pia mater and the dura mater.

The space between the arachnoid and the pia mater is called the *subarachnoid space* and contains cerebrospinal fluid (CSF). This fluid originates in the choroid plexuses of the ventricles and finally escapes through the foramina in the roof of the fourth ventricle to reach the subarachnoid space. Ultimately, the fluid is absorbed in the arachnoid granulations of such major sinuses as the superior sagittal sinus.

Increased Intracranial Pressure

Effects. The rigid, bony enclosure of the brain is a necessary protective shield; its presence, however, has some attendant disadvantages. Any lesion that causes the brain to expand tends to cause a rise in intracranial pressure, which in turn increases the pressure in the veins. Initially CSF and venous blood are displaced, but in due course there is a marked rise in intracranial pressure and a rise in CSF pressure. The increased venous and capillary pressure combined with hypoxia leads to cerebral edema, which further increases the volume of the brain. The rise in intracranial pressure tends to reduce cerebral blood flow, but it activates reflexes that counteract this effect by raising the systemic blood pressure. An increase — sometimes to very high levels — in blood pressure is an important sign of raised intracranial pressure. In its turn, it reflexly slows the heart rate. *Routine care of a patient with a*

---

*A Babinski sign means that when the sole of the foot is stroked, the big toe dorsiflexes and there is fanning of the toes. Normally the toe moves down (plantarflexes).

suspected intracranial lesion therefore involves monitoring of the blood pressure and the heart rate.

Raised intracranial pressure is characterized by *headaches,* often severe, that are probably caused by stretching of the meninges. *Vomiting* is common and is due to stimulation of the medullary centers. Progressive mental impairment may also occur. Traction on the cribriform plate, through which the optic nerve fibers leave the eye, causes compression of the nerves, thereby obstructing the normal flow of axoplasm to the brain. The result is swelling of the optic disc, termed *papilledema,* which can be seen with an ophthalmoscope. Papilledema is an extremely important sign of increased intracranial pressure, and it is also serious because if allowed to persist it causes atrophy of the optic nerve and ultimately blindness.

Causes

1. Edema of the Brain. Generalized edema of the brain is a feature of a raised arterial P_{CO_2} and of encephalitis. Localized edema is a feature of injury and infarction of the brain.

2. Obstruction of the Flow of CSF. Any obstruction of the flow of CSF from the choroid plexuses in the ventricular system to the superior sagittal sinus causes an increase in the intracranial pressure. Blockage of the aqueduct of Sylvius, obstruction of the foramina in the roof of the fourth ventricle, and adhesions in the subarachnoid space (such as may occur following meningitis) are examples of such obstruction.

3. Meningitis. Any form of meningitis causes an increase in exudation of fluid into the CSF. In addition, there is obstruction due to the formation of fibrinous and subsequent fibrous adhesions, particularly at the base of the brain.

4. Space-occupying Lesions. *Hemorrhage* into the brain, the formation of a *hematoma* (whether within the brain, subdural space, or extradural space), and the formation of an *abscess* or *tumor* are all examples of space-occupying lesions that ultimately cause an increase in intracranial pressure.

Apart from the generalized consequences of raised intracranial pressure, space-occupying lesions have additional effects. A lesion of one cerebral hemisphere causes such swelling that part of the hemisphere is pushed beneath the falx cerebri to the other side. *This is an example of herniation* (see Fig. 44–6). Furthermore, in such a supratentorial lesion, the expanded brain pushes downward through the orifice of the tentorium cerebelli in such a way that the midbrain is forced downward and part of the cerebrum (the unci of the temporal lobes) herniates. This has several effects, which are described in the following paragraphs.

(a) There is pressure on the third nerve. The nerve affected first is on the same side as the lesion, and this leads to dilatation of the pupil. *A fixed, dilated pupil is an important sign of the herniation and occurs first on the same side as the cerebral lesion. Careful and frequent examination of the eyes is therefore an important part of the care of patients with suspected cerebral lesions, e.g.,* a head injury.

(b) Downward movement of the brain stem tears small blood vessels. Compression of, or bleeding into, the midbrain and pons causes serious effects. When the upper brain stem is affected, there is loss of consciousness. With lower brainstem damage, there is respiratory arrest and death.

(c) An expanding lesion of one cerebral hemisphere may force the midbrain to one side in such a way that a cerebral peduncle is pressed against the tentorium. This causes damage to the pyramidal fibers on the side opposite the cerebral lesion; since these fibers cross over in the medulla, there is *an upper motor-neuron paralysis of the body on the same side as that of the cerebral lesion.*

Increased intracranial pressure can force the medulla into the foramen magnum together with the tonsils of the cerebellum. *Cerebellar herniation compresses the medulla, causing respiratory arrest and death. It can be precipitated by performing a lumbar puncture on a patient with a markedly raised intracranial pressure.* This procedure is therefore contraindicated under these circumstances.

Traumatic Lesions of the Central Nervous System

An injury involving the jaws is sometimes accompanied by a much more important injury to the brain. Blows on the head produce damage to the region beneath the injury and to the brain at the opposite pole; this is the so-called *contrecoup injury.* Minor injuries cause petechial hemorrhages and traumatic inflammatory edema, whereas more severe injuries may actually tear (*lacerate*) the brain, and hemorrhage may be of sufficient magnitude to cause death.

Subdural Hemorrhage.   Sometimes following an injury one of the poorly supported bridging veins that pass from a venous sinus to a cerebral vein is torn, and a subdural hematoma forms. Less commonly a venous sinus itself is disrupted, as when there is a fracture of the base of the skull. If the hematoma is large, it organizes at the periphery and remains fluid in the center. The cyst that is formed imbibes fluid and enlarges to form a *chronic subdural hematoma* that acts as a space-occupying lesion. The injury that causes this type of lesion is often relatively mild, and in an elderly or alcoholic patient it may be completely overlooked. Weeks later, headaches and other signs and symptoms of raised intracranial pressure appear.

Extradural Hemorrhage.   This form of hemorrhage occurs when the *middle meningeal artery* is torn; it is usually in association with a fracture of the skull involving the temporal region. Unconsciousness may occur immediately after the injury, but the patient often recovers and feels well for a few hours. This *lucid interval* is deceptive. Presently, as the bleeding proceeds, increasing signs of raised intracranial pressure appear; this is followed by coma and death. It is evident that *all cases of head injury, except the most trivial, should be observed carefully for 24 hours.* This word of caution applies particularly to persons suspected of being drunk — a state that may be mimicked by the combination of medicinal brandy given by a well-wisher and an extradural hemorrhage.

Nontraumatic Cerebrovascular Disease

Subarachnoid Hemorrhage.   This condition is not uncommon in persons between the ages of 20 and 50 years. The hemorrhage stems from a ruptured aneurysm of one of the major cerebral arteries in the area of the circle of Willis. The aneurysms lie in the subarachnoid space and are from 0.5 to 1.0 cm in diameter; because of this size, they are often called *berry aneurysms* (Figs. 44–1 and 44–2). They are thought to arise at the site of congenital defects in the elastic coat of the arteries. Sometimes they are multiple.

Cerebral Hemorrhage, Thrombosis, and Embolism.   Atherosclerosis and hypertension both predispose to *cerebral hemorrhage* (sometimes called *cerebral apoplexy*). Commonly, the site is from a branch of the middle cerebral artery. The area of brain affected is in the region of the basal ganglia, the external and the internal capsule. The immediate effects of hemorrhage tend to be more severe than those produced by thrombosis. In both there is the clinical picture commonly called a "stroke."

With *hemorrhage* there is usually sudden loss of consciousness. As blood disrupts the substance of the brain, coma deepens and death ensues. This course is not inevitable, however, and the bleeding may stop.

Figure 44–1.   Berry aneurysm. An unruptured aneurysm (An) is seen to be arising from the left vertebral artery. Note the following normal structures: FL, frontal lobe; TL, temporal lobe; Olf, olfactory nerve; Opt, optic nerve; MB, mamillary body; P, pons; M, medulla oblongata; SC, spinal cord; Cb, cerebellum; CbT, cerebellar tonsil; and Uncus. (Courtesy of Dr. N. B. Rewcastle.)

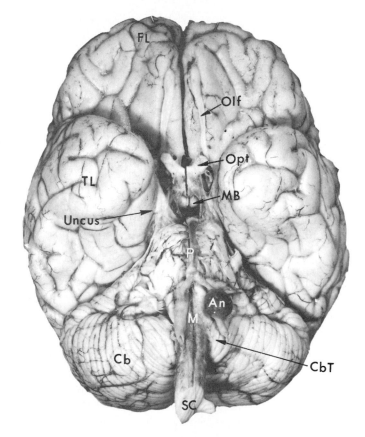

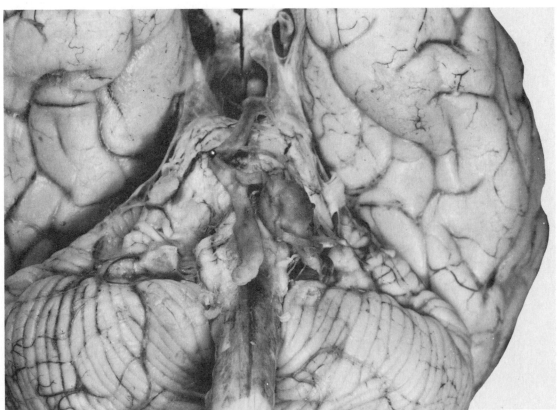

Figure 44–2.   Berry aneurysm. This is the same specimen as in Figure 44–1, but the aneurysm has been lifted up to show its connection with the vertebral artery. (Courtesy of Dr. N. B. Rewcastle.)

With *thrombosis* the patient may experience prodromal or warning signs (*e.g.*, transient hemiplegia, blindness in one eye, speech defect, or confusion) before the onset of the stroke. The stroke itself often occurs during sleep; although consciousness may be lost, this effect is not invariable. Sometimes evidence of progressive damage may be apparent over a period of several days. Apparently, this is due to spread of the thrombosis and hence is called a *thrombotic stroke in evolution.* Thrombosis causes *infarction,* which can itself lead to later hemorrhage in the damaged area (Fig. 44–3).

The infarct caused by thrombosis is usually pale; in those patients who survive, the area softens (a process called *colliquative necrosis*). The microglial cells enlarge, become phagocytic, and appear as large, foamy macrophages. The damaged nerve fibers are not replaced, and the area heals by proliferation of astrocytes, which produces a *glial scar.* The area of brain thus collapses, and sometimes a central cyst remains where once there was brain tissue. Note that any nerve cells destroyed are not replaced.

Infarcts are sometimes found in the absence of detectable thrombosis of a cerebral artery. The explanation is generally to be found in the extracranial arterial supply to the brain — the carotid and vertebral arteries. Severe stenosis of these vessels can seriously imperil the blood supply to the brain. Under these circumstances, infarction is to be found in the "watershed" areas that are at the boundary zones where the vascular territories of two cerebral vessels join.

Cerebral embolism is a common cause of stroke. The embolus generally originates from the heart, and the onset of the stroke is sudden.

Clinical Features of Stroke. In cerebral hemorrhage, thrombosis, and embolism, the clinical picture depends on the size and location of the area of

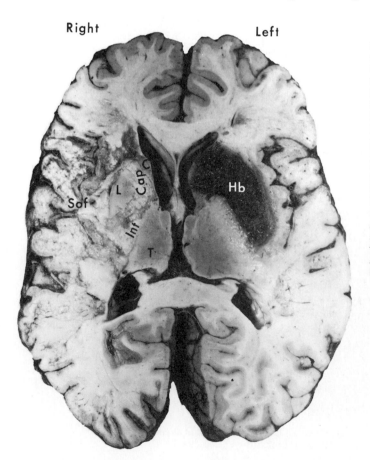

Right   Left

Figure 44–3. Cerebral softening and hemorrhage. The brain has been sectioned horizontally and is viewed here from below. There is severe damage. On the right-hand side there is extensive softening (Sof). Note the shrunken appearance of the affected area, which extends outward to involve the gray matter of the cerebral cortex. The internal capsule (Int Cap) is severely affected. It lies between the lentiform nucleus (L) and the caudate nucleus (C) anteriorly and between the lentiform nucleus and thalamus (T) posteriorly. Loss of its corticospinal fibers leads to an upper motor neuron lesion of the opposite side of the body. The patient had had a stroke three months before death. This attack, which had been attributed to a cerebral thrombosis, left the patient with a left hemiplegia. She subsequently had another stroke involving the opposite side. Note the extensive hemorrhage (Hb) that has occurred into the area of softening on the left side. (Courtesy of Dr. N. B. Rewcastle.)

brain affected. With a severe stroke, consciousness is lost, but recovery gradually sets in, and consciousness then returns. At first, speech is often impaired, but as time passes, it returns to normal. The neurological findings depend upon the area of brain affected. Commonly, the long cerebrospinal tracts in the internal capsule are destroyed, and the picture is that of *hemiplegia* — loss of voluntary movement on the side of the body opposite to that of the cerebral lesion (upper motor neuron lesion). Destroyed neurons are never replaced and lost axons are never regenerated. Nevertheless, considerable clinical recovery can be expected following a stroke. Good nursing and physical therapy can do much to tide the patient over the severe initial period. For example, during this time bedsores and urinary tract infections should be prevented. Good oral hygiene and maintenance of adequate fluid and food intake are also important. Finally, encouragement and physical exercises can do much to minimize the effects of the ultimate paralysis or other neurological losses.

Quite apart from acute episodes of thrombosis or infarction, cerebral atherosclerosis can lead to multiple, bilateral ischemic lesions in the brain. The characteristic mental deterioration of old age is one effect of the lesions, but if they are extensive, there may be severe bilateral damage to the corticospinal tracts. When bilaterally innervated muscles such as those of the tongue and pharynx are affected, the condition is called *pseudobulbar palsy*.

Infections of the Central Nervous System

Pyogenic Bacterial Infections

Pyogenic bacteria may produce a diffuse infection of the subarachnoid space, a condition that is called *meningitis*, or they may produce a localized suppuration in the brain substance, a condition called *cerebral abscess*.

Pyogenic Meningitis

Mode of Infection.   Two routes are common:

Blood-borne.   *Hemophilus influenzae* and the meningococcus gain entry to the blood, presumably from an infection in the upper respiratory tract. The route is probably via the choroid plexuses, where the organisms are filtered out of the blood during the course of a septicemia. The infection spreads through the ventricular system and reaches the subarachnoid space in the region of the basal cisterns. It is here that the most severe effects are seen. The pia mater and the arachnoid are acutely inflamed, and there is a massive polymorphic and fibrinous exudate into the subarachnoid space. With modern chemotherapy the patients often survive, but even then the exudate may undergo organization, and the foramina in the roof of the fourth ventricle may become blocked. Cerebrospinal fluid accumulates in the ventricular system, which expands accordingly; this is one mechanism by which *hydrocephalus* develops. In the young child the pressure exerted on the developing bones leads to a tremendous enlargement of the vault of the skull.

Local Spread.   Meningitis may follow the spread of infection from the middle ear or mastoid air cells — sites of infection that are common in childhood. It is also a complication of a fractured skull in cases in which the wound is exposed to the exterior or to the nasal cavity. Fracture of the cribriform plate of the ethmoid bone is followed by an escape of cerebrospinal fluid into the nose (a condition called *cerebrospinal rhinorrhea*). Meningitis may follow.

Clinical Features.   Fever, severe headache, disorders of consciousness, and convulsions (particularly in children) are the outstanding symptoms. Stiffness of the neck and resistance to forward bending are the outstanding signs. The diagnosis is made by performing a lumbar puncture (recall the dangers of this procedure in a patient with raised intracranial pressure). The

Right   Left

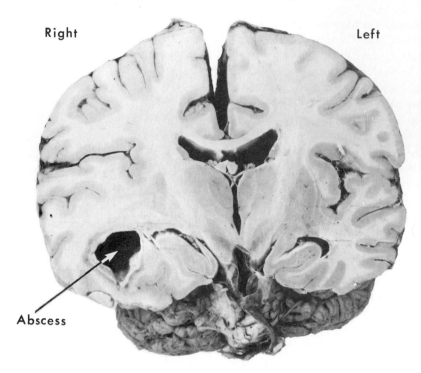

Abscess

Figure 44–4. Cerebral abscess. Sagittal section of the brain showing a large abscess in the right temporal lobe. When the brain was sectioned, pus drained from the abscess, which now appears to be empty. Owing to chronic otitis media, the patient had a chronic discharge from his right ear. He developed headaches and stiffness of the neck but was moribund by the time he reached the hospital. Necropsy revealed an extradural abscess overlying the roof of the right middle ear. Infection had spread into the brain. (Courtesy of Dr. N. B. Rewcastle.)

pressure of the fluid is increased, as is its protein content. The glucose level is low, because the organisms ferment the sugar. Numerous polymorphs are present, and organisms can be demonstrated either directly on a smear or by culture.

Cerebral Abscess

Mode of Infection.   As with meningitis, there are two modes of infection.

Blood-borne.   Patients with chronic chest infections (empyema, lung abscess, and bronchiectasis) sometimes develop a cerebral abscess. Presumably, the infection is blood-borne; an alternative explanation is that spread occurs from an infected nasal air sinus — a common accompaniment of chronic chest suppuration.

Local Spread.   As with meningitis, local spread occurs from an infected middle ear or nasal air sinus (Fig. 44–4).

Viral Infections   **Viral Meningitis (Aseptic Meningitis).**   Poliovirus, coxsackie viruses, ECHO viruses, and mumps virus are among the many agents that can cause meningitis. The symptoms are similar to those of pyogenic meningitis, but they are less severe. The cerebrospinal fluid contains lymphocytes rather than polymorphs. An important point of differentiation is that *the glucose level is normal.*

Viral Encephalitis.   The syndrome of encephalitis resembles that of aseptic meningitis, but to it is added evidence of cerebral damage: coma, cranial nerve paralysis, and hemiplegia, for example. Some of the causative agents are described in Chapter 12.

Diseases Affecting the Myelin Sheath   The major nerve fibers both within the central nervous system and in the peripheral nervous system have a myelin sheath, which acts as an insulating covering, thereby aiding in transmission of impulses in the axon. Damage to the myelin sheath leads to impaired conduction, even though the axon itself remains intact. Two groups of disorders are recognized:

1. The *demyelinating diseases,* of which multiple sclerosis is by far the most frequent.

2. The *dysmyelinating diseases* or *leukodystrophies,* in which myelin formation is impaired.

Multiple Sclerosis

Multiple sclerosis, or disseminated sclerosis as it is also called, is a chronic disease characterized by exacerbations and remissions that often extend over many years. The brain and spinal cord show the development of well-circumscribed foci (plaques) of demyelination (Fig. 44–5). These plaques occur in all parts of the central nervous system, but they are more frequent in certain areas. During the acute phases there is an inflammatory reaction and severe impairment of nerve conduction. The nerve axons are generally preserved, and a considerable degree of functional recovery occurs after each phase. Depending on the site of damage, multiple sclerosis first manifests itself as sudden impairment of vision, inability to speak clearly (dysarthria), cerebellar dysfunction, or paralysis due to pyramidal tract damage. Alteration in emotional state and bladder dysfunction also occur. Each acute episode is followed by recovery, occasionally complete, but more frequently there is some residual damage, so that with the passage of years the patient ultimately becomes quite disabled.

Other Demyelinating Diseases

Several diseases are known that resemble multiple sclerosis but are more acute. Demyelination is also a feature of the encephalitis that occasionally follows certain viral infections, such as following vaccination for smallpox and rabies, as well as following certain naturally occurring viral diseases such as rubella.

The Leukodystrophies

The leukodystrophies constitute a group of rare diseases in which there is a defect in the formation of myelin. Usually manifested during infancy or childhood, they are familial.

Figure 44–5. Multiple sclerosis. Horizontal section of the brain showing many areas of demyelination (arrows). Since it is the myelin sheaths of nerve fibers that give the white matter its color, areas of demyelination appear gray and superficially resemble the gray matter. (Courtesy of Dr. N. B. Rewcastle.)

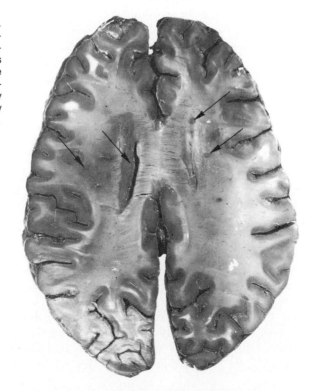

**Toxic,
Deficiency, and
Metabolic
Disorders**

The brain is a very active metabolic organ. Although it represents about 2 per cent of the body weight, it is responsible for 20 per cent of the body's resting oxygen consumption. It is not surprising, therefore, that it can easily be affected adversely by many agents that interfere with metabolism. A few of these are listed below.

1. Poisons. Lead and arsenic are examples of agents that can cause permanent brain damage. Likewise, poisoning by carbon monoxide can cause necrosis of the basal ganglia and can lead to extrapyramidal syndromes, which are described later.

2. Deficiency of Oxygen (Hypoxia). The brain is extremely sensitive to oxygen deprivation. Even short periods of hypoxia can produce permanent damage.

3. Vitamin Deficiencies

Vitamin B₁ (Thiamine) Deficiency. In some patients vitamin B₁ deficiency causes focal areas of necrosis in the brain. In North America the condition is usually associated with alcoholism. Several syndromes can occur. For example, in *Wernicke's disease* there is impaired mentation and unsteadiness, which, when severe, makes the patient unable to stand or walk without help. Paralysis of the external eye muscles resulting in double vision (*diplopia*) is common, as is polyneuritis. Wernicke's disease may be combined with *Korsakoff's psychosis*, in which there is grave mental impairment with inability to learn new facts and severe loss of memory (*amnesia*). The patient may fill in memory gaps by fictitious stories, a condition known as *confabulation*.

Pellagra Encephalopathy. This condition is described in Chapter 23.

Subacute Combined Degeneration of the Spinal Cord. This condition is due to vitamin B₁₂ deficiency and accompanies pernicious anemia.

4. Metabolic Encephalopathies

Hepatic Encephalopathy. Degeneration of neurons is responsible for the mental deterioration encountered in chronic liver disease (Chapter 33).

Chronic Alcoholism. The pathetic state of some chronic alcoholics is a combined effect of alcohol, vitamin deficiency, and liver damage.

Hypoglycemia. Poisoning with insulin causes hypoglycemia, coma, convulsions, and death. Permanent neuronal loss can occur in those who survive; the changes resemble those of hypoxia. At one time, insulin convulsions were used as a treatment for certain psychiatric conditions, but this practice has now been abandoned.

**Degenerative
Nervous
Diseases**

There are many diseases of the nervous system in which neuronal degeneration occurs for no known reason. In some of these conditions there is a strong hereditary factor, whereas in others the degeneration is probably due to slow virus infection (*e.g.,* in kuru and Creutzfeldt-Jakob disease; see Chapter 12). A few common examples of degenerative nervous diseases will be described.

1. Alzheimer's Disease. Deterioration of intellectual capacity (called dementia) is one of the great problems facing modern society, since it places a great financial as well as emotional burden on the family, the health services, and society as a whole. Dementia affects one person in every six over the age of 65 years, and the most common cause is Alzheimer's disease. Early signs are inability to learn new material and loss of short-term memory. In due course there is relentless loss of intellect, mental ability, and physical capability. This results in death from intercurrent infection or other complication of the bedridden state. Pathologically the brain shows loss of neurons and in addition "senile plaques," which include microscopic deposits of amyloid material. The cause of Alzheimer's disease is unknown, and among the many suggested possibilities are chronic poisoning with aluminum and infection with some slow virus.

2. Senile Dementia.   Cerebral atrophy with compensatory dilatation of the ventricles is a common event in old age and is the second most common cause of dementia. Sometimes it is combined with Alzheimer's disease.

3. Parkinson's Disease.   This common disease is due to selective degeneration of neurons in the substantia nigra. Axons from this part of the brain pass to the basal ganglia and influence them by releasing dopamine. Release of the basal ganglia from this influence results in the symptoms of Parkinson's disease. The patient's muscles become rigid, the face is expressionless, and movement becomes difficult. A fine tremor completes the picture; "pill rolling" movements of the fingers are characteristic. As noted by Parkinson in his original description in 1817, the patient tends to bend forward, so that when walking he or she has a tendency to change to a running pace. The senses and intellect remain unimpaired. The whole picture is termed the *extrapyramidal syndrome* and is also seen following encephalitis (postencephalitic parkinsonism), vascular ischemic episodes, and poisoning with carbon monoxide.

4. Huntington's Chorea.   Patients with this disease exhibit basal ganglia degeneration as well as cortical neuronal loss. Bizarre grimacing and uncontrolled irregular jerking movements (*chorea*) are combined with progressive dementia in this disease, which is inherited as a mendelian dominant trait.

5. Motor Neuron Disease.   Primary degeneration of the pyramidal tracts, the anterior horn cells, and their cranial equivalents can occur either singly or in combination to produce a variety of syndromes.

Epilepsy

The term epilepsy comes from the Greek and means a seizure. Epilepsy should be regarded as a syndrome rather than a disease entity because it is a symptom of an underlying brain disorder. It occurs in about 1 per cent of the population, and only about 5 per cent of the sufferers are mentally subnormal.

Epilepsy consists of a sudden, uncoordinated burst of impulses from a group of nerve cells. The seizure that results may be limited to a particular part of the brain, and this constitutes *partial,* or *focal, epilepsy.* On the other hand, the seizure may cause loss of consciousness and may be accompanied by widespread brain dysfunction; this is *generalized epilepsy.*

Focal Epilepsy

There are many areas of the brain in which epileptic discharges may originate, and there are therefore many clinical variations of local fits. If the temporal lobe is affected, the patient experiences hallucinations, which may be of taste, smell, hearing, or sight. Sometimes there is a feeling of great familiarity of the surroundings — this constitutes the "déjà vu phenomenon." In *jacksonian epilepsy* the motor areas of the brain are affected, and the patient experiences muscular twitching confined to a particular area (*e.g.,* the lips or a hand), and the twitching slowly extends to involve adjacent areas, *e.g.,* the whole limb or even the whole body. Sometimes after recovery from a jacksonian fit the affected part remains paralyzed — this is known as Todd's paralysis. In any type of partial epilepsy the focal discharging area may steadily extend its effect, so that the initial local disturbances progress to involve a wide area, and the condition then becomes an example of generalized epilepsy.

Generalized Epilepsy

In generalized seizures there is loss of consciousness; two major types are described.

Grand Mal Seizures. There may be a *prodromal phase* lasting several hours or even days when the patient becomes aware that an attack is imminent. Often a change of mood is the forerunner of the attack itself. Grand mal seizures may commence with some sensory manifestation (a strange taste or feeling, or seeing flashes of light) or some motor activity (movement of one part of the body), which is described as the *aura*. This precedes loss of consciousness by a few seconds. Then follows the generalized convulsion. At first the muscles exhibit *tonic contraction*, and as the chest muscles contract the patient may emit a characteristic cry as air is forced past the glottis. The tonic phase is followed by a *clonic phase*, in which the muscles exhibit powerful jerking movements. Movement of the jaw and tongue causes saliva to froth at the mouth, and at this stage, which lasts about half a minute, the tongue may be bitten and the patient may sustain damage. The final phase is one of relaxation, and the patient passes from a comatose state into normal sleep. As consciousness returns the patient may pass into a *postictal state* characterized by fatigue, headache, confusion, or automatic behavior. Transient neurological signs such as hemiplegia or other paralyses may be a feature. Amnesia for the period of the seizure and the postictal state is usual. During the tonic and clonic phases the patient is often incontinent of urine and less frequently of feces also.

Petit Mal Seizures. In petit mal seizures, sometimes described by the patient as "fainting turns" or "dizzy spells," there is a transient loss of consciousness. The patient develops a staring expression, and there may be an upward rolling of the eyes. A child engaged in some activity will discontinue it for a few seconds, and then resume the action when the seizure is ended as though nothing had happened. Petit mal is most common in children, and attacks may cease at puberty.

Causes of Seizures

Seizures can be induced in anyone if a powerful enough stimulus (*e.g.*, an electric current) is applied. There is indeed a threshold level for each individual, and any stimulus above this will result in an epileptic fit. In subjects with a "normal" threshold there are many conditions (*e.g.*, hypocalcemia) that will induce seizures. Sometimes a local brain lesion will lower the threshold, and this results in epilepsy. When such lesions can be recognized, the disease is labelled *symptomatic epilepsy*. When no cause can be identified, resort must be made to the term *idiopathic epilepsy*.

Diseases Causing Symptomatic Epilepsy. Among the numerous organic causes of epilepsy the following should be noted:

Cerebral Tumors. This is the commonest cause of symptomatic epilepsy, and in 10 per cent of the cases a seizure is the initial sign of the tumor. Glioma or metastatic carcinoma should always be considered as a likely cause of fits commencing in patients over the age of 40 years.

CASE HISTORY I. (See Figure 44–6.) The patient had had no previous history of epilepsy; he suffered his first attack at the age of 58 years. It started with twitching of the left foot, and then the involuntary movements spread to involve the whole leg, the left arm, and finally the whole body. With the onset of a generalized convulsion, the patient lost consciousness. This type of focal motor seizure that steadily extends to involve adjacent areas is called Jacksonian epilepsy. Examination of the patient at this time revealed no abnormal neurological signs. Radiography and electroencephalography showed no evidence of a focal brain lesion. Although a diagnosis of carcinoma of the lung was considered, sputum examination was negative for malignant cells, and a chest radiograph was normal. Nevertheless, the epileptic attacks continued. On several occasions the patient bit his tongue and was incontinent. Three months after the first attack, the patient suddenly developed a left-sided hemiplegia. Carotid artery thrombosis was considered, but arteriography failed to confirm the diagnosis. Radiographs, however, showed deformity of the right lateral ventricle. The patient died suddenly. A necropsy revealed a glioblastoma multiforme (see Fig. 44–6).

Cerebral Trauma.   Trauma may cause seizures immediately or after a period of time; in the latter event it is presumed that scarring of the brain is the cause.

Cerebrovascular Disease.   Fits may occur in cerebral hemorrhage and infarction.

Cerebral Infections.   Brain abscess and encephalitis may precipitate a seizure.

Metabolic Diseases.   Hypoglycemia (insulin overdose), hypocalcemia (tetany), uremia, and hypoxia are examples of metabolic disorders that may cause seizures.

Sun Stroke.   See Chapter 22.

Drug Intoxication.   Certain drugs such as strychnine cause convulsions, but seizures may also follow the withdrawal of a drug (*e.g.,* alcohol or barbiturates) in addicts.

Miscellaneous Brain Diseases.   There are many diseases associated with seizures, for example, cerebral palsy.*

Convulsions are more common in infants, presumably owing to the fact that the nervous system is immature and more unstable. Many children have convulsions during the eruption of teeth or with a sudden onset of fever. Hence, convulsions are encountered in children with pneumonia, otitis

---

*Cerebral palsy is a popular term for a condition in which there is a major disturbance of motor function that is generally nonprogressive and has been present since infancy. Upper motor neuron damage with spasticity is the dominant feature. Cerebral palsy is not a distinct entity, but is the end-result of many processes — inherited defect, infection, birth trauma, etc. The term has been adopted by fund-raising societies (*e.g.,* the United Cerebral Palsy Associations in the United States and the Spastics Society in the United Kingdom) and is unlikely to disappear readily from medical terminology.

Figure 44–6. Glioma of cerebral hemisphere. Sagittal section through the brain to show a large tumor in the right cerebral hemisphere. The center of the tumor is necrotic, and it shows dark areas that result from bleeding. Note that the tumor is not encapsulated and that its growth has distorted the lateral ventricles, particularly the one on the right-hand side. The expanding tumor has caused herniation of the hemisphere beneath the falx cerebri (arrow). The falx itself has been removed. (Courtesy of Dr. N. B. Rewcastle.)

Right   **Left**

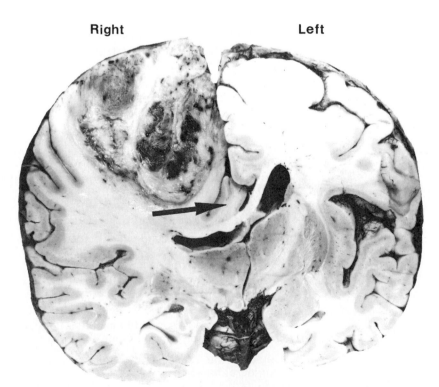

media, and the common viral infections. Such convulsions may be an isolated incident due presumably to some metabolic defect, or they may be the forerunner of more persistent seizures in later life. Seizures may occur following general anesthesia, and patients prone to epilepsy require supervision for several hours postoperatively.

Idiopathic Epilepsy.   When no morphological or biochemical cause of the seizures can be found the disease must be labelled idiopathic. Often when attacks begin in childhood no cause can be found, and it is possible that there is some specific genetic defect in cerebral metabolism. Patients with epilepsy may have their seizures precipitated by a variety of circumstances. Thus, hyperventilation can cause a fit, as may a flickering light or an emotional disturbance. If such triggers can be recognized, then both idiopathic and symptomatic seizures may be averted.

In the treatment of epilepsy a variety of drugs are in use. One of the commonest is phenytoin (Dilantin), and an important complication of the administration of this drug is gingival hyperplasia. Indeed, this occurs in about 50 per cent of patients taking this medication. Good oral hygiene reduces the effect; if marked hyperplasia occurs, the advisability of using some other drug should be considered.

Tumors of the Central Nervous System

Primary Tumors.   The most common type of primary tumor of the central nervous system is derived from glial tissue and is called a *glioma;* several types are described, the one occurring most frequently being derived from astrocytes (Fig. 44–6). Well-differentiated astrocytomas invade slowly, but the poorly differentiated tumors (Grades III and IV astrocytoma, also called glioblastoma multiforme) are more malignant and kill rapidly. Although all gliomas are locally invasive and may metastasize within the central nervous system, one curious feature of these tumors is that *none of them ever produces distant metastases.* In spite of this, the prognosis is usually poor, because gliomas are difficult to remove surgically.

The *meningioma* is a benign tumor arising from the meninges; it is therefore not a tumor of the brain itself. It is included here because the effects produced are very similar to those of a cerebral tumor. Meningiomas usually grow slowly and produce pressure atrophy of the underlying brain. They may remain symptomless, and it is not uncommon to encounter a meningioma as an incidental finding in an autopsy performed on a patient who has died of some other disease. Nevertheless, when symptoms occur the tumor should be removed. Occasionally growth is more rapid, and it may kill the patient by reason of its location or because of increased intracranial pressure.

Secondary Tumors.   Secondary tumors are common and may be responsible for the presenting symptoms of a disease. Carcinoma of the lung in males and carcinoma of the breast in females are the common primary tumors in these cases.

Review Questions

1. A patient is suspected to have an intracranial lesion such as a tumor or brain damage following a head injury. Explain why it is important to monitor each of the following:
   - (a) the level of consciousness
   - (b) the blood pressure
   - (c) the pulse rate
   - (d) the size of the pupils

2. Classify the causes of increased intracranial pressure. Explain why it can be dangerous to perform a lumbar puncture.

3. Compare the causes and effects of a subdural hemorrhage with those of an extradural hemorrhage.

4. List the common causes of a stroke. Distinguish them according to the differences in clinical presentation.

5. A child has fever and convulsions. Describe the symptoms that would suggest a diagnosis of meningitis. Discuss how the diagnosis may be confirmed.

6. Compare the causes and effects of grand mal seizures with those of petit mal seizures.

7. Name two common malignant tumors of the brain in males over the age of 40 years. Outline the possible effects of a tumor situated in the right frontal lobe.

Selected Readings

Escourolle, R., and Poirier, J.: Manual of Basic Neuropathology. 2nd ed. Translated and adapted by L. J. Rubinstein. Philadelphia, W. B. Saunders Company, 1978.

Leading Article: Chronic subdural hematoma. British Medical Journal, *1*:433–434, 1979.

Leading Article: Alzheimer's disease. British Medical Journal, *281*:1374–1375, 1980.

Schoene, W. C.: The nervous system. *In* Robbins, S. L., and Cotran, R. S. (Eds.): Pathologic Basis of Disease. 2nd ed. Philadelphia, W. B. Saunders Company, 1979, Chapter 31.

Simpson, J. A., and Mawdsley, C.: Diseases of the nervous system. *In* Macleod, J. (Ed.): Davidson's Principles and Practice of Medicine. 13th ed. Edinburgh, Churchill Livingstone, 1981, pp. 649–744.

Index

Numbers in *italics* denote illustrations; t denotes tables.

Abdomen, acute, 478–479, 497
  diseases of, 476–479
  distention of, in intestinal obstruction, 478
  hernias of, 477–478
  pain in, in toxemia of pregnancy, 536–537
Aberrance, 219
ABO blood groups, 369
Abortion, 537
  chromosomal abnormality and, 47
  syphilis and, 116
Abruptio placentae, 308–309, *309*, 506, 538
Abscess(es), 74
  amebic, 209
  cerebral, 630, *630*
  chronic, 108, 110
    apical, bacteremia and, 447
  in acute appendicitis, 475
  of lung, *442*, 424
  peritoneal, 476
  pyemic, 291
  subphrenic, *456*, 476
  with pancreatitis, 498
Acantholysis, 600, 601
Acanthosis, 592, *593*
Acetaminophen, toxic effects of, 53
Achalasia of cardia, 450
Acholuric jaundice, 355, 485
Achondroplasia, 41, 577
Acid(s), 273
  ascorbic, 302. See also *Vitamin C.*
  nucleic, role of, 27–28, *28*
  viral, 176–177
Acid-base balance, 273–276
  regulation of, kidneys and, 502–503
Acidemia, 274–275
Acidosis, 275
  diabetic, keto acids in, 270, 275
  hyperchloremic, 275
  lactic, 270, 275
  metabolic, 275–276
    in shock, 307
    with renal failure, 508
  renal tubular, 275
  respiratory, 275
Acinus, formation of, in normal gland, 17
  of liver, 480, *481*
  of lung, 415
Acne rosacea, 602
Acne vulgaris, 602
  in Cushing's syndrome, 557
Acrodermatitis enteropathica, 328–329
Acromegaly, 554, 555
ACTH. See *Adrenocorticotropic hormone (ACTH).*
Actin, 26
Actinic keratosis, 605
  in squamous cell carcinoma of external ear, 618
Addison's disease, 518–519, 556–557, *556*

Adenine arabinoside, in viral infections, 181
Adenocarcinoma, 241, *242, 243*
Adenohypophysis, 552, 553–555
Adenoids, swelling of, otitis media and, 619
Adenolymphoma, of parotid gland, 453
Adenoma(s), 230
  excess aldosterone secretion from, 615
  of adrenal, 557
  of bronchus, 438, *438*
  of kidney, 517
  of large intestine, 472, 473
  of liver, 494
Adenomyosis, 536
Adenosine diphosphate (ADP), platelet aggregation and, 282
Adenosine 3':5'-cyclic phosphate. See *Cyclic AMP.*
Adenosine triphosphate (ATP), energy storage by, 24, *25*
Adenosis, sclerosing, of breast, 542
Adenovirus, *178*, 185
  HeLa cells with, *179*
  sore throat due to, 446
ADH. See *Antidiuretic hormone (ADH).*
Adhesions, fibrous, 72
  in Crohn's disease, 467, 468
  peritoneal, 476–477
  uveal tract, 616
  with otitis media, 619
Adhesive mediastinopericarditis, 401
Adhesiveness, of cells, 21
Adipocytes, hyperplasia of, 323
ADP, platelet aggregation and, 282
Adrenal cortex, 556–559
  hypersecretion by, 557
  insufficient secretion by, 556–557
    with glucocorticoid therapy, 559
Adrenal glands, 554–559
  histoplasmosis of, *556*
  metastases to, 239
Adrenal glucocorticoids, 356, 558–559
Adrenal medulla, 555
Adrenocorticotropic hormone (ACTH), 551, 553
  Cushing's syndrome and, 557, 558, *558*
  ectopic syndrome, 557
  in Addison's disease, 556–557
Adrenogenital syndrome, 557
Adult hyaline membrane disease, 428–429
Adult respiratory insufficiency syndrome, 428–429
Aflatoxin, liver carcinoma and, 248
African trypanosomiasis, 213, 213t
Agenesis, 219
Agglutination, 119, *120*
Agglutinins, 119
Agranulocytosis, 359, 362
  in acute leukemia, 362
Air hunger, 275

Albers-Schönberg disease, 577
Albinism, 42
Albumin, 340–341
    separation of, 338, 339, *339, 340*
    tagging of, 65
Albuminuria, in glomerulonephritis, 509
    in toxemia, of pregnancy, 536, 537
Alcoholic hepatitis, 487
Alcoholism, and heart failure, 400
    and pancreatitis, 497, 498
    central nervous system in, 632, 635
    fat accumulation in, 53, 56, *56, 57*
    fat embolism in, 574
    liver in, 53, *489, 489*
    vitamin deficiency in, 327, 328
Aldosterone, 556
    excess secretion, in Conn's syndrome, 557
    sodium and water regulation and, 271, *271*
Alimentary tract, upper, diseases of, 444–453
Alkalemia, 274–275
Alkaline, phosphatase, bones and, 570
Alkalosis, 274–275, *276*
    metabolic 276
    respiratory, 275
Allele, definition of, 40
Allergic contact dermatitis, 131, 593, 594, *595*
Allergic encephalomyelitis, 139
Allergic granulomatosis, progressive, 375–376
Allergic reactions, to blood transfusion, 370
Alloantibodies, 356, 369
Allografts, 132–134
Allophenic animals, 256
Alopecia in chronic discoid lupus
    erythematosus, 373
Alpha particles, 260, 261
Alpha-1-antitrypsin deficiency, 431
Alpha-fetoprotein, 254, 526
Alveolar-arterial gas exchange, impaired, 418,
    418
Alveolus, of lung, 415, *415, 416*
Alveolitis, 425–429, *428*
Alzheimer's disease, 225, 632–633
Amantadine, in viral infections, 181
Amebiasis, 209–210
Amenorrhea, 534
Ames test, 249
American leishmaniasis, 214t, 215
Ammonia, liver and, 483, 486
Amniocentesis, in detection of fetal
    abnormality, 12–13, 50
Amniotic fluid embolism, 292
AMP, cyclic, in cholera, 462
Amphotericin-B, for fungal infections, 198
Ampulla of Vater, 499
    carcinoma of, 501
Amylase, 496
    blood level of, in pancreatitis, 497
Amyloid, 343–345, *343, 344*
    composition of, 345
Amyloidosis, 343–345
    in rheumatoid arthritis, 586
Anabolic phase, following injury, 302
Analgesic nephropathy, 514–516
Anaphase, 36
Anaphylactic shock, 124–125
Anaphylatoxins, 121
Anaphylaxis, 124–125
Anaplasia, 234, *235*
Anasarca, 276
Anastomoses, porta-systemic, 482–483
Anastomotic channels, 286

Anchorage dependence, loss of, in tumors,
    255
Ancylostoma duodenale, 205
Ancylostomiasis, 205
Anemia(s), 251–257, 252t
    bone marrow inadequacy, 357
    cardiac output and, 400
    classification of, 353
    clinical features of, 351–352
    fever with, 316
    hemolytic, 355–357
        penicillin and, 126
    high output heart failure in, 400
    in leukemia, 362
    in malabsorption syndrome, 470
    in myocardial infarction, 388
    iron deficiency, *350*, 353
        in Plummer-Vinson syndrome, 450
    leukoerythroblastic, 363
        from osteopetrosis, 577
        with bone marrow tumors, 585
    megaloblastic, 353–354
        bone marrow smear in, *354*
    pathological effects of, 351–352
    pernicious, 354
        degeneration of spinal cord with, 632
    postgastrectomy, 458–459
    posthemorrhagic, 303–304, 353
    sickle cell, 45, 355
    tumors and, 233
    with renal failure, 508
Anesthesia, heat-regulating mechanism and,
    318
Anesthetics, chronic bronchitis and, 433
Aneurysm, *407*, 411–412, *412*
    aortic, atheromatous, 407–408, *407*
        dissecting, 411–412, *412*
        syphilitic, 408, *409*
        thrombosis in, 283
        types of, *412*
    arteriovenous, 411
    berry, 626, *627*
    causes of, 411
    effects of, 411
    of left ventricle, 390
Angina pectoris, 286, 387
Angioedema, 279, 597–598
Angiogenic factor in tumors, 230
Angiomas, cherry, 604
Angiosarcoma, 243
Angiotensin, 297, 503
Angular stomatitis, 82, 83, 195, 327
Aniline dye workers, bladder carcinoma in,
    522
Anion gap, 270
Anions, plasma, 271t
Anisocytosis, 349, 354
Ankylosing spondylitis, 586–587
Ankylosis, bony, 585
    fibrous, 585
Ankylostoma duodenale, 205, 301t
Ankylostomiasis, 205
Anomalies, developmental, 218–222
Anorexia nervosa, 322, 555, 623
Antepartum hemorrhage, 537
Anthracosis, 437, *439*
Antibiotics, bacterial resistance to, 46
Antibodies, 115–128. See also
    Immunoglobulins.
    monoclonal, 118
    production of, theories of, 136–137

Antibody-dependent cell-mediated cytotoxicity, 124
Antibody-forming tissues, 113–114
Antidiuretic hormone (ADH), 503–504, 553
  fluid balance and, *271*
  water deficiency and, 272
Antigen(s), 113
  Australia, 189, 190
  identification of, *119*
  immunological tolerance to, 137–138, *138*
  of blood groups, 369
  transplantation, 134
    in tumors, 255
Antigen-antibody interaction, in acute inflammation, 64. See also *Immune-complex reactions.*
Antihistamine drugs, 75, 458
Antiseptics in slow wound healing, 100–101
Antistreptolysin O (ASO) titer, 383
Antitetanic serum (ATS), 152
Antitoxins, 112, 121
Anuria, 506
  vs. urethral obstruction, 520
Anxiety, heart failure and, 401
Aorta, aneurysm of, 411–412, *412*
    dissecting, 411–412, *412*
    syphilitic, 408, *409*
    thrombosis in, 238
    types of, *412*
  atheroma of, 404, *405, 407*
  atherosclerosis of, 404–408, *405–407*
  coarctation of, 381, 382
Aortic stenosis, calcific, 386
Aortic valve disease, 392–393, 408
Aortitis, syphilitic, 166
  aneurysm from, 408, *409*
Aphthous ulcers, 445
Aplasia, 224
  bone marrow, 362
Apocrine glands, 591
Apocrine metaplasia, in mammary dysplasia, 542
Apoferritin, 350, *352*
Apoplexy, cerebral, 626, 627–628
Appendicitis, acute, *67, 74,* 475–476, *475*
    infected emboli with, 291
Appendix, disorders of, 472–476
  mucocele of, 476
APUD system, of cells, 566
Aqueous humor, 613
Arachnoid, 624
Arboviruses, 186
Arbovirus encephalitis, 186
Argentaffin cells, 566
Arm, lymphedema of, 278
Arsenic, brain damage due to, 632
Arterial thrombosis, 286
Arteriolar sclerosis, 404
Arteriolosclerosis, 404
Arteriosclerosis, 403–404
  heart disease and, 387–390
Arteriovenous aneurysm, 411
  high-output heart failure and, 400
Arteritis, giant-cell, 409
  in polyarteritis nodosa, 375
  infective, 408
  rheumatoid, 408
  syphilitic, 408, *409*
  thrombosis due to, 285
Artery(ies). See also name of specific artery.
  diseases of, 403–412

Artery(ies) (*Continued*)
  hardening of, 403–404. See also *Arteriosclerosis.*
  obstruction of, ischemia due to, 290
  spasm of, 295–296
  structure of, 403
  thrombosis in, 286
Arthritis, 585–587
  chronic hepatitis and, 491
  in gout, 336
  rheumatoid, 585–586, *586*
    amyloidosis in, 344
    glucocorticoids for, 558
    necrobiosis in, 61
  suppurative, 585
  tuberculous, 585
Arthropods, as vectors of disease, 81
Arthus reaction, 126–127, *127*
  small vessel damage and, 410–411, *410*
Asbestos, cancer and, 267
Asbestosis, 437
  and pulmonary neoplasms, 438, 440
Ascaris lumbricoides, 201t, 205
Aschoff's nodule, 383
Ascites, 276
  in cirrhosis, 493–494
  with papillary cystadenocarcinoma of ovary, 531
Ascorbic acid, 326
Aseptic meningitis, 630
Aspergillus species, 198, 434
  otitis externa from, 618
Aster, in mitosis, 37
Asthma, bronchial, 433–434, *434*
    glucocorticoids for, 558
  bronchial obstruction with, 436
  cardiac, 398, 435–436.
  in carcinoid syndrome, 468
Astrocytomas, 636
Atheroma, 404, *405, 407.* See also *Atherosclerosis.*
Atherosclerosis, 404–408, *405–407*
  cerebral, 629
  effects of, 407–408
  etiology and pathogenesis of, 405–407
  lipoproteins and, 342
  peripheral vascular disease and, 411
  thrombosis due to, 286
  with diabetes, 335
Athlete's foot, 195
Atom(s), description of, 259–260, *260*
Atomic number, 159, 260
Atopic dermatitis, 126, 594–595
Atopy, 126
Atresia, 219
Atrial fibrillation, 393–394, *394*
Atrial flutter, *394,* 395
Atrial septal defects, 380, *381*
Atrial tachycardia, paroxysmal, 393
Atrophy, 223–225, *225*
  pressure, tumors and, 232
Auditory meatus, 618
Auditory nerve, schwannoma of, sensorineural deafness due to, 621
Auditory tube, 619
Australia antigen, 139, 190
Autoantibody(ies), formation of, 138–140
  in chronic hepatitis, 491
  in collagen vascular diseases, 374
  red cells and, 355–356
Autografts, 132

Autoimmune diseases, 137–141
  glucocorticoids for, 558
Autoimmunity, 138–141
Autolysis, 55, 58
Autophagosomes, 25, *27*, 57
Autoradiography, 12, *13*
Autosomes, 31
Axial regeneration, 91
Azotemia, 502

B cells, 114–118, *118*
  failure of development of, 134–135
  immunoglobulin production by, 115–118
Babinski sign, 624
Bacillary dysentery, 464, 470
Bacilli, acid-fast, 153
  gram-negative intestinal, 149
    anaerobic, 152–153
  tubercle, 153
Bacillus Calmette-Guérin (BCG), 123
  for cancer, 257
Backache, in osteoporosis, 579
  in pancreatitis, 497
Bacteremia, 84
  chronic apical abscess and, 447
  sequelae of, 88
Bacteria,
  putrefactive, in gangrene, 60
Bacterial pyrogens, 318
Bacteriolysins, 121
Bacteriophage, entry into bacterial cell of,
  175, *175*
Bacteroides, description of, 152–153, 153t,
  161
Bamboo spine, 586
Bancroft's filariasis, 207
Barr body, 31–32, *32*
Basal-cell carcinoma of skin, 244, *245*, *606*
Basal metabolic rate, 313
Base. See also *Acid-base balance*, 273
Basement membrane, IgG antibody in, *140*
Basophil, 358
Bedsores, 100, 410
Bee sting, 125
Behçet's syndrome, 445
Bence Jones protein, 583
Bends, 292
Beriberi, 326
Berry aneurysm, 626, *627*
Beta particles, 260, 261
Bicarbonate, 270, 270t
Bicarbonate-carbonic acid buffer system, 274
Bile canaliculi, *26*
Bile duct(s), 499
  obstruction of, 484–485
Bilharziasis, 201–202
Biliary cirrhosis, 494
Biliary colic, 500
Biliary tract, carcinoma of, 501
  disorders of, 499–501
Bilirubin metabolism, 352t, 483–484, 484t
Biochemical lesions, 53, 262
Biochemical profile, 19
Biological materials, chemical and physical
  analysis of, 19
Biopsy, 5
Birth-control pill, adenomas of liver and, 494
  vitamin B$_6$ deficiency with, 328
Bittner virus, breast carcinoma and, 251, 543
Blackhead, in acne vulgaris, 602
Blackwater fever, 212

Bladder, carcinoma of, 521–522, *521*
  diverticulum of, 520
  dysfunction, in multiple sclerosis, 631
  inflammation of, 515
  neurogenic, 520
  papilloma of, benign, 522
Blast transformation, 131–132
Blastema, in wound healing, 91
Blastomyces dermatitidis, 197
Blastomycosis, North American, 197
  of lung, *197*
  South American, 197
Bleeding, See also *Hemorrhage*.
  disorders, 365–367, 368t
    tests in, 367, *368*, 369
  during pregnancy, 537–538
  from cervical polyps, 533
  from nose, in lethal midline granuloma,
    375
  from papilloma of breast, 542
  from rectum, in intussusception, 477
  functional uterine, 533
  in diverticular disease, 472
  in dysentery, 470
  in portal hypertension, 482
  in stomach carcinoma, 460
  in ulcerative colitis, 470
  irregular vaginal, in carcinoma of
      endometrium, 536
    with uterine fibroids, 535
  spasm and, 295
  with carcinoma of cervix, 533
  with hydatidiform mole, 538
  with peptic ulcer, 456
  with stomach ulceration, 459–460
Bleeding time, 367
Blind loop syndrome, 469
Blindness, due to conjunctivitis, 612
  due to giant-cell arteritis, 409
  due to glaucoma, 613
  due to Graves' disease, 562
  due to Paget's disease, 581
  due to vitamin A deficiency, 325
  increased intracranial pressure and, 625
  night, 325
  with diabetes, 614–615
Blisters, 592, 599
  in bullous pemphigoid, 602
  in pemphigus vulgaris, 600–601, *600*
Block, heart, 395
Blood, calcium level of, 571
  capillaries, occlusion of, 409–411
  cells, red, 348–357. See also *Red cells*.
    white, 357–362. See also *White cells*.
  changes in, following hemorrhage, 304
  circulation of. See *Circulation*.
  clotting mechanism, 363–365, *364*
    defects in, 366–367
  creatinine level, 502
  disorders, 347–371
  fibrinolytic system, *282*
  flow, disturbances of, inflammation and,
      64–65, *65*
    thrombosis due to, 282–284, *285*
  flukes, 200–203
  groups, 369
    inheritance of, 40
    transfusion and, 369–370
  loss. See *Bleeding* and *Hemorrhage*.
  pH of, 274
  abnormalities of, 274–276
    maintenance of, 274
  shunting of, portal-systemic, 482–483

Blood (*Continued*)
  sludging of, 302, 308, 342
  spread of infection in, 88–89
  supply, in wound healing, 100
    poor, with fractures, 576
  urea level of, 502
  volume, restoration of, following
    hemorrhage, 303–304, *304*
Blood pressure, high. See *Hypertension.*
  intracranial lesion and, 624–625
  regulation of, hemorrhage and, 303
    kidneys and, 503
Blood transfusion, 370–371
  cross matching, 370
  hazards of, 370–371
  indications, 370
Blood urea nitrogen (BUN), 504–505, *505*
Blood vessels, abnormalities of, thrombosis
    due to, 285
  diseases of, 403–413
  small, diseases of, 409–411
  spread of infection in, 84, 88–89
Blue babies, 382
Blue bloaters, 433
BMR, 313
Body, fluids in, mechanism of control,
    276–279
  temperature of, abnormalities of, 314–320
    regulation of, 312–314, *314*
Boil, 84, 144, *145*
Bone(s), abnormalities of, developmental,
    576–577
    due to metabolic disorders, 577–579
  development of, 568–569
  fractures of, 574–576, *575*
  infections of, 572–574
  irradiation damage of, 264, 266
  ischemic disease of, 574
  metabolic functions of, 571–572
  metastases to, 239, *546*, 583–585, *584*
  osteomyelitis of, 572–573, *573*
  osteoporosis of, 574, 579, *580*
  Paget's disease of, 579, 581
  scan, technetium, 11, *11*, 12
  structure of, 569–570
  syphilis of, 574
  tuberculosis of, 573
  tumors of, 581–585, *582–584*
Bone marrow, aplasia of, 362
  inadequacy anemia of, 357
  irradiation of, 266
  tumors of, 582–583, *584*
Bony ankylosis, 585
Borrelia vincentii, 160, 166t
Botulism, 79
Bowel. See *Intestine(s).*
Bowen's disease, 252
  squamous-cell carcinoma in, 606
Boyden chamber, 68
Bradykinin, 76
Brain, abscess, from otitis media, 620
  damage to, due to metabolic disorders, 632
    fever with, 316
    pulmonary edema with, 436
  edema of, 625
  hypoxia and, 632
  in malignant hypertension, 298
  increased intracranial pressure, 624–626
  metastases to, 239, 636
  stroke and, 626–629, *628*
  structure and function of, 623–624
  trauma to, 626
  tumors of, *635*, 636

Breast, diseases of, 540–549
  dysplasia of, 541–542
  enlargement of, 541
  fat necrosis of, 541
  male, 548
  mastitis of, 541
  Paget's disease of, 547, *548*
  structure and development of, 540–541
  supernumerary, 541
  tumors of, benign, 542
    malignant, 542–547, *544, 545, 546*
Breath, fecal odor of, in liver disease, 483
Breathing, normal function, 415
  rate and depth of, 418–419
Brill-Zinsser disease, 171
Broad casts, in urine, 506
Brode's abscess, 573
Bronchial asthma, 433–434, *434*
  glucocorticoids for, 558
  vs. cardiac asthma, 397–398
Bronchiectasis, *422*, 424, 436
  bronchopneumonia due to, 422
  with carcinoid tumor of bronchus, 438, *438*
  with chronic lung infection, *424*
  with lung carcinoma, 438, *439*
Bronchitis, chronic, 429–430
  bronchopneumonia due to, 73, 422
Bronchopneumonia, 421–425, *422, 423*
  coliform, 149
  endogenous, 421–424
  exogenous, 424–425
  following bronchial obstruction, 436
  pneumococcal, 146–147, 420–421
  staphylococcal, 422
  streptococcal, 146
  tuberculous, 156, *157*
  with carcinoma of bronchus, 438
Bronchoscopy, in lung carcinoma, 439
Bronchospasm, in anaphylaxis, 125
Bronchus, carcinoid tumor of, 438, *438*
  obstruction of, 436–437
Brown tumors of osteitis fibrosa cystica, 578
Brucellosis, fever in, 315
Buerger's disease, 409
Buffer systems, in blood, 274
Bullae, of skin, 592
  in vesiculobullous diseases, 599–602
Bullous pemphigoid, 445, 602
BUN, 502, 504–505, *505*
Burkitt tumor, 244
Burns, thermal, shock following, 306–307
Burning on passing urine in urinary tract
  infection, 516
Burr cells, 349
Bursa of Fabricius, in lymphoid tissue
  development, 114, *114*
Butterfly rash in lupus erythematosus, 373

C cells, of thyroid, 559
Cachexia, malignant tumors and, 235
Calcific aortic stenosis, 386
Calcification, dystrophic, 59
  in pancreatitis, 497
  metastatic, 578
  with atherosclerosis, 405
Calcitonin, 571–572
Calcium, in malabsorption syndrome, 470
  metabolism of, and bone absorption,
    571–572
  normal blood level of, 571–572

Calculus, dental, 447
 urinary, 523
Calor, in acute inflammation, 63
Callus, 575
Campylobacter, food poisoning due to, 464
Canal of Schlemm, *611,* 612
Canaliculi, bile, 26
Cancer, 229. See also *Carcinoma* and
   Tumor(s).
 development of, 252–253
 fever in, 316
 immunological aspects of, 255
 incidence and causes of, 246–257
 migrating thrombophlebitis with, 288
 nature of, 253–255
 treatment of, 257
Cancer en cuirasse, 544
Candida albicans, 195
 in endocarditis, 385
 in stomatitis, 82, 83
Candidiasis, 195
Canker sores, 445
Capillaria philippinensis, 208
Capillaries, occlusion of, 409–411
Capillary fragility test, 367
Capillary hemangioma, 604
Capsid, 174, *174*
Capsomeres, 174–175, *174, 175*
Capsule, of joints, 585
Carbohydrate metabolism, disturbances of, in
   liver disease, 486
Carbon monoxide poisoning, 632
Carbonic acid, 272
Carbuncle, 144, *145*
Carcino-embryonic antigen (CEA), 254
Carcinogenesis, 54, 246–247
 theories of, 255–257
Carcinogens, chemical, 247–249
 physical, 249–266
 ultimate, 248
Carcinoid syndrome, 468
Carcinoid tumor, of bronchus, 438, *438*
 of small intestine, 468
Carcinoma. See also *Cancer* and *Tumor(s).*
 basal-cell, 244, *245, 606*
 bronchial obstruction from, 436
 definition of, 233
 dermatomyositis and, 375
 embryonal, of testis, 525
 epithelial, glandular, 240–241, *242, 243*
 mammary dysplasia and, 542
 mucoid, 241
 of ampulla of Vater, 501
 of biliary tract, 501
 of breast, 542–547, *544–546*
 of cervix, 533–534
 of colon, 472, *473, 474*
 of endometrium, 536
 of esophagus, 451
 of gallbladder, 501
 of kidney, 518–519, *518*
  fever with, 316
 of lips, *236,* 446
 of liver, *492,* 494–495, *494*
 of lung, 235, 438–440, *439, 441*
 of pancreas, 498–499
 of skin, basal-cell, 244, *245, 606*
  squamous-cell, 240, *241,* 605–607
 of stomach, 460, *460, 461*
 of thyroid gland, 565–566, *565*
 of tongue, 446–447
 of urinary tract, 521–522, *521*
 pathological fracture and, 575

Carcinoma (*Continued*)
 squamous-cell, 240, *241*
 transitional-cell, 241
 with ulcerative colitis, 471
Carcinoma-in-situ, 226, *232,* 253, *254*
 dysplasia of oral epithelium and, 446
Carcinomatous syndromes, 235
Cardia, achalasia of, 450
Cardiac asthma, 435–436
Cardiac output, relationship of to venous
   filling pressure, 396, *397*
Cardiac reserves, 395
Cardiac sphincter, 449
 impaired function of, 450
Cardiogenic shock, 388
Cardiomegaly, 223, *224*
Cardiomyopathy, 400
Caries, 447
Carotinoid pigments, 485
Caseation in tuberculosis, 154–155, *155*
Casts, in urine, 505–506
Cat-scratch disease, 109
Cataracts, 612
 with diabetes, 377
Catarrhal inflammation, 71
Cations, in plasma, 271t
Cavities, teeth and, 447
Celiac disease, 469
Cell(s), abnormal growth of, 215
 chromatin positive, 32
 connective tissue, 17–19
 culture of, 12–14
 damage to, 53–58
 death of, 57–58
 degeneration of, 54
 differentiation of, abnormalities of, 225–226
 division of, 36–37
 effect of virus on, 177–178
 embryology of, 16
 epithelial, 17, *20*
 epithelioid, 108–109
  in tuberculosis, 154, *154,* 155
 foam, 60
 germ, of ovary, 54
 giant, formation of, foreign bodies and, 108,
   109
  multinucleate, 31
 HeLa, with adenovirus, *179*
 LE, 374
 normal, structure of, *20,* 21–33
 plasma, development of, 114–115, *114*
  in inflamed gum, *110*
 pus, 73
 radiation and, 261–262
 red, 347–351. See also *Red cells.*
 small round, 110
 spheroidal, 241
 stable, 92
 stem, tumors of, 243–244
 totipotent, 19
 white. See *White cells.*
Cell membrane, 21–22
Cell receptors, 22
Cell transformation, 251
Cellulitis, 146
Central nervous system, 623–637
 degenerative diseases of, 632–633
 demyelinating diseases of, 631, *631*
 in cerebrovascular disease, 626–629, *628*
 in epilepsy, 633–636
 increased intracranial pressure and,
   624–626
 infarction in, 628–629, *628*

Central nervous system (*Continued*)
  infections of, 629–630, *630*
  meninges and, 624
  mctabolic disorders and, 632
  motor system and, 624
  poisons and, 632
  structure and function of, 623–624
  traumatic lesions of, 626
  tumors of, 636
  vitamin deficiencies and, 632
  wound healing in, 104
Central venous pressure, rise in, 396, *397*
Centrilobular emphysema, 430–431, *430–432*
Centromere, 36
Cercariae, 202, *202*
Cerebellar dysfunction in multiple sclerosis, 631
Cerebellar herniation, 626
Cerebral abscess, 630, *630*
Cerebral arteries, aneurysm of, ruptured, 626, *627*
Cerebral embolism, 384, 628
Cerebral hemorrhage, 626–629, *628*
Cerebral palsy, 635
Cerebral thrombosis, 627–629
Cerebrospinal fluid (CSF), 624
  in meningitis, pyogenic, 629–630
    viral, 630
  increased intracranial pressure and, 624–625
Cerebrospinal rhinorrhea, 629
Cerebrovascular disease, 626–629, *630*
Ceruminous glands, 618
Cervicitis with cervical erosion, 533
Cervix, cancer of, 533–534
  disorders of, 533–534
Cestoda, 200, 200t
Cestodes, 203–205, *203*
Chagas' disease, 213, 400
Chalones, 104
Chancre of syphilis, 162–163, *163*
Cheilosis, 327
Chemotactic factor, 67–68, 129
Chemotaxis, 67, 68, 76
Chemotherapy, viral, 181
Cherry angiomas, 604
Chickenpox, 186
  oral mucosa in, 445
Children, chronic renal disease in, 578
  cystic fibrosis in, 497
  epilepsy in, 636
  fever in, 317
  intussusception in, 477
  osteomyelitis in, 572
  otitis media in, 619
  protein-calorie malnutrition in, 322
Chinese liver fluke, 201
Chlamydia, 170
Chloramphenicol, pancytopenia due to, 362
Chloride, 270, 270t
Chlorothiazide, potassium depletion with, 273
Chlorpromazine, agranulocytosis from, 363
Cholangiocarcinoma, 495
Cholangitis, 494
  ascending, 501
Cholecystitis, 501
Cholecystokinin, 499
Cholelithiasis, 499–501, *500*
Cholera, 462, 464
Cholera infanticum, 463
Cholestasis, 485
Cholesteatoma, epidermoid, 620

Cholesterol, atherosclerosis and, 406
Cholesterol granuloma, 620
Chondrosarcoma, 581
Chorea, Huntington's, 633
Chorioadenoma destruens, 538
Choriocarcinoma, of placental tissue, 246, 539
  of testis, 526
Chorionic gonadotropin, 526
  with hydatidiform mole and choriocarcinoma, 539
Choroid, 611, *614*
  melanomas in, *615*, 616
Choroiditis, 616
Christmas disease, 366
Chromatids, 36
Chromatin, 27, 31
Chromosomes, 31–33, 36
  abnormalities of, diseases associated with, 47–50
  number of, alteration in, 48–50
  Philadelphia, 50
  ring, 38
  sex, 31
  structure of, abnormalities of, 50
Chyme, 455
Cicatrization, in chronic inflammatory lesion, 110
  of skin wounds, 102
  with peptic ulcer, 456–457
Cigarette smoking, effects of, 387, 405, 429–431, 446, 499, 522
Ciliary body, 610, *611*
Cimetidine, 458
Circle of Willis, berry aneurysm of, 626, 627
Circulation, collateral, 286
  disorders of, 280–298
  normal, 280
  overloading, pulmonary edema from, 436
    with blood transfusion, 370
  peripheral, failure of, 308
Cirrhosis, biliary, 494
  cryptogenic, 491
  hepatitis and, 490
  high-output heart failure in, 400
  micronodular vs. macronodular, 491
  of liver, 44, *488*, *489*, 491–494, *492–494*
    carcinoma and, 494–495, *494*
Cistron, 28
Claudication, intermittent, 286
  in peripheral vascular disease, 411
Clone, definition of, 13
  forbidden, 137
Clonorchis sinensis, 201, 201t
Clostridia, 150–151
  in gangrene, 60
  shock with, 306
Clostridium botulinum, food contamination by, 79
Clostridium difficile, 150, 467
Clostridium perfringens, 55, 151, 153t
Clostridium sporogenes, 151
Clostridium tetani, 151, 153t
Clostridium welchii, 55, 151, 153t
  hemolytic anemia from, 356
Clot, in phlebothrombosis, propagation of, 286–287, *287*
  vs. thrombus, 283
Clotting factors, liver disease and, 486
  platelets and, 281–282, 363–369
Clotting mechanism, 281, 363–365, *364, 365*
  defects in, 366–367
Clotting time, 367
Cloudy swelling, 56, *56*

Clubbing, of fingers and toes, in tetralogy of Fallot, 382
Coagulation, 281, 363–367, *364*, *365*
  disseminated intravascular, 356–357, 537
    small vessel damage in, 410
Coagulative necrosis, 58–59
Coarctation of aorta, 50, *381*, 382
Cobalamin. See *Vitamin B₁₂*.
Coccidioides immitis, 197
Coccidioidomycosis, 197
Cochlea, *619*, 623
Codons, 28
Coin lesion, of lung, 196, *197*, 220
Cold. See *Hypothermia*.
Cold antibodies, 356
Cold injury in infants, 319
Cold sores. See *Herpes simplex*.
Colic, biliary, 500
  renal, 522
Colitis, ulcerative, 470–471
    potassium depletion in, 273
  with renal failure, 508
Collagen, 17–18, *18*, *19*, 34–36, *36*
  changes in, 61
  elastosis of, 61
  formation of, in wound healing, 97–98
Collagen vascular diseases, 373–376
Collapsed lung, 436–437
Collateral circulation, 286
Colliquative necrosis, 59, 628
Colloid osmotic pressure, 276
Colon, adenomas of, 472, *473*
  carcinoma of, *242*, *243*, 472, *473*, *474*
  disorders of, 470–472
  diverticular disease of, 471–472, *471*, *472*
  in bacillary dysentery, 464
  in ulcerative colitis, 470–471
Coma, diabetic, 334
  hyperosmolal, 334–335
Comedo, 602
Compact bone, *569*, *570*
Complement, activation of, 67, 76, 119–121, *120*
  cleavage products of, 76, *120*, 121
  deficiency of, in angioedema, 597–598
  fixation of, 121, *122*
Complement-fixing antibodies, 119–121, *122*
Conductive deafness, 620
Condylomata acuminata, 605
Condylomata lata, 164
Congenital disease, definition of, 50
Congestive heart failure, 396, 398, 400
  bronchopneumonia following, 423
Conjugation, of bacteria, 46
Conjunctivitis, 612
  gonococcal, 147
  inclusion, 170
Connective tissue, cells of, 16–19
  metaplasia of, 226
  regeneration in, 130
  tumors of, benign, 230, 232
    malignant, 242–244
Conn's syndrome, 557
Consolidation of lung, *73*, *198*, *420*, *421*, *422*
Constipation, in carcinoma of large intestine, 472
  in Crohn's disease, 467
  in intestinal obstruction, 478
Constrictive pericarditis, 402
Contact dermatitis, 593–594
Contact inhibition, 98, 104
  and cancer, 255

Contraction, in wound healing, 92–93, *93*
Contracture of chronic inflammatory lesions, 110
Contrecoup injury, 626
Convalescence, following injury, 300–302
Convulsions, in eclampsia, 537
  in epilepsy, 633–636
  insulin, 635
Coombs test, 356
Cor pulmonale, 391–392, 433
Cornea, 611, *611*
  conjunctivitis of, 612
  dystrophy of, 612
Coronary arteries, spasm of, 388
  stenosis of, 387
  thrombosis of, 387
Corpus luteum, 530
Cortical necrosis, renal, *390*, 507, 537
Corticoids, 556
  overproduction of, 557
Corticospinal tract, damage to, 624
Corticotropin-releasing factor (CRF), 551
Cortisol, 556
Corynebacterium acnes, 602
Corynebacterium diphtheriae, 84, 149
Cotton-wool spots, 614
Cough, whooping, lymphocytosis in, 360
Coxiella burnetii, 172
Coxsackie viruses, 181
Cradle cap, 596
Creatine phosphokinase, 389
Creatinine, excretion of, 502
Creatinine clearance, 504
Creeping substitution, 133
Crescent formation, in glomerulonephritis, 512, 513, *513*
Cretinism, 561, *562*
Creutzfeldt-Jakob disease, 193
CRF, 551
Cri du chat syndrome, 50
Crisis, 315
  in lobar pneumonia, 421
Crohn's disease, 467–468, *467*, *468*
Cross-infection, 81–82
Cross-matching, for blood transfusion, 370
Cryoglobulin(s), 339
  precipitated, occlusion by, 410
Cryoglobulinemia, 339
Cryostat, 6
Cryosurgery, 320
Cryptococcosis, 196, 558
Cryptococcus neoformans, 196
Cryptogenic cirrhosis, 491
Cryptorchidism, 525
CSF. See *Cerebrospinal fluid (CSF)*.
Culture, tissue, 12–14
Cushing's syndrome, 557, 558
  from glucocorticoid therapy, 558
Cutaneous leishmaniasis, 214t, 215
Cyanide poisoning, 289
Cyanosis, central, in tetralogy of Fallot, 382
  in lung disease, 418
  peripheral, 330, 396
Cyclic AMP, 22, *22*
  cholera and, 462
Cyclical periodic edema, 279
Cyclitis, 616
Cyclopia, trisomy 18 in, *48*
Cyst(s), dermoid, 222
  developmental, 222
  epidermoid, *606*
  hydatid, *204*, 205

Cyst(s) (*Continued*)
  ovarian, 246, 531
  sebaceous, 606
  thyroglossal, 222
Cystadenocarcinoma, papillary, of ovary, 531,
  532
Cystadenoma, 230
  papillary, of ovary, 531
Cystic disease, of breast, 541–542
  of pancreas, 42, 496–497
Cystic fibrosis, 496–497
Cysticercosis, 204
Cysticercus, 204
Cystitis, 515
Cytolysosomes, 25, 27, 27, 57
Cytoplasm, 22–26
Cytosine arabinoside, in viral infections, 181
Cytotoxic drugs, gout and, 336
  pancytopenia due to, 362

Dandruff in seborrheic dermatitis, 596
Dane particle, 190, 190
Dark ground illumination, 5
Deafness, conductive, 620–621
    from earwax, 618
  from Ménière's disease, 621
  from otitis media, 619
  from otosclerosis, 620
  in Paget's disease, 581
  sensorineural, 621
Decompression syndrome, 292
Decontamination, 83–84
Defibrination syndrome, 366–367
Degeneration, Wallerian, 103
Deglutition, 444–445
  muscles of, paralysis of, 451
Dehiscence of wound, 101–102
Deletion, of chromosomes, 38
Dementia, in pellagra, 328
  senile, 633
Demolition phase, of wound healing, 97, 99
Demyelinating diseases, 630–631, 631
Dengue, 186
Density dependence, of cell growth, 105
  in cancer, 255
Dental calculus, 447
Dental plaque, 447
Deoxyribonucleic acid (DNA), chemical
    structure of, 27, 28
  in genetic engineering, 45–47, 47
  reduplication of, 37, 37
  tritiated thymidine incorporation into, 12,
    13
de Quervain's thyroiditis, 565
Dermatitis, 592–597, 593–596
  contact, 593–594
  in malabsorption syndrome, 470
  in pellagra, 328
  otitis externa and, 618
  seborrheic, riboflavin deficiency and, 327
  stasis, with varicose veins, 595–596
  x-ray, 214, 263
Dermatographism, 76
Dermatomyositis, 374–375
Dermatophytes, 194
Dermis, 591
  inflammatory reaction in, 597–598
Dermoid cyst, 222
Desert fever, 197
Desquamative interstitial pneumonia (DIP),
  427

Deuterium, 260, 260
Dextrocardia, 380
Diabetes insipidus, 504, 553
  in diseases of hypothalamus, 552
  water deficiency in, 272
Diabetes mellitus, 331–335
  clinical types of, 332–334
  complications of, 334–335
  hypoglycemia due to, 336
  polyuria in, 333, 504
  potassium depletion in, 273
  retinopathy in, 614–615
  surgery and, 335
  tuberculosis and, 158
  with hyperpituitarism, 554
Diabetic acidosis, keto acids in, 270, 275
Diabetic coma, 334
Diabetic microangiopathy, 335
Diarrhea, chronic, potassium depletion with,
    273
  in bacillary dysentery, 464
  in carcinoid syndrome, 468
  in carcinoma of large intestine, 472
  in cholera, 464
  in Crohn's disease, 467–468
  in inflammation of colon, 470
  in pellagra, 328
  in typhoid fever, 85
  in ulcerative colitis, 470–471
  infantile, 465
  metabolic acidosis with, 275
  pathogenesis of, 461–463
  renal failure and, 506
  traveller's, 465
Dicumarol anticoagulants, bleeding disorders
    due to, 366
Diet, fatty liver and, 489
  hyperlipoproteinemia and, 341–342
Diethylstilbestrol, vaginal carcinoma and,
    248, 250
Differentiation, 16
  loss of ability for, 19
Diphtheria, 84, 149–150
  shock in, 307
Diphtheroids, skin protection by, 83
Diphyllobothrium latum, 201t, 204
Diplopia, in myasthenia gravis, 589
Disaccharidases, 461
Dislocation, 585
Dissecting aneurysm of aorta, 411–412, 412
Disseminated intravascular coagulation,
    356–357, 537
  small vessel damage in, 410
Disseminated sclerosis, 631, 631
Distomes, 200, 201, 201t
Diuresis, osmotic, in diabetes mellitus, 333
Diuretics, potassium depletion with, 273
Diverticular disease of colon, 471–472, 471,
  472
Diverticulitis, 471–472
Diverticulum, of bladder, 520
DLE. See under Lupus erythematosus.
DNA. See Deoxyribonucleic acid (DNA).
DNA viruses, 176–177
Dolor in acute inflammation, 63
Domains, of immunoglobulins, 116, 117
Dormancy, of malignant tumor, 240
Down's syndrome, 49, 49
Dracunculiasis, 208
Dracunculus medinensis, 201t, 208
Dressler's syndrome, 401
Dropsy, 276

Drug(s), adverse reaction to, fever with, 316
    bone marrow aplasia from, 362, 363
    cytotoxic, gout and, 336
        pancytopenia due to, 362
    for shock, 310
    hemolytic anemia and, 355, 356
    hepatocellular dysfunction and, 486
    hypersensitivity to, 125–126
    interstitial nephritis from, 514
    interstitial pneumonia from, 427
    intrinsic asthma due to, 434
    megaloblastic anemia from, 354
    obstructive jaundice from, 485
    photodermatitis from, 594
    sensorineural deafness due to, 621
    skin eruptions caused by, 598
    toxic erythema from, 598
    vitamin B_6 deficiency with, 328
Dry beriberi, 327
Dry gangrene, 60–61
Ductular carcinoma, of breast, 543
Ductus arteriosus, patent, *381*, 382
Dumping syndrome, 459
Duodenum, 460
    ulcers of, 455–459. *456, 457*
Dura mater, 624
Dust, hypersensitivity to, 125
    inhalation of, pneumoconioses from, 437
Dwarf, achondroplastic, 577
    renal, 578
Dysarthria in multiple sclerosis, 631
Dyscrasia, 226
Dysentery, bacillary, 464, 470
    chronic amebic, 209
Dysmenorrhea, in pelvic endometriosis, 536
    in pelvic inflammatory disease, 532
Dysmyelinating diseases, 631
Dysphagia, 445
    causes of, 451–452
    from aneurysm, 411
    in Plummer-Vinson syndrome, 450
    with carcinoma of esophagus, 451
    with esophageal webs, 450
Dysplasia, 226, 252–253
    mammary, 541–542
    of cervix, carcinoma and, 533–534
    of oral epithelium, 446
    of skin, *252, 253*
Dyspnea, 418–419
    in rheumatic heart disease, 383
    paroxysmal nocturnal, 395–396, 435–436
    wheezing, in bronchial asthma, 433–434
Dysrhythmias, 393–395, *393, 394*
    heart failure and, 401
Dystrophic calcification, 59, 405, 497
Dystrophy, 226
    corneal, 612

Ear. See also *Deafness.*
    components of, 618, *619*
    external, 618
    glue, 620
    inner, 621
    Ménière's disease, 621
    middle, 149, 618–619
    otitis externa, 618
    otitis media, 619–620
    otosclerosis, 620
Eardrum, 618, *619*
Earwax, otitis externa from, 618

Ebb phase, following injury, 299
Eburnation, 587
Eccrine glands, 591
Echinococcus granulosus, 201t, 205
ECHO viruses, 181
Eck shunt, 486
Eclampsia, 537
Eclipse phase of viral reproduction, 176
Ectasia, of arteries, 407
Ectoderm, 16
Ectopia, 219
Ectopic beats, 393, *394*
Ectopic pregnancy, 537
    ruptured, fever with, 316
Eczema. See *Dermatitis.*
Eczema vaccinatum, 183–184
Edema, 276–279, *277*
    cardiac, 278, 397
    cyclical periodic, 279
    from hepatocellular dysfunction, 485–486
    from hypoalbuminemia, 341
    in anaphylaxis, 125
    in glomerulonephritis, 278, 512
    in myxedema, 561
    in nephrotic syndrome, 278, 509
    in toxemia of pregnancy, 536, 537
    lymphatic, 278
    nutritional, 278–279
    of brain, 625
    of optic disc, 614, 627
    of starvation, 322
    pitting, 278
    pulmonary, 435–436. See also under
        Lung(s).
    types of, 276–279
    with renal failure, 278, 507
    with varicose veins, 413
Ehlers-Danlos syndrome, 61
Elastic fibers, 18, 36
Elastosis of collagen, 61
Electrocardiogram, abnormal, *394*
    in myocardial ischemia, 388, *394*
    normal, *393*
Electrolyte(s), 270–271. See also *Fluid and
    electrolyte balance.*
    concentration of, 271t
Electromagnetic radiation, 261
Electron microscope, 8–10
Electrophoresis, 339, *339*
Elephantiasis, 207, 278
Embolism, 290–292
    amniotic fluid, 292
    cerebral, 384, 628
    fat, 292, 574
    following myocardial infarction, 390
    gas, 291–292
    infected, 291
    peripheral vascular disease and, 411
    phlebothrombosis and, 287
    pulmonary, 290–291, *291*
    saddle, *291*
    systemic, 291
    tumor, 292
    types of, 290–292
    with atherosclerosis, 408
Embryology of human body, 16–21
Embryonal carcinoma of testis, 525
Emigration of white cells, 66
Emotional state, alteration in, in multiple
    sclerosis, 631
Emphysema, pulmonary, 430–433, *430, 431,
    432*

Empyema thoracis, 108, 441, *442*
Enanthem, 183, 445
Encephalitis, viral, 630
Encephaloid carcinoma, 241, 544
Encephalomyelitis, allergic, 139
  postvaccinal, 184
Encephalopathy(ies), hepatic, 486–487, 632
  metabolic, 632
  Wernicke's, 326, 632
Endarteritis obliterans, 110, 404, 408
Endocarditis, bacterial, fever in, 317
    pulpitis and, 447
  in rheumatic fever, 383
  infective, 385–386, *385*
  nonbacterial thrombotic, 384
  Streptococcus viridans, glomerulonephritis
    and, 512
Endocervix, 533
Endochondral ossification, 569
Endocrine glands, 17. See also *Hormones*.
  disorders of, 550–567
Endocytosis, 21, 176
Endoderm, 16
Endogenous pyrogens, 69, 70, 318
Endometriosis, hormonal aspects of, 530
Endometrium, abnormalities of, changes in
    menstruation from, 534–535
  carcinoma of, 536
  hyperplasia of, menorrhagia and, 534
    ovarian tumors and, 535
Endoplasmic reticulum, 23–24, *24*
  proliferation of, phenobarbital in, 54, *54*
Endorphins, 22, 553
Endothelium, pavementation of, 65
Endotoxic shock, 307
Energy production, 24–25, *25*
Enkephalin, 553
Entamoeba histolytica, 209–210
Enteritis, 462–465
  regional, 467–468, *467, 468*
Enterobius vermicularis, 201t, 205–206
Enterococci, 146
Enterokinase, 460
Enteropathy, gluten-induced, 460, *469*
  protein-loss, hypoalbuminemia with, 341
Enteroviruses, 181–182
Envelope, of virus, 174, *174, 178*
Enzymes, induction of, by drugs, 54, *54*
  lysosomal, 25, 69
Enzyme-deficient red cells, 355
Eosinophil, 71, 111, 125, 302, *350*, 358, *358,
  359*
Eosinophil-chemotactic factor of anaphylaxis,
  125
Eosinophilia, 361
  in tissue necrosis, 58–59
Ependyma, 623
Epidermis, 590
  dysplasia of, 252–253, *252–254*
  hyperplasia of, 223
  in prevention of infection, 82–83
  tumors of, 230, *232*, 240, *241*, 604–607
Epidermoid cholesteatoma, 620
Epidermoid cyst, *606*
Epididymis, infections of, 525
Epigenetic theory, of neoplasia, 256
Epilepsy, 633–636
  jacksonian, 633
Epinephrine, 331, 550, 555
  pulmonary edema from, 435
Epithelial cells, 16–17, *20*
Epithelial nevus, 604

Epithelial pearl, 240, *241*
Epithelioid cells in tuberculosis, 154, *154,
  155*
Epithelium, changes in, vitamin A deficiency
    and, 323
  germinal, of ovary, 530
    tumors of, 531
  healing of, 95–96, *95, 98*, 102–103
  metaplasia of, 225–226
Epitopes, 113
Epstein-Barr virus, 188, 251
  infectious mononucleosis and, 188, 251,
    360
Ergot poisoning, arterial spasm with, 296
Erosions, cervical, 533
  of stomach, 459–460, *459*
Eruptions, drug, 598
  papulosquamous, 592, 597
Erysipelas, 146
Erythema, in urticaria, 597
  toxic, 598
Erythema multiforme, 601–602, *601*
Erythroblastosis fetalis, 356
Erythrocyte, 348. See also *Red cells*.
Erythrocyte sedimentation rate (ESR), 117,
  342–343
Erythroderma, hypothermia in, 319
Erythropoiesis, regulation of, kidneys in, 503
Erythropoietin, 351
Escherichia coli, 149, 149t
  gastroenteritis due to, 463, 465
  in acute appendicitis, 475
  urinary tract infection from, 514
Esophageal obstruction, water deficiency in,
  272
Esophagitis, 451
  with hiatus hernia, 451
Esophagus, disorders of, 449–452
  lower, ulceration of, with hiatus hernia,
    450–451
  tumors of, 451
  varices of, 482, *482, 483*
  webs of, 450
Espundia, 215
ESR, 117, 342–343
Estrogen, breast cancer and, 287
  effects of, 529, 530
  receptors of, 547
Ethionine, in proliferation of endoplasmic
    reticulum, 54
Eustachian tube, 619
Exanthem, 183, 445, 598
Exchange surface, of cell membrane, 21
Excoriations, 592
Exocervix, *533*
Exoerythrocytic stage in malaria, 210, *211*
Exons, 30, 31
Exophthalmos in Graves' disease, 562, *563*
Expressivity, in genetics, 42–43
Extradural hemorrhage, 626
Extrapyramidal syndrome, 633
Exudate, 316, 491
  cellular, functions of, 68–70
    variability of, 70–71
  formation of, 65–68, 277
Eye(s). See also *Blindness* and *Vision*.
  cataracts in, 612
  conjunctivitis in, 612
  development of, 610–612, *611*
  disorders of, due to vitamin A deficiency,
    325
    in diabetes, 614–615

Eye(s) (*Continued*)
  effect of raised intracranial pressure on, 625
    glaucoma in, 612–613
    in Graves' disease, 562, 563
    in rheumatoid arthritis, 583
    in shock, 309
    structure of, 611
Eyeworm, 201t, 208

F factor, in bacteria, 46
Face, moon, 557
  periodic flushing of, in carcinoid syndrome, 468
Faint, 305
Fallopian tubes, development of, 532
  inflammatory disease of, 532–533
Fallot, tetralogy of, 380, *381*, 382
Falx cerebri, 624
Famine edema, 278
Fasciola hepatica, 201, 201t
Fasciolopsis buski, 201, 201t
Fat, accumulation of, in cell, 56, *56*, 57
Fat embolism, 292, 574
Fat necrosis of breast, 541
Fatty casts, in urine, 506
Fatty change, in cells, 56, *56*
Fatty liver, *57*, 489
Fava bean, hemolytic anemia from, 355
Fc receptors, 116
Fecalith, in acute appendicitis, 475
Feces. See also *Constipation* and *Diarrhea*.
  in bacillary dysentery, 464
  in cholera, 460
  in Crohn's disease, 467
  in diverticular disease of colon, 471
  in intestinal secretory diarrhea, 460
  in malabsorption syndrome, 470
  in obstructive jaundice, 485
  in peptic ulcer, 456
  in ulcerative colitis, 470
  mass of, in acute appendicitis, 475
Feminization, with gynecomastia, with interstitial cell tumor, 526
Fernandez reaction, 159
Ferritin, 350, 352t
Fetal alcohol syndrome, 218–219
Fever, 314–319. See also *Temperature*.
  following injury, 302
  in aged patient, 315
  of unknown origin (FUO), 316–318, *317*
  pathogenesis of, 69, 318–319
  relapsing, 161
  rheumatic, 383
  scarlet, 446
  with blood transfusion, 370
Fibers, collagen, 34–35, *36*
  connective tissue, 17–18
  elastic, 36
  reticulin, 34, *35*
Fibrillation, atrial, 393, *394*
  ventricular, 393
Fibrin, 281, 363, *364*, 365
  formation of, 363, *364*, 365
  in acute inflammation, 66
Fibrinogen, 281, 338, 363–365, *364*, *365*
Fibrinoid necrosis, 61, 375
Fibrinolytic system, blood, 281, *282*

Fibrinous inflammation, 70, *71*
Fibroadenoma of breast, 542
Fibroblasts, in chronic inflammation, 110
  in granulation tissue, 94–95
Fibroid of uterus, 535–536, *535*
Fibroleiomyoma of uterus, 535–536, *535*
Fibrosarcomas, 242–243
Fibrosing alveolitis, 427
Fibrosis, 61
  in chronic inflammation, 110
  radiation, *265*
  replacement, 286
Fibrous ankylosis, 585
Filaments, intermediate, 26
Filariasis, 207–208, *201*
  lymphangitis with, 278
Fingers, clubbing of, in hypertrophic osteodystrophy, 581
  in tetralogy of Fallot, 382
Fistula, cardiac output and, 400
Flare in triple response to histamine, 75, *76*
Flashing lights in retinal detachment, 613
Fleas, as vectors of infection, 81, 171
Floaters in retinal detachment, 613
Floppy valve syndrome, 62
Flora, local, alteration of, 90
  resident, 83
Fluid(s), 271–272
  mechanism of control, 276–277
Fluid and electrolyte balance, disorders of, 269–276
Fluid compartments of body, 269–270, *270*
Fluid exudate, 65–66
Flukes, 200–203, 201t, *202*, *203*
5-Fluorouracil, action of, 53
Flutter, atrial, 395
Foam cells, 60
Focal glomerulonephritis, 513
Folic acid, deficiency of, megaloblastic anemia from, 353
  for red cell formation, 351
Follicle-stimulating hormone (FSH), 529, *552*, 553
Folliculitis, 84, 144, *145*
Fomites, definition of, 80
Food, hypersensitivity to, 125–126
Food poisoning, 465
  staphylococcal, 79, 145
Foreign bodies, as emboli, 292
  bronchial obstruction from, 436
  giant cell formation around, 108, *109*
  in wound, slow healing with, 100–101
Forme fruste, definition of, 43
Fractures, 574–576
  healing of, stages in, 575, *575*
  of skull, extradural hemorrhage from, 626
  pathological, 235, 575
Free radicals, 55
Freund's adjuvant, 131
Frigidity, 623
Fröhlich's syndrome, 552
Frostbite, 320
  small vessel damage from, 409–410
Frozen section technique, advantages of, 6, 7
FSH, 529, *552*, 553
Fungi, classification of, 194
Fungus diseases, 194–198
  with glucocorticoid therapy, 558
FUO, 316–318, *317*
Furuncle, 144, *145*
Fusobacterium fusiforme, in gangrene, 60

Galactorrhea, 554
Galactosemia, 42, 44, 53
Gallbladder, diseases of, 499–501
    distention of, in carcinoma of pancreas, 498
Gallstones, 499–501, *500*
Gametocytes of *Plasmodium falciparum, 212*
Gamma rays, 260–261
Gammopathy, monoclonal, *339, 340,* 341
    polyclonal, *339, 340,* 341
Ganglioneuroma, 246, 556
Gangrene, 60–61
    dry, 60–61
    gas, pathogenesis of, 85, 150–151
        shock with, 307
    in peripheral vascular disease, 411
    in thromboangiitis obliterans, 409
    of fingers, *295*
    wet, 294
    with diabetes, 335
Gangrenous inflammation, 60, 71
Gargoylism, 62
Gas emboli, 291–292
Gas gangrene, 85, 150–151
    shock with, 307
Gastrectomy, effects of, 458–459
Gastric juice, 454, 457–458
    components of, 455
Gastric ulcer, bleeding from, 455–460
Gastrin, 457
Gastritis, with renal failure, 508
Gastroenteritis, 463–465
Gastrointestinal tract, bleeding into, fever
        with, 316
    disorders of, 454–479
        defective iron absorption with, 353
        hypoalbuminemia with, 341
        with renal failure, 508
    irradiation damage to, 266
Gene(s), 28–31, *30*
    cloning of, 45–47, *47*
    codominant, 40
    definition of, 27
    derepression of, in tumors, 254
    dominant, 40–41, *41*
    histocompatibility of, 44
    mapping of, 14, 45
    mode of action of, 44–45
    polymorphism of, 45
    recessive, 40–42, *42*
    sex-linked, 42–43
    structural, 30
General paralysis of insane (GPI), 166
Genetic code, 28
Genetic counseling, 50
Genetic engineering, 45–47, *47*
Genetic theory, of carcinogenesis, 256
Genome, definition of, 44
Genotype, 40
Germ cells of ovary, 530
German measles, 185
    developmental anomalies and, 218
Germinal epithelium of ovary, 530
    tumors of, 531
GH, *552,* 554
Ghon focus, 156, *157*
GHRF, 551
Giant cell(s), formation around foreign
        bodies, 108, 109
    Langhans type, 154
    multinucleate, 31
Giant-cell arteritis, 409
Giant-cell tumor of bone, 581, *582*

Giardia lamblia, 210
Giardiasis, 210
Giddiness, in Ménière's disease, 621
Gigantism, 220, 554
Gingiva, normal, *448, 449*
Gingivitis, 447–448, *449*
    in herpes simplex, 445
    ulcerative, 60, 161
Gingivostomatitis, herpetic, 445
Glands, formation of, 17. See also names of
        specific glands, e.g., *Adrenal glands.*
Glaucoma, 612–613
    vs. iridocyclitis, 616
Glioblastoma multiforme, 636
Glioma, *635,* 636
Gliosis, replacement, 286, 628, *628*
Globulins, 341–342
    separation of, 338, 339, *339, 340*
Glomerular filtration rate, blood urea and,
        504–505, *505*
Glomerulonephritis, 509–513
    antigen-antibody complexes in, 140
    streptococcal, 146, 509
    types of, 511–513
Glomerulus, normal, 510, *513*
Glossitis, atrophic, in Plummer-Vinson
        syndrome, 450
    in malabsorption syndrome, 470
    in vitamin deficiency, 327, 328
Glucagon, 331
Glucocorticosteroids, 556, 558–559
    fat embolism and, 574
    for shock, 310
    in opportunistic infections, 90, 558
    wounds and, 93, *93*
Gluconeogenesis, 330
Glucose metabolism, 24, *25,* 330–331
Glucose tolerance test, 330
Glucose-6-phosphate dehydrogenase (G6PD),
        deficiency of, 42, 45
    anemia from, 355
Glue ear, 620
Gluten-induced enteropathy, 469, *469*
Glycocalyx, 32, 461
Glycogen oxidation, 24, *25*
Glycogen storage diseases, 57
Glycogenolysis, 330
Glycolysis, *25*
Glycoproteins, 34, 339
Glycosuria, 331, 503
    in diabetes mellitus, 333
    renal, 503
Goiter, 560, *560*
    in Graves' disease, 562
    in Hashimoto's disease, 564–565, *564*
    nodular colloid, 560, 561
    toxic nodular, 564
Goldblatt, 297
Golgi complex or apparatus, 25–26, *27*
Gonad(s), irradiation damage to, 263
Gonadotropin, 529
    chorionic, 530
        with hydatidiform mole and
            choriocarcinoma, 539
    deficiency, 554–555
    pituitary, *552, 553*
Gonadotropin-releasing factors (GRF), 551
Gonococcal epididymo-orchitis, 525
Gonococcal salpingitis, 532
Gonococcus, description of, *147,* 149t
Gonorrhea, 147–148, *148*
    prostatitis with, 526

Goodpasture's syndrome, 126, 509, *510*, 513
Gout, 108, 326
    fever with, 316
    urate stones with, 522
Graafian follicle, 530
Grading of tumors, 239
Graft(s), allogeneic, 132
    homovital vs. homostatic, 133
    syngeneic, 132
    tissue, 132–134
        rejection of, 132–133
Graft vs. host reaction, 138
Gram-negative coliforms, shock from, 306,
    307
Gram-negative intestinal bacilli, 149, 149t
    anaerobic, 152–153
    urinary tract infection from, 514–516
Grand mal seizures, 634
Granular casts, 505–506
Granulation tissue, formation of, 93–95, *96*,
    97–99, *97*
        in chronic inflammation, 107t, 108,
        109–110
    protection against infection, in wound
        healing, 99
Granulocytes, 358. See *White cells.*
Granuloma, 108–109
    cholesterol, 620
    lethal midline, 375
    noncaseating tuberculoid, 108–109, *154*
    paracoccidioidal, 197
Granulomatosis, progressive allergic, 375–376
    Wegener's, 376
Granulomatous disease, chronic, 70
Granulomatous inflammation, 108–109
Graves' disease, 562–564, *563*
GRF, 551
Griseofulvin for fungal infection, 195
Ground substance, 33–34
    changes in, 61–62, 66
Growth, disorders of, 215–226
Growth hormone (GH), 331, *552*, 554
    hyperpituitarism and, 554
    hypopituitarism and, 554
Growth hormone-releasing factor (GHRF),
    551
G6PD deficiency, anemia from, 42, 45, 355
Guinea worm, 208
Gummas in syphilis, 165
Gynecomastia, 49, 526, 548

Hageman factor, clotting mechanism and,
    363–364, *364*, 365
Hair, loss of, in chronic discoid lupus
    erythematosus, 373
Hair follicles, 591
Halitosis, 447
Halos around lights in glaucoma, 613
Halothane, liver damage from, 487
Hamartomas, 220–222, *220*, *221*
    melanotic, 603–604, *603*, *604*
    vascular, 604
Hansen's disease, 159–161. See also *Leprosy.*
Haptens, 113
Haptoglobin, 351, 352t
Harvey, William, 280
Hashimoto's disease, 139, 564–565, *564*
Haversian systems, 569, *569*
Hay fever, 126
Head. See also *Central nervous system.*
    injury to, 626

Headache, in meningitis, 629
    in Paget's disease, 581
    in toxemia, 536
    with increased intracranial pressure, 625
Healing, by primary intention, 95, 97–98, *98*
    by secondary intention, 98–100, *98*
Heart
    in calcareous aortic stenosis, 386
    in endocarditis, infective, 385–386
        thrombotic, 384
    in myocardial infarction, 387–390, *389*, *390*,
        394. See also *Myocardial infarction.*
    in shock, 308
    rate, intracranial lesion and, 324–325
    regeneration in, 103
    reserves, 395–396
    Starling's law of, 396
    thrombosis in, 288, *384*, 390, *390*
    valves, in carcinoid syndrome, 468
        in infective endocarditis, 385–386, *385*
        in rheumatic fever, 383, *384*
        prosthetic, endocarditis with, 386
    ventricle, left, aneurysm of, 390
Heart arrest, ischemia due to, 290
    metabolic acidosis with, 275
Heart attack, 379. See also *Myocardial
    infarction.*
Heart block, 395
Heart diseases, 379–402
    arteriosclerotic, 387–392
    congenital, 379–382, *381*
    rheumatic, 383, *384*
    valvular, 392–393, 398, 400
Heart dysrhythmias, 393–395, *394*
Heart failure, 379, 395–401, *399*
    congestive, 398, 400
    from hypertension, 298
    from myocardial disease, 400
    high output failure in, 400
    in myocardial infarction, 388
    left ventricular, 397–398
    pulmonary edema with, 435–436
    right ventricular, 396–397
        chronic bronchitis, 433
Heartburn, in esophagitis, 451
Heat cramps, 315
Heat exhaustion, 315
Heat loss, areas of, 313
Heat stroke, 314
Heat-regulating mechanisms, 313–314, *314*
Heberden's nodes, 587
HeLa cells, 14, 176, 179
    with adenovirus, *179*
Helix of virus, 174–175, *175*
Helminths, classification of, 200, 201t
Helper cells, 130, 135
Hemangioma, 220, *220*, 221
    capillary, 604
    of liver, 481, 494
Hemarthrosis, 302
    in hemophilia, 366
Hematemesis, 302
    from esophageal varices, 482
    in cirrhosis, 491
    in portal hypertension, 482
    with peptic ulcer, 456, 459
Hematocele, 526
Hematocrit reading, 348–349, 349t
Hematoma, 302
    fracture repair and, 575, *575*
    of central nervous system, 625
    subdural, 626
Hematopoiesis, 347

Hematoxylin and eosin (H & E), 5
Hematuria 302, 505
  fat embolism and, 292
  from calcium oxalate stones, 522
  in benign prostatic enlargement, 527
  in carcinoma of kidney, 518
  in glomerulonephritis, 509, 512
  in schistosomiasis, 201–202
  in urinary tract infection, 516
Heme formation, 350, 352t
Hemianopsia, bitemporal, with pituitary
  tumors, 554
Hemiplegia, arteriosclerosis and, 298
  with stroke, 629
Hemoconcentration, thrombosis due to, 286
Hemoglobin, buffering and, 274
  metabolism of, 350, 351, 352t
  variants of, 45
Hemoglobin C, anemia from, 355
Hemoglobinemia, 351, 352t, 505
Hemoglobinopathies, 44–55, 355
Hemoglobinuria, 351, 352t
Hemolymph nodes, electron micrograph of,
  9, 10
Hemolysin, 121
Hemolysis, acute, fever with, 316
Hemolytic anemia, 355–357
Hemolytic disease of newborn, 348, 356
Hemolytic jaundice, 485
Hemolytic uremic syndrome, 357
Hemopericardium, 302
Hemoperitoneum, 302
Hemophilia, 366
Hemophilus influenzae, meningitis due to,
  629
  otitis media due to, 619
Hemophilus pertussis, 123
Hemoptysis, 302
  in heart failure, 398
  in lung carcinoma, 438, 439
  in mitral stenosis, 383
Hemorrhage. See also *Bleeding.*
  acute, causes of, 302–303
    effects of, 303–304, *304,* 306, *306*
  anemia from, 352t, 353
  antepartum, 537
  cerebral, 626–629, *628*
  extradural, 626
  fever with, 316
  from hypertension, 297
  from ruptured aneurysm, 411
  in ectopic pregnancy, 537
  into brain, 625
  petechial, fat embolism and, 292
    vasculitis and, 410–411
    with small vessel disease, 409
  shock following, 305–306
  subarachnoid, 626
  subdural, 626
  tumors and, 235
  with atherosclerosis, 404
  with brain injuries, 626
  with peptic ulcer, 456, 459
Hemorrhagic disease of newborn, 366
Hemorrhagic fevers, 186
Hemorrhagic inflammation, 70
Hemorrhagic shock, 305–306
Hemosiderin, Prussian blue reaction for, 6–7,
  7
Hemosiderosis, transfusional, 371
Hemostatic plug, 365
Hemothorax, 302

Hepatectomy, partial, liver regeneration after,
  102
Hepatic artery, 480
Hepatic encephalopathy, 486, 636
Hepatic necrosis, 487–488, *487, 488*
Hepatitis, alcoholic, 489
  chronic, 490–491
  lupoid, 491
  viral, 189–192, *190, 191,* 490
Hepatization of lung in lobar pneumonia, 421
Hepatocellular failure, 485–487
Hepatocellular jaundice, 485
Hepatoma, 495
Hepatorenal syndrome, 487
Hercules, infantile, 557
Hernia, 477–478
  hiatus, 450, *450*
  incisional, 102
  inguinal region and, 524
Herniation, central nervous system, 625–626,
  635
Herpes simplex, 8–10, 87, 178, *178,* 188
  latent, 178
Herpes viruses, 186–188
  carcinoma of cervix and, 251, 533
Herpes zoster, 186–188, *187*
  glucocorticoids for, 558
Herpetic whitlow, 188
Herxheimer reaction, 164
Heterografts, 134
Heteroplasia, 219–220
Heterotopia, 219
Heterozygote, 40
Hexose monophosphate shunt, 25, 70
Hiatus hernia, 450, *450*
Histamine, in acute inflammation, 75
  in anaphylactic shock, 124–125
Histiocytic lymphoma, 244
Histochemistry, 6
Histocompatibility (HLA) genes, 134
Histopathology, 4
Histoplasma capsulatum, 196
Histoplasmin test, 196
Histoplasmosis, 196–197, *197,* 518–519
  of adrenal glands, 556
Hives, 597–598
HL-A system, 134
Hodgkin's disease, 243–244
  fever with, 316
  tuberculosis in, 158
Homeostasis, acid-base balance and, 274
  glucose metabolism and, 330
  temperature maintenance and, 312
Homografts, 132–134
Homozygote, 40
Hookworm disease, 205
Hormones, 550. See also name of specific
    hormone.
  breast carcinoma and, 543, 547
  mode of action of, 550–551
  oversecretion of, tumors and, 233, 236
  tumors dependent upon, 250
Hospital infection, 81–82
Host, definitive vs. intermediate, 200
Human chorionic gonadotropin (HCG), 530,
  539
Humor, aqueous, 611–612, *611*
Hunger, air, 275
Huntington's chorea, 633
Hurler's syndrome, 62
Hyaline, in cellular degeneration, 57
Hyaline casts, 505

Hyaline membrane, in lung, 419, 426, *426*, 428

Hyaline membrane disease, in adults, 426, *426*

in newborn, 419

Hyalinization, 61

Hyaluronic acid, 34

Hyaluronidase, 34, 89

Hybridization of cells, 14

Hybridoma, 14, 118

Hydatid disease, *204*, 205

Hydatidiform mole, 538, *538*

Hydrocele, 526

Hydrocephalus, pyogenic meningitis and, 629

Hydrochloric acid, gastric, 83, 455, 457

Hydrocortisone (cortisol), 556. See also *Glucocorticosteroids.*

Hydrogen isotopes, 259–260, *260*

Hydronephrosis, 519, 520, *521*

in ureteric reflux, 520

Hydropericardium, 276

Hydrophobia, 191

Hydropic degeneration, 56, *56*

Hydrosalpinx, 532

Hydrothorax, 276, 440

Hydroureter, 519

in ureteric reflux, 520

Hydroxyapatite, 569

Hydroxybutyrate dehydrogenase (HBD), in blood, 58

Hydroxyproline, in collagen, 35

5-Hydroxytryptamine (5-HT), platelet adhesiveness and, 282

Hyperalbuminemia, 341

Hypercalcemia, 577, 578

calcitonin and, 572

from hyperparathyroidism, 577, 578

from vitamin D, 571

urinary calculi with, 522

Hypercalciuria, 571, 577

from vitamin D, 571

Hypercapnia, 417

Hyperchloremic acidosis, 275

Hyperchlorhydria, 458

Hypercholesterolemia, and atherosclerosis, 406

in obstructive jaundice, 485

Hyperchromatism, in malignant tumors, 234, 235

Hyperemesis gravidarum, 536

Hyperemia, 64

Hypergammaglobulinemia, 341

in chronic hepatitis, 490

in lepromatous leprosy, 160

Hyperglycemia, following injury, 299–300, 300t

in Cushing's syndrome, 557

in diabetes mellitus, 333

Hyperkalemia, in Addison's disease, 557

with renal failure, 508

Hyperkeratosis, 592, *594*

Hyperlipoproteinemia, 341–342

Hypernephroma, 518–519, *518*

Hyperosmolal coma, in diabetes mellitus, 334–335

Hyperparathyroidism, 522, 577–578

bone abnormalities due to, 578

Hyperphosphatemia, in chronic renal disease, 578

Hyperpigmentation, of skin, in Addison's disease, 557

in Nelson's syndrome, 554

radiation and, 163

Hyperpituitarism, 554

Hyperplasia, 222–223

Hyperpnea, 418

Hyperpyrexia, 314

malignant or fulminating, 318–319

Hypersensitivity, 112, 124–128, 130–132

cell-mediated, 130–132

immunoglobulins and, 124–128, *127–128*

in chronic inflammation, 106–137

Hypersplenism, 363

in portal hypertension, 483

Hypertension, systemic, 296–298

arteriolosclerosis with, 404

effects and complications of, 297–298

from pheochromocytoma, 555–556

gout and, 336

in Cushing's syndrome, 557

in toxemia of pregnancy, 536, 537

kidneys and, 508

malignant, 298

pathogenesis of, 296–297

portal, 482–483

pulmonary, 380, 382, 391–392

renal lesions of, 514

types of, 296

with glucocorticoid therapy, 559

with pyelonephritis, 516

with chronic renal failure, 508

Hypertensive retinopathy, 297, 614

Hyperthyroid storm, 562

Hyperthyroidism, 562–564, *563*

Hypertrophic osteoarthropathy, 581

Hypertrophy, 223, *224*, 527

of breast, 541

Hyperuricemia, 336

Hyperventilation, hysterical, 622

respiratory alkalosis and, 275

Hyphae, 194

Hypoalbuminemia, 340–341

erythrocyte sedimentation rate and, 342

in nephrotic syndrome, 508

with hepatocellular dysfunction, 485–486

Hypocalcemia, 497

vs. respiratory alkalosis, 275

Hypofibrinogenemia, 366

Hypoglycemia, 233, 336

encephalopathy due to, 632

following gastrectomy, 459

in Addison's disease, 556–557

in hypopituitarism, 554

Hyponatremia, in Addison's disease, 557

Hypophysis, disorders of, 552–555

Hypopituitarism, 554–555

hypothermia in, 319

Hypoplasia, 219, 224

Hypoproteinemia, in nephrotic syndrome, 508

Hypostatic pneumonia, 423

Hypotension, in Addison's disease, 556, 557

in myocardial infarction, 388

Hypothalamus, 551–552

cycling center in, 530

relationship with pituitary gland, *552*

temperature-sensitive area of, 313

Hypothermia, 319–320

in adults, 319

in infants, 319

in skin diseases, 319

induced, 320

local, 320

with starvation, 322

Hypothyroidism, 560–561, 562

Hypoventilation, respiratory acidosis and, 275

Hypoxemia, 436
Hypoxia, 288–289
  brain damage due to, 632
  chronic, polycythemia secondary to, 357
  erythropoietin and, 351
  ischemia due to, 289
  with hypercapnia, 416–417
  without hypercapnia, 418
Hypoxic spells, in tetralogy of Fallot, 382
Hysterical hyperventilation, 622

Icterus, 483. See also *Jaundice.*
Idiopathic, definition of, 4
IgA, 118, *118*
IgD, 118, *118*
IgE in anaphylaxis, 115, *118*
IgG, 117, *118*
IgM, 118, *118*
Ileum, 466
Ileus, 478
  meconium, 479
Illumination, dark ground, 5
Immersion hypothermia, 319
Immobilization, effects of, on bone, 574
Immune adherence, 121
Immune complex disease, glomerulonephritis in, 508
Immune-complex reactions, 126–128, *127, 128*
  urticaria, 597, 598
Immune response, 112–142
  cell-mediated, 28–132
  functional steps in, 135–136
  in cancer, 255
  in chronic inflammation, *110,* 111
  to tuberculosis, 158
  to viral infections, 180
Immunization, active vs. passive, 123
  against living organisms, 123
  for poliomyelitis, 182
  for rabies, 192
  for smallpox, 183–184
Immunoblasts, 131
Immunoelectrophoresis, 339, *340*
  countercurrent, 119
Immunofluorescence, in renal disease, 510
Immunoglobulin(s), 115–121
  actions of, 119–121, *120*
  against cancer, 255
  classes of, 117–118, *118*
  detection of, 119–121, *119, 120,* 122t
  domains of, 116, 117
  effects of, 122–128
  in graft rejection, 132–133
  organ-specific vs. non–organ-specific, 139, 140
  structure of, 115–118, *116, 117, 118*
Immunological deficiency diseases, 135–135
Immunological memory, 115
Immunological tolerance, 137–138, *138*
Immunoperoxidase technique, 7–8
Impetigo, staphylococcal, 144, *145*
  streptococcal, 146
Impotence, 623
Inborn errors of metabolism, 44
Incarcerated hernia, 477
Incision, healing of, 95–98, *98*
Inclusion body, 177
Inclusion conjunctivitis, 170
Incus, 619, *619*

Infant(s), beriberi in, 327
  congenital heart disease in, 379–382
  defective iron absorption in, 353
  diarrhea in, 463, 464, 465
  hemolytic jaundice in, 485
  hypothermia in, 319
  scurvy in, 325
  starvation in, 322
Infantile eczema, 595–596
Infantile Hercules, 557
Infarction, 286, 292–294, *293, 294*
  definition of, 59
  fever with, 316
Infection(s), 79–90
  anaerobic, 150–153
    of wound, 153t
  body defenses against, 82–84
  chlamydial, 170–171
  clostridial, 150–152
  congenital, 80
  definition of, 80
  diabetes mellitus and, 335
  fever due to, 315
  fungal, 194–198
  gonococcal, 147–148
  helminthic, 200–208
  hepatic, 481
  hospital, 81–82
  meningococcal, 148
  mycobacterial, 153–161
  mycoplasmal, 169
  nosocomial, 81–82
  opportunistic, 90, 198
  patterns of, 84–87
  pneumococcal, 146–147
  protozoal, 209–216
  pyogenic, 143–149, 149t
  rickettsial, 171–172
  shock from, 306, 307
  sources of, 80–81
  spread of, 81–90, 87
  staphylococcal, 144–146, *145*
  streptococcal, 146
  tuberculous, 153–158
  tumors and, 235
  viral, 173–193. See also *Viral infections.*
  with blood transfusion, 370
Infectious mononucleosis, lymphocytosis in, 360
  sore throat due to, 446
Infective endocarditis, 385–386, *385*
Inflammation, acute, 63–78
  causes of, 63–64
  chemical mediators of, 75–78
  sequelae of, 72–75, 72
  variations of, 70–71
  chronic, 75, 106–111
  causes of, 106–107
  components of, 107t
  suppurative, 71
  types of, 127–131
  definition of, 75
  granulomatous, 108–109
  in necrosis, 59
  ionizing radiation, 263
  shock with, 347
Influenza, 184–185
Infundibular stem, 553
Inheritance, intermediate, 43
  Mendel's laws of, 40
  of dominant disease, 40–41, *41*
  of recessive disease, 41–42, *42*

Initiation, in carcinogenesis, 274
Injury, changes following, 299–311
Inotropic effect, 396
Inspissation, 74
Instructional theory of antibody production, 136
Insulin, convulsions, 635
  overdosage, hypoglycemia due to, 336
  overproduction, by tumor, 233
  secretion and action of, 331
Insulin-dependent diabetes mellitus, 331–333, 334t
Insulin-independent diabetes mellitus, 333–334, 334t
Intercellular space, 33
Interferon, 130, 180–181, 319
  use in cancer therapy, 257
Intermediate tumors, 244
Intermittent claudication, 286, 411
Interstitial cell tumor of testis, 526
Intestinal angina, 466
Intestine(s). See also *Gastrointestinal tract.*
  gangrene of, 60
  in shock, 309
  large, disorders of, 470–472. See also *Colon.*
    resident flora, 83
    obstruction of, 478
    in pelvic inflammatory disease, 532
  small, Crohn's disease of, 467–468, *467, 468*
    disorders of, 460–470
    in cholera, 462, 463, 464
    in malabsorption syndrome, 468–470, *469*
    inflammations of, 463–465
    normal mucosa of, 17, *18,* 462
    tumors of, 468
    ulceration of, in typhoid fever, 85
    volvulus of, 471
Intoxication, infection vs., 79
  meat, 486
  water, 272
Intracranial pressure, increased, 624–626
Intraepidermal vesicles, 600–601
Intrinsic factor, 351, 455
Introns, *30,* 31
Intussusception, 477
Involucrum, 572, *573*
Involution, 224
Iodine deficiency, goiter due to, 560
  hypothyroidism due to, 561
5-Iodo-2-deoxyuridine (5-IDU), in viral infections, 181
Ionizing radiation(s), 259–268
Iridocyclitis, 616
Iris, 610, *611*
Iritis, 616
Iron, for red cell formation, 350, 350t
Iron deficiency anemia, 353
  blood film in, 350
  in Plummer-Vinson syndrome, 450
Irreversible shock, 308–309
Irritants, insoluble particulate, chronic inflammation and, 106
Ischemia, 289–290
  causes of, 289–290
  from aneurysms, 411
  myocardial. See *Myocardial infarction.*
  of intestine, 465–467, *466*
Ischemic bowel disease, 465–467, *466*
Islets of Langerhans, *19, 225,* 331
  tumors of, hypoglycemia due to, 336

Isoenzymes, 58, *59*
Isolation, reverse, definition of, 82
Isoniazid, vitamin B$_6$ deficiency with, 328
Isotopes, 259–260, *260*
  radioactive, 10–12
Itching, 592. See also *Pruritus.*
  in atopic dermatitis, 595
  in biliary cirrhosis, 494
  in neurodermatitis, 596
  in obstructive jaundice, 485
  in urticaria, 597
  with drug eruptions, 598

Jacksonian epilepsy, 633
Jaundice, 483–485
  acholuric, 355, 485
  hemolytic, 485
  hepatocellular, 485
  obstructive, 484–485
    in carcinoma of pancreas, 498
    malabsorption due to, 485
    with gallstones, 500
Jejunum, 460
Joint(s), ankylosing spondylitis of, 587
  arthritis of, 585–586. See also *Arthritis.*
  diseases of, 585–587, *586*
  osteoarthritis of, 587
Joint-mice, 587
Junctional nevus, 603, *603*

Kala-azar, 214–215, 214t, *214*
  hypergammaglobulinemia with, 341
Kallikrein, 76, *282*
Kaposi's varicelliform eruption, 184, *184*
Karyolysis, *56,* 58
Karyorrhexis, *56,* 58
Karyotype, *47*
  changes in, in neoplasia, 255
Keloid formation, 102
Keratic precipitates, 616
Keratitis, 612
Keratoacanthoma, 607
Keratomalacia, 325
Keratosis, actinic, 605, *606*
    in squamous-cell carcinoma of external ear, 618
  seborrheic, 604, *605*
Kernicterus, 485
Keto acids, 270, 333
Ketone bodies, 275, 333
Ketosis, 275
  diabetic, 333, 334
Kidney(s), amyloidosis of, 343–344
  carcinoma of, fever with, 316
  cortical necrosis of, *309,* 507, 537
  disorders of, 502–523
    hyperparathyroidism with, 578
    hypertension with, 297, 298
    manifestations of, 506–509
    metabolic acidosis and, 275
    metastatic calcification with, 578
    with diabetes, 335
  effect of urinary obstruction on, 520, *521*
  end-stage, 516–517
  failure of, acute, 506–507
    chronic, 507–508
    in gout, 336

Kidney(s) (*Continued*)
 fluid balance and, 272
 function, 502–503
   defective, water and sodium balance
     with, 272
   tests of, 504–505, *505*
 in glomerulonephritis, 509–513, *510, 513,
   516*
 in interstitial nephritis, 514
 in lupus nephritis, *512*, 514
 in malignant hypertension, 514
 in nephrosclerosis, 514
 in shock, 308
 mechanism of urine formation in, 503–504
 normal ultrastructure of, 511
 protein-losing, 508–509
 regeneration of, 103
 stones in, 522
   osteoporosis and, 579
 tubular necrosis in, 507
 tumors of, 517–519, *518*, 521–522
Killer cells, 116
Kinetoplast, *214*
Kinins, in acute inflammation, 76, 77
 in kidney, 503
Klinefelter's syndrome, 49, 548
Koch phenomenon, 130–131
Koplik's spots, of measles, 185, 445
Korsakoff's psychosis, 227, 632
KP, 616
Krebs cycle, 24–25, *25*
Kuru, 193
Kwashiorkor, 279, 322
Kyphosis, 573
Kyphoscoliosis, 573

Labyrinth, 621
Labyrinthitis, from otitis media, 621
Laceration, of brain, 626
Lactate dehydrogenase (LDH), in blood, 58,
 59
Lactation, 530, 540
Lactic acid, 275
 in shock, 270, 275
Lactic acidosis, 270
Lactogen, placental, 530
Lactotroph cells, 553
Lamellar bone, 569, *569*
Langerhans, islets of, tumors of,
 hypoglycemia due to, 336
Langhans giant cells, *109*, 154, *155*
Laparotomy, 5
Lazy leukocyte syndrome, 70
LE cells, 374
Lead poisoning, brain damage due to, 632
 gout due to, 336
Legionella pneumophila, 123, 425
Legionnaire's disease, 425
Legs, in peripheral vascular disease, 411
 in phlegmasia alba dolens, 413
 phlebothrombosis of, 286–287, *287*
   edema with, 278
 stasis dermatitis on, 595–596
 ulcer of, *94*
 varicose veins of, 413
 vascular disease of, with diabetes, 335
Leiomyoma, of small intestine, 468
Leiomyosarcoma, 243
Leishman-Donovan bodies, 213, *214*
Leishmania braziliensis, 214t, 215

Leishmania donovani, 214t, 215
Leishmania tropica, 214t, 215
Leishmaniasis, 213–215, *214*, 214t
Lens, 610, 612
Lentigo maligna, *607*, 608
Lepromin reaction, 159
Leprosy, 159–161, *160*
 lepromatous, 159
 tuberculoid, 159
Leptospirosis, 161, 162, 166t
Lesions, biochemical, 3, 53
Lethal midline granuloma, 375
Lethal synthesis, 53
Leukemia(s), 244, 361–362
 acute, 361–362
 chronic lymphocytic, lymphocytosis in, 361
 chronic, myelocytic, 50, 361
Leukemoid blood picture, 360
Leukocytes, 357–362. See also *White cells*.
 polymorphonuclear. See *Polymorph(s)*.
Leukocytosis, 359
Leukodystrophies, 631
Leukoerythroblastic anemia, 363, 577, 585
Leukopenia, 359
Leukoplakia, 445
Leukorrhea, 533
LH, 530, 552
Lichen planus, oral mucosa in, 445, 446
Lichen simplex chronicus, 596
Lichenification, 592, *596*
Light, ultraviolet. See *Ultraviolet light*.
Light microscopy, 4–8
 of collagen, 34–35
Limb-girdle muscular dystrophy, 588
Limbs, gangrene of, 60–61
 in peripheral vascular disease, 411
Linitis plastica, 460
Linkage, in genetics, 43, 44
Lip(s), carcinoma of, 446
 inflammation of, riboflavin deficiency and,
   327
Lipase, 496
Lipids, atherosclerosis and, 406–407
Lipochromes, 485
Lipoproteins, 26, 339, 341–342
 in nephrotic syndrome, 509
 synthesis, 26, 56
Liposarcoma, 243
Lipping, 587
Liquefaction, in necrosis, 59
 in tuberculosis, 154–155
Liver, acinus of, 480, 481
 alcohol and, 57, *57*
 amebic abscess of, 209
 amyloidosis of, 343, *344*
 blood supply of, 529, 531
 cell of, 27
 chronic venous congestion of, 398, 399
 cirrhosis of, 44, *488, 489*, 491–494, *492–494*
   carcinoma and, *492*, 494–495, *494*
 disorders of, 480–495
   chronic, encephalopathy due to, 486–487,
     632
   jaundice in, 483–485. See also *Jaundice*.
 failure of, bleeding disorders due to, 366
   terminal manifestations of, 487
 fatty, 489
 flukes, 201
 function, 480–482
 hemangioma of, 481
 hepatocellular failure, 485–487
 in amyloidosis, 343, *344*

Liver (*Continued*)
  in heart failure, 398, *399*
  in hepatitis, 487–489, *487, 488*. See also
    Hepatitis.
  in portal hypertension, 482–483
  in schistosomiasis, 202
  metastases to, 238–239, *239*
  necrosis of, 487–489, *487–489*
  normal, 20, *24*, 480–481, *481*
  regeneration of, 102–103
  tumors of, *492*, 494–495, *494*
  with shock, 308
Loa loa, 201t, 208
Lobar pneumonia, 420–421, *420*
Lobes, breast, 540
Lobular carcinoma, of breast, 543
Lobules, breast, 540
Lockjaw, 35, 151–152
Locus, in genetics, 40
Loiasis, 201(t), 208
Louse, body, as vector of infection, 81, 166t,
  171
Lumbar puncture, contraindication to, 626
Lumps, breast, in carcinoma, 545
    in fat necrosis, 541
    in mammary dysplasia, 542
Lung(s). See also *Pulmonary.*
  allergic disease of, 434–435
  blastomycosis of, *198*
  brown induration of, with chronic venous
    congestion, 398
  carcinoma of, *235*, 438–440, *439, 441*
    hypertrophic osteoarthropathy in, 581
  collapsed, 436–437
  congestion of, in heart failure, 397–398
  cystic fibrosis of, 424
  dysfunction of, respiratory failure from
    415–418
  edema of, 435–436
    bronchopneumonia due to, 423
    with left ventricular failure, 370, 391–398
  embolism in, 290–291, *291*
  flukes in, 201
  hamartoma of, 220, *221*
  hypoventilation of, 275
  impaired alveolar-arterial gas exchange,
    418, *418*
  in bronchial asthma, 433–435, *434*
  in bronchial obstruction, 436–437
  in bronchopneumonia, 421—425
  in chronic interstitial lung disease, 429–433
  in emphysema, 430–431, *430–432*
  in interstitial pneumonia, 425–429, *426*,
    428t
  in lobar pneumonia, 420–421
  in pneumoconiosis, 437–438, *437*
  in shock, 428–429
  in tuberculosis, 156, *157*, 158
  infarction of, 293, *293*
  irradiation damage to, 264, *265*
  metastases to, 239
  normal structure and function of, 414–415,
    415–417
  progressive fibrosis of, with
    bronchopneumonia, 424
  tumors of, 438–440
Lupoid hepatitis, 491
Lupus erythematosus, 140, 373–374, 616
  chronic discoid (DLE), 373
  fever with, 316
  systemic (SLE), 373–374
    hypergammaglobulinemia with, 341

Lupus nephritis, *512*, 514
Luteinizing hormone (LH), 530, 533
Lymph nodes, *114*
  as defense against infection, 84
  in lung carcinoma, *439*, 440
  metastases to, *237, 238*
    in breast carcinoma, 544
Lymphadenitis, 84
Lymphadenopathy, 223
Lymphangitis, 84
Lymphatic(s), metastases of, 237, *237*
  spread of infection in, 88
Lymphatic edema, 317
Lymphatic leukemia, 360
Lymphatic permeation, 271
Lymphoblastoid cells, 14
Lymphoblasts, 406
Lymphocytes, B, 114
  blast transformation of, 131–132
  culture of, 13, *47*
  in acute inflammation, 68
  in immune response, 113–115, *114*
  T, 113, 128
Lymphocytosis, 359, 360
  in chronic lymphatic leukemia, 361
  relative, 359
Lymphogranuloma venereum, 109, 170
Lymphokines, 68, 77, 129–130
Lymphoma, 233–234, 267
  Burkitt, 244
  malignant, hypergammaglobulinemia with,
    341
Lymphopenia, 389
Lymphoreticular system, 33
  malignancy of, hypergammaglobulinemia
    with, 341
Lymphosarcoma, 244
Lymphotoxin, 129
Lyon hypothesis, 32
Lysogenic, definition of, 177
Lysogenic viruses, 177–178
Lysosomes, 25–26, *26*, 27
Lysozyme, 83–84

M protein, *340*, 341
Macrocyte, 349, 351
Macroglobulin, 339
Macroglobulinemia, erythrocyte
  sedimentation rate and, 342
Macrophages, 33, *34*, 70, *73*
  accumulation of, in chronic inflammation,
    109
  in immune response, 135
  in wound healing, 97, 99
  secretory function of, 70
Macrophage-activating factor, 129
Macule, 591
Madura foot, 198
Maduromycosis, 198
Major histocompatibility complex, 134
Malabsorption syndrome, 468–470
  in cystic fibrosis, 497
  in obstructive jaundice, 483
  in pancreatitis, 498
  iron deficiency anemia in, 353
  megaloblastic anemia with, 354
  osteoporosis in, 579
  vitamin A deficiency in, 325

Malaria, 210–212, *211, 317*
    fever in, 315
    malignant, 316–317
Malformations, causes of, 218–220, 222
    congenital, of heart, 379–380, 382
    types of, 219, 220, 222
Malignancy, hypergammaglobulinemia with, 342
Malignant exophthalmos, 562
Malignant hypertension, 298
Malleus, 619
Mallory's trichrome stain, 35
Malnutrition, protein-calorie, in childhood, 322
Malpighi, 280
Mammary dysplasia, 541–542
Mammoplasty, reduction, 541
Mantoux test, 131
Marasmus, nutritional, 322
Marrow, bone, 570
    tumors of, 582–585
Masculinization, in adrenogenital syndrome, 557
    ovarian tumors and, 531
Mass number, 295, *296*
Mastectomy, radical, 545–546
    simple, 546
Mastitis, 541
Mastoiditis, 620
Maternal deprivation syndrome, 552
Maturation, of cells, 16
Mean corpuscular hemoglobin (MCH), 349
Mean corpuscular hemoglobin concentration (MCHC), 349
Measles, 185, 193
    Koplik's spots of, 210, 445
Meat intoxication, 486
Meconium, 497
Meconium ileus, 497
Mediastinoscopy, in lung carcinoma, 389–399
Medullary carcinoma, 242, 544
Megakaryocytes, 363
Megaloblast, 351
Megaloblastic anemia, 353–354
    bone marrow smear in, 354
Meiosis, 37–38
Melanocyte, 603
Melanocyte-stimulating hormone (MSH), 552
Melanoma, malignant, 246, 607–609, *607, 608*
    of uveal tract, *615,* 616
Melanotic hamartomas, 603–604, *603, 604*
Melena, 302
    with chronic peptic ulcer, 509
Membrane bones, 569
Membranoproliferative glomerulonephritis, 512
Membranous glomerulonephritis, 511, *513*
Mendel's laws of inheritance, 40
Ménière's disease, 621
Meningeal artery, middle, extradural hemorrhage and, 626
Meninges, 624
Meningioma, 636
Meningitis, 148, 625, 629–630
    cryptococcal, 196
    from otitis media, 620
    pyogenic, 629–630
    tuberculosis with, 155
    viral, 630
Meningococcus, description of, 148, 149t
Menorrhagia, 534
    iron deficiency anemia from, 353

Menorrhagia (*Continued*)
    with uterine fibroids, 535
Menstrual cycle, endometrial changes in, 584
Menstruation, abnormalities of, 534–535
Mental retardation, 44
Mesangiocapillary glomerulonephritis, 512
Mesenchyme, 17–19, 568
Mesenteric artery, occlusion of, 286
Mesenteric vein, superior, obstruction of, 288
Mesoderm, 16
Mesothelioma, pleural, 442
Mesothelium, re-formation of, 103
Metabolic acidosis, 275–276
    with renal failure, 508
    with shock, 307
Metabolic alkalosis, 276
Metabolic encephalopathies, 632
Metabolic functions of bone, 629–630
Metabolism, acid-base balance and, 273–274
    bilirubin, 483–484, *484*
    carbohydrate, disturbances of, in liver disease, 486
    changes in, during starvation, 321–322
    during shock, 307
    glucose, 300–301
    heat produced by, 313
    hemoglobin, 350, 351, *352*
    inborn errors of, 44–45
    protein, liver and, 485–487
    purine, 336
Metaphase, 36
Metaplasia, 225–226, 325
Metastases, 229
    dormancy of, 240
    tumor spread by, 237–239
Metastatic calcification, 578
Methemalbumin, 351, 352t
Metrorrhagia, 534
Micelles, 499
Microangiopathic hemolytic anemia, 357
Microangiopathy, diabetic, 335
Microfilariae, 207, *207*
Microglia, 19, 33
Microscopy, 4–10
    electron, 8–10
    light, 4–8
    phase contrast, 5
    resolving power in, 4
    units of measurement in, 4
Microtome, rotary, 6
Microtrabecular lattice, 10, 22–23, *23*
Microtubules, 23, *23,* 26
Micturition, frequency of, in urethral obstruction, 519–520
    in urinary tract infection, 516
Midgetism, 554
Migration-inhibition factor, 129, *129*
Milk, witch's, 541
Mineralocorticoids, 556
Minimal-change glomerulonephritis, 511, *513*
Miracidia, 202
Miscarriage, 537
Mites, as vectors of infection, 171, 172
Mitochondria, 24–25, *24*
Mitogenic factor, 130
Mitosis, *13,* 16, 26, 36–37
    effects of radiation on, 262
    triradiate, 234
Mitral regurgitation, 390, 392
Mitral stenosis, atrial fibrillation in, 393–395
    due to rheumatic disease, 383, *384*
Mitral valve, diseases of, 392

Mitsuda reaction, 159
Molds, 194
Moles, hydatidiform, 538, *538*
  melanotic, 603–604, *603, 604*
Molecular disease, 45
Molluscum contagiosum, *183*
Mönckeberg's medial sclerosis, 403–404
Mongolism, 49, *49*
Moniliasis, 195
Monoblasts, 358, *358*
Monocyte, 358, *358, 359*
  in inflammatory exudate, 60
Monocytosis, 360
Mononuclear phagocytic system, 33
Mononucleosis, infectious, fever in, 317
  lymphocytosis in, 360
Monospot test, for infectious mononucleosis, 360
Moon face, 557
Morbilli. See *Measles.*
Morning sickness, 536
Morphea, 375
Mosquitos, as vectors of infection, 81
Motor neurons, 623
  degenerative disease of, 633
  in paralysis, 624
Motor system, 624
Mouth, blisters in, in pemphigus vulgaris, 445, 600
  disorders of, 444–447
  gangrene of, 60
  in iron deficiency anemia, 353
  inflammation of, riboflavin deficiency and, 327
  resident flora of, 83
mRA, 27, *29*
MSH, 552
Mucocele, of gallbladder, 500
Mucocutaneous leishmaniasis, 214t, 215
Mucoid carcinoma, 544
Mucopolysaccharidosis, 62
Mucoproteins, 34
  excessive accumulation of, with myxedema, 561
Mucormycosis, 198
Mucoviscidosis, pancreas in, 496–497
Müllerian ducts, 532
Multifactor inheritance, 43
Multinucleate giant cells, 31
Multiple endocrine adenopathy syndrome, 566
Multiple sclerosis, 630, *630*
Mumps, 185, 452
  orchitis with, 185
Mural thrombosis, following myocardial infarction, 390, *390*
Murmurs, in tetralogy of Fallot, 382
Muscle, diseases of, 587, 589
  hypertrophy of, 223
  striated, regeneration of, 103
  tumors of, 589
  types of fibers in, 587
  unstriated, regeneration of, 103
  weakness of, in Graves' disease, 562
Muscular dystrophy, 588–589
Mutation, ionizing radiation and, 266
  somatic, 37
Myasthenia gravis, 589
Mycelium, 194
Mycobacteria, description of, 153
Mycobacterium leprae, 159
Mycobacterium tuberculosis, 153

Mycoplasma pneumoniae, 169
Mycoplasmal infections, *169,* 170
Mycosis, superficial, 194–196
  superficial deep, 196–198
Mycosis fungoides, 244
Myelin sheath, diseases affecting, 630–631
Myeloblast, 358, *358*
Myelocyte, 358, *358, 359*
Myelocytic leukemia, chronic, 50, 361
Myeloma, multiple, 582–583, *584*
Myeloproliferative disorder, 363
Myocardial fibrosis, 286, 390
Myocardial infarction, 387–390, *389, 390, 394*
  clinical features of, 388
  complications of, 388, 390
  dysrhythmias in, 387, 388
  effects of, 388–390
  fever with, 316
  heart failure and, 400
  serum enzyme levels following, 58, 388–390
Myocarditis, 400
Myoepithelial cells, 452, 530
Myofibroblasts, 93–95
Myometrium, 534
Myosin, 26
Myositis ossificans, 576
Myringotomy, 619
Myxedema, 561
  anemia in, 351
  coma in, 561
  hypothermia in, 319
  pretibial, *563*
Myxomatous degeneration, 62
Myxovirus, *177,* 184–185

Nails in iron deficiency anemia, 353
Nausea, in pregnancy, 536
Necator americanus, 201, 205
Neck, stiffness of, in meningitis, 629
Necrobiosis, 61
Necropsy, 5
Necrosis, 57–59
  colliquative, 59, 628
  definition of, 58
  diagnosis of, by biochemical means, 58
  papillary, of kidney, 514, *515,* 516
  piecemeal, in hepatitis, *491*
  renal cortical, *309,* 507, 537
  renal tubular, 506
  structured vs. structureless, 59
  types of, 58–59
Necrotizing papillitis, of kidney, 514, *515,* 516
Negri body, *177,* 192
Nelson's syndrome, 554
Nemathelminthes, 200, 201t
Nematodes, 205–206
Neomycin, use of, in hepatic failure, 487
Neoplasia. See *Tumor(s).*
Nephritis, interstitial, 514
  lupus, *512,* 514
Nephroblastoma, 246, 519
Nephropathy, analgesic, 514, *515,* 516
Nephrosclerosis, 297, 404, 514
Nephrosis, 511
Nephrotic syndrome, 278, 335, 508–509
  glomerulonephritis with, 509
Nerve(s), healing of, 103–104
  spread of infection in, 89

Nerve cells, 623
Nervous system, central. See *Central nervous system.*
  peripheral, wound healing in, 103–104
Neuroblast, 623
Neuroblastoma, 246, 256–257, *556*
Neurodermatitis, 596, *596*
Neurofibroma, 236
Neurofibromatosis, multiple, 41, *41*, 220–222
Neurogenic bladder, 520
Neuroglia, 623
Neurohypophysis, 552–553
Neurological manifestations of renal failure, 508
Neurons, 622
  motor, degenerative disease of, 633
    paralysis of, 624–626, 629
Neuropathy, in malabsorption syndrome, 470
  with diabetes, 335
Neuropsychiatric manifestations of liver disease, 486–487
Neurosyphilis, parenchymatous, 166
Neurotubules, 26
Neutropenia, 360
Neutrophil, 348, 358, 359
Neutrophil count, regulation of, 360
Neutrophilia, 359–360
Nevocellular nevi, 603, *603*, 604
Nevus(i), epithelial, 604
  melanoma and, 604, 607
  melanotic, 603–604, *603*, *604*
  nevocellular, 603–604, *603*, *604*
  vascular, 604
Newborn, hemolytic disease of, 348, 356
  hemorrhagic disease of, 366
Niacin, 327
Night blindness, with vitamin A deficiency, 325
Nitrogen, decompression syndrome and, 292
Nitrogen balance, following injury, 300–301
  from chronic renal failure, 508
  from urethral obstruction, 520
Nodular colloid goiter, 560, 561
Nodular melanoma, 608, *608*
Nondisjunction, 38
Norepinephrine, 555
Normoblast, 348, *358*
North American blastomycosis, 197, *198*
Nosocomial infection, 81–82
Nuclear imaging, for detecting myocardial infarction, 390
Nucleic acid, of latent virus, 177
  role of, 27–28, *29*
  viral, 174, 176–177
Nucleolus, 31
Nucleus, 27–33
Nummular eczema, 595
Nutmeg liver, 398, *399*
Nutritional edema, 278
Nutritional marasmus, 322
Nystatin, for fungal infections, 198

Oat-cell carcinoma of lung, 267, 440, *441*
Obesity, 322–324, 551
  diabetes and, 334
  effects of, 324
  pathogenesis of, 323
Oddi, sphincter of, 499
Oliguria, 506
  with acute renal failure, 507

Omentum, greater, peritonitis and, 476
Onchocerca volvulus, 201, *207*
Onchocerciasis, 207, *207*
Oncogene, 252
Oncogenic viruses, 250–252
Operator gene, 30, *30*
Operon, 28, 30, *30*
Ophthalmia neonatorum, 612
Ophthalmitis, gonococcal, 147
Opportunistic infection, 90
  fungi causing, 198
  pneumocystosis in, 215
  strongyloidiasis in, 206
Opsonins, 68, 121
Optic chiasma, compression of, in pituitary tumors, 554
Optic disc, edema of, 298, 614
  with increased intracranial pressure, 625
Optic nerve, 610
Optic nerve cupping, 613
Oral cavity. See also *Mouth.*
  tumors of, 446–447
Oral epithelium, dysplasia of, 446
Oral mucosa, lesions of, 445–446
Orcein stain, 36
Orchitis, 525
  in leprosy, 160
  in mumps, 452
Organ culture, 14
Organelles, 23
Oriental sore, 214, 215
Ornithosis, 170–171
Orthomyxoviruses, 185
Osmoreceptors, 553
Osmosis, 269–270
Osmotic diuresis, in diabetes mellitus, 333
Osmotic pressure, of plasma proteins, 276
Ossification, endochondral, 569
Osteitis deformans, 579–581
Osteitis fibrosa cystica, 578
Osteoarthrits, 587
Osteoarthropathy, hypertrophic, 581
Osteoblasts, 569, 570
Osteoclasts, 569, 570
Osteoclastoma, 581, 582
Osteodystrophy, renal, 578
Osteogenesis imperfecta, 41, 576–577
Osteoid, 570
Osteolysis, 570
Osteolytic secondaries, 584
Osteomalacia, 571, 579
  hyperparathyroidism with, 577–578
Osteomyelitis, 572–573, *573*
  Salmonella and, 573
  trauma and, 88
  with fractures, 576
Osteopenia, 570
Osteopetrosis, 577
Osteophytes, 587
Osteoporosis, 570
  generalized, 579–581, *580*
  in Cushing's syndrome, 577
  in peripheral vascular disease, 411
  localized, 574
  with glucocorticoid therapy, 558
Osteosarcoma, 12, 243, 582, *583*
  with Paget's disease, 581
Osteosclerosis, 579
Otitis externa, 618
Otitis media, 146, 619–620
  acute, 619
  chronic, 619–620

Otitis media (*Continued*)
  complications of, 620
Otosclerosis, 620
Ovary, development of, 530
  diseases of, 530–531, 532
  dysgenesis, 49–50
  hormones secreted by, 529–530
  irradiation damage of, 263
  teratoma of, 246, *247*
Overeating, fatty liver from, 489
Ovulation, 530
  rise in temperature with, 312
Oxidation of glycogen, 24, *25*
Oxidative phosphorylation, in Krebs cycle,
    24, *25*
Oxygen deficiency, brain damage due to, 632
Oxygen toxicity, 428, 429
Oxytocin, 530, 553

Packed cell volume (PCV), 348–349, 349t
Paget's disease, alkaline phosphatase in, 570
  of bone, 579, 581
  of breast, 547, *548*
Pain, acute abdominal, 478–479
  in abruptio placentae, 592
  in achalasia of cardia, 450
  in acute inflammation, 66, 76
  in appendicitis, 475
  in bacillary dysentery, 470
  in cholecystitis, 501
  in cholelithiasis, 500
  in ectopic pregnancy, 537
  in esophagitis, 451
  in glaucoma, 613
  in infections of testis, 525
  in intestinal obstruction, 478
  in myocardial infarction, 388
  in osteoarthritis, 587
  in osteosarcoma, 581, 582
  in otitis media, 619
  in pancreatitis, 497
  in pelvic endometriosis, 536
  in pelvic inflammatory disease, 532
  in peripheral vascular disease, 411
  in pleurisy, 441
  in penumothorax, 441
  in rheumatoid arthritis, 585
  in stomach carcinoma, 460
  in toxemia, 536–537
  in ulcerative colitis, 470.
  in urinary tract infection, 516
  tissue tension in, 66
  with bone marrow tumors, 583
  with peptic ulcer, 455
  with torsion of testis, 524
  with urinary calculi, 522
Painful white leg, in pregnancy, 413
Pallor, in anemia, 351
Palsy, pseudobulbar, 629
Pancreas, atrophy of, 225, *225*
  carcinoma of, 498–499
    migrating thrombophlebitis with, 288
  cystic fibrosis of, 42, 496–497
  development and function of, 496
  diseases of, 496–499
  diabetes with, 332
  malabsorption due to, 497, 498
  epithelial cells of, *19*
  in pancreatitis, acute, 497–498
    chronic, 498
  in shock, 309

Pancreatitis, acute, 497–498
  chronic, 498
Pancytopenia, 362–363
Panencephalitis, subacute sclerosing, 193
Panlobular emphysema, 430–431, *432*
Pannus, 585
Panophthalmitis, 616
Pap smear, 253, 533–534
Papillary cystadenocarcinoma of ovary, 531,
  532
Papillary cystadenoma, of ovary, 531
Papillary cystadenoma lymphomatosum, 453
Papillary muscle, rupture of, 390, 392
Papillary necrosis, of kidney, 514, *515*
Papilledema, 298, 614
  with increased intracranial pressure, 625
Papilloma(s), 230, *232*
  of bladder, 522
  of breast, 542
  Shope, 251
  squamous-cell, 604–605, *605*
Papovaviruses, *178*, 188–189
Papules, 592
Papulosquamous eruptions, 592, 597
Paracoccidioidal granuloma, 197
Paracoccidioides brasiliensis, 197
Paraffin section, 5
Paragonimus westermani, 201, 201t
Parainfluenza viruses, 185
Parakeratosis, 253, *254*, 592, *594*
Paralysis, due to pyramidal tract damage, in
    multiple sclerosis, 631
  facial, in Paget's disease, 581
  infantile, 182
  motor neurons in, 624, 633
  of muscles of deglutition, 451
  seventh nerve, from otitis media, 620
Paralytic ileus, 478
Paramyxoviruses, 185
Parasite, definitive, 200
Parathyroid hormone, 571, 577
  bone metabolism and, 571, 577–578
Paresthesia, 623
Parkinson's disease, 633
Parotid gland, acute suppurative
    inflammation of, 452
  tumor of, 452–453, 453
Parotitis acute, 452
  in mumps, 452
Paroxysmal nocturnal dyspnea, 397–398,
    435–436
Paroxysmal tachycardia, 393
Partial prothrombin time (PT), *365*, 367
Partial thromboplastin time (PTT), *365*, 367
Patch, definition of, 592
Patent ductus arteriosus, *381*, 382
Pathogen, definition of, 80
Pathogenesis, definition of, 3
Pathological fracture, 575
Paul-Bunnell test for infectious
    mononucleosis, 360
Pavementation, of endothelium, 65
PCV, 348–349, 349t
Peau d'orange, 544
Pellagra, 327
Pelvic endometriosis, 536
Pelvic inflammatory disease (PID), 147, 532
Pemphigoid, bullous, 602
Pemphigus vulgaris, 445, 600–601, *600*
Penetrance, in genetics, 42–43
Penicillin, action of, 53
  anaphylaxis and, 125

Pepsin, 455
Peptic ulcer, chronic, 455–460, *455–457*, 459
  with glucocorticoid therapy, 559
Perforation, in acute appendicitis, 475
  in peptic ulcer, 456
Pericarditis, 71
  following myocardial infarction, 390, 401
  in rheumatic fever, 383
  in systemic lupus erythematosus, *71*
  tuberculous, *107*
Pericardium, diseases of, 401–402
    constrictive, 402
Periodontitis, 447–448, *449*
Peripheral nervous system, wound healing
  in, 103–104
Peripheral vascular disease, 411
Peritoneal adhesions, 476–477
Peritoneum, metastases to, 239
  spread of infection in, 88
Peritonitis, 476
  in pelvic inflammatory disease, 532
Perlèche, 327
Pernicious anemia, 400
  degeneration of spinal cord with, 632
Petit mal seizure, 634
pH, of blood, abnormalities of, 274–276
  · maintenance of, 274
Phagocytosis, 25, 68–70, *69*
Pharyngotympanic tube, 619, *619*
Pharynx, disorders of, 444–446
  tumor of, 446
Phase content microscopy, 5
Phenobarbital, in proliferation of
  endoplasmic reticulum, 54, *54*
Phenotype, 40
Phenylalanine in phenylketonuria, 44
Phenylbutazone, agranulocytosis from, 363
Phenylketonuria, 42, 44
Pheochromocytoma, 555–556, 566
  hypertension with, 296
Philadelphia chromosome, 50
Phlebitis, 144, 287–288, 412
Phleboliths, 288
Phlebothrombosis, 286–287
  edema with, 278
  pathogenesis of, *287*
  propagation of clot in, 287, *287*
Phlegmasia alba dolens, 413
Phocomelia, 218
Phosphate in bone, 569
Photoallergic dermatitis, 594
Photodermatitis, 594
Phototoxic dermatitis, 594
Phthisis, 315
Phytohemagglutinin, 132
Pia mater, 624
Picornaviruses, 181
PID, 147, 532
Pigmentation, increase in, Addison's disease,
  557
Pink puffers, 433
Pinna, 618
Pinworm, 205–206
Pituitary gland, disorders of, 552–555
  hypersecretion of ACTH, adrenal
    overactivity secondary to, 557
  in shock, 309
  relationship with hypothalamus, *552*
  tumors of, 554
Pituitary gonadotropins, 553
Pituitary growth hormone, 554
Pityriasis rosea, 597

Placenta, premature separation of, 350, 592
Placenta previa, 537–538
Placental hormones, 530
Plane warts, 604
Plantar wart, 604
Plaques, dental, 447
  of skin, 592
Plasma, normal, composition of, 271t
Plasma cells, *18*, *110*
  development of, 114–115, *114*
  in inflamed gum, *110*
Plasma cell mastitis, 540
Plasma membrane, 21–22, *21*
Plasma proteins, 274, 338–342
  liver and, 534
  methods of separation of, 338–339
  osmotic pressure of, 277
Plasmatic zone, 64
Plasmids, 45–46
Plasmin, 281, *282*
Plasmodium, 210, *211*, *212*
Platelet(s), 281–282, *348*, 363
  adhesiveness of, 282
  aggregation of, 282
  aplasia of, 362
  clotting factors and, 363–369, 368t
  deficiency, bleeding due to, 366
  in thrombosis, 282–285
Platelet count, 367, 368t
Platelet factor 3, 282, 364–365, *364*
Platelet release reaction, 282
Platyhelminthes, 200, 201t
Pleomorphic adenoma, of salivary gland,
  452–453, *453*
Pleomorphism, in tumors, 234, *235*
Pleura, diseases of, 440–442
  metastases to, 274
Pleural effusion, 440
Pleural rub in lobar pneumonia, 421
Pleurisy, 440–441
Pleuritis, 440–441
Plummer-Vinson syndrome, 450
  cancer of tongue in, 446
Pneumococci, description of, 146–147, 149
Pneumoconioses, 437
Pneumocystis carinii, 215
Pneumocystosis, 215
Pneumocytes, 415
Pneumonia, 419–429
  hypostatic, 423
  interstitial, 425–427
  lobar, 420–421, *420*
  unresolved, in lung carcinoma, 438–439
Pneumonitis, 420
Pneumothorax, 441
Podocytes, 511
Poikilocytosis, *348*, 358
Poikiloderma, 263, *264*
Poison(s), brain damage due to, 632
  degenerative conditions of liver from, 487
  heart and, 400
  renal tubular necrosis from, 507
Poison theory of radiation damage, 262
Poisoning, cyanide, 289
  ergot, arterial spasm with, 296
  food, 465
  gastroenteritis due to, 463
  lead, gout and, 336
  pulmonary edema in, 435
Poliomyelitis, 182
Poliovirus, 182
  antibody response to, 180

Pollen, hypersensitivity to, 125
Polyarteritis, microscopic, 375–376
  glomerulonephritis in, 513
Polycystic kidney, 517, *517*
Polycythemia, 357
  gout, secondary to, 336
  in renal disease, 503
  in tetralogy of Fallot, 382
  thrombosis due to, 286
  with COLD, 433
  with right ventricular failure, 397
Polycythemia vera, 357
Polydactyly, 220
Polydipsia, in diabetes insipidus, 504, 552
  in diabetes mellitus, 332, 504
Polymorph(s), *348, 358, 359*
  biologically active components of, 76
  in inflammatory exudate, 66–70, *67, 69*
Polymorphism, 45
Polyneuropathy in dry beriberi, 327
Polyoma virus, 251
Polyp(s), 230
  cervical, 533
Polyploidy, definition of, 31
Polyposis coli, 250, 472, *473*
Polysomes, 23, *23*
Polyuria, 504
  in diabetes insipidus, 504, 553
Pontiac fever, 425
Portal hypertension, 482–483
Port-wine stain, 604
Postmortem change, 58
Postpericardiotomy syndrome, 401
Postsinusoidal pressure, 482
Potassium, 270
  balance, disturbances of, 273
  metabolism of, following injury, 302
  retention of, with renal failure, 508
Pott's disease, 572
Poxviruses, 182–184
Precipitin, 119, *119*
Precocious sexual development, 526
Prednisone, 558
Pre-eclampsia, 536
Pregnancy, anemia in, 351
  bleeding during, 537–538
  cholelithiasis and, 499
  choriocarcinoma in, 539
  ectopic, 537
  false, 623
  heart failure and, 401
  hormonal aspects of, 530
  hydatidiform mole in, 538–539, *539*
  hyperemesis gravidarum in, 536
  megaloblastic anemia in, 353
  osteomalacia and, 637
  painful white leg in, 413
  renal tubular necrosis and, 560
  toxemia of, 536–537
  varicose vein formation in, 413
Presbyopia, 611
Presinusoidal pressure, 482
Pressure, blood. See *Blood pressure*.
  central venous, rise in, 396
  intracranial, increased, 624–626
  mechanical, malignant tumors and, 234,
    438, *439*
  postsinusoidal, 482
  presinusoidal, 482
  pulmonary venous, rise in, 397–398
Pressure atrophy, benign tumors and,
    232–233
  of bone, 574

Pretibial myxedema, *563*
PRF, 551
Progesterone, 530
Prognathism, in acromegaly, *555*
Progressive systemic sclerosis, 275
Prolactin, 584, 612
Prolactin-releasing factor (PRF), 551
Prolactinoma, 554
Proliferative glomerulonephritis, *510,*
  511–512
Promyelocyte, 358, *358*
Pronormoblasts, 348, 358
Properdin, 121
Prophase, 36
Proptosis, *563*
Prostacyclin, in thrombosis, 285
Prostaglandins, 76–77
Prostate, 526–528
  benign enlargement of, 519–520, 526–527,
    527
    urethral obstruction from, 519
  carcinoma of, 580–581, 250, 527–528
Prostatitis, 525, 526
  epididymo-orchitis following, 525
Protein(s), 269–270
  abnormal, synthesis of, 45
  antigenicity of, alteration in, 139
  Bence Jones, 583
  cytoplasmic, denaturation of, 58
  in renal disease, 503
  in wound healing, 101
  M, 341
  metabolism, liver and, 485–486
  myeloma, 583
  plasma, 274, 338–346. See also *Plasma
    proteins*.
  synthesis, 28, *29*
    ribosomes in, 23
  translation-inhibiting, 180
Protein-calorie malnutrition in childhood, 322
Protein-losing enteropathy, hypoalbuminemia
  with, 341
Protein-losing kidney, 508–509
Proteinuria, 503
  in nephrotic syndrome, 508
Proteus, 149, 149t
  hospital infection by, 82
  urinary tract infection from, 514
Prothrombin time (PT), *365*, 367
Purozone phenomenon, *120*
Prurigo nodularis, 596
Pruritus, 592. See also *Itching*.
  in obstructive jaundice, 485
Pruritus ani, 205–206
Pruritus vulvae, 335
Prussian blue, reaction for hemosiderin, 6–7,
  7
Pseudobulbar palsy, 629
Pseudocyesis, 623
Pseudocyst formation, with pancreatitis, 498
Pseudohyphae, 194
Pseudomembranous inflammation, 71, 84
Pseudomonas, 149, 149t
  enterocolitis from, 466–467, 466
  hospital infection by, 82
  urinary tract infection from, 514
  and vasculitis, 376
Pseudomyxoma peritonei, 476, 531
Psittacosis, 170–171
Psoriasis, 597, *598, 599*
Psoriatic arthritis, 586
Psychosis, Korsakoff's, 327, 632
  with glucocorticoid therapy, 559

PT, *365*, 367
PTT, *365*, 367
Puberty, delayed and precocious, in diseases
    of hypothalamus, 552
  in female, 529–530
Puerperal sepsis, 146
Pulmonary. See also *Lung(s)*.
Pulmonary embolism, 290–291, *291*
Pulmonary emphysema, 430–431, 430–432
Pulmonary hypertension, 380, 382, 390–392
Pulmonary stenosis, 380, *381*
Pulmonary tuberculosis, fever in, 156, *157*,
    158
Pulmonary valve disease, 393
Pulmonary venous pressure, rise in, 396
Pulpitis, 447
PUO, 316–318
Pupil, dilated, with cerebral lesion, 625
Purine metabolism, 336
Purpura, *302*, 366
Pus, 73
  tuberculous, 155
Pus cells, 73
Pustules, 592
Pyelitis, 515
Pyelonephritis, 88, 514–516
Pyemia, 89, 145, 290, 620
  in infective endocarditis, 385–386
Pyknosis, 56, 58, 348
Pyloric stenosis, metabolic alkalosis in, 276
  with peptic ulcer, 456–457
Pyoderma, 144
Pyogenic infections, 143–144
Pyogenic membrane, 74, 110
Pyogenic meningitis, 629–630
Pyonephrosis, 515
Pyosalpinx, 532
Pyramidal tract, damage to, 624–626
Pyrexia, 302, 312, 314–319. See also *Fever*.
  heart failure and, 401
  of unknown origin, 316–318
Pyridoxine, 328
Pyrogens, bacterial, 318
  endogenous, 69–70, 318

Q fever, 172

R factor, in bacteria, 46
Rabies, 177, 192
Rachitic rosary, 578
Radiation, electromagnetic, 261
  ionizing, acute inflammation and, 62
    cancer and, 249
    effects of, 259–268, 427
    wound contraction inhibition by, 93, *93*
  particulate, 260–261
  types of, 260
Radiation syndrome, 264–266
Radioactive isotopes, 10–12
Radiodermatitis, 263, *264*
Radionuclides, 11
Radiosensitivity factors in, 267
Radiotherapy, 257, 266–267
  cure rate of, 267
Rapidly progressive glomerulonephritis,
  512–513, *513*
Rash(es), description of, terminology for,
  591–592
Raynaud's phenomenon, arterial spasm with,
  4, 296, 374, 375

Receptors, cell, 22
Recombinant DNA, 31, 181
Rectum, carcinoma of, 472
Red cells, 348, *348*
  autoantibodies and, 355–356
  blood groups and, 369
  development of, 348
  disposal of, 351, *352*
  electron micrographs of, 9, 10
  enzyme deficient, 355
  examination of, 348–349
  formation of, requirements for, 350–351,
    350t
  in hemolytic anemia, 355, 357
  in iron deficiency anemia, 353
  in megaloblastic anemia, 354
  in polycythemia, 357
  normal, characteristics of, 349t
  occlusion of capillaries by, 410
Red-cell fragmentation syndrome, 356–357
Reed-Sternberg cells, 243–244
Reflux, ureteric, 515, 520
Regeneration, in chronic inflammatory
    lesions, 110
  in connective tissue, 103
  in wound healing, 91–92
  mechanism of, 104–105
  of epithelium, 102–103
Regional enteritis, 467–468, *467, 468*
Regulator gene, 30, *30*
Relapsing fever, 161, 166t
Renal. See also *Kidney(s)*.
Renal colic, 522
Renal edema, 278
Renal glycosuria, 503
Renal osteodystrophy, 508, 578
Renal vasoconstriction, 506–507
Renin, 297, 503
Repair, in wound healing, 92
Reproductive system, female, 529–539
  male, 524–528
Resolution, following acute inflammation, 72
Resolving power, of microscope, 4
Respiratory acidosis, 275, 417
Respiratory alkalosis, 275
Respiratory distress syndrome of newborn,
  419
Respiratory failure, 415–418
Respiratory syncytial virus (RSV), 185
Respiratory tract, diseases of, 414–443
  normal structure and function, 414–415,
    415, 416, 417
  viruses of, 184–186
Restrictive endonucleases, 46
Reticulin, 35, *35*
Reticulocyte, 348
Reticulocyte count, in hemolytic anemia, 357
Reticulocytosis, 348, 357
Reticuloendothelial (RE) system, 33
  as defense against infection, 84
  hyperplasia of, 111
Retina, 610
  detachment of, 610, 613, *615*
  diseases of, 614–615
  normal, 614
Retinoblastoma, 246, 250, 615
Retinol, deficiencies and excesses of, 324–325
Retinopathy, 614–615
  diabetic, 614–615
  hypertensive, 297, 614
Reverse transcriptase, 176, 251, 252
Rh-hemolytic disease of newborn, 356
Rhabdomyoma, 589

Rhabdomyosarcoma, 589
Rhabdovirus, causing rabies, 192
Rhesus blood system, 369
Rheumatic endocarditis, chronic, 383, *384*
Rheumatic fever, 146, 383
Rheumatic heart disease, 383–384
  atrial fibrillation in, 394–395
Rheumatoid aortitis, 408
Rheumatoid arthritis, 427, 585–586, *586*
  amyloidosis with, 344
  necrobiosis in, 61
Rheumatoid factor, 586
Rhinitis, allergic, 125
Rhinorrhea, cerebrospinal, 629
Rhinoviruses, 185–186
Rhodopsin, vitamin A in, 326
Riboflavin, deficiency of, 327
Ribosomes, 23, *24*
Rickets, 571, 578
  hyperparathyroidism with, 577–578
Rickettsia mooseri, 171
Rickettsia prowazeki, 171
Rickettsia rickettsii, 171
Rickettsiae, 171–172
Rigor, 315
Ring chromosomes, 38
Ringworm, 194–195
  vs. psoriasis, 195
RNA, messenger, 27, *29*
  transfer, 28, *29*
  viruses, 176
Rocky Mountain spotted fever, 171
Rodent ulcer. See *Basal-cell carcinoma.*
Romanowsky stain, 348
Rotaviruses, *178*, 182
Rouleaux formation, 342
Roundworms, 205–206
Rous virus, 250–251
Rubber industry, bladder carcinoma and, 522
Rubella, 185, 821
Rubor in acute inflammation, 63
Runt disease, *138*

Sabin vaccine, 182
Saddle embolus, *291*
Sago spleen, *343*
Salivary glands, disorders of, 452–453
  pleomorphic tumor of, 452, *453*
Salk vaccine, 180, 182
Salmonella, gastroenteritis due to, 464
  osteomyelitis due to, 573
Salmonella typhi, 85
Salpingitis, 532
  acute, 147, 532
Salt, deficiency and excess of, 272–273
Sarcoidosis, hypergammaglobulinemia with, 341
Sarcoma, definition of, 232, 242–243
  melanotic, 246
  spindle-cell, 243
Scalded skin syndrome, 145
Scalp, seborrheic dermatitis of, 596
Scanning electron microscope, 10, *10*, 462
Scar, formation of, in chronic inflammatory lesions, 110
  wounds and, 97–100, *98*, *99*
  normal skin vs., 100
  weak, 102
Scar tissue, 92, 95
Scarlet fever, 146, 446
Schick test, 150
Schistosoma hematobium, 201–202, 201t, *202*
Schistosoma japonicum, 202
Schistosoma mansoni, 202
Schistosomiasis, 201–203, 201t, *203*
  bladder carcinoma and, 522
Schlemm, canal of, *611*, 612
Schwann cells in nerve wound healing, 103–104
Schwannoma of vestibulocochlear nerve, sensorineural deafness due to, 621
Scirrhous carcinoma, 241–242, 543–544, *545*
Sclera, *611*
Scleroderma, 374
Sclerosing adenosis of breast, 542
Scoliosis, 573
Scrapie, 192
Scrub typhus, 172
Scurvy, 326
Sebaceous cyst, *606*
Sebaceous glands, 591
  hyperplasia in rosacea, 602
Seborrheic dermatitis, 596
  riboflavin deficiency and, 327
Seborrheic keratosis, 604, *605*
Secretin, 497
Seizures, 633–636
Selective theory, of antibody production, 136
Sella turcica, enlargement of, with pituitary tumors, 554
Seminoma, 525
  cryptorchidism and, 526
Senile dementia, 633
Sensorineural deafness, 621
Sepsis, puerperal, 146
Septal defects, of heart, 380, *381*
Septic emboli, 291
Septic infarct, 291
Septicemia, 84
Sequestrum, 572, *573*
Serous inflammation, 70
Serum glutamic oxaloacetic transaminase (SGOT), 58, 389
Serum glutamic pyruvate transaminase (SGPT), 58
Serum sickness, 126, *127*, 128
  glomerulonephritis in, 509
Seventh nerve paralysis from otitis media, 620
Sex chromosomes, 31
Sex hormones. See *Estrogen* and *Progesterone.*
Sexual characteristics, secondary, development of, 530
Sexual development, precocious, 526
Sheehan's syndrome, 555
Shigella, bacillary dysentery due to, 464
Shingles, 186–188, *187*
Shivering, 313, 315
  with fever, 358
Shock, 299, 305–310
  anaphylactic, 124–125
  endotoxic, 483
  in myocardial infarction, 388
  irreversible, 308–309
  lactic acid in, 270
  lung in, 428–429
  metabolic acidosis with, 275, 307
  metabolic upset during, 307
  pathogenesis of, 305–308
  treatment of, 309–310
  types of, 305–307
Shope papilloma, 288
Shwartzman phenomenon, 306
SI units, 270

Sialoadenitis, 452
Sialolithiasis, 452
Sickle cell, 349, 355
Sickle cell anemia, 355
Sight. See *Blindness; Eye(s); and Vision.*
Sigmoid sinus thrombosis, 620
Silicosis, 437, *437*
Simmond's disease, 555
Skin, acne vulgaris of, 602
    basal-cell carcinoma of, 244, *245,* 606
    dermatitis of, 592–596, *593–596*
    diseases of, 591–609
        terminology in, 591–592
    drug eruptions of, 598, *599*
    eczema, in Paget's disease of breast, 547
    erythema multiforme of, 601–602, *601*
    hamartomas of, melanotic, 603–604, *603,*
        604
        vascular, 220, *220, 221,* 604
    in lupus erythematosus, 373–374
    in scleroderma, 375
    papulosquamous eruptions of, 597
    radiation effects of, 263, *264,* 266
    rashes on, See *Rash(es).*
    resident flora of, 83
    squamous-cell carcinoma of, 240, *241,*
        606–607
    staphylococcal infections of, 144–145, *145*
    stasis dermatitis of, with varicose veins, *94,*
        595–596
    toxic erythema of, 598
    tumors of, benign, 604–605, *605*
        malignant, 605–609, *606–608*
    urticaria of, 597–598
    vesiculobullous diseases of, 599–602, *600*
    wounds of, healing of, 95–100
Skin reactive factor, 129
Skull, fracture of, extradural hemorrhage
       from, 626
    in Paget's disease, 579–580
SLE. See under *Lupus erythematosus.*
Sleeping sickness, 213
Slough, 74
Slow reacting substance of anaphylaxis, 125
Slow virus infection, degenerative nervous
    diseases due to, 192–193
Sludging, 302, 308, 342
Smallpox, 183–184
Smoking. See *Cigarette smoking.*
Sodium, 270, 271t
    balance, disturbances of, 272–273, *271*
        mechanisms which regulate, 271–272,
        271
        with reduction in blood volume, 301, *301*
Sodium pump, 22, 155
Somatic mutation, 37
Somatomedins, 554
Somatostatin, 331
Somatotroph cells, 554
Somatotropin, 554
Somnolence in diseases of hypothalamus, 551
Sore(s), canker, 445
    pressure, 410
Sore throat, streptococcal, 446
        glomerulonephritis following, 509
        rheumatic fever and, 383
South American blastomycosis, 197
South American trypanosomiasis, 213, 213t
Spasm, arterial, 295–296, 388
    intestinal obstruction due to, 478
    venous, 294
Spermatogenesis, 524

Spherocytes, 349
Spherocytosis, hereditary, 355
Spinal cord, anterior horn cells of, damage to,
    624, 633
Spine, bamboo, 586
    tuberculosis of, 573
Spirochetes, 161–167, 166t
Spleen, in amyloidosis, *343*
    infarction of, 293, *294*
Splenomegaly, congestive, in portal
    hypertension, 482
Spondylitis, ankylosing, 586–587
Spongiosis, 594, *595*
Spotted fever, 148
Sprain, 585
Sprue, malabsorption syndrome from, 469
Squamous cell carcinoma, of esophagus, 451
    of external ear, 618
    of lips, 446
    of lung, 440
    of skin, 606
    of tongue, 446–447
Squamous-cell papilloma, of skin, 604–605,
    605
Squatting in tetralogy of Fallot, 382
Staging of tumors, 239–240
Stain, hematoxylin and eosin, 5
    Ziehl-Neelsen, 153
    Stapes, 619, *619*
Staphylococcus albus, 83, 144, 149t
Staphylococcus aureus, bronchopneumonia
       from, *422,* 424
    gastroenteritis due to, 463
    infective endocarditis from, 385
    lesions produced by, 144–146, *145,* 149t
    mastitis from, 541
    osteomyelitis from, 572
    otitis media due to, 619
    skin infection with, 73–74
Starling's law of heart, 396
Starvation, 321–322
    edema in, 278–279
    fatty liver from, 489
    hypoalbuminemia with, 340
    malignant tumors and, 235
    metabolic changes during, 275, 321–322
    water deficiency and, 272
Stasis, in acute inflammation, 64
Stasis dermatitis, 595–596
Stasis ulcers, *94,* 595–596
Status asthmaticus, 434
Steatorrhea, 470
    in disorders of pancreas, 498
Stein-Leventhal syndrome, 530–531, 535
Stem cells, 33
    tumors of, 243–244
Sterility, from mumps orchitis, 525
    in mucoviscidosis, 497
    with pelvic inflammatory disease, 147, 532
Steroids. See *Glucocorticosteroids.*
Stevens-Johnson syndrome, 602
    oral mucosa in, 445
Stiffness of neck in meningitis, 629
Stokes-Adams attacks, 395
Stomach, carcinoma of, 460, *460, 461*
    disorders of, 454–461
        megaloblastic anemia from, 353–354
    inflammation of, in enteritis, 463
    ulcers of, 455–460, *455, 456, 457*
Stomal ulcer, 458
Stomatitis, angular, 195, 327
    Candida albicans and, 82, 83

Stones, gallbladder, 499–501, *500*
  urinary, 522
Stools. See also *Feces.*
  rice-water, in cholera, 461
Strangulated hernia, 477
Strawberry nevus, 604
Streptococcal sore throat. See *Sore throat.*
Streptococcus(i), anaerobic, 153
  types of, 146
Streptococcus pyogenes, bronchopneumonia
    from, 425
  glomerulonephritis and, 511–512
  lesions produced by, 146, 149t
  otitis media due to, 619
  sore throat due to, 446
Streptococcus viridans, 83, 146, 149t
  endocarditis from, 386
    glomerulonephritis and, 512
Streptomycin, sensorineural deafness due to,
  621
Stress, acute reaction to, 340
  diseases aggravated by, 624
  endocrine reactions to, 299
Stroke, cerebral hemorrhage and, 626
  clinical features of, 628–629
  from cerebral embolism, 384, 628
  heat, 314
  thrombotic, 626, 628, *628*
Stroma, of ovary, 267, 530
Strongyloides stercoralis, 201t, 206
Stye, 144
Subacute sclerosing panencephalitis, 193
Subarachnoid hemorrhage, 626
Subarachnoid space, 624
  pyogenic bacterial infection of, 629–630
Subcutaneous nodules in rheumatoid
  arthritis, 586
Subdural hemorrhage, 626
Subepidermal vesicle, 601–602
Subluxation, 585
Subphrenic abscess, *456, 457,* 476
Succus entericus, 460
Suicide with glucocorticoid therapy, 559
Sulfonamides, action of, 53, hemolytic
  anemia from, 356
  pancytopenia due to, 362
Sulfones for leprosy, 161
Sun stroke, 314
Sunlight, effects of, *606.* See also *Ultraviolet
  light.*
Superinfections, 90
Supernumerary breast tissue, 541
Suppressor cells, 130, 135
Suppuration, 71, 73–75, *74*
Surfactant, 416
  in hyaline membrane disease, 419
Surgery, diabetes mellitus and, 335
  hypoalbuminemia with, 340
SV-40 viruses, 251
Svedberg units, 117, 339
Swallowing, 444–445
  difficulty in, 451–452. See also *Dysphagia.*
Swan-Ganz catheter, use of, 310
Sweat glands, 591
  in cystic fibrosis, 497
Sweating, 313
  with fever, 315
Swiss cheese, pattern of endometrium, 535
Syncope, 305
Syndactyly, 219, *219*
Syndrome, definition of, 4
Synechiae, 616

Synovial fluid, 585
Synovial joint, 585. See also *Joint(s).*
Synovitis, 585
Synovium, 585
Synthesis, lethal, 53
Syphilis, 162–167, *163, 165,* 166t
  arteritis in, 166, 408, *409*
  congenital, 166–167
  of bone, 574
  secondary, vs. pityriasis rosea, 597
  standard tests for, 162
  testicular gumma in, 525
  Wasserman reaction for, *122*
Systemic sclerosis, 427
Systole, 395

T_3, 559
T_4, 559
T cells, 113, *114,* 115, 128–132
  immunity to viral infections and, 180
  in leprosy, 160
  in tuberculosis, 158
  failure of development of, 135
Tabes dorsalis, 166
Tachycardia, effects of, 395
  paroxysmal, 393
Tachypnea, 418
Taenia saginata, 201t, 204
Taenia solium, 201t, 204
Tamm-Horsfall mucoprotein, 505
Tapeworms, 200, 201t, 203–205
Target cells, 349
Target theory of radiation damage, 262
Tartar, 447
Tay-Sachs disease, 112
Technetium, 10–11
Teeth, disorders of 447–448, *448, 449*
Telangiectasia, 592
  in rosacea, 602
  radiation and, 263
Telophase, 37
Temperature. See also *Fever.*
  failure to maintain, in diseases of
    hypothalamus, 552
  measurement of, 312
  normal, 312
  regulation of, 313–314, *314*
  wound healing and, 101
Temporal arteritis, 409
Temporal bone, injury to, sensorineural
  deafness due to, 521
Tendons, regeneration of, 103
Tenesmus, 462
Tentorium, 624
Teratogen, definition of, 218
Teratoma, 246, *247*
  of ovary, *247,* 531
  of testis, 525
Testes,
  atrophy of, in myotonic muscular
    dystrophy, 588
  disorders of, 524–526
  irradiation damage of, 263
  teratoma of, 525
Tetanus, 85, 151–152
Tetany, with alkalosis, 275, 276
  with hypocalcemia, 297
Tetracycline, use in acne vulgaris, 602
Tetralogy of Fallot, 380, *381,* 382
Thalassemia syndromes, 355

Thalidomide, 50, 218
Thermal burns, shock following, 306–307
Thiamine, 326–327
    deficiency, 53, 632
Thiouracil, agranulocytosis from, 363
Thirst, 272
    in diabetus insipidus, 553
    in diabetes mellitus, 504
Thoracotomy, use of 5
Thread worm(s), 205–206
Thrombin, 363, *364*
    autocatalytic action of, 365
Thromboangiitis obliterans, 409
Thrombocytopenia, in bleeding disorders,
    366
Thrombocytopenic purpura, 366
Thrombophlebitis, 287–288
    migrating, 288
    septic, 88–89
    with blood transfusion, 371
Thrombosis, 282–288, *283, 284, 285*
    arterial, 286
    cardiac, 288
    causes of, 285–286
    cerebral, 626, 628–629
    coronary artery, myocardial infarction due
        to, 387
    from aneurysms, 411
        aortic, 283
    in giant-cell arteritis, 409
    in thromboangiitis obliterans, 409
    in vasculitis, 410–411
    mural, following myocardial infarction, 390,
        390
    peripheral vascular disease and, 411
    pathogenesis of, 282–286
    sigmoid sinus, 620
    vascular abnormalities leading to, *285*
    venous, 286–288, *287*
    with atherosclerosis, 406, 407
Thrombotic endocarditis, nonbacterial, 384
Thromboxane A2 (TXA2), role of, in
    thrombosis, 284–285
Thrombus, 282–286, *283, 284*
    fate of, 288, *289*
Thrush, 195
Thymidine, tritiated, incorporation into DNA,
    12, 13
Thymoma, in myasthenia gravis, 589
Thymus in lymphoid tissue development,
    114, *114*
Thyroglobulin, 559
Thyroglossal cyst, 222
Thyroid gland, 559–566
    goiter, 560, *561*
    hormones, action of, 559–560
    in Hashimoto's disease, 564–565, *564*
    in hyperthyroidism, 562–564, *563*
    in hypothyroidism, 560–561
    in subacute thyroiditis, 565
    tumors of, 266, 565–566, *565*
Thyroiditis, subacute, 565
Thyroid-stimulating hormone (TSH), 553, 559
Thyroid-stimulating immunoglobulin, 563
Thyrotoxicosis, 539, 562–564, *563*
    cardiac output and, 400
Thyrotroph cells, 553
Thyrotropin, 553
Thyrotropin-releasing factor (TRF), 551
Thyrotropin-releasing hormone (TRH), 551
Thyroxine (T$_4$), 559
Tick(s), as vectors of infection, 81, 166t, 171

Tinea, 195
Tinnitus, in Ménière's disease, 621
Tissue, antibody-forming, 131–114, *114*
    connective. See *Connective tissue.*
    embryology of, 16–21
    granulation. See *Granulation tissue.*
Tissue culture, 12–14
Tissue grafts, 132–134
Tissue tension, 276–277
    in pain, 66
Titer of antibody, *120*
TNM classification of tumors, 240, 547
Todd's paralysis, 633
Toes, clubbing of, in tetralogy of Fallot, 382
    gangrene of, in thromboangiitis obliterans,
        409
Tongue, atrophic, in Plummer-Vinson
        syndrome, 450
    carcinoma of, 446–447
    in vitamin deficiency, 327, 328
    inflammation of, in malabsorption
        syndrome, 470
Tonofilaments, 26
Tonsillitis, 146, 446
Tophi, 336
Torsion of testis, 524–525
Toxemia, of pregnancy, 536–537
Toxic erythema, 598
Toxic megacolon, acute, 471
Toxic nodular goiter, 564
Toxic shock syndrome, 145–146
Toxoid, 122
Toxoplasma gondii, 212
Toxoplasmosis, 212–213
Trabecular meshwork, *611*, 612
Trace elements, 328–329
Trachoma, 170
Trachoma-inclusion conjunctivitis (TRIC),
    170
Transcription, 27, *30*
Transfer factor, 129, 130, 131
Transformation of cells, 13–14, 176
Transfusion, blood, 369–371
Transfusional hemosiderosis, 371
Translation, 28
Translation-inhibiting protein (TIP), 180
Translocation of chromosomes, 38
Transmission electron microscope, 8–10
Transplants. See *Graft(s).*
Transplantation antigens, 134
    in tumors, 255
Transposition of great vessels, 380
Transudate, 277, 440
Trauma, effects of, 299–311
Traumatic myositis ossificans, 576
Traumatic shock, 306
Traveller's diarrhea, 210, 465
Trematoda, 200, 201t
Trematodes, 200–203, 201t, *202*
Trench mouth, 60, 161
Treponema pallidum, 162, 166t
Treponema pertenue, 162, 166t
Treponemal immobilization (TPI) test, 162
TRF, 551
Trichinella spiralis, 201t, 206
Trichinosis, 206
Trichomonas vaginalis, 215
Trichomoniasis, 215
Trichuris trichiura, 201t, 206
Tricuspid valve disease, 392
Triiodothyronine (T$_3$), 559
Triple response, 75, *76*

Triploidy, 47
Trisomy, 48, *48*
Tritium, 260, *260*
tRNA, 28, *29*
Tropocollagen, 35, *36*
Trousseau, 288
Trypanosomes, description of, 213
Trypanosomiasis, 213, 213t
Trypsin, 496
Tryptophan, deficiency of, 327
Tsetse fly, as vector of infection, 81
TSH, 553, 559
Tuber cinereum, 553
Tubercle bacilli, 153
Tubercle follicle, 154, *154, 155*
Tuberculin, 131
Tuberculoid reaction, 108
    caseating vs. suppurative, 109
Tuberculosis, 153–157, *154, 155, 156, 157*
    Addison's disease due to, 556
    bovine, 155–156
    generalized miliary, 155
    meningitis accompanying, 155
    metastatic, 158
    of bone, 573
    of breast vs. plasma cell mastitis, 541
    of urinary tract, epididymis in, 525
    pulmonary, 156–158, *156, 157*
        fever in, 315, 317
    with glucocorticoid therapy, 558
Tuberculosis arthritis, 585
Tuberculous salpingitis, 533
Tubular necrosis, renal, 507
Tumor(s), 228–258. See also *Carcinoma.*
    benign, 230–233
        definition of, 229
        effects of, 232–233
    classification of, 229–230, 231t
        difficulties in, 245–246
    connective tissue, benign, 230, 232
        malignant, 242–244
    definition of, 229
    embryonic, 246
    epithelial, benign, 230, *232*
        malignant, 240–242
    fever with, 316
    hormone-dependent, 250
    incidence and cause of, 246–257
    intermediate, 244–245
    malignant, 233–244
Tumor emboli, 292
Tumor specific transplantation antigens, 255
Turner's syndrome, 50
Twitching with renal failure, 508
Tympanic membrane, 618
Typhoid fever, fever in, 315
    pathogenesis of, 85–86, *86*
Typhus, 171–172

Ulcer(s), 74
    acute, of stomach and duodenum, 459–460,
        459
    aphthous, 445
    carcinomatous, of colon, 472, *473*
    gastric, acute, 459–460
    mucosal, 74
    of genital mucosa, canker sores and, 445
    of lower esophagus, with hiatus hernia, 450
    of small intestine, in typhoid fever, 85
    peptic, chronic, 455–459, *455, 456, 457*

Ulcer(s) (*Continued*)
    rodent, 244, *245*
    stasis, 94, 413, 495–496
Ulcerative colitis, 470–471
    potassium depletion in, 273
Ultracentrifuge, for plasma protein
        separation, 339
Ultraviolet light, acute inflammation and, 63
    basal cell carcinoma of skin and, 605
    cancer and, 249, 605, *606*
    effect on skin, *606*
    photodermatitis from, 594
Underdevelopment, in tetralogy of Fallot,
    382
Urea, excretion of, 502
Urea clearance test, 504
Uremia, 507–508
Ureter, obstruction of, 519
Ureteric reflux, 520
Urethra, obstruction of, 520
    stricture of, 147
Urethritis, non-gonococcal, 170
Urgency, of micturition, in urinary tract
        infection, 516
Uric acid in gout, 326
Urinalysis, 505–506
Urinary tract, calculi in, 522
    infection, 149, 514–516
        fever in, 315
        prostatitis with, 526
        shock following, 307
    lower, diseases of, 519–522
        obstruction of, 519–520
        tumors of, 521–522, *521*
    tuberculosis of epididymis in, 525
Urine, burning on passing, in urinary tract
        infection, 516
    casts in, 505–506
    examination of, 505–506
    in obstructive jaundice, 485
    mechanism of formation, 503–504
Urobilinogen, 484, *484*, 485
Uropathy, obstructive, 519–520
Urticaria, 597–598
Uterus, body of, disorders of, 534–536
    cervix of, disorders of, 533–534
    double, 532, *532*
    leiomyoma of, *233*, 535–536, *535*
Uveal tract, 610
    diseases of, 615–616
    tumors of, 616
Uveitis, 615–616
    canker sores and, 445

Vaccination, for hepatitis B, 191
    for poliomyelitis, 182
    for smallpox, 183–184
Vaccine, 123
Vaccinia, generalized, 184
    progressive, 184
Vaccinia virus, 183
Vacuolar degeneration, 56, *56*
Vacuoles, autophagocytic, 25
Vagabond disease, 171
Vagina, carcinoma of, diethylstilbestrol and,
        248, 250
    discharge from, in carcinoma of cervix, 533
        in trichomoniasis, 215
        with cervical erosion, 533
    double, 532
    rhabdomyosarcoma of, 589

Valley fever, 197
Valvular diseases of heart, 392–393
Varicella, 186, 187
Varices, esophageal, 482, *482, 483*
     encephalopathy with, 486–487
Varicose veins, 413
     slow wound healing and, 93, *94*
     stasis dermatitis with, 413
     ulcer with, *94*
Variola, 183–184
Vascular abnormalities, thrombosis due to,
     285
Vascular disease, bleeding due to, 367
     peripheral, 411
     with diabetes, 335
Vascular hamartomas, of skin, 604
Vascular occlusion, ileus due to, 478
Vascular spasm, 294–296
Vasculitis, 410
     Arthus reaction and, 126–127, *127*
     gonococcal, 410
     necrotizing, 376
Vasodilatation, 64
Vasomotor nephropathy, 506–507
Vasopressin, 553. See also *Antidiuretic
     hormone.*
Vasovagal attack, 305
Vater, ampulla of, 499
     carcinoma of, 501
Vegetations, in endocarditis, infective, 385,
     385
     nonbacterial thrombotic, 384
     in heart, 288
     in rheumatic fever, 383
Veins, diseases of, 412–413
     inflammation of, 287–288
     obstruction, edema with, 278
       ischemia due to, 290
     spasm of, 294
     thrombosis in, 286–288
       stasis dermatitis following, 595–596
     varicose, 413
       stasis dermatitis with, 413, 595–596
Venereal disease research laboratory (VDRL)
     test, 162
Venipuncture, spasm following, 294
Venospasm, 294
Venous obstruction, edema in, 278
Venous pressure, central, rise in, 396
Ventilation, failure of, 416–417
     of lung, 415
Ventricle, left, aneurysm of, 390
     septal defects, 380, *381*
     thrombosis, 288, 390, *390*
Ventricular fibrillation, 395
Ventricular tachycardia, paroxysmal, 393
Verruca vulgaris, 188, 230, *232*
Vertebral column, tuberculosis of, 573
Vertigo in Ménière's disease, 621
Vesicle(s), 592
     intraepidermal, 600–601
     subepidermal, 601–602
Vesicoureteric reflux, 515, 520
Vesicular virus diseases, 601
Vesiculobullous diseases, 599–602
Vestibular apparatus, 618
Vestibulocochlear nerve, schwannoma of,
     sensorineural deafness due to, 621
Vibrio cholerae, 89, 464
Vibrio parahaemolyticus, 463, 464
Vincent's infection, 60

Vinyl chloride, cancer and, 248
Viral diseases, vesicular, 601
Viral encephalitis, 630
Viral exanthems, 598
Viral hepatitis, 189–192, *190, 191,* 490
Viral infections, 68, 173–193
     cancer and, 250–252
     demyelination with, 631
     fever in, 319
     gastroenteritis due to, 464–465
     immunity to, 180–181
     oral mucosa in, 445
     slow, degenerative nervous disorders and,
        46, 192–193
     sore throats due to, 446
     types of, 181–193
Viral interference, 180
Viral meningitis, 630
Virchow's triad, 285
Virilism, 557
Virion, 174, *174*
Virus(es), bronchopneumonia due to, 425
     classification of, 179–180
     cytopathic effects of, 177, 179
     electron microscopy of, 8, 10
     latent, 177
     oncogenic, 250–252
     properties of, 174–181, *175*
     slow, 46, 192–193
Visceral leishmaniasis, 214–215, *214,* 214t
Vision. See also *Blindness* and *Eye(s).*
     blurring of, in glaucoma, 613
       in toxemia, 536
       in uveitis, 616
     impairment of, in multiple sclerosis, 631
     loss of, in Graves' disease, 562
Vitamin(s), 324–328, 324t
     deficiencies, central nervous system
        disorders due to, 632
       in malabsorption syndrome, 470
     for red cell formation, 351
Vitamin A, deficiencies and excesses of,
     324–326, 497
Vitamin B complex, 326–328
Vitamin B$_6$, 328, 324t
Vitamin B$_{12}$, 324t
     for red cell formation, 350t, 351
     spinal cord degeneration and, 354
Vitamin C, 302, 326
     deficiency, slow wound healing and, 101
     for collagen formation, 35
     for red cell formation, 351
Vitamin D, 326
     deficiency, bone abnormalities due to,
        578–579
     in regulating blood calcium level, 571
Vitamin E, 55, 326
Vitamin K, 326, 366
     deficiency, bleeding disorders due to, 366
Volvulus, 477
Vomit, coffee-ground, in stomach carcinoma,
     460
Vomiting, in intestinal obstruction, 478
     in pregnancy, 536
     metabolic alkalosis with, 276
     renal failure and, 508
     with increased intracranial pressure, 625
     with pyloric stenosis, peptic ulcer and, 456
     von Recklinghausen's disease, 220–222
       of bone, 578
Vulvovaginitis, 147

Wallerian degeneration, 103–104
Warm antibodies, 356
Warthin's tumor, 453
Warts, 188, 230, *232*, 605
Wassermann antibody, 162
Wassermann reaction, 121, *122*
Waste products, removal of, failure of, 330
Water accumulation of, in cell, 56, *56*
    as component of body, 269, *270*
    balance, disturbances in, 272–273
Water intoxication, 272
Waterhouse-Friderichsen syndrome, 559
Waxy casts, in urine, 506
Webs, esophageal, 450
Wegener's granulomatosis, 376
Weight gain, in toxemia, 536, 537
Weight loss, in stomach carcinoma, 460
Weil-Felix reaction, 172
Weil's disease, 161
    renal tubular necrosis in, 507
Wen, *606*
Wernicke's encephalopathy, 327, 632
    in hyperemesis gravidarum, 536
Westergren method, 342
Wet beriberi, 327
Wet gangrene, 294
Wheal, 597
    in triple response to histamine, 75, *76*
Wheezing dyspnea in bronchial asthma, 433
Whipworm, 201t, 206
White cells, 358–363
    development of, 358, *358*, 360
    emigration of, 66
    in leukemia, 361–362
    normal count and variations, 358–359
White leg, painful, in pregnancy, 413
Whitlow, herpetic, 188
Whooping cough, lymphocytosis in, 360
Widal reaction, 86, *86*
Willis, circle of, berry aneurysm of, 411, 626, 627
Wilms' tumor, 246, 519

Winter vomiting disease, 465
Wintrobe method, 342
Witch's milk, 541
Worms, classification of, 200, 201t
Wound(s), contraction of, 92–93, *93*
    dehiscence of, 101–102
    infections of, 82, 144, 149, *153*
    tensile strength of, 97
Wound healing, 91–105
    by primary intention, 95–98, *98*
    by secondary intention, 98–100, *99*
    complications of, 101–102
    factors influencing, 100–101
    of skin, 95–100
Woven bone, 569
Wuchereria bancrofti, 201t, 207

Xanthomas, 485
Xenografts, 134
Xeroderma pigmentosum, 249
Xerophthalmia, 325

Y body, 32–33, *32*
Yaws, 162
Yeasts, 194
Yellow fever, 186
    renal tubular necrosis in, 507
Yersinia enterocolitica, 463, 464

Ziehl-Neelsen stain, 153
Zinc, in acrodermatitis enteropathica, 328–329
    in wound healing, 101
Zonula adherens, *20*
Zonula occludens, *20*
Zymosan, in phagocytic vacuoles, *69*